Pharmacy Practice
for Technicians

Mastering Community and Hospital Competencies

Fourth Edition

Don A. Ballington, MS
Robert J. Anderson, PharmD

Paradigm PUBLISHING

St. Paul • Los Angeles • Indianapolis

Acquisitions Editor	Alison Brown Cerier
Senior Developmental Editor	Christine Hurney
Production Editor	Donna Mears
Cover and Text Designer	Jaana Bykonich
Photo Researcher	Terri Miller, E-Visual Communications, Inc.
Production Specialists	Jack Ross and Ryan Hamner
Production Services	Publication Services, Inc.

Care has been taken to verify the accuracy of information presented in this book. However, the authors, editors, and publisher cannot accept responsibility for Web, e-mail, newsgroup, or chat room subject matter or content, or for consequences from application of the information in this book, and make no warranty, expressed or implied, with respect to its content.

Trademarks: Some of the product names and company names included in this book have been used for identification purposes only and may be trademarks or registered trade names of their respective manufacturers and sellers. The authors, editors, and publisher disclaim any affiliation, association, or connection with, or sponsorship or endorsement by, such owners.

Photo Credits: Following the index.

We have made every effort to trace the ownership of all copyrighted material and to secure permission from copyright holders. In the event of any question arising as to the use of any material, we will be pleased to make the necessary corrections in future printings. Thanks are due to the aforementioned authors, publishers, and agents for permission to use the materials indicated.

ISBN 978-0-76383-458-6 (Text)
ISBN 978-0-76383-460-9 (Text + Study Partner CD)

© 2010 by Paradigm Publishing, Inc., a division of EMC Publishing, LLC
875 Montreal Way
St. Paul, MN 55102
E-mail: educate@emcp.com
Web site: www.emcp.com

Printed in the United States of America

18 17 16 15 14 13   13 14 15 16 17 18

Brief Contents

Contents

Unit 2
Community Pharmacy 149

Chapter 8
Nonsterile Pharmaceutical Compounding

Unit 3
Institutional Pharmacy

Chapter 9
Hospital Pharmacy Practice

Chapter 13
Human Relations and
Communications

Chapter 14
Your Future in Pharmacy Practice

Preface

Pharmacy Practice for Technicians, Fourth Edition teaches the techniques and procedures to prepare and dispense medications in community, institutional, and other pharmacy settings. This text offers the tools to achieve the pharmacy technician competencies defined by the American Society of Health-System Pharmacists (ASHP). Through studying this text, students learn how to count, measure, and compound drugs using both sterile and nonsterile pharmacy techniques. The text covers reading the prescription or medication order in the hospital pharmacy; preparing, packaging, and labeling the medication; and maintaining the patient profile. In addition to teaching basic drug knowledge, the text supports practical skills related to billing and inventory management. The activities of the pharmacy technician are very important to the quality of patient care. Throughout, the text reinforces the fact that the support provided by the technicians in all pharmacy settings allows the pharmacist to spend more time counseling patients and monitoring the quality and effectiveness of drug therapies.

Chapter Features: A Visual Walk-through

Chapter features are designed to help students learn how to fulfill the responsibilities of the pharmacy technician to work safely and effectively. Take a look at the key features beginning with those on the chapter opener as shown below.

1

LEARNING OBJECTIVES establish clear goals and help focus chapter study.

2

IMPORTANT TERMS are bolded and defined in context. Students are encouraged to preview the chapter terms on the Study Partner CD at the start of each chapter. Chapter terms are also listed at the conclusion of each chapter for quick reference.

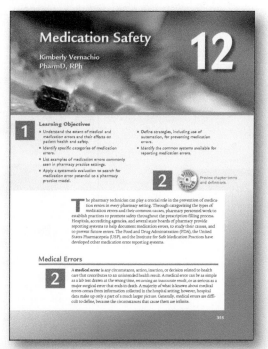

3

SAFETY NOTES
highlight rules and guidelines for preventing medication errors.

4

PHOTOS, TABLES, AND FIGURES visually reinforce the information taught in the chapter.

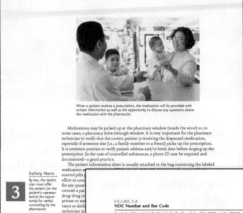

5

CHAPTER TERMS lists the important terminology with definitions.

6

CHAPTER SUMMARY provides an overview of the key points of the chapter.

7

CHECK YOUR UNDERSTANDING questions provide a quick way for students to check their comprehension of the chapter's objectives. Students are encouraged to study additional quiz questions on the Study Partner CD.

8

THINKING LIKE A PHARMACY TECH questions challenge students to apply the chapter topics to hands-on pharmacy scenarios.

9

COMMUNICATING CLEARLY activities provide engaging topics for discussion and practice of communication skills.

10

RESEARCHING ON THE WEB exercises invite students to investigate topics further on the Internet.

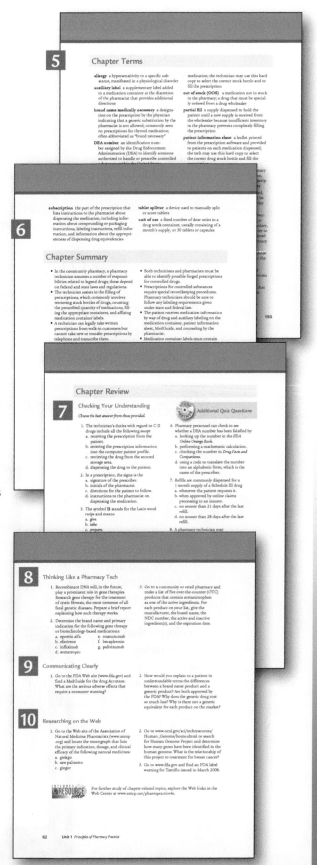

Resources for the Student

In addition to the chapter content, students have access to several print and electronic resources to help them master essential skills for the pharmacy technician role.

Appendixes

The appendixes provide valuable reference material, including a list of the most commonly prescribed drugs and their drug categories (Appendix A), a list of look-alike and sound-alike medications and recommendations from the Institute for Safe Medication Practices (ISMP) (Appendix B), and a group of common pharmacy practice terms and phrases translated into Spanish (Appendix C).

Study Partner CD

The Study Partner CD included with each textbook offers the following tools to support student learning:

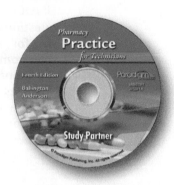

- Chapter Terms and Flash Cards
- Matching Activities
- Quizzes in Practice or Reported Modes
- Link to Internet Resource Center

Chapter Terms and Flash Cards The Study Partner CD includes chapter terms and definitions with audio support and an image bank of key illustrations and photographs from the text-book. The CD also includes flash cards to help students learn these important terms.

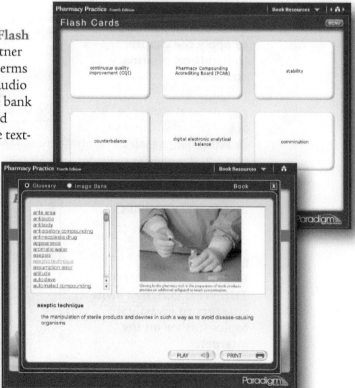

Matching Activities The Study Partner CD also includes interactive matching activities that require the student to demonstrate an understanding of chapter content.

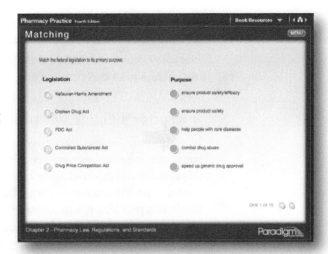

Quizzes The Study Partner CD includes a rich bank of multiple-choice quizzes available in both Practice and Reported modes. In the Practice mode, the student receives immediate feedback on each quiz item and a report of his or her total score. In the Reported mode, the results are e-mailed to both the student and the instructor. Both book-level and chapter-specific quizzes are available.

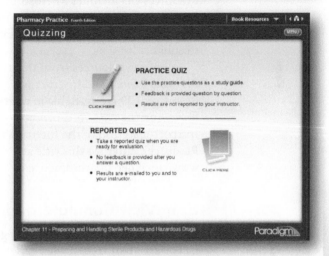

Internet Resource Center

The Internet Resource Center for this title at www.emcp.net/pharmpractice4e provides additional resources, chapter study notes, and interactive flash cards for learning the generic and brand names of the most-prescribed drugs.

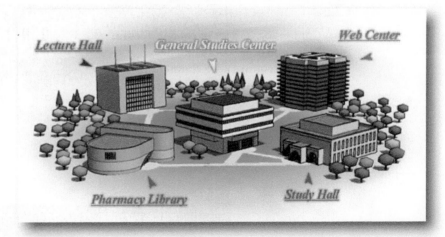

Resources for the Instructor

Pharmacy Practice for Technicians, Fourth Edition, is supported by several tools to help instructors plan their course and assess student learning.

Instructor's Guide with Instructor Resources CD

In addition to course planning tools and suggested syllabi, the *Instructor's Guide* provides answers for all end-of-chapter exercises and chapter-specific teaching hints. The *Instructor's Guide* also provides ready-to-use chapter tests and midterm and final examinations. Available with each print *Instructor's Guide*, the Instructor Resources CD includes Microsoft® Word documents of all the resources in the print *Instructor's Guide* as well as PowerPoint® presentations to enhance lectures.

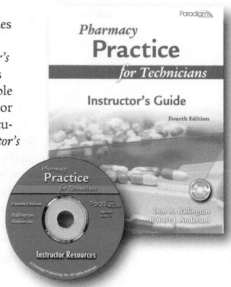

All of the resources from the print *Instructor's Guide* and Instructor Resources CD are available in electronic format on the password-protected Instructor section of the Internet Resource Center for this title at www.emcp.net/pharmpractice4e.

ExamView Computerized Test Generator

A full-featured computerized test generator on CD offers instructors a wide variety of options for generating both print and online tests. The test bank provides 50 questions for each chapter. Instructors can create custom tests using the chapter item banks and edit questions or add new items of their own design.

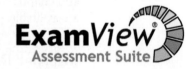

Class Connections

Class Connections is a set of content files for Blackboard and other course management systems. Content includes chapter outlines, PowerPoint presentations, and quizzes.

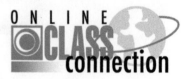

Textbooks in the Pharmacy Technician Series

In addition to *Pharmacy Practice for Technicians, Fourth Edition*, Paradigm Publishing, Inc. offers other titles designed specifically for the pharmacy technician curriculum:

- *Pharmacology for Technicians, Fourth Edition*
- *Pharmacology for Technicians Workbook, Fourth Edition*
- *Pharmacy Calculations for Technicians, Fourth Edition*
- *Pharmacy Labs for Technicians*

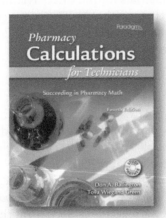
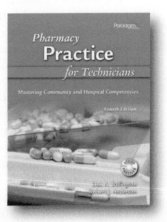

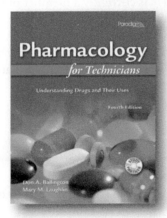
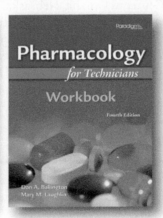
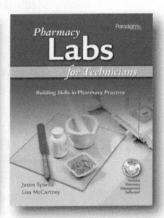

About the Authors

Don A. Ballington, MS, served as program coordinator of the pharmacy technician training program at Midlands Technical College in Columbia, South Carolina, for 27 years. He has also served as president of the Pharmacy Technician Educators Council and in 2005 received the council's Educator of the Year award. Mr. Ballington has conducted site visits for pharmacy technician accreditation and helped develop the American Society of Health-System Pharmacists model curriculum. He has also been a consulting editor for the *Journal of Pharmacy Technology*. Over the course of his career at Midlands Technical College, he developed a set of high-quality training materials for pharmacy technicians. These materials have been made available in three textbooks: *Pharmacology for Technicians, Pharmacy Calculations for Technicians,* and this title, *Pharmacy Practice for Technicians*. All are now available in fourth editions.

Robert J. Anderson, PharmD, is a professor emeritus at the Southern School of Pharmacy at Mercer University in Atlanta, Georgia, with over 30 years of experience in academia and practice. He is also a part-time community pharmacist in both independent and chain community pharmacies and is president of RJA Consultants, LLC. He has been a guest lecturer in clinical pharmacology at both Georgia State University in Atlanta, Georgia, and North Georgia University in Dahlonega, Georgia. Dr. Anderson has been a clinical pharmacy specialist at Kaiser Permanente, Southeast Region, in Atlanta. He has also been an associate director for the Department of Pharmaceutical Services at the University of Nebraska Medical Center in Omaha, Nebraska. He is currently a member of the United States Pharmacopeia (USP) Expert Committee. In addition to serving as co-author on the third and fourth editions of *Pharmacy Practice for Technicians*, he has written chapters in *Clinical Pharmacology and Therapeutics* and *Handbook of Nonprescription Drugs*, and has served on the editorial boards of *Family Practice Recertification* and *American Journal of Managed Care Pharmacy*.

Acknowledgments

The quality of this body of work is a testament to the feedback we have received from the many contributors and reviewers who participated in *Pharmacy Practice for Technicians, Fourth Edition*.

Robert W. Aanonsen, CPhT
Platt College
Tulsa, Oklahoma

Cheryl Aiken, BS Pharm, PharmD, RPh
Hotel Pharmacy, Inc.
Brattleboro, Vermont

Donald Becker, CPhT
San Jacinto College–North Campus
Houston, Texas

Danika Braaten, RPhT, CPhT
Northland Community and
  Technical College
East Grand Forks, Minnesota

Verender Gail Brown, CPhT
High-Tech Institute
Orlando, Florida

Linda M. Calvert, CPhT
Front Range Community College
Westminster, Colorado

Debborah G. Cummings, CPhT
Southeast Technical Institute
Sioux Falls, South Dakota

Andrea N. Curry, BS, CPhT
Concorde Career College
Memphis, Tennessee

Jennifer Danielson, PharmD, RPh,
  MBA, CDE
University of Washington
  School of Pharmacy
Mill Creek, Washington

Cathy Dunne
North Orange County Community
  College District
Anaheim, California

Donna E. Guisado, RDA, BSOM
North-West College
West Covina, California

Carla May, RPh
Vance Granville Community College
Henderson, North Carolina

Michelle C. McCranie, CPhT
Ogeechee Technical College
Statesboro, Georgia

Andrea R. Redman, PharmD, BCPS
Emory University Hospital
Atlanta, Georgia

Ann Oberg, BS, CPhT
National American University
Sioux Falls, South Dakota

Rebecca Schonscheck, CPhT
High-Tech Institute
Phoenix, Arizona

Kimberly Vernachio, PharmD, RPh
Aetna Pharmacy Management
CVS Pharmacies
Canton, Georgia

In addition, we would like to say a special thank you to Cheryl Aiken for her skillful and careful review of the content of the textbook and all of the quiz questions and matching exercises on the Study Partner CD. We also thank Andrea Redman for her thorough review of the textbook and the writing of the test bank questions.

The authors and editorial staff invite your feedback on the text and its supplements. Please reach us by clicking the "Contact us" button at www.emcp.com.

Unit

1

Principles of Pharmacy Practice

The Profession of Pharmacy

1

Learning Objectives

- Describe the origins of pharmacy.
- Differentiate among the various kinds of pharmacies.
- Describe four stages of development of the pharmacy profession in the twentieth century.
- Enumerate the functions of the pharmacist.
- Discuss the educational curriculum for today's pharmacy student.

- Explain the licensing requirements for pharmacists.
- Identify the duties and work environments of the pharmacy technician.

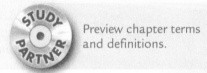

Preview chapter terms and definitions.

From its ancient origins in spiritualism and magic, pharmacy has evolved into a scientific pursuit involving not only compounding and dispensing but also the dispensing of information about medications. With 4 billion prescriptions filled each year and more expected with our aging population, a number of new pharmacy schools have opened in the past decade to address expected pharmacist shortages. The annual U.S. drug cost in 2016 is predicted to be almost $500 billion, an increase of 82% from 2006. To address projected pharmacist shortages and in order for the pharmacist to fulfill modern-day roles, the pharmacy technician will be increasingly needed to provide essential services.

The Origins of Pharmacy Practice

In early civilization, disease was thought to be caused by evil spirits, demons, or evil forces. This belief that sickness was due to spiritual forces called for the priest, sorcerer, or medicinal healer to first identify the evil spirit before determining the appropriate remedy. Predictably, early recipes for drug preparations were freely mixed with prayers, chants, incantations, rituals, and imitative magic.

The use of drugs in the healing arts by all cultures is as old as civilization. Modern archaeologists, exploring the five-thousand-year-old remains of the ancient city-states of Mesopotamia (near modern-day Iraq and Iran), have unearthed clay

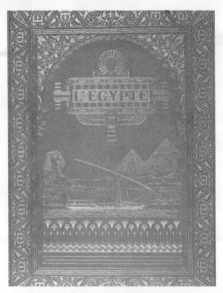

The Ebers papyrus is an early collection of recipes for natural medicinal agents from Egypt that was used for centuries.

tablets listing hundreds of medicinal preparations from various sources, including plants, animals, and minerals. The ancient Egyptians compiled lists of drugs, known as *formularies, dispensatories,* or *pharmacopeias.* The most famous of the lists was the Ebers papyrus, which was written about 1500 B.C. and included a collection of recipes. This list marked the early beginnings of a more empirical and rational approach to medicine.

In the Far East a similar mixture of natural sources of medicine and magic existed. The botanical basis for pharmacy may trace its early origins to China. To this day the people of China and India rely heavily on natural herbs to treat common ailments. An example of a common herb from the Far East that is widely used in Western culture today is ginseng for energy. Many remedies all over the world were discovered by trial and error with the herbs over many centuries.

To the ancient Greeks we owe the beginnings of a more scientific approach to the practice of medicine. The word *pharmacy* comes from the ancient Greek word *pharmakon,* meaning *drug or remedy.* Hippocrates, traditionally viewed as "the father of medicine," believed that illness had a rational and physical explanation and was not the result of possession by evil spirits or disfavor with the gods. Hippocrates is credited with using scientific principles to identify, determine the cause of, and treat disease. Today, Hippocrates is best remembered for the Hippocratic oath, by which physicians pledge "to do no harm."

The greatest of the ancient pharmaceutical texts, however, was *De Materia Medica (On Medical Matters),* written by Dioscorides in the first century A.D. Although a Greek physician, he served in the Roman army during the rule of Nero and traveled widely, gathering knowledge of medicinal herbs and minerals. His text included descriptions of herbal remedies and their usage, side effects, quantities, dosages, and storage. *De Materia Medica* served as the standard text on drugs for 15 centuries.

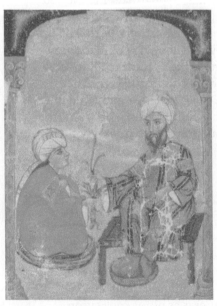

De Materia Medica (On Medical Matters), written by Dioscorides, is a collection of knowledge of natural medicinal agents used in medicine and pharmacy practice for 15 centuries.

Another ancient Greek physician, Galen (130–200 A.D.), organized six centuries of medical and pharmaceutical knowledge and observation since Hippocrates and conducted animal experiments to further his knowledge of the human body. He is best known for producing a systematic classification of drugs for the treatment of various pathologies that was unchallenged for nearly a century. The term *galenical pharmacy* was used to describe the process of creating extracts of active medicinals from plants (once a major activity of the pharmacist). Galen, though a physician, is considered to be the "father of pharmacy."

In the early Middle Ages, pharmacy practice was evolving in both Europe and the Persian Empire. The Arabic people are generally credited with developing the first list of drugs introducing various dosage formulations (pills, syrups, extracts) and identifying the pharmacist as a qualified and licensed health professional. Based on influence from ancient Greek and Arabic peoples, the apothecary concept developed in western Europe in the eleventh and twelfth centuries along with the creation of professional guilds. These guilds existed primarily to maintain a monopoly and control of the training and length of apprentice-

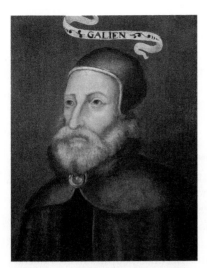

Galen is considered "the father of pharmacy" for classifying, identifying, and extracting active ingredients from natural sources.

ships. The guilds were early forerunners of state boards of pharmacy as well as the growth of professional organizations and formal education at universities.

The Greek, Roman, and Arabic influences on the development of pharmacy practice were questioned in Europe during the Renaissance (1350–1650 A.D.). This period saw the rise of alchemy and the use of chemicals. **Alchemy** combined elements of chemistry, metallurgy, physics, and medicine with astrology, mysticism, and spiritualism all as parts of one greater force. In one common example of the application of their trade, the alchemists would attempt to change common metals into silver and gold.

Exotic new drugs and spices were also arriving from the New World and added to the list of available medicinal agents. The pharmacist was now becoming a chemist as well as a botanist. The practice of pharmacy varied greatly between countries. The Renaissance also experienced the emergence of pharmacies and hospitals run by religious orders. These monastic facilities served the larger communities by providing free medicine to the poor. These pharmacies are the origin of today's community healthcare clinics, health departments, and hospitals.

In the seventeenth century, the emergence of science and publishing led to advances in the practice of pharmacy. At the beginning of the scientific revolution, in the Renaissance, most scholars in western Europe were deeply learned in the Greek and Latin classics, and so it is not surprising that, when inventing new terms to describe their discoveries and observations, they borrowed bits and pieces of these ancient languages. Such word coinage, based on Greek and Latin word prefixes and suffixes, remains at the heart of the scientific naming of many medical terms today (see the Greek and Latin Word Parts reference in the Pharmacy Library section of this text's Internet Resource Center at www.emcp.net/pharmpractice4e).

Rudimentary testing and research to determine the efficacy of botanical drugs was initiated, and this effort was a forerunner of pharmacology and pharmacognosy. Each major city in Europe published its own pharmacopeia or drug list, which later became a country drug list. Created in Great Britain in the seventeenth century, the *Martindales Pharmacopoeia* is still considered a well-respected and useful pharmacy reference. Also during this time, the pharmacist was becoming recognized as a provider of health care, though many apothecaries in Europe were still being operated by physicians.

There were very few pharmacists among the early colonists of the United States. Predictably, the profession followed the European model, albeit at a much slower pace. Pharmacists in the colonies could be doctors, druggists, merchants, or storekeepers. Until the nineteenth century, it was commonplace for a physician to own the dispensary that distributed drugs to patients. However, gradually the professions separated and the pharmacy or apothecary shop became an independent entity owned and operated by the pharmacist.

The United States developed its own pharmacopeia of drug standards in 1820. Revisions of the United States Pharmacopeia (USP) exist today and provide national drug standards. The American Pharmaceutical Association (APhA) was organized in 1852 initially to address adulteration of imported drugs. The APhA has traditionally focused on the scientific basis of the profession whereas a later organization, the National Association of Retail Druggists (NARD), focused more on the business side of the profession. These organizations exist today and reflect the schism of pharmacy—is it primarily a business or a profession?

With the development of new synthetic drugs and an explosion of new research and access to information on drugs, the profession of pharmacy has grown concurrently with that of medicine. Over centuries the profession has transitioned from dispensing crude natural products of questionable efficacy to dispensing highly complex synthetic chemicals that are both efficacious and potentially toxic.

The Pharmacy Workplace of Today

Pharmacy technicians are employed in most of the same settings as pharmacists, including community pharmacies (i.e., drugstores), hospital pharmacies, home healthcare, and long-term care facilities. Figure 1.1 illustrates the market share of prescription sales in the various types of pharmacy distribution outlets. Pharmacists and technicians work in clean, well-lit, and well-ventilated environments. For the most part, their work requires standing, often for long hours. Because people's health needs continue beyond the traditional workday, both pharmacists and pharmacy technicians may be on call or work days, nights, weekends, and holidays. At any time, 24 hours a day, some number of the estimated 275,000 certified pharmacy technicians are on the job. With the ongoing approval of lifesaving drugs and an increase in the aging population in the United States, the need for both pharmacists and pharmacy technicians is expected to continue for the foreseeable future.

Community Pharmacies

Three-fifths of all pharmacists in the United States work in a **community pharmacy**, also called a *retail pharmacy*. Most community pharmacies are divided into a restricted prescription area offering prescription merchandise and related items and a front area offering over-the-counter (OTC) drugs, dietary supplements, medical supplies, and other merchandise. There are many types of community pharmacies that dispense the majority of prescriptions. Some of these pharmacies are independently owned small businesses, others are part of large retail chains, and still others are smaller franchise operations. However, the recent trend is toward fewer independent pharmacies, especially in metropolitan areas, because these small pharmacies have difficulty competing with the large-scale operations of chain pharmacies.

FIGURE 1.1
U.S. Prescription Market Share by Type of Pharmacy

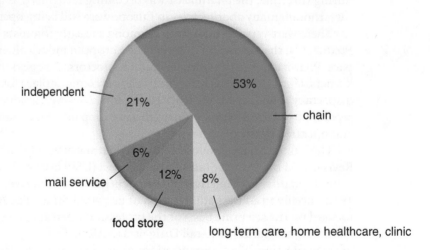

independent 21%

53% chain

mail service 6%

food store 12%

8% long-term care, home healthcare, clinic

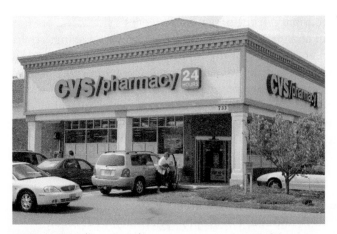

Many metropolitan areas have one or more community pharmacies that provide pharmacy services 24 hours a day, 7 days a week.

The staff of a typical community pharmacy will consist of several pharmacists with Bachelor of Science (BS) or Doctor of Pharmacy (PharmD) degrees and several pharmacy technicians including those who have passed the certification examination. Some pharmacists will have additional education, training, and experiences in business and clinical practice. The ratio of pharmacy technicians allowed to practice with pharmacists differs in each state and is under the auspices of the state board of pharmacy.

A **chain pharmacy** may be national or regional and may be found in department stores (e.g., Wal-Mart, Target), grocery stores (e.g., Kroger, Publix), or typical corner drugstores (e.g., Walgreens, CVS, Rite-Aid). Most chain pharmacies are strategically located to allow for large-volume dispensing with heavy use of both pharmacy technicians and automation. Many of the administrative decisions in chains are made at the corporate level.

An **independent pharmacy** is a community pharmacy that is owned and usually operated by one pharmacist or a group of pharmacists rather than a corporation as in the case of a chain pharmacy. Most compounding of prescriptions is done in this type of pharmacy, in addition to dispensing of prescriptions. Some independent pharmacies have evolved into compounding pharmacies. A **compounding pharmacy** specializes in the preparation of nonsterile and sterile preparations that are not commercially available. A pharmacist owner of an independent pharmacy makes his or her own decisions regarding the practice of pharmacy, with more attention and time spent on improving customer service.

A **franchise pharmacy** combines characteristics of an independent business and a large retail chain. Franchise agreements vary, but typically they involve a franchisor that grants exclusive use of the company name and rights to sell company products to an owner/operator of a drugstore, the franchisee. To be successful in winning customers most franchise pharmacies sell only medication and health-related products and services and are commonly called *apothecaries*.

An example of such a franchise operation is Medicine Shoppe International, Inc., owned by Cardinal Health Company. It is the largest franchisor of independent community pharmacies in the United States. Franchise pharmacies attempt to provide more personalized health care than their competition.

Somewhat related to retail pharmacy is the **mail-order pharmacy**, which is run by a centralized operation using both automation and pharmacy techs to dispense and mail large volumes of prescriptions every day. Each year more and more prescriptions are being filled by mail-order pharmacies, which are often located out-of-state. Because of economies of scale, mail-order pharmacies can acquire drugs at lower cost and pass on some of the savings to insurers and customers. Many health insurance companies encourage enrollees to use mail-order pharmacies to save money. Insurance company agents called pharmacy benefit managers (or PBMs) control costs through generic prescribing, formularies, prior authorizations, and tiered pricing.

Most studies have not been able to document the cost savings of mail-order pharmacies. Despite their apparent cost savings, they have certain limitations. For example, most prescriptions for chronic disease must be filled with a 3 month supply when ordered through a mail-order pharmacy. If the patient experiences a side effect or adverse reaction or the physician changes the medication, then the drug savings could be offset by drug wastage. Another trade-off for the supposedly lower cost is that medication counseling is limited to a printout or calling a toll-free number. Concerns also exist about the time delay patients experience when waiting for needed mail-order medication(s) such as antibiotics or chronic disease medications, which typically should be taken immediately upon prescribing or on a regular basis, respectively. Also, there are safety, storage, and legal issues of delivering medications through the mail.

Institutional Pharmacies

Broadly defined, an **institutional pharmacy** is a pharmacy associated with any organized healthcare delivery system. Traditionally, a hospital pharmacy is the most common example. However, home healthcare, long-term care facilities, managed-care organizations, and nuclear pharmacies are more recent examples of places where institutional pharmacies can be found.

Hospital Pharmacies One-fourth of all pharmacists work in a hospital setting. Similar to a community pharmacy, the **hospital pharmacy** carries out the functions of maintaining drug treatment records and ordering, stocking, compounding, repackaging, and dispensing medications and other supplies. The hospital pharmacist prepares, or supervises the preparation of, a unit dosage system (i.e., a 24–72 hour supply of medication for a patient), sterile IV medications, and an extensive floor stock inventory (see Chapter 9, *Hospital Pharmacy Practice*).

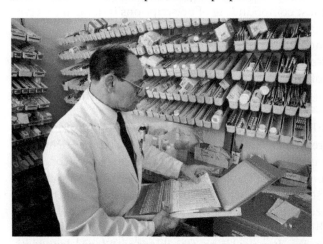

The pharmacy provides an important service to the hospital. Here, a pharmacist reviews a patient's medication administration record (MAR).

Many hospitals provide sufficient staffing to cover these services 7 days per week, 24 hours per day. The staff of the typical hospital pharmacy may include administrators with master's degrees (e.g., Master of Business Administration [MBA]) or PharmD degrees, staff pharmacists with BS degrees, staff and clinical pharmacists with PharmD degrees, and certified pharmacy technicians.

To ensure a sterile environment and minimize infectious disease, many pharmacy technicians in the hospital (and some in a compounding pharmacy) work in a clean room under specialized ventilation cabinets, called laminar flow hoods, where they prepare sterile preparations and hazardous drugs. Gowns, masks, hairnets, bootees, and gloves are needed in this environment to prevent the spread of infection. Infection control and preparation of sterile and hazardous products will be discussed in more detail in Chapter 10, *Infection Control*, and Chapter 11, *Preparing and Handling Sterile Products and Hazardous Drugs*.

Home Healthcare Systems **Home healthcare** is the delivery of medical, nursing, and pharmaceutical services and supplies to patients who remain at home. Treating patients at home is generally less costly than round-the-clock care in the hospital. Many hospitalized patients are discharged as soon as possible to continue their recovery at home with IV fluids and medications. The home healthcare market continues to grow because of our aging society and as an alternative to the higher cost of hospitalizations.

Pharmacists and pharmacy technicians working in a **home healthcare pharmacy** provide IV and oral medications and often must be available on a 24 hour basis for emergencies. The pharmacy tech prepares and dispenses medications which, after final check by the pharmacist, are then delivered to the patient's home. A pharmacist or nurse is responsible for educating the patient or the patient's caregiver on the appropriate and safe use of these medications and equipment.

Long-Term Care Facilities A **long-term care facility** such as an extended-care facility (ECF) or nursing home provides institutional services predominantly to older adults or disabled "residents" who can no longer provide for routine or medical care for themselves, including adults who suffer from chronic (long-lasting) diseases or such debilitating illnesses as stroke or Alzheimer disease. Both medical care and residential care are provided for a length of time appropriate for the resident's needs.

A skilled-care facility (SCF) is limited to patients requiring more round-the-clock nursing care (such as IV infusions) or recovery after a recent hospitalization (most patients are discharged from an SCF to home or to an ECF when they have adequately recovered). An SCF or an ECF generally provides a higher level of nursing care than home healthcare. Other examples of long-term care facilities include facilities that treat patients with acute or chronic psychiatric disorders or rehabilitation facilities for those with serious traumatic brain or spinal cord injuries.

Some long-term care facilities have an in-house pharmacy on their premises, whereas others either contract with a community pharmacy or allow each resident (or the resident's family) to choose his or her pharmacy.

In-house pharmacies typically provide a 7 day supply of medication for the long-term care residents in blister packs. Community pharmacies that provide medications to nursing homes will generally fill medication carts or trays with a 30 day supply of medication, because medication orders infrequently change in this environment.

Managed-Care Pharmacy Services **Managed care** has grown dramatically over the past 40 years. One of the first managed-care organizations was Kaiser Permanente, a nonprofit private venture started in California in the 1930s. A **health maintenance organization (HMO)** is an organization that provides health insurance using a managed care model. Most HMOs are outpatient clinics, but some may own hospitals. The responsibility of a technician in an HMO is similar to that of a technician working in a community pharmacy.

The philosophy guiding the care provided by an HMO is that keeping patients of all ages healthy or their disease(s) controlled decreases hospitalizations and emergency room visits and therefore lowers expenses to the healthcare system. HMOs encourage their patients to take an active role in their own health care by eating right, exercising often, and avoiding negative life style choices such as smoking and alcohol abuse. HMOs encourage patients to have annual checkups, to get all their immunizations on schedule, and to get necessary laboratory tests (like a cholesterol or sugar test) and screening tests (like a Pap smear or mammogram) to detect early diseases, which may be surgically correctible.

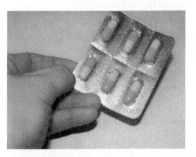

A blister-packed medication in unit dosage form makes it easier for nursing homes to dispense medications to patients.

Most HMOs have their own staff physicians who are on salary; some private practice physicians have a contractual agreement with an HMO. If patients would like to see a specialist, they often are required to first get a referral from their HMO primary care physician to control access and costs. The primary care physician serves as the "gatekeeper" to healthcare. HMOs have been successful in slow-

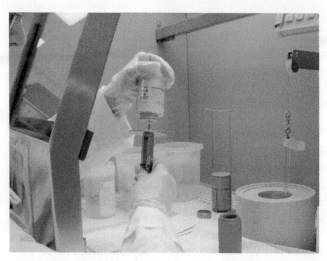

A pharmacy technician with special certification prepares a sterile radioactive medication using special equipment and protective shields.

ing the pace of the inflationary increases in the costs of health care without compromising the quality of care. As a result, many employers now include an HMO option in their health plan.

Most HMOs are centralized primary-care clinics (i.e., they serve adult, pediatric, and obstetric-gynecology [ob-gyn] patients with pharmacy, X-ray, and laboratory departments under one roof). An HMO, like a hospital, usually has an approved drug list or **formulary** that has been recommended by a pharmacist and approved by the medical staff. The formulary plus the use of low-cost generic drugs allows the organization to volume-purchase select drugs to lower operational and patient costs.

After the patient sees the physician, the patient may go to the HMO pharmacy to fill a prescription. As with many community pharmacies, patients seeking refills of prescription medication may call an automated telephone number to expedite processing and reduce waiting times. Besides reducing waiting time by the patient, this call-in system also allows the pharmacist to spend more time reviewing the computerized medication profile, which is an important part of the prescription preparation process. The system also allows the pharmacist time to provide counseling to the patient. The additional time in reviewing profiles and counseling patients will hopefully lead to fewer medication errors.

Many HMO pharmacies have a tiered pricing plan so that patients pay one price for a generic drug, a higher price for a "preferred" brand name drug, and an even higher price for a "nonpreferred" brand name product. An HMO pharmacy generally has a lower inventory of brand name drugs than a community pharmacy due to the presence of a more restricted drug formulary and tiered pricing plan. Many insurance companies have adopted a restricted formulary and tiered pricing plan for covering drug insurance claims in the community pharmacy. Needless to say, tiered pricing gives the patient incentive to choose generic or preferred brand name drugs whenever possible.

Nuclear Pharmacies A **nuclear pharmacy** is a specialized practice that compounds and dispenses sterile radioactive pharmaceuticals for over 100 diagnostic or therapeutic uses. Specialized equipment and training and certifications in radiation safety are required to practice in such an environment. Staff must wear badges to monitor exposure to radiation. A nuclear pharmacy is commonly located off-site and managed by one of several specialty pharmaceutical manufacturers.

The Pharmacist

The role of the modern-day **pharmacist** has evolved from compounder and dispenser of natural medicines to dispenser of synthetic products and medication information. In the last two decades the pharmacist has become more intricately involved in the prevention of medication-related problems relating to dose, adverse reactions, and safe combinations of drugs. The profession of pharmacy exists today primarily to safeguard the health of the public. The pharmacist can impact patient safety by recognizing an error in the dosing of a medication, a problematic combination of drugs, or a dangerous use of a drug such as in the case of a drug that might cause a birth defect when taken by a pregnant woman. Prescription medications can cure illness and prevent and control disease. However, adverse reactions and interactions with other medications and foods can occur and cause costly hospitalizations or even death.

Evolution of the Pharmacist's Role

During the twentieth century the pharmacy profession evolved through four stages:

1. Traditional era—dominated by the formulation and dispensing of drugs from natural botanical sources such as plants
2. Scientific era—dominated by the development of drugs and scientific testing of the effects of drugs on the body and mass production of synthetic drugs
3. Clinical era—evolved in the 1960s and combined traditional roles of the pharmacist with a new role as dispenser of drug information to the patient and physician
4. Pharmaceutical care era—expanded the mission statements of the profession to include responsibility for ensuring positive outcomes for drug therapy

During the traditional era the job of the pharmacist or apothecary consisted almost entirely of preparing and dispensing drugs. In the 1920s, for example, 80% of all prescriptions were compounded individually by the pharmacist; today less than 1% are. A nineteenth-century apothecary not only sold drugs but also often gathered plant botanicals and created or manufactured medicines from them. The soda fountain was also a unique feature of most pharmacies in this era due to the pharmacist's knowledge of mixing and compounding syrups, carbonation, and chemistry; Coca Cola and Pepsi were developed by pharmacists.

Unlike today, at the turn of the century a pharmacist-in-training would spend more time as an apprentice in a pharmacy than as a full-time student in the university. During this time the study of pharmacognosy was emphasized in academic studies. **Pharmacognosy** is the knowledge of the medicinal functions of natural products from animal, plant, or mineral origins, and galenical pharmacy is the knowledge of the techniques for preparing medications from such sources.

The emergence of the pharmaceutical industry in the twentieth century ("scientific era") created a crisis for the profession. During this scientific era after World War II, pharmaceutical manufacturers developed many new drugs and dosage forms such as tablets and capsules that were synthesized, developed, and mass-produced more economically and with better quality than by the indi-

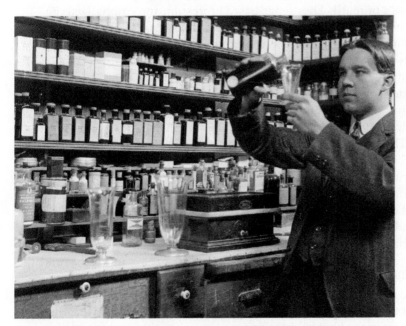

Dr. Emil King prepares medicine in his pharmacy in Fulda, Minnesota, in 1905. Many physicians owned pharmacies in the early nineteenth century and prepared their medications from natural sources.

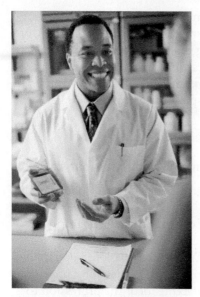

The pharmacist, with the support of the pharmacy technician, works to ensure positive outcomes for drug therapy through careful medication monitoring and patient counseling.

vidual pharmacist. Antibiotics, hormones, vaccines, and other drugs were synthesized and brought to the market. As the manufacturing of drugs moved from the apothecary shop to the assembly lines of the pharmaceutical manufacturers, the pharmacist increasingly became more a retail merchant selling premanufactured products. To counter this trend and keep up with the many scientific advances, educational institutions increased the emphasis on the sciences and expanded the curriculum. A 5 year (including 2 years of prepharmacy coursework) Bachelor of Science degree was required in 1960. **Pharmacology**, the scientific study of drugs and their mechanism of action including side effects, became an increasing part of the pharmacy curriculum, along with physics, medicinal chemistry, and physiology.

The clinical era began in the early 1960s. Additional basic science courses were developed including **pharmaceutics**, which studied the release characteristics of the drug dosage form. By this time many pharmacy students and practitioners began to feel that their training had shifted too far in the direction of basic scientific knowledge and had strayed too far from the actual practice of pharmacy. Pharmacists constituted a highly knowledgeable, scientifically trained professional class with vast knowledge of drugs; yet they were often underutilized and devoted the bulk of their energies to completing routine tasks, running a business, and dispensing drugs rather than sharing information on drugs and interacting with patients and other professionals. In fact, up until 1969 it was *not ethical* for a pharmacist to label the medication vials with the drug name or discuss potential side effects with the patient.

In 1973 the American Association of Colleges of Pharmacy (AACP) established a study commission under Dr. John S. Millis to reevaluate the mission of the pharmacy profession. The 1975 Millis Commission report, titled *Pharmacists for the Future*, defined pharmacy as a primarily knowledge-based profession and emphasized the *clinical* role of pharmacists in sharing their knowledge about drug use.

The Millis Commission report led to a new emphasis in the profession called *clinical* or *patient-oriented pharmacy*. Curriculums were again changed, and more colleges of pharmacy eventually adopted 6-year Doctor of Pharmacy (PharmD) degree programs. New courses were developed, such as **pharmacokinetics** (individualizing doses of drugs based on absorption, distribution, metabolism, and elimination from the body), biochemistry (applying chemistry to biological processes), therapeutics, and pathophysiology. **Therapeutics** is the study of applying pharmacology to the treatment of illness and disease states, whereas **pathophysiology** is the study of disease and illnesses affecting the normal function of the body. In addition, laboratories were moved from the university to more patient-oriented pharmacy practice settings, such as the hospital and community pharmacy. Interdisciplinary experiences with physicians, residents, and interns in the university hospital became a standard practice.

In 1990 Drs. Charles Hepler and Linda Strand built on the Millis Report with a new framework defined as **pharmaceutical care**, which further expanded the role of the pharmacist to include appropriate medication use to achieve positive outcomes with the prescribed drug therapy. The mission statements of many pharmacy organizations now reflect this new philosophy. During this pharmaceutical care era, the patient-oriented focus in the hospital began to move more to the community pharmacy setting. Patient counseling and medication monitoring and management by the pharmacist are becoming more accepted by physicians and consumers.

The Role of the Pharmacist

In the traditional era the primary duty of the pharmacist was compounding, the mixing of herbs and chemicals to create tablets, capsules, ointments, and solutions; however, today compounding in pharmacy is nearly a lost art (see Chapter 8, *Nonsterile Pharmaceutical Compounding*). The advanced education and training of pharmacists have prepared them to assume more patient care responsibilities and liability. Today the pharmacist still compounds and dispenses drugs but increasingly spends more time doing the following:

- gathering information and inquiring about the medical, medication, and allergy histories of patients
- checking age-appropriate dosing for medications and avoiding duplications of therapy
- counseling on possible side effects and adverse reactions
- checking computer screens to monitor for drug interactions with other prescription drugs, over-the-counter (OTC) drugs, and diet supplements
- screening patients for minor illnesses that can be safely self-medicated
- providing information and making recommendations about OTC medications, as well as vitamins, minerals, herbs, and diet supplements
- providing drug information to physicians, physician assistants, nurse practitioners, and nurses
- providing advice about home healthcare supplies (e.g., home test kits, insulin needles, support hose) and medical equipment (e.g., home monitors to check blood sugar, wheelchairs, crutches, walkers, canes)
- monitoring drug response in patients with chronic diseases such as high blood pressure, diabetes mellitus, high cholesterol, and asthma
- monitoring the safe use of controlled substances such as narcotics
- vaccinating high-risk adults

Today's community pharmacist now has a broader scope of practice that includes not only dispensing drugs for existing disease but also creating patient care initiatives to prevent or identify disease. Because of their accessibility, many pharmacists are now trained to administer immunizations such as influenza (i.e., "flu") and pneumonia shots to the high-risk older adult population in the community and nursing home where state law permits. Other pharmacists are active in screening for and educating their patients about high blood pressure, diabetes, cholesterol, or osteoporosis before these diseases can damage the body. Pharmacists also can be trained to assist and support motivated patients to quit smoking. Other educational trends for the pharmacist include assisting patients to take better care of themselves with healthier lifestyle choices and advising them about the selection of OTC drugs, vitamins, minerals, herbs, and diet supplements.

The successful pharmacist practicing in an independent pharmacy must

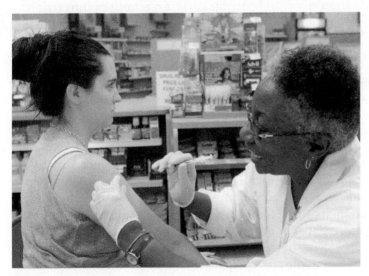

The pharmacist's role has continued to evolve, and now many pharmacists provide services to promote public health. For example, many pharmacists administer flu vaccines each fall season.

also be a businessperson and entrepreneur, offering needed but as yet unmet services to the community. The pharmacist commonly functions as a small businessperson through the following activities:

- hiring and supervising employees
- evaluating insurance contracts
- reconciling unpaid insurance claims
- maintaining and ordering sufficient inventory
- selling merchandise not directly related to health
- managing the retail operation

In larger university hospitals, more specialization exists among advanced-trained pharmacists (i.e., pediatrics, neonatal, internal medicine, critical care, cancer, transplant, nutrition, surgery), who often accompany physicians on their morning rounds, advise them on appropriate medication use, and monitor patients for adverse effects or drug interactions. These pharmacists are often responsible for educating and counseling patients about their drugs and diseases when they are discharged from the hospital. Other typical tasks for the hospital pharmacist include providing drug information, recommending drug formulary changes, educating nurses, developing departmental policies and procedures, dispensing investigational and hazardous drugs, purchasing drugs and medical supplies, monitoring narcotic and antibiotic use, and providing medications to each unit of the hospital, including carts of medicines to be used in medical emergency situations.

The pharmacist who works in a home healthcare pharmacy may prepare medications and IVs, including IV nutrition and antibiotics, for home use for patients of all ages, as well as chemotherapy and pain medications for cancer patients. Pharmacists practicing in a long-term care facility or nursing home often provide the following services:

- establish recordkeeping systems related to controlled substances
- review the drug regimens of residents, reporting irregularities related to drug treatments or controlled substances
- monitor the on-site repackaging and storage of pharmaceuticals
- ensure that medications are uncontaminated and have not expired
- call attention to medication errors and possible adverse reactions or interactions
- educate residents and sometimes their family members regarding drug therapies and self-medication
- provide medications to outpatients or residents on weekend leave

In many of these areas the pharmacist may also play a crucial role in ensuring regulatory compliance by the long-term care facility. For example, the consultant pharmacist must perform a monthly check of each patient drug profile in a long-term care facility. The professional organization for "geriatric" consultant pharmacists is the American Society of Consultant Pharmacists (ASCP).

In addition to dispensing prescriptions in an HMO pharmacy, many advanced-trained clinical pharmacists work closely with primary-care physicians to better control chronic disease by educating, monitoring, and, if necessary, adjusting the dosages of medications per physician-approved protocols. The pharmacist may be more involved in monitoring the response of drugs to better control chronic diseases such as high blood pressure, diabetes, asthma, high cholesterol, and clotting disorders.

The specific responsibilities of the pharmacist will vary somewhat depending on the work environment; however, considerable overlap exists. For example, the community pharmacist may now be responsible for preparing sterile intravenous (IV) medica-

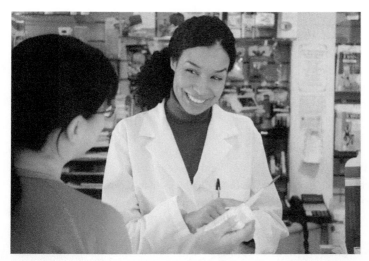

The pharmacist plays an important role in dispensing medications, as well as instructing patients about side effects of medications, food and drug interactions, and dosing schedules.

tions for the home healthcare patient or sending medications to a nursing home. The hospital pharmacist may counsel patients on their discharge medications. The pharmacist works closely with the healthcare team to optimize therapy and improve patient care in nearly all practice settings.

Thus the modern-day pharmacist in all practice settings carries out the important role of monitoring response to therapy, as well as educating patients and dispensing prescription drugs, in part, to prevent costly hospitalization from preventable adverse reactions and interactions. In addition, the pharmacist serves as a reliable source of drug information for the other healthcare professionals.

Education and Licensing Requirements for Pharmacists

During the growth and development of pharmacy in the United States many "pharmacists" were actually dispensing physicians. In the early 1800s the Philadelphia College of Pharmacy became the first school to offer courses in materia medica, pharmacy, and pharmaceutical chemistry and to grant pharmacy-specific diplomas. Landgrant universities, starting with the University of Michigan in 1868, started offering formal education and degree programs. It was not until the late 1800s that the American Pharmaceutical Association (APhA) encouraged exams and licensure to be required and the profession to be regulated by the state government. Up until 1920 formal education was not required in order to take an examination to become a pharmacist; prior to this time applicants could complete a 3 or 4 year apprenticeship before taking the exam.

With the advancement of the sciences, the control of the profession moved from apprenticeships under the pharmacist's guidance to more formal education of students within the university. Students took internships with practitioners that were remnants of the apprenticeship program. One indication of the rising professional status of pharmacy is the stringent licensing and educational requirements placed on practitioners. Over the past 80 years the curriculum in pharmacy has expanded from 2 to 6 years because of the complexity of new drugs and expanded roles for the pharmacist.

All colleges of pharmacy now offer the Doctor of Pharmacy (PharmD) degree, which is usually the equivalent of a 6-year program. Most colleges of pharmacy require 2 years of prepharmacy education, including calculus, chemistry, physics, microbiology, and biology. Many colleges require applicants to take the Pharmacy College Admission Test (PCAT), and most colleges require an on-site interview. Acceptance into a pharmacy school has become extremely competitive in recent years. The typical successful applicant has a prior degree, grade point average (GPA) of 3.5/4.0, experience in pharmacy and community service projects, and excellent communication skills and self-motivation. Many pharmacy students started out working as pharmacy technicians in a community or hospital pharmacy and gained valuable experience that helped shape their career goals.

At this time, I vow to devote my professional life to the service of all humankind through the profession of pharmacy.

I will consider the welfare of humanity and relief of human suffering my primary concerns.

I will apply my knowledge, experience, and skills to the best of my ability to assure optimal drug therapy outcomes for the patients I serve.

I will keep abreast of developments and maintain professional competency in my profession of pharmacy.

I will maintain the highest principles of moral, ethical, and legal conduct.

I will embrace and advocate change in the profession of pharmacy that improves patient care.

I take these vows voluntarily with the full realization of the responsibility with which I am entrusted by the public.

Source: Courtesy of the American Association of Colleges of Pharmacy.

Once accepted at a university, pharmacy students find that the coursework is extremely challenging. Basic science courses include anatomy and physiology, pathophysiology of disease, biochemistry, immunology, pharmaceutics, pharmacokinetics, pharmacology, and therapeutics. Practice or internship time in community and hospital pharmacies is interspersed throughout the curriculum. The last year in the PharmD program is spent in various practice settings such as hospitals, clinics, community pharmacies, home healthcare, and nursing homes to expose and better prepare the student to practice all functions of pharmacy. At graduation, it is tradition for all graduates to recite the Pharmacist's Oath (see Table 1.1).

In the United States, all states require pharmacists to be licensed. Obtaining a license involves graduating from an accredited college of pharmacy, passing a state board certification examination, and serving an internship under a licensed pharmacist either during or after formal schooling. In addition, in most states, pharmacists must meet continuing education requirements to renew their licenses. Most states have reciprocal agreements recognizing licenses granted to pharmacists in other states. Licensing and professional oversight governing the practice are carried out by state pharmacy boards in each state. Some pharmacy graduates will go on to pursue further education and higher degrees, residencies, or fellowships; others will enter specialty fields such as managed care or work in mail-order pharmacies, home healthcare, long-term care, nuclear pharmacy, or academia, as well as in drug information, sales, marketing, or research.

The Pharmacy Technician

The modern-day role of the pharmacist would not be possible without the assistance of well-trained and educated pharmacy technicians. A **pharmacy technician**, also called the pharmacy tech, is an individual working in a pharmacy who, under the direct supervision of a licensed pharmacist, assists in all pharmacy activities that do not require the professional judgment of a pharmacist.

The number of prescriptions filled increases each year as our population ages and lives longer. The pharmacy technician can assume routine functions that allow the pharmacist to spend more time reviewing the computerized profile, counseling the patient, or communicating with the physician. Regardless of practice setting, the pharmacy tech can assist with workload by entering patient and prescription information into the computer, preparing the medication to be dispensed, and providing customer service. The pharmacist provides the final check on the original prescription with the medication bottle and label prior to counseling the patient.

Evolution of the Pharmacy Technician's Role

The expansion of the pharmacist's role has created an increasing need in the workforce for educated, well-trained pharmacy technicians. Without pharmacy technicians, pharmacists would not have sufficient time to counsel patients, review medication profiles, monitor for side effects and adverse reactions, screen patients for disease, and discuss cost-effective drug therapy options with the prescriber. Without pharmacy techs, the risk of preventable and costly medication errors may increase.

The role of the pharmacy technician has evolved over the past four decades. Originally, many pharmacy techs were trained as medics in the military and returned after service to our country to take positions in hospitals where they could better use their training and experience. In the hospital, the technician was trained to participate in drug delivery systems and the compounding of sterile preparations. In more recent times the role of the pharmacy tech has slowly evolved from that of a part-time clerk or cashier to more of a pharmacist's assistant in the community pharmacy. In the early nineteenth century a category of registered pharmacy assistants was recognized; these individuals were commonly apprentices without formal education but served as predecessors for today's pharmacy technicians.

Technician activities may range from ordering, stocking, and inventorying drugs to preparing the IV order to assisting in the dispensing process (e.g., gathering and entering patient and prescription information in the computer, retrieving the medication, dispensing and preparing a label for the medication). In addition to providing the final check on the medication order, the pharmacist is also responsible for patient counseling or giving specific advice to the patient on prescription or nonprescription medications. Only the pharmacist typically can discuss prescription changes with the physician or nurse and counsel patients. The technician functions in strict accordance with standard written procedures and guidelines, especially in the hospital setting.

A central defining feature of the technician's job is accountability to the pharmacist for the quality and accuracy of his or her work. Although the technician carries out many of the duties traditionally performed by pharmacists, the pharmacist must always check the technician's work. Medication errors such as entering incorrect data from the prescription or selecting the wrong drug, dose, or dosage form can cause serious and sometimes life-threatening reactions if not detected. As a paraprofessional (defined as a skilled assistant to a professional person), the pharmacy technician bears a relationship to the pharmacist similar to that of an X-ray technician to a radiologist or a medical technologist to a pathologist. The pharmacist, in turn, takes final responsibility (and liability) for the technician's actions. It is important to note that the essential differences in the duties of a pharmacist and a technician involve accountability and making decisions about the patient's health care.

The Role of the Pharmacy Technician

Nearly everywhere a pharmacist practices there will be one or more pharmacy techs also working. As will be discussed later in Unit 2, pharmacy technicians employed in a community pharmacy typically do the following:

- enter prescription information into the computerized patient database
- aid the pharmacist in the filling, labeling, and recording of prescriptions

Safety Note

Rather than working independently, the pharmacy technician works under the direction of the supervising pharmacist.

Safety Note

Pharmacy technicians play a valuable role in reducing the risk of medication errors.

- operate and assume responsibility for the pharmacy cash register
- stock and inventory prescription and over-the-counter (OTC) medications (those not needing a prescription)
- maintain computerized patient records
- bill online insurance claims
- order and maintain parts of the front-end stock

The pharmacy technician in a hospital setting may take part in these and other functions involving delivering, stocking, or inventorying medications anywhere in the hospital. In addition, the pharmacy technician may operate manual or computerized robotic dispensing machinery. In both the hospital and home healthcare setting, technicians will be involved in the preparation of sterile and sometimes hazardous products. Unit 3 contains more discussion on the role of the pharmacy technician in the hospital setting.

The pharmacy technician's duties in long-term care or nursing home settings have characteristics of his or her duties in both community and hospital pharmacies. Under supervision by the pharmacist, in a long-term care facility, a tech may do the following:

- log prescriptions and refill orders via computer
- prepare online billings
- maintain drug boxes or trays for emergencies
- package and label medications
- deliver medications to the nursing home
- maintain records, retrieve patient charts, and organize them for the pharmacist's review
- conduct regularly scheduled inspections of drugs in inventory and in nursing stations to remove expired or recalled medications
- repackage drugs in unit doses labeled for each patient

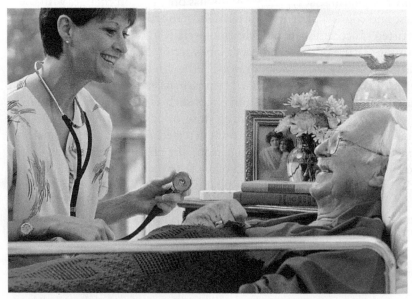

Pharmacy technicians also work in HMO settings and perform functions similar to those in the community pharmacy, with the exception that insurance billing and cashiering are minimal. Automation is more likely to be used in a large-volume mail-order operation, and medications may be filled 24 hours per day, 7 days a week.

Pharmacists and pharmacy technicians work with home healthcare workers who provide services to homebound patients.

Education and Licensing Requirements for Pharmacy Techs

Most state boards of pharmacy now recognize the existence and importance of the pharmacy technician. The American Pharmaceutical Association (APhA) supports state regulation of technicians by either registration or licensure. Most state boards of pharmacy regulate the activities and even the ratio of pharmacy techs to pharmacists within a pharmacy.

In the past, on-the-job training was sufficient for the tech working in a pharmacy. To better assist the pharmacist in providing patient care, formal technician training programs have been developed in order to better train pharmacy technicians for their expanded roles in the pharmacy. Initially these programs were centered in the hospitals to better train their staff in the necessary functions of the hospital pharmacy. Today, some programs remain hospital-based, but many more are being developed in community colleges and technical schools to meet the increasing personnel needs, especially in the community pharmacy setting.

The American Society of Health-System Pharmacists (ASHP) developed a model curriculum as a guide to meet the needs of technicians in all practice settings. Academic-based programs vary in curriculum and length. In some states pharmacy technicians must be certified to practice. (See more on certification in Chapter 14, *Your Future in Pharmacy Practice*.) Many hospital and community pharmacies may require that pharmacy technicians be initially certified or become certified within a specified period of time. Some pharmacy employers encourage technicians to become certified by paying for the certification exam and giving salary increases to those who pass it.

In a specialized area of practice such as sterile and nonsterile compounding and nuclear pharmacy, the pharmacy technician requires additional training and certifications. The Professional Compounding Centers of America (PCCA) provides didactic courses and laboratories in which pharmacy technicians learn the latest innovations in compounding unique dosage forms in the hospital and community pharmacy. To receive certification as a nuclear pharmacy technician (NPT), one must complete a rigorous 300 hours of online self-study and supervised instruction in addition to experiential training with nuclear pharmacists serving as preceptors. With additional training, certifications, and responsibilities, an increase in salary can be expected.

Formal education programs are designed to better prepare the student to pass the certification exam and start a challenging career as a certified pharmacy technician. In many states technicians are required to attend seminars to keep their knowledge and skills current for continuing certifications and/or licensure. In addition to education, registration, licensure, and certification, a pharmacy technician must possess other personal characteristics to successfully contribute to patient care in a pharmacy. The importance of communication skills and professional attitudes and behaviors is discussed in Chapter 13. Similar to the Pharmacist's Oath, a code of ethics for the pharmacy technician is an important aspect of professional recognition and is discussed further in Chapter 14.

Chapter Terms

alchemy the European practice during the Middle Ages that combined elements of chemistry, metallurgy, physics, and medicine with astrology, mysticism, and spiritualism such as turning ordinary metals into silver and gold

chain pharmacy a community pharmacy that consists of several similar pharmacies in the region (or nation) that are corporately owned

community pharmacy any independent, chain, or franchise pharmacy that dispenses prescription medications to outpatients; also called a *retail pharmacy*

compounding pharmacy a pharmacy that specializes in the preparation of nonsterile (and sometimes sterile) preparations that are not commercially available

formulary a list of drugs that have been pre-approved for use by a committee of health professionals; used in hospitals, in managed care, and by many insurance providers

franchise pharmacy a small chain of professional community pharmacies that dispense and prepare medications but are independently owned; sometimes called an *apothecary*

health maintenance organization (HMO) an organization that provides health insurance using a managed care model

home healthcare the delivery of medical, nursing, and pharmaceutical services and supplies to patients at home

home healthcare pharmacy a pharmacy that dispenses, prepares, and delivers drugs and medical supplies directly to the home of the patient

hospital pharmacy an institutional pharmacy that dispenses and prepares drugs and provides clinical services in a hospital setting

independent pharmacy a community pharmacy that is privately owned by the pharmacist

institutional pharmacy a pharmacy that is organized under a corporate structure, following specific rules and regulations for accreditation

long-term care facility an institution that provides care for geriatric and disabled patients; includes extended-care facility (ECF) and skilled-care facility (SCF)

mail-order pharmacy a large-volume centralized pharmacy operation that uses automation to fill and mail prescriptions to a patient

managed care a type of health insurance system that emphasizes keeping the patient healthy or diseases controlled in order to reduce healthcare costs

nuclear pharmacy a specialized practice that compounds and dispenses sterile radioactive pharmaceuticals to diagnose or treat disease

pathophysiology the study of disease and illnesses affecting the normal function of the body

pharmaceutical care a philosophy of care that expanded the pharmacist's role to include appropriate medication use to achieve positive outcomes with prescribed drug therapy

pharmaceutics the study of the release characteristics of specific drug dosage forms

pharmacist one who is licensed to prepare and dispense medications, counsel patients, and monitor outcomes pursuant to a prescription from a licensed health professional

pharmacognosy the study of medicinal functions of natural products of animal, plant, or mineral origins

pharmacokinetics individualized doses of drugs based on absorption, distribution, metabolism, and elimination

pharmacology the scientific study of drugs and their mechanisms of action

pharmacy technician an individual working in a pharmacy who, under the supervision of a licensed pharmacist, assists in activities not requiring the professional judgment of a pharmacist; also called the *pharmacy tech* or *tech*

therapeutics the study of applying pharmacology to the treatment of illness and disease states

Chapter Summary

- The profession of pharmacy has ancient roots, dating to the use of drugs for magical and curative purposes.
- Pharmacy has evolved over the past 50 years from preparing natural medications to dispensing synthetic medications.
- The primary mission of pharmacy is to safeguard the public and help patients achieve favorable outcomes with their prescribed medication(s).
- Today, pharmacists are highly educated professionals who are licensed to practice in a wide variety of practice settings.
- The pharmacist is responsible for dispensing the medication to patients, as well as the necessary information to appropriately use the products.

- Pharmacists in all settings provide a readily available resource to healthcare professionals on information related to drug therapy.
- The pharmacy technician is a paraprofessional who, under the direct supervision of a pharmacist, carries out a wide range of duties in order for the pharmacist to effectively carry out his or her professional responsibilities.
- Formal educational training programs and opportunities to become a certified pharmacy technician are becoming more important in all practice settings.
- Because of our aging population and the subsequent need for prescription medications required for many people to live longer and better lives, pharmacists and pharmacy technicians are in great demand.

Chapter Review

Checking Your Understanding

Choose the best answer from those provided.

1. A list of *approved* drugs in ancient Egypt was also known as a
   a. formulary.
   b. dispensatory.
   c. pharmacopeia.
   d. All of the above

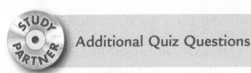 Additional Quiz Questions

2. The profession of pharmacy exists today to
   a. distribute prescription drugs to the public.
   b. control narcotic drug use by the public.
   c. provide necessary OTC and herbal medications to the public.
   d. safeguard the health of the public.

3. Knowledge of the medicinal functions of natural products from animal, plant, or mineral origins is known as
   a. pharmacognosy.
   b. pharmacology.
   c. nuclear pharmacy.
   d. clinical pharmacy.

4. The emergence of the pharmaceutical industry threatened to reduce the role of the pharmacist to that of a
   a. compounder of medications.
   b. pharmaceutical scientist.
   c. drugstore operator.
   d. toxicologist.

5. The work that heralded the emergence of modern clinical pharmacy was the
   a. Ebers Report.
   b. Millis Commission Report.
   c. Report of the President's Commission on Controlled Substances.
   d. Kefauver-Harris Amendment to the Food, Drug, and Cosmetic (FDC) Act of 1938.

6. Another name for a community pharmacy is a
   a. retail pharmacy.
   b. long-term care facility.
   c. home healthcare pharmacy.
   d. health maintenance organization (HMO).

7. The primary role of a clinical pharmacist is to
   a. dispense medications.
   b. compound medications.
   c. develop a drug formulary.
   d. provide information about medications and monitor drug therapy to ensure optimal patient outcomes.

8. Licensing and professional oversight of pharmacists and pharmacy technicians is carried out by the
   a. colleges of pharmacy.
   b. American Pharmacists Association.
   c. United States Pharmacopeial Convention (USP).
   d. state pharmacy boards.

9. A pharmacy technician can do all the following *except*
   a. counsel a patient.
   b. enter information into the computer.
   c. prepare a label.
   d. return drug stock to the shelf.

10. The final responsibility for the accuracy of the pharmacy technician's work is the
    a. pharmacy technician himself or herself.
    b. another pharmacy technician.
    c. supervising pharmacist.
    d. store manager.

Thinking Like a Pharmacy Tech

1. Go to the library and find a copy of the latest edition of the federal government's *Occupational Outlook Handbook*. Using information from this handbook, prepare a short report on the work conditions, duties, training, salaries, and job outlook for pharmacy technicians.

2. Call a local drugstore and hospital pharmacy and arrange to interview two practicing pharmacy technicians about their job duties. Compare your findings with the description you researched in Exercise 1. Prepare an oral report for your class.

3. Contact the program director of a pharmacy technician training program in another state. Request (or view online) a copy of the program's curriculum. Based on the information that you receive, contrast this curriculum with your current program.

Communicating Clearly

1. Explain why you think it is important for patients to play an active role in their own health care. How can the pharmacist's role be adapted to meet this need?

2. The pharmacist has been at or near the top of many surveys that rank the public's trust. Pharmacists and those who work in a pharmacy strive to behave in a professional manner and communicate effectively with the patients they serve. Make a list of five things that you have noticed about the profession of pharmacy and/or a particular pharmacist that make you feel the trust is warranted.

3. Review the most recent National Association of Boards of Pharmacy (NABP) *Survey of Pharmacy Law* and discuss the status of pharmacy technicians in your state. Where else might you find this information?

Researching on the Web

Exercises in this section focus on Web research and information retrieval. The information you access on the Internet needs to be thoughtfully reviewed and evaluated. As you complete the Internet questions in this and later chapters, use the following questions to help determine the reliability and validity of information:

- Who created this site, and who are the sponsors of the site? From whose perspective is the material written?
- Who is the intended audience of the site?
- What special knowledge do the site authors and contributors have?
- Is the material factual, or does it seem biased? Can the information be validated by a secondary source?
- When and how often is the Web site updated?
- Is this site easy to navigate? Can you find new information quickly and efficiently?
- Will you bookmark this site and use it regularly?

1. Visit one of the many online news services such as Microsoft Network (MSN), Cable News Network (CNN), American Broadcasting Company (ABC), Reuters, or medical online news services such as Medscape, WebMD, or Mayohealth. Search these sites and find at least three recent news items about a medical treatment or new drugs. Print and summarize the articles and present them to the class.

2. Visit a healthcare organization (e.g., American Heart Association, American Cancer Society, American Diabetes Association) and list three lifestyle changes that can prevent or minimize disease.

3. Go to jointcommission.org and enter the key words "medication errors." Identify the five most common causes of medication errors with older adults in the hospital.

4. Visit www.ascp.com and review the guidelines on the various roles of pharmacy technicians in long-term care.

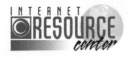 For further study of chapter-related topics, explore the Web links in the Web Center at www.emcp.net/pharmpractice4e.

Pharmacy Law, Regulations, and Standards

2

Learning Objectives

- Distinguish among laws, regulations, professional standards, and ethics.
- List and describe the major impacts on the profession of pharmacy by major pieces of statutory federal drug law in the twentieth century.
- Discuss the roles of the Food and Drug Administration, the Drug Enforcement Administration, the Occupational Safety and Health Administration, and the national and state boards of pharmacy.

- Enumerate the duties that may legally be performed by pharmacy technicians in most states.
- Explain the potential for tort actions under the common law related to negligence and other forms of malpractice.
- Discuss the importance of drug and professional standards.

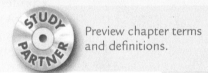

Preview chapter terms and definitions.

A variety of mechanisms control the practice of pharmacy including common, statutory, and regulatory laws passed by federal, state, and local government entities. In addition, standards are established by professional organizations. Laws have been passed to limit the abuse potential of controlled substances, mandate pharmacist counseling, and provide drug insurance for Medicare patients. Technicians must be aware of laws and regulations, as violations may result in lawsuits and loss of employment. The complex system of interrelated laws, regulations, and standards helps to ensure that the marketing and dispensing of medications is carried out safely and in the public interest.

The Need for Drug Control

In the United States, the laws related to pharmacy practice are generally stricter than those in other countries. For example, in some countries you may be able to get many medications, including antibiotics, without a prescription. To persons working in pharmacy in the United States today, such laxity of control over drugs seems astonishing when one considers the possibility of inappropriate use, adverse reactions, and interactions with other drugs. Issues related to our drug laws and regulations are being debated publicly because of the illegal importation of drugs from Canada and Mexico by many U.S. citizens.

The contemporary pharmacy is subject to many kinds of control at the federal, state, and local levels. Various groups and organizations, including the following, exercise controls on contemporary pharmacy:

- courts
- federal, state, and local legislative bodies such as the U.S. Congress, state legislatures, and municipal governing councils
- federal and state regulatory agencies
    - Food and Drug Administration (FDA), with general authority to regulate the manufacture and sale of drugs
    - Drug Enforcement Administration (DEA), with enforcement authority over controlled substances
    - Occupational Safety and Health Administration (OSHA), with authority over workplace safety
    - Federal Trade Commission (FTC), with authority over business practices
    - Health Care Financing Administration (HCFA) of the Department of Health and Human Services (DHHS) and Center for Medicare Services (CMS), with authority over reimbursement under the Medicare and Medicaid programs
    - state health and welfare agencies
    - state boards of pharmacy, with licensure and regulatory authority over pharmacy practice at the state level
- United States Pharmacopeia (USP), which publishes the compendia setting standards for drug formulation, dosage forms, and compounding standards
- professional organizations
    - American Pharmacists Association (APhA)
    - American Association of Colleges of Pharmacy (AACP)
    - National Association of Boards of Pharmacy (NABP)
    - the Joint Commission, formerly the Joint Commission on Accreditation of Healthcare Organizations (JCAHO)
    - American Society of Health-System Pharmacists (ASHP)
    - Academy of Managed Care Pharmacy (AMCP)
- individual institutions such as community pharmacies, hospitals, long-term care facilities, and home healthcare organizations

Due to the importance of drugs in our society, their control and the profession of pharmacy are governed by both state and federal laws, regulations, and professional standards within the industry.

Laws

A **law** is a rule that is passed and enforced by the legislative branch of government. Combined, laws are a system of rules that reflects the society and culture out of which they arise. The law offers a *minimum* level of acceptable standards. The legislature represents consumers in passing and enforcing laws that are designed to protect the public. Violations in laws may result in damages, fines, probation, loss of licensure, or even incarceration in extreme cases.

Regulations

A **regulation** is a written rule and procedure that exists to carry out a law of the state or federal government. For example, the Food and Drug Administration (FDA) has published regulations on the drug approval process, generic drug substitution, patient counseling, and adverse reaction reporting systems. The Drug Enforcement Agency (DEA) has rules regulating the distribution, storage, documentation, and filling of controlled substances. For example, when dispensing and billing prescriptions, pharmacists and technicians must follow Medicare Part D and Medicaid regulations. The state board of pharmacies has regulations that must be followed with regard to the practice of pharmacy within that state. Where there is conflict between federal and state laws or regulations, the more strict law or regulation applies.

Standards

A **standard** is a set of criteria to measure product quality or professional performance against a norm. Standards exist for both drug products and individual professional behavior. For example, the United States Pharmacopeia (USP), with input from scientists, sets standards or criteria for drug quality that must be met by pharmaceutical companies before their new products are submitted to the FDA. The USP also has set national standards for all pharmacies preparing sterile and nonsterile preparations.

The Joint Commission provides a higher standard of care in hospitals and other healthcare facilities through a rigorous inspection in its accreditation process. Receiving accreditation from the Joint Commission is the healthcare equivalent of getting the *Good Housekeeping* Seal of Approval. Although accreditation is voluntary under the law, many insurance carriers require it for reimbursement when providing services for its members.

While laws represent a minimum level of standards, ethics provide for the standards of personal conduct within a profession. Ethics are standards of behavior that pharmacists and technicians are encouraged to follow. Ethical standards for pharmacy technicians are discussed in Chapter 14. If there is ever a legal challenge, the behavior of the professional is compared to the standards of other professionals practicing in the community. The concept of "standards of care" is discussed later in the chapter.

History of U.S. Statutory Pharmacy Law

During the nineteenth century, drugs in the United States were unregulated. Medicines did not have to prove to be either safe or effective in order to be marketed. The highly addictive drug opium was popularized by the Chinese laborers working on the transcontinental railroad and was widely available without a prescription and abused. Boisterous charlatans would take their traveling medicine shows from town to town in the West to proclaim the latest "miracle cure." There were no regulations on labeling these so-called medicines and no research to support any of the claims. Most of these potions contained a high content of alcohol that usually made the customer "feel better." Occasionally, some of these potions were not so innocuous and caused injury or death to those who consumed them. At the turn of the nineteenth century, there were also major concerns regarding the purity of drugs that were imported from other countries. As a result, statutory laws were established to protect the public from the dangers of unregulated drug manufacturing, marketing, and use. Statutory laws are laws passed by legislative bodies at the federal, state, and local

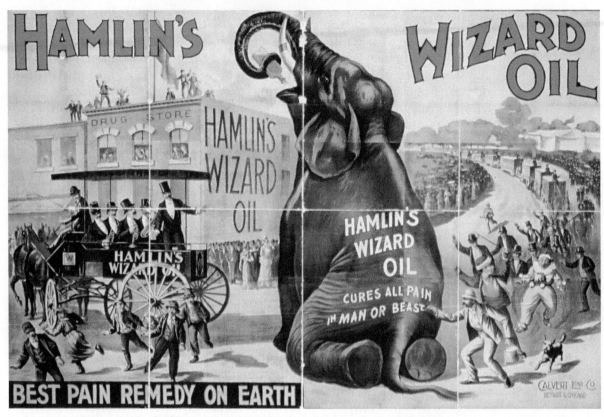

In the late 1800s there was no control on the sale of pharmaceutical products. Thus consumers were not protected.

levels. The following sections highlight the major statutory laws impacting the profession of pharmacy in chronological order.

Pure Food and Drug Act of 1906

To combat real-life abuses in drug formulation, labeling, and market claims, the U.S. Congress passed the first of a series of landmark twentieth-century laws to regulate the development, compounding, distribution, storage, and dispensing of drugs. The purpose of the Pure Food and Drug Act of 1906 was to prohibit the interstate transportation or sale of adulterated and misbranded food and drugs. This act required that the labels not contain false information about the drugs' strength and purity. The act, although amended, proved unenforceable, and new legislation was later required.

Food, Drug, and Cosmetic Act of 1938

Newly developed manufactured drugs were more powerful and potentially dangerous; thus new laws were needed. In 1937 the need for new legislation was tragically demonstrated by 107 deaths resulting from the sale of a sulfa drug product that contained diethylene glycol, a toxic chemical that is used today as antifreeze for automobile radiators. The Food, Drug, and Cosmetic (FDC) Act of 1938 is one of the most important pieces of legislation in pharmaceutical history. It created the FDA and required pharmaceutical manufacturers to file a **new drug application (NDA)** with each new drug before marketing. Manufacturers needed to prove that the product was *safe for use* by humans. In addition to proving safety, each new prescription and nonprescrip-

TABLE 2.1   Definitions of Adulterated and Misbranded Drugs

Adulterated Drugs

- consisting "in whole or in part of any filthy, putrid, or decomposed substance," ones "prepared, packed, or held under unsanitary conditions"
- prepared in containers "composed, in whole or in part, of any poisonous or deleterious substance"
- containing unsafe color additives
- purporting to be or represented as drugs recognized "in an official compendium" but differing in strength, quality, or purity from said drugs

Misbranded Drugs

- containing labeling that is "false or misleading in any particular"
- in packaging that does not bear "a label containing (1) the name and place of business of the manufacturer, packer, or distributor and (2) an accurate statement of the quantity of the contents in terms of weight, measure, or numerical count"
- not conspicuously and clearly labeled with the information required by the act
- that are habit forming but do not carry the label "Warning—May Be Habit Forming"
- that do not contain a label that "bears (1) the established name of the drug, if any, and (2) in case it contains two or more ingredients, the established name and quantity of each active ingredient, including the quantity, kind, and proportion of any alcohol, and also including, whether active or not, the established name and quantity" [of certain other substances listed in the act]
- that do not contain labeling with "adequate directions for use" and "adequate warnings against use in those pathological conditions or by children where its use may be dangerous to health, or against unsafe dose or methods or duration of administration or application"
- that are "dangerous to health when used in the dose or manner, or with the frequency or duration prescribed, recommended, or suggested in the labeling"

tion drug had to be approved by the FDA. Pharmaceutical manufacturers were required to conduct and submit the results of toxicological studies on animals followed by clinical trials with human beings to determine degree of toxicity and the effect of the drug in humans, respectively. The NDA must detail the chemical composition of the drug and the processes used to manufacture it. The FDC Act of 1938 also extended and clarified the definitions of adulterated and misbranded drugs. These definitions are provided in Table 2.1. This act also defined the relevant "official compendia" as the *United States Pharmacopeia* and the *National Formulary*.

Under this act, the FDA had the power not only to approve or deny new drug applications (NDAs) but also to conduct inspections of manufacturing plants to ensure compliance. The Supreme Court later held that the act applied to interstate transactions, as well as to intrastate transactions, including those within pharmacies. Unfortunately, the act required only that drugs be safe for human consumption, not that they be effective or useful for the purpose for which they were sold.

Durham-Humphrey Amendment of 1951

The Durham-Humphrey Amendment of 1951 stated that drug stock containers do not have to include "adequate directions for use" as long as they bear the legend "Caution: Federal Law Prohibits Dispensing without Prescription." The dispensing of the drug by a pharmacist with a label giving adequate directions for use from the prescriber meets the law's requirements. The amendment thus established the distinction between so-called legend, or prescription, drugs and over-the-counter (OTC), or nonprescription, drugs. (These types of drugs will be explained in more detail in Chapter 3, *Pharmacology in Practice*.) The amendment also authorized the taking of prescriptions verbally, rather than in writing, and the refilling of prescriptions. However, the refilling of prescriptions subject to abuse was limited. Under the amendment, prescriptions for such substances could not be refilled without the expressed consent of the prescriber.

Kefauver-Harris Amendment of 1962

The Kefauver-Harris Amendment of 1962 was passed in response to the birth of thousands of infants—mostly in Europe—with severe congenital abnormalities whose mothers had taken a new tranquilizer called *thalidomide*. It extended the FDC Act of 1938 to require that drugs not only be safe for humans but also be *effective*. The amendment requires drug manufacturers to file with the FDA an investigational new drug application (INDA) before initiating a clinical trial in humans. After extensive trials in which a product is proved both safe and effective, the manufacturer may then submit an NDA that seeks approval to market the product. The clinical testing to prove both safety and efficacy in humans takes an average of 7–10 years before reaching the marketplace; in order to compensate for innovation and research costs, the government allows "patent" protection for brand name products for a length of time.

Comprehensive Drug Abuse Prevention and Control Act of 1970

The Comprehensive Drug Abuse Prevention and Control Act of 1970, commonly referred to as the **Controlled Substances Act (CSA)**, was created to combat and control drug abuse and to supersede previous federal drug abuse laws. The act classified drugs with potential for abuse as controlled substances and ranked them into five categories, or schedules. A description of the five schedules of drugs is outlined in Table 2.2. Schedule I drugs are not commercially available.

A **controlled substance** is defined as a drug with a risk for abuse and physical or psychological dependence. The agency made primarily responsible under this act is the Drug Enforcement Administration (DEA), an arm of the Department of Justice. The DEA is charged with enforcement and prevention related to the abuse of controlled substances such as the many narcotic pain medications on the market.

Schedule I drugs are not legally dispensed in the United States due to their high potential for abuse and addiction. Schedule II narcotics are the most highly regulated, and sudden increases in usage in a particular pharmacy (or prescribed by a particular doctor) may cause the DEA to investigate. Schedule II drugs have no refills. Schedule III, IV, and V drugs have less abuse and addiction potential than Schedule II drugs and have limits on refills. Often upon recommendation from the manufacturer and the FDA, the DEA classifies new drugs into a schedule and will even reevaluate drugs that have been on the market for some time to determine whether they warrant being changed to a "scheduled" drug. For example, there is concern about the overuse of hydrocodone combination products; the DEA is considering reclassifying this drug from Schedule III to Schedule II.

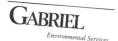
Drug Schedules under the Controlled Substances Act of 1970

	Manufacturer's Label	Abuse Potential	Accepted Medical Use	Examples
	C-I	highest potential for abuse	for research only; must have license to obtain; no accepted medical use in the United States	heroin, lysergic acid diethylamide (LSD)
Schedule II	C-II	high possibility of abuse, which can lead to severe psychological or physical dependence	dispensing severely restricted; cannot be prescribed by telephone except in an emergency; no refills on prescriptions	morphine, oxycodone, meperidine, hydromorphone, fentanyl, methylphenidate, dextroamphetamine
Schedule III	C-III	less potential for abuse and addiction than C-II	prescriptions can be refilled up to five times within 6 months if authorized by physician	codeine/hydrocodone with aspirin, codeine/hydrocodone with acetaminophen, anabolic steroids
Schedule IV	C-IV	lower abuse potential than C-II and C-III; associated with limited physical or psychological dependence	same as for Schedule III	benzodiazepines, meprobamate, phenobarbital
Schedule V	C-V	lowest abuse potential	some sold without a prescription depending on state law; if so, purchaser must be over 18 and is required to sign log and show driver's license	liquid codeine combination cough preparations, diphenoxylate/atropine

Poison Prevention Packaging Act of 1970

To prevent accidental childhood poisonings from prescription and nonprescription products, the Poison Prevention Packaging Act was passed in 1970. This act is enforced by the Consumer Product Safety Commission and requires that most over-the-counter (OTC) and prescription drugs be packaged in a **child-resistant container** that cannot be opened by 80% of children under 5 but can be opened by 90% of adults.

The law provides that on request by the patient, the pharmacist or pharmacy technician as his or her agent may dispense a drug in a non-child-resistant container. The patient, but not the prescriber, may make a blanket request that all drugs dispensed to him or her be in noncompliant containers. Many older patients and those with severe rheumatoid arthritis will request a non-child-resistant container. It is important to

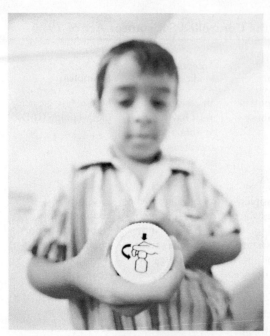

Unless specifically requested by the customer, medications are dispensed in child-resistant containers to prevent accidental poisoning.

remind such patients to childproof their homes when young children visit. The antibiotic azithromycin (or Z-pak) is an example of a common medication that can be dispensed in a non-childproof package. Other exceptions provided for by the law are detailed in Table 2.3.

Drug Listing Act of 1972

The Drug Listing Act of 1972 gives the FDA the authority to compile a list of currently marketed drugs. Under the act, each new drug is assigned a unique and permanent product code, known as a National Drug Code (NDC), consisting of 10 characters that identify the manufacturer or distributor, the drug formulation, and the size and type of its packaging. The FDA requests, but does not require, that the NDC appear on all drug labels, including labels of prescription containers. Using this code, the FDA is able to maintain a database of drugs by use, manufacturer, and active ingredients and of newly marketed, discontinued, and remarketed drugs. The bar coded information is also widely used today to double-check the accuracy of prescriptions filled by automation. The NDC will be described more thoroughly in Chapters 3, 4, and 6.

Orphan Drug Act of 1983

An **orphan drug** is one that is intended for use in a few patients with a rare disease or condition affecting less than 200,000 people. Developing and marketing such a drug

---

TABLE 2.3   Exceptions to the Requirement for Child-Resistant Containers Pursuant to the Poison Prevention Packaging Act of 1970

- single-time dispensing of product in noncompliant container as ordered by prescriber
- single-time or blanket dispensing of product in noncompliant container as requested by the patient or customer in a signed statement
- one noncompliant size of an OTC product for older adults or handicapped users, provided that the label carry the warning "This Package for Households without Young Children" or, if the label is too small, "Package Not Child Resistant"
- drugs dispensed to institutionalized patients, provided that these are to be administered by employees of the institution
- certain drugs and packaging exempt
- common examples of specific drugs:
   - inhalation aerosols (ProAir, Proventil HFA)
   - methylprednisolone (Medrol) tablets with no more than 85 mg per package
   - oral contraceptives to be taken cyclically, in manufacturer's dispensing packages
   - potassium supplements in unit dosage form
   - powdered anhydrous cholestyramine or colestipol
   - prednisone tablets with no more than 105 mg per package
   - sublingual nitroglycerin (tablets to be taken by dissolving beneath the tongue)

would be prohibitively expensive. The Orphan Drug Act of 1983 encourages the development of orphan drugs by providing tax incentives and allowing manufacturers to be granted a time for exclusive licenses to market such drugs. Orphan products often receive expedited review and accelerated approval because they are for serious or life-threatening disease. Over 250 orphan drugs have been approved by the FDA for marketing.

For example, Wilson disease is a rare progressive genetic disorder characterized by excess copper stored in various body tissues that can lead to organ dysfunction and premature death. The incidence is approximately 1 in 30,000. Early diagnosis and treatment may prevent serious long-term disability and life-threatening complications. Treatment is aimed at reducing the amount of copper that has accumulated in the body and maintaining normal copper levels thereafter. The research costs for developing treatments for such a rare disorder would be prohibitive to a pharmaceutical manufacturer without financial incentives, patent and legal protections, and accelerated approvals.

Drug Price Competition and Patent-Term Restoration Act of 1984

During the 1950s and 1960s there were many anti-substitution laws passed by the states due to "counterfeit" drugs on the market. Thus, brand name drugs were primarily used and generic drugs were limited to drugs on the market prior to 1938. By the 1980s there was political pressure by both the government and pharmacists to reduce healthcare costs by dispensing more generic drugs. A given drug typically has several names, including its chemical name and its official **generic name** or nonproprietary name, both of which are given in official compendia, and one or more **brand name** or proprietary names given by manufacturers. See Table 2.4 for a listing of the different names for one drug. The generic or trade name is commonly used on prescriptions.

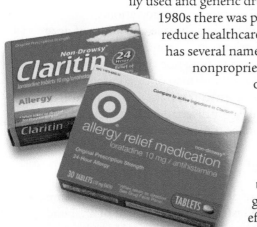

The rise in availability of cheaper, generic name drugs was due in part to the Drug Price Competition and Patent-Term Restoration Act of 1984.

Generic drugs are comparable to their brand name counterparts in dosage form, safety, strength, route of administration, quality, performance, and intended use. Generics do not go through the same rigorous scientific review on safety and effectiveness as brand name drugs; they must, however, demonstrate bioequivalence to the brand name product; this will be further discussed in Chapter 4. A generic drug can be substituted (under regulations now existing in every state) for the brand name drug in prescriptions.

The Drug Price Competition and Patent-Term Restoration Act (also known as the Waxman-Hatch Act) encouraged the creation of both generic drugs and innovative new drugs by streamlining

TABLE 2.4 Different Names for One Drug

Type of Name	Drug Name
chemical name	p-isobutylhydratropic acid
generic name	ibuprofen
brand name	Advil, Motrin, Motrin IB

the process for generic drug approval and by extending patent licenses as a function of the time required for the NDA approval process. The patent license was extended to allow the manufacturer of the brand name drug who completed the NDA to recoup research and development costs, as well as to provide an incentive to research new drugs for the marketplace. Once the original patent expires, any manufacturer is allowed to market a generic drug, which will be less costly than the brand name counterpart. The growth and expansion of generic manufacturers can be traced to this act. Today more than 60% of prescriptions in community pharmacies are dispensed with generic drugs.

Prescription Drug Marketing Act of 1987

Passed in response to concerns over safety and competition issues raised by secondary markets for drugs, the Prescription Drug Marketing Act of 1987 prohibits the re-importation of a drug into the United States by anyone except the manufacturer. This has become a major political and economic issue as many seniors travel across the border or receive their prescriptions through the mail at presumed substantial savings especially from Canada. Pharmaceutical manufacturers have threatened to reduce the supply of drugs to Canada if the practice of illegal re-importation continues. Canada is concerned that re-importation may create a shortage of medications for its own citizens. The United States has elected not to enforce the private contraband of individuals but clearly discourages its practice and hopes that the new Medicare Modernization Act of 2003 (discussed later in the chapter) will minimize re-importation.

The act also prohibits the sale or trading of drug samples, the distribution of samples to persons other than those licensed to prescribe them, and the distribution of samples except by mail or by common carrier. This action was taken in response to prescription drug samples being illegally diverted and distributed by a few unethical pharmaceutical sales representatives.

Anabolic Steroid Act of 1990

Anabolic steroids are a synthetic version of the human hormone called testosterone. The abuse of anabolic steroids by many prominent sports athletes has been widely reported in the media. Though with vigorous training there may be some short-term benefits, these drugs have a long list of serious adverse side effects and can cause permanent damage to the body. Many of these drugs are illegally manufactured, imported, and sold on the black market in the United States. The potency, purity, and strength are not regulated, and therefore it is almost impossible for users to know how much they are taking.

Responding to increasing illicit traffic, Congress passed the Anabolic Steroid Act of 1990, which identifies anabolic steroids as a Schedule III class of drugs and allows the FDA to enforce the law for legal drugs as well as illegal imports. Because anabolic steroids are classified as Schedule III drugs, prescriptions for ana-

Rafael Palmiero had over 3000 hits including 569 home runs in his 20 year career. He was suspended from baseball after testing positive for anabolic steroids and retired shortly thereafter.

bolic steroids like Androgel, Androderm, and Testim can be refilled a maximum of five times or for up to 6 months from the date written, whichever comes first, similar to prescriptions for many potent narcotic analgesics and sleep medications.

Omnibus Budget Reconciliation Act of 1990

The Omnibus Budget Reconciliation Act of 1990 (OBRA-90) requires that, as a condition of participating in the state Medicaid reimbursement program, states must establish standards of practice for drug utilization review (DUR) by the pharmacist. Among other provisions, the act requires "a review of drug therapy before each prescription is filled or delivered to an individual . . . typically at the point of sale . . . . The review shall include screening for potential drug therapy problems due to therapeutic duplication, drug-disease contraindications, drug-drug interactions (including serious interactions with nonprescription over-the-counter drugs), incorrect drug dosage or duration of treatment, drug-allergy interactions, and clinical abuse/misuse." Today the pharmacist reviews the patient profile on each new prescription and refill utilizing computer software.

Under the law a pharmacist, or the technician acting on the pharmacist's behalf, must also make an offer to counsel the patient or customer, but this person may refuse such counseling. The pharmacy technician usually has the patient sign a book or registry (or make a notation in the computer or message prompt at the cash register), which documents that the offer to counsel was made and accepted or refused. Otherwise, the pharmacist must offer to discuss and review with the patient the following:

- name and description of medication
- dosage form
- dose
- route of administration
- duration of drug therapy
- action to take after a missed dose
- common severe side effects or adverse effects
- interactions and therapeutic contraindications, ways to prevent the same, and actions to be taken if they occur
- methods for self-monitoring of the drug therapy
- prescription refill information
- proper storage of the drug
- special directions and precautions for preparation, administration, and use by the patient

OBRA-90 uses the possibility of loss of Medicaid participation to enforce the clinical practices of screening prescriptions and counseling patients and caregivers. It also requires state boards of pharmacy or other state regulatory agencies to provide for the creation of DUR boards for prospective and retrospective review of drug therapies and educational programs for training physicians and pharmacists with regard to the use of medications. The law also requires that manufacturers rebate to state Medicaid programs the difference between the manufacturer's best price for a drug (typically the wholesale price) and the average billed price. Most state boards of pharmacy now require counseling for all patients. Unfortunately, no additional reimbursement is provided for mandatory counseling.

Dietary Supplement Health and Education Act of 1994

One area in which the FDA is permitted limited oversight is in the diet supplement market, which includes vitamins, minerals, herbs, and nutritional supplements. The Dietary Supplement Health and Education Act (better known as *DSHEA*) was passed in 1994 and provided definitions and guidelines on diet supplements. Unlike prescription and OTC drugs, manufacturers are not required by this law to prove safety, efficacy, or standardization to the FDA. Because diet supplements are sold with nonprescription products, many consumers are unaware of the subtle difference in regulatory oversight of diet supplements.

The FDA may only review "false claims" advertisements and monitor safety. Manufacturers of these dietary supplements are not permitted to make claims of curing or treating ailments; they may only state that the products are supplements to support health. If health claims are made, the FDA can then require manufacturers to provide the research and proof to back up those claims similar to requirements for prescription and nonprescription drugs.

If the FDA wants to remove a dietary supplement from the market for safety reasons, it may do so; however, it must then hold public hearings, and the burden of proof is shifted to the FDA to prove that the dietary supplement is unsafe. For example, the drug ephedra, or its herbal equivalent ma huang, contained in many weight-loss products was removed from the market in 2004 by the FDA as a result of multiple reports of serious adverse reactions and some deaths; however, the lower courts overruled the FDA's action in 2005. In 2006 the Court of Appeals upheld the FDA action, thus removing all ephedra products from the market.

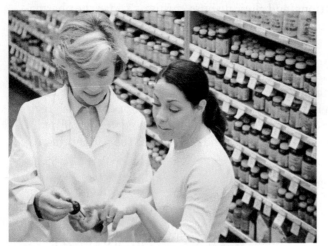

A patient often requests the counseling of a pharmacist when purchasing diet supplements since labeled information is quite limited.

Health Insurance Portability and Accountability Act of 1996

The Health Insurance Portability and Accountability Act (HIPAA) of 1996 had many provisions that have directly impacted all healthcare facilities, including pharmacies. One provision was the "portability" of moving health insurance from one employer to another without denial or restrictions. In the past, an employer could refuse to provide a new employee with health insurance or restrict coverage. For example, if the employee had a preexisting medical condition like diabetes, then the employer could exclude any expenses related to that condition for 6 months or a year or more; pregnancy was considered a preexisting condition with medical expenses not covered for 12 months. In addition, if an employee leaves his or her current employment, then the former employer must offer COBRA (Consolidated Omnibus Budget Reconciliation Act of 1985) benefits. These benefits allow the employee to continue current medical coverage for up to 18 months but at his or her own expense.

HIPAA mostly affects the confidentiality of patient medical records including prescription records. With more and more electronic submission of personal data to health professionals, insurance companies, and pharmaceutical manufacturers, HIPAA has placed safeguards to protect patient confidentiality. All healthcare facilities must provide information to the patient and document on how they protect the patient's health information. In pharmacy, this may include any transmission of prescription data to anyone other than the patient and the healthcare professional, or it may include an area designed for private counseling. Every pharmacy must have a training program in place for its employees with annual renewals. For pharmacy technicians, this means they must, under penalty of law, not reveal any information on any patient outside the pharmacy. Violations would also be grounds for immediate termination. The ramifications of HIPAA are covered in more detail in Chapter 13, *Human Relations and Communications.*

Food and Drug Administration Modernization Act

The Food and Drug Administration Modernization Act was passed to update the labeling on prescription medications. Products labeled with "Caution: Federal Law Prohibits Dispensing without a Prescription" were changed to read "[prescription symbol] only." As mentioned earlier, *legend* is the term formerly used to indicate whether a drug was available by prescription or over the counter (OTC). The new labeling requirements were implemented in 2004. The law also authorizes fees, to be paid by the applicant drug manufacturer, to be added to a new drug application (NDA) to provide additional resources to the FDA to process and accelerate the review and approval of new drugs.

Medicare Prescription Drug, Improvement, and Modernization Act of 2003

The Medicare Modernization Act (MMA), better known as Medicare Part D, became effective January 1, 2006, providing prescription drug coverage to patients eligible for Medicare benefits. This is a voluntary insurance program, not an automatic government benefit. This program provides some drug coverage, especially for those patients with economic hardships or those on high-cost medications. Patients are required to pay an extra premium (with their Medicare insurance) and are usually subject to a deductible (depending on insurance selected) before benefits are realized. Patients may be penalized if they elect not to join when they are eligible. The details of Medicare Part D insurance programs are further discussed in Chapter 7, *The Business of Community Pharmacy.*

For patients on high-cost medications or with certain health conditions, a pharmacist may provide (and get reimbursed for) medication management therapy services (MMTS) or an annual in-depth review of the patient's medication profile. The purpose of this review is to add a safety feature to prevent adverse reactions and drug interactions and to look at ways to reduce the patient (and insurance) cost.

A lesser-known provision of the MMA includes the development of health/savings accounts (HSAs). This act provides a health insurance option for patients under the age of 65 years. Under an HSA the patient, or his or her family, agrees to pay a monthly premium and carry a high deductible. In return the premium is fully tax deductible, and whatever amount is not used during that calendar year carries over to the next year. This is an example of a consumer-driven health insurance program (CDHP) that is becoming more popular as health insurance costs skyrocket. The individual (rather than the insurance provider) decides which physician to see, which prescriptions to fill and where, and which surgical procedures to accept from his or her premiums. The CDHP plans take advantage of lower negotiated medical expenses from their insurer in return for accepting more risk with a higher deductible. If the person should have a serious illness with catastrophic healthcare costs, then insurance would be provided after the deductible is met.

Combat Methamphetamine Epidemic Act of 2005

In response to the diversion and illegal manufacture of OTC products into the manufacture of the highly addictive stimulant methamphetamine, new legislation was passed. This act was initially passed in 2005, was incorporated into the Patriot Act in 2006, and took effect in September 2006. The act reclassifies all products containing the chemicals pseudoephedrine, phenylpropanolamine, and ephedrine and restricts the amount that can be purchased in any 30-day period. In addition, all of the products must be stored "behind the counter," the purchaser must present legal identification for purchase, and a log must be kept for all sales. Each pharmacy must also document that all employees have completed a training program. The DEA is responsible for enforcement. Chapter 7 contains additional information and procedures for the pharmacy technician to legally sell these OTC products.

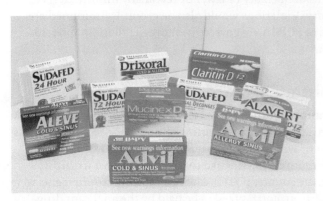

The Combat Methamphetamine Epidemic Act of 2005 was designed to reduce the availability of drugs used to illegally produce methamphetamine.

Regulatory Law—Role of National Oversight Agencies

The laws, acts, and amendments discussed in this chapter provide the minimum level of acceptable standards. The FDA and DEA have used the laws, acts, and amendments passed in the twentieth century to address a broad scope of issues and provide a basic structure for the safe use of drug products and for the practice of pharmacy.
Regulatory law is the system of rules and regulations established by governmental bodies such as the Food and Drug Administration (FDA) and state boards of pharmacy that exist to carry out the laws of the state or federal government.

Food and Drug Administration (FDA)

The **Food and Drug Administration (FDA)** is under the Department of Health and Human Services (HHS) and consists of five centers: Drug Evaluation and Research (CDER), Food Safety and Applied Nutrition, Veterinary Medicine, Devices and Radiological Health, and Biologics (Vaccinations) Evaluation and Research. The profession of pharmacy is most impacted by CDER. This center is primarily involved in the following:

- new drug development and review
- generic drug review
- over-the-counter drug review
- post–drug approval activities

The FDA has the primary responsibility and authority to enforce the law; however, the FDA has no legal authority over the practice of pharmacy in each state. The FDA has the ability to create and enforce regulations that will assist in providing the public with safe drug products. The FDA requires all manufacturers to file applications for investigation studies and approval of new drugs, provides guidelines for packaging and advertisement, and oversees the recall of products that are deemed dangerous.

For example, a manufacturer has very strict FDA guidelines as to how the product may be packaged, labeled, advertised, and marketed to physicians (and now the public). A manufacturer may not make speculative or false claims about the potential of the product, and it must also disclose the side effects, adverse reactions, and contraindications. The FDA has been known to ask a manufacturer to cancel advertising campaigns and even to instruct the manufacturer to present a new advertising campaign to clear up any misconceptions. Even OTC-marketed medications undergo this same level of scrutiny from the FDA, and the labels of OTC products must conform to a preferred format to make all of the information "understandable and readable" to the layperson.

The FDA is also responsible for the annual publishing (available online) of *Approved Drug Products with Therapeutic Equivalence Evaluations*, better known as the FDA Orange Book. This reference identifies all drugs approved by the FDA based on both their safety and their effectiveness in compliance with the FDA Act of 1938 and the Kefauver Amendments of 1962. This reference is used in the pharmacy primarily to make sure that generic products can be safely substituted for brand name products. The Orange Book is discussed further in Chapter 3.

Drug Enforcement Administration (DEA)

The **Drug Enforcement Administration (DEA)** is the primary agency responsible for enforcing the laws regarding both legal and illegal addictive substances. Although this agency directs most of its funds and personnel toward the illegal trafficking of drugs, it also has the responsibility to supervise the legal use of narcotics and other scheduled or controlled substances.

Inspection of all medical facilities, including pharmacies, is a function of the DEA and is usually limited to facilities where suspicious activity has been detected. The DEA works closely with the state drug and narcotic agencies that are responsible for annual physical inspections and local investigation of unsafe prescribing, dispensing, or forging of controlled drug prescriptions. Remember that laws vary from state to state. If the state law is more stringent, it will be followed; if federal law is more stringent, then it will be followed.

The DEA has established an audit trail to allow the agency to track the flow of narcotics from manufacturer to warehouse to pharmacy to patient. Special forms and procedures must be completed and documented in all medical facilities for both the ordering and the disposal of narcotic drugs (see Chapter 7). Many pharmacies use a "perpetual inventory" (or tablet-by-tablet records) for complete accountability of narcotic drugs. All prescriptions for Schedule II drugs must be filed separately and be available for inspection.

Registration with the Drug Enforcement Administration Through the **Controlled Substances Act (CSA),** every individual, institution, or business involved with manufacturing, distribution, dispensing, research, instructional activities, detoxification programs, importing, exporting, or compounding of controlled substances must be registered with the DEA. The DEA issues a license to medical practitioners that enables them to write prescriptions for scheduled drugs (or controlled substances) and to each individual pharmacy to order scheduled drugs from wholesalers. A hospital will register with coverage for both inpatient and outpatient dispensing. Registrations will vary from 1 to 3 years in length. Most pharmacies are issued a 3 year registration.

Prescriber The CSA defines who may prescribe controlled substances. The DEA can determine and monitor which physicians prescribe scheduled drugs. Practitioners are authorized to prescribe controlled substances by the jurisdiction in which they are licensed. Examples of practitioners include physicians, nurse practitioners, dentists, veterinarians, and podiatrists. The prescription must be written for a legitimate medical purpose in the course of the physician's professional practice activities. For example, a dentist may write a narcotic prescription for dental pain but not for back or cancer-related pain. Physician assistants cannot write Schedule II prescriptions, because they are not licensed with the DEA; in these cases the physician must write the prescription. Except in emergencies, the prescription must be written (no telephone or fax) to minimize fraudulent use and maintain a record-tracking system if necessary. The increasing adoption of electronic prescribing may minimize forged prescriptions for controlled drugs.

Occupational Safety and Health Administration (OSHA)

The Occupational Safety and Health Administration (OSHA) is under the Department of Labor. Its primary mission is to ensure the safety and health of America's workers by setting and enforcing regulations and standards; providing training, outreach, and education; establishing partnerships; and encouraging continual improvement in workplace safety and health. OSHA uses its resources effectively to stimulate management commitment and employee participation in comprehensive workplace safety and health programs. Its place in pharmacy is to protect against inadvertent needle sticks and safe disposal of syringes to prevent the transmission of hepatitis and HIV; in hospitals, home healthcare, and compounding pharmacies that prepare hazardous substances, OSHA is responsible for overseeing policies and procedures to protect the employee from unnecessary drug exposures. This will be discussed further in Chapter 11.

National Association of Boards of Pharmacy (NABP)

The **National Association of Boards of Pharmacy (NABP)** is the only professional organization that represents all fifty of the state boards of pharmacy. Unlike the FDA or DEA, the NABP has no regulatory authority. One of the primary roles of the NABP is to develop a national pharmacist examination for licensure that is administered by local state boards of pharmacy. The NABP also coordinates the reciprocation of pharmacists practicing in different states. **Reciprocation** is the administrative process of ensuring that pharmacists are eligible for relicensure in another state.

The NABP also provides guidance to the state boards of pharmacy by verifying the licensure legality of online pharmacies via its registered Verified Internet Pharmacy Practice Sites (VIPPS) program. It also helps to coordinate the issuing of provider identification numbers administered by the National Council for Prescription Drug Programs (NCPDP) called NCPDP Provider ID numbers. The NCPDP provides over 70,000 pharmacies with a unique identifying number for interactions with the FDA, the DEA, and many third-party processors of prescription claims.

Individual states have differing laws regarding the practice of pharmacy. Because many of the states developed laws pertaining to pharmacy over many years as acts and then amendments, the laws seem to have been put together in an unorganized fashion. A need for a common model developed, and the NABP developed the Model State Pharmacy Practice Act (MSPPA). Individual states can then model their practice acts on the MSPPA and individualize certain aspects of the regulation as needed within the given state. The MSPPA, along with various other recommendations, is often used as the "backbone" for the state regulation that the state board of pharmacy puts into place.

State Boards of Pharmacy

Each state has its own state board of pharmacy. The state-specific boards of pharmacy are all organized under the National Association of Boards of Pharmacy (NABP). The state board reviews applications, administers examinations developed by the NABP, licenses qualified applicants, and regulates the practice of licensees throughout the state. State boards of pharmacy consist of leaders from the pharmacy community and a consumer member that are appointed by the governor. The pharmacists often represent community, hospital, and other areas of pharmacy practice within the state.

Each state board of pharmacy maintains a database of all active pharmacist licenses and inspects all new pharmacies. This state agency is also responsible for developing and administering the pharmacy law exam for licensure or reciprocation from another state. In many states, this agency records the registration or certification of pharmacy technicians. The board has the authority to suspend or revoke the license or registration of a pharmacist or technician with evidence of violations of state or federal laws.

State boards of pharmacy provide regulations regarding refilling of prescriptions, both scheduled and nonscheduled drugs. Although most states have similar laws regarding prescription refills, each state must provide its own regulation because a national "law" does not exist. Typically, nonscheduled drug prescriptions are refillable for up to 1 year from the date written. Medications categorized as Schedule III, IV, and V drugs are refillable for up to 6 months from the date written. Although the law regarding refills on narcotics is covered by the CSA Amendments issued by the federal government, most states have a law that duplicates the federal law. However, some states may or may not recognize "emergency prescriptions" of Schedule II narcotics or may require a written prescription for any scheduled drug in which the state deems abuse is a problem.

Each state may also regulate whether certain drugs are OTC or require a prescription. Some insulins, for example, are available without a prescription, although it is not advisable for a patient to use insulin without the current care of a physician. Some states require a prescription for insulin syringes or require that accessibility of syringes be limited to discourage illicit drug use.

Legal Duties of Pharmacy Personnel

A statutory federal definition of the role of the pharmacy technician does not exist, and no uniform definition of the role and duties of the pharmacy technician is found from state to state. Definitions of the roles and duties of the pharmacy technician are under constant review and change as pharmacists are called upon to perform more clinical functions. Some states require licensure or registration with the board, whereas others may require passing national certification exams. (See Chapter 14, *Your Future in Pharmacy Practice*, for more on national certification.)

Some states specifically authorize the scope of practice by technicians, whereas others define what a technician may or may not do by detailing what the pharmacist must do. Many states limit numbers of pharmacy technicians in all practice settings by specifying a ratio of techs to pharmacists. By default, duties not required by law or regulation to be done by the pharmacist may be carried out by the technician. Table 2.5 lists duties that are typically performed by pharmacists and may not be performed by technicians; Table 2.6 lists duties that typically may be performed by technicians. Because of variations from state to state, these tables may not be completely accurate for every state or a given practice site. In all practice locations, however, all technicians' duties listed, if allowable, must be carried out under the direct supervision of a licensed pharmacist.

It is important that a technician become familiar with the applicable statutes and regulations of the state in which he or she practices. In most states, for example, technicians may compound solutions for intravenous (IV) infusion under the supervision of a pharmacist. In some states, however, only the pharmacist may do such compounding. A hospital pharmacy has a written manual of policies and procedures to dictate the respective duties of the technician and the pharmacist.

A detailed analysis of state laws and regulations that affect the practice of pharmacy technicians is beyond the scope of this book, but technicians in training are urged to contact knowledgeable professionals in training institutions and/or state boards of pharmacy to learn about state-specific statutes and regulations, particularly

---

TABLE 2.5 Duties Typically Performed by Pharmacists

A. Dispensing, Recordkeeping, and Pricing
  - receiving a verbal, or oral, prescription in person or by telephone
  - preparing the written form of the verbal prescription from a doctor's office or another pharmacy
  - interpreting and evaluating prescriptions
  - reviewing patient profile (e.g., medication history, duplication of medications, allergies, drug interactions)
  - verifying and certifying records
  - transferring prescriptions to another pharmacy

B. Preparing Doses of Precompounded Medications
  - checking/verifying finished prescriptions

C. Preparing Doses of Extemporaneously Compounded, Nonsterile Medications
  - checking and verifying that drugs were selected properly
  - calculating weights and measures
  - verifying that weighing and measuring were done properly
  - verifying finished product

D. Preparing Doses of Extemporaneously Compounded, Sterile Medications
  - verifying that drugs were selected properly
  - calculating weights and measures
  - verifying use of aseptic equipment and procedures
  - verifying that weighing and measuring were done properly
  - checking and verifying finished product

E. Transporting Medications to and from Floors/Units in a Hospital (especially controlled substances)
  - checking and verifying delivery records
  - examining returned medications for integrity and reusability
  - emptying returned medications into stock containers

F. Replenishing Floor Stocks (especially controlled substances)
  - checking and verifying
  - replenishing stocks
  - certifying and checking drug stations
  - disposing of unused items and discontinued medications

G. Verifying Finished Product against Original Order or Prescription

---

TABLE 2.6   Duties Typically Performed by Pharmacy Technicians

A. Dispensing, Recordkeeping, and Pricing
- receiving written prescriptions and conveying them to the pharmacist
- answering and properly directing telephone calls
- preparing records, including patient profiles and billing records
  (Note: Some states allow certified pharmacy technicians to accept prescriptions over the telephone.)

B. Preparing Doses of Precompounded Medications
- retrieving medications from shelf or supply cabinet
- selecting containers
- preparing labels
- counting or pouring medications
- reconstituting prefabricated medications
- pricing prescriptions

C. Preparing Doses of Extemporaneously Compounded, Nonsterile Medications
- retrieving medications from shelf or supply cabinet
- selecting equipment for the compounding operation
- weighing and measuring
- compounding
- preparing labels
- selecting containers
- packaging
- maintaining and filing of records extemporaneous compounding
- cleaning area and equipment

D. Preparing Doses of Extemporaneously Compounded, Sterile Medications
- retrieving medications from shelf or supply cabinet
- selecting equipment for the compounding operation
- using aseptic equipment and procedures
- weighing and measuring
- admixing parenteral products
- preparing labels
- selecting containers
- packaging
- maintaining and filing records of extemporaneous compounding
- cleaning area and equipment

E. Transporting Medications to and from Floors/Units
- preparing cart, tray, or other means of conveyance
- delivering controlled drugs
- maintaining delivery records
- distributing medications to wards
- organizing medications for administration to patients
- retrieving, reconciling, and recording credit for medications not administered
- returning unused medications to unit dose bins and injectables to stock
  (Note: Some states allow a "tech check tech" system in which one technician is allowed to check another technician's work preparing unit dose carts.)

F. Replenishing Floor Stocks
- Checking for expiration dates
- Removing overstocks

those related to registration and/or certification by the state, as well as to the specification of those duties that the technician may lawfully undertake. Other references that are useful in comparing duties from state to state include the following:

- the *Pharmacy Law Digest*
- the annual NABP *Survey of Pharmacy Law*
- the Pharmacy Technician Certification Board Web site

Violation of Laws and Regulations

When certain violations occur under any level of law—local, state, or federal—a prosecutor or public representative may bring a case against the party who violated the law or regulation. Examples include tax evasion, driving under the influence of alcohol, and more serious cases such as manslaughter and murder. Such a crime or violation against the state (or federal government) is filed using terms such as *State vs. John K. Smith,* and it is the prosecutor's duty to see that society is protected from individuals who violate the law.

When cases are filed in court, the party or person filing the case is called the **plaintiff**, and the party being sued or that the case is against is called the **defendant**. The plaintiff is responsible for proving his or her case; this is referred to as burden of proof. The burden of proof in a case involving crimes against the local, state, or federal government is referred to as *reasonable doubt*. This means that the prosecutor or plaintiff must provide convincing evidence that the party committed the act, beyond any "reasonable" doubt of a normal person. If the party is found guilty, then the punishment may be monetary fines, probation, or incarceration.

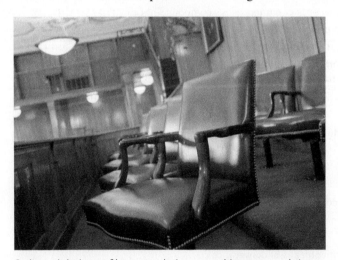

If the defendant in a case is a licensed (or registered) healthcare provider (i.e., physician, nurse, pharmacist, technician), then the appropriate state board may examine the case and determine whether the party's license should be revoked or suspended. The license may be revoked on ethical grounds, or the board may have a specific regulation that allows it to revoke a license in the event the person is convicted of a felony. If evidence of alcohol or drug abuse is proven, the state board may require successful completion of a drug rehabilitation program before the license can be reinstated.

Serious violations of laws, regulations, or ethics may result in suspension or revocation of professional licenses.

Civil Laws

Civil law is the term given to areas of the law that concern the citizens of the United States and the wrongs they may commit against one another but not generally against the local, state, or federal government and their respective laws and regulations. Civil law in the United States is derived from the precepts of common law used in England and brought here by the settlers. This law covers issues such as wrongs against one another and contracts. **Common law** is the system of precedents established by decisions in cases throughout legal history.

Occasionally, a crime is committed in violation of a state or federal law, and the party is prosecuted. In these cases the victim or his or her family may also sue the party in civil court for monetary damages. In that case the person may be tried two times, facing two separate plaintiffs. In the criminal case, the defendant might face monetary fines, probation, or prison. The civil case might result in monetary awards to the plaintiff.

Torts

In the context of civil law, a **tort** refers to personal injuries. Torts relate to wrongs that one citizen commits against another. In the case of a tort, the injured party sues the party that caused the injury (*Tom Jones vs. Dave's Drugstore and Dave the Registered Pharmacist [RPh]*). The local, state, and federal governments do not take part in a lawsuit such as this, because the crime was between two citizens and not against the government and/or its laws and regulations. The simplest is the "broken" contract.

Other examples of torts include negligence, malpractice, slander (using spoken words to speak falsely of another), libel (using written words to falsely represent another), assault (threatening another with bodily harm), and battery (causing bodily harm to another). For example, if a pharmacist or technician speaks unkindly to a customer about the professional competence of another health professional, that pharmacist or technician may be found guilty of slander.

The most common tort in the medical arena is **negligence** (i.e., not providing the minimum standard of care). **Malpractice** is a form of negligence in which the standard of care was not met. **Standard of care** is the level of care expected to be provided by various healthcare providers. Standard of care, when used to judge the type of care provided to a patient, is based on (1) comparisons to the actions of other healthcare professionals in the same situation; (2) compliance with existing written guidelines, protocols, or policies and procedures; and (3) expert testimony of health professionals provided by the plaintiff or the defense.

When considering standard of care, two criteria are always taken into account: the (1) level of training of the healthcare provider and (2) normal practices for the geographic area in which the healthcare provider works. Only those healthcare providers who work in the same geographic area and have the same level of training would be compared. For example, a pharmacist in Denver would not be compared with a pharmacist in Boston, because local practices and written protocols may differ by geographic area. A pharmacist with advanced education and training would be held to a higher standard in a court of law.

In addition, a pharmacy technician and a pharmacist would not be held to the same standard, because they have a different level of training. A pharmacy technician is not expected to provide the same service or standard of care to a patient as the pharmacist; similarly, a cardiologist would be expected to provide a different service or standard of care than that of a nurse practitioner in the cardiologist's office. The actions of a technician, however, could be compared to those of another technician. In the event of a serious medication error, a certified technician would be held to a higher standard than one not certified.

When a case of negligence or malpractice is brought, the burden of proof is on the plaintiff to prove what is known as the *four Ds of negligence:* duty, dereliction, damages, and direct cause. The plaintiff must first prove the defendant had a duty to provide care or there was a contract for care between the two parties. The plaintiff must then prove that the defendant was derelict in his or her duty, that this dereliction caused actual damages to the plaintiff, and that the damages were a direct cause of the defendant's dereliction.

The burden of proof in civil court is lower than in a criminal case. The plaintiff must prove his or her case by a "preponderance of the evidence," which means that it is more likely than not that the defendant is guilty of the accused act. If the defendant is found guilty, then he or she may be ordered to pay an award of money to the plaintiff. It is not possible for the defendant to be incarcerated, because the crime was not committed against the state but rather against another citizen. All pharmacies, most practicing pharmacists, and some pharmacy technicians carry professional liability insurance to protect their business and personal assets from a lawsuit.

Several levels of negligence or malpractice may be determined during an investigation and subsequent trial. If two or more causes are a factor in the negligence and personal injury to the patient, then a case of contributory negligence may be determined. For example, if the physician and pharmacist were both responsible for the injury to a patient, then each may be found guilty. The award to the plaintiff may then be broken down according to the judge's or jury's assessment of the comparative negligence. If the physician was more responsible than the pharmacist, then the award may be broken down by a percentage, where the physician must pay 70% of the damages award and the pharmacist must pay 30% of the damages award. Cases even exist where the patient is found to have contributed to his or her own injury (e.g., not taking medication as directed) and thus found to be comparatively negligent. In this case his or her total award may be reduced by a certain percentage, depending on the judge's or jury's determination.

Law of Agency and Contracts

The **law of agency and contracts** is based on the Latin term *respondeat superior,* which translates to "let the master answer." This law is a general principle that applies to the employee-employer relationship. The employee is in effect an "agent" for his or her employer and may enter into contracts on the employer's behalf. This is important in health care, because in the medical office the nurse may act as an agent for the physician, and in the pharmacy the technician may act as an agent for the pharmacist. This means not only that a contract may be made but also that it is just as valid as if the physician or the pharmacist made that contract.

An example of how the contract is made in the pharmacy is as simple as the technician receiving a prescription from the patient at the window and agreeing to get the prescription filled. By doing this, an implied contract now exists, and the pharmacy and pharmacist are obligated to provide the patient with a service. If a mistake is made, then the pharmacy and/or pharmacist may be held liable, even though he or she was not the one who entered into the contract to provide service. The pharmacist (or pharmacy in the case of a chain) must therefore "answer" for all of the acts of his or her employees. However, a pharmacy technician can be sued if it can be proven that the technician overstepped the limitations of the job such as dispensing a prescription drug without a check by the supervising pharmacist.

Invasion of privacy may be another violation that results in a lawsuit. Medical and prescription records, including those generated and filed in the pharmacy, are considered the physical property of the facility that generates them; however, the intellectual property contained in the medical record is the property of the patient. This information may not be divulged to another without the consent of the patient or by subpoena (i.e., a legal order). The pharmacy is held responsible for the actions of its personnel if a violation occurs. Privacy of medical information is now covered by federal law under HIPAA of 1996 as discussed earlier in the chapter. Violations of HIPAA may carry heavy personal fines and immediate termination. Confidentiality of medical information is further discussed in Chapter 13.

Drug and Professional Standards

In addition to laws and regulations of the FDA, the DEA, and state boards of pharmacy, national standards for drug products and professional standards exist. **Professional standards** are guidelines of acceptable behavior and performance established by professional associations. National professional pharmacy organizations help advance the profession by setting high professional standards that are well above what is required by laws and regulations.

United States Pharmacopeia

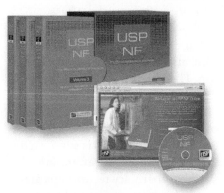

The *United States Pharmacopeia–National Formulary* is an important reference for pharmacists and pharmacy technicians.

The **United States Pharmacopeia (USP)** is an independent scientific organization that is responsible for setting official quality standards for all prescription drugs, OTC drugs, and dietary supplements sold in the United States. The mission of the USP is to promote the public health by developing and disseminating quality drug standards and information for medicines, healthcare delivery, and related products and practices. The USP develops authoritative, unbiased information on drug use and disseminates this information to healthcare professionals. The FDC Act of 1938 designated the USP to develop the official compendia for drugs marketed in the United States. The USP publishes the *United States Pharmacopeia–National Formulary (USP–NF)*, a book that contains standards for medicines, dosage forms, drug substances, excipients or inactive substances, medical devices, and dietary supplements. A manufactured drug product must conform to these standards to avoid possible charges of adulteration and misbranding and to be approved by the FDA.

USP Chapters 795 and 797 set standards that involve the storage, packaging, and preparation of nonsterile and sterile compounded preparations. These standards were developed by a council of experts of the USP. They have been adopted by many accrediting agencies, including the state boards of pharmacy and the Joint Commission. The standards are discussed in more detail in Chapters 8 and 10, respectively. Examples of 797 standards that may affect the practice of pharmacy include the following:

- specifications for "clean room" and filters to prepare sterile preparations
- recommendations for personnel cleansing and gowning
- expiration or "beyond use" dates and storage conditions for IV nutrition, single and multidosage vials, and ampules
- safety precautions and practices for handling hazardous drugs including radioactive pharmaceuticals that are compounded sterile products
- sterility and pyrogen or bacterial testing for all at-risk sterile products

Professional Organizations

Various professional organizations encourage setting the bar for a higher standard of pharmacy practice. For example, the American Pharmacists Association (APhA), the American Society of Health-System Pharmacists (ASHP), and the American Society of Consulting Pharmacists (ASCP) all have established standards for a postgraduate residency training program. These national pharmacy organizations have set standards and seek membership and input from pharmacy technicians.

The National Council for Prescription Drug Programs (NCPDP) has established industry standards to facilitate online electronic billing to third-party insurance carriers. Under the auspices of the National Association of Boards of Pharmacy (NABP), the National Institute for Standards in Pharmacist Credentialing (NISPC) has established standards and a national certification exam for pharmacists in specialty practice areas. As discussed earlier, NABP also accredits Internet pharmacies for consumers through its Verified Internet Pharmacy Practice Sites (VIPPS) program. To be VIPPS-accredited, a pharmacy must comply with the licensing and inspection requirements of its state and of each state to which it dispenses medications. In addition, it must meet VIPPS criteria, which address such issues as the patient's right to privacy, authentication and security of prescription orders, adherence to a recognized quality assurance policy, and provision of meaningful consultation between patients and pharmacists.

Pharmacists that are members of professional organizations are generally assumed to support the mission statement and policies of that organization. For example, the mission statement of APhA is "to serve society as the profession responsible for the appropriate use of medications, devices, and services to achieve optimal therapeutic outcomes." All organizations profess to advance the practice of pharmacy. These mission statements provide a standard of care that is above and beyond the minimum of what is required by federal and state pharmacy laws and regulations.

Pharmacy technicians also have professional organizations that focus on acquiring advanced knowledge and skills leading to certification. The Pharmacy Technician Certification Board or PTCB has the support of national pharmacist organizations. Its mission is to develop, maintain, promote, and administer a high-quality certification and recertification program for pharmacy technicians across various practice settings. Similarly, the Institute for Certification of Pharmacy Technicians (ICPT) is supported by national retail pharmacy organizations. The certification process and exams are discussed in more detail in Chapter 14. With certifications, pharmacy technicians are able to work more effectively with pharmacists to offer better patient care and service.

Chapter Terms

brand name the name under which the manufacturer markets a drug; also known as the *trade name*

child-resistant container a medication container with a special lid that cannot be opened by 80% of children but can be opened by 90% of adults; a container designed to prevent child access in order to reduce the number of accidental poisonings

civil law the areas of the law that concern U.S. citizens and the crimes they commit against one another

common law the system of precedents established by decisions in cases throughout legal history

controlled substance a drug with potential for abuse; organized into five schedules that specify the way the drug must be stored, dispensed, recorded, and inventoried

Controlled Substances Act (CSA) laws created to combat and control drug abuse

defendant one who defends against accusations brought forward in a lawsuit

Drug Enforcement Administration (DEA) the branch of the U.S. Justice Department that is responsible for regulating the sale and use of drugs with abuse potential

Food and Drug Administration (FDA) the agency of the federal government that is responsible for ensuring the safety and efficacy of food and drugs prepared for the market

generic name a common name that is given to a drug regardless of brand name; sometimes denotes a drug that is not protected by a trademark; for example, acetaminophen is the generic drug name for Tylenol

law a rule that is designed to protect the public and usually enforced through local, state, or federal governments

law of agency and contracts the general principle that allows an employee to enter into contracts on the employer's behalf

malpractice a form of negligence in which the standard of care was not met and was a direct cause of injury

National Association of Boards of Pharmacy (NABP) an organization that represents the practice of pharmacy in each state and develops pharmacist licensure exams

negligence a tort for not providing the minimum standard of care

new drug application (NDA) the process through which drug sponsors formally propose that the FDA approve a new pharmaceutical for sale and marketing in the United States

orphan drug a medication approved by the FDA to treat rare diseases

plaintiff one who files a lawsuit for the courts to decide

professional standards guidelines of acceptable behavior and performance established by professional associations

reciprocation the administrative process for relicensure of pharmacists in another state

regulation a written rule and procedure that exists to carry out a law of the state or federal government

regulatory law the system of rules and regulations established by governmental bodies

standard a set of criteria to measure product quality or professional performance against a norm

standard of care the usual and customary level of practice in the community

tort the legal term for personal injuries that one citizen commits against another in a lawsuit

United States Pharmacopeia (USP) the independent scientific organization responsible for setting official quality standards for all drugs sold in the United States as well as standards for practice

United States Pharmacopeia–National Formulary (USP–NF) a book that contains U.S. standards for medicines, dosage forms, drug substances, excipients or inactive substances, medical devices, and dietary supplements

Chapter Summary

- Governments and professional organizations have a right to exercise control over the manufacture, dispensing, and use of drugs to ensure quality and prevent harm to others because of the misuse or abuse of medications.
- Controls over the use of drugs are embodied in laws, regulations, and drug standards.
- Statutory laws and amendments passed by the U.S. Congress such as the Food, Drug, and Cosmetic (FDC) Act, Durham-Humphrey Amendment, and Kefauver-Harris Amendments have improved public safety by classifying drugs and ensuring their safety and efficacy.
- The Comprehensive Drug Abuse Prevention and Control Act is another example of statutory law that established schedules for controlled substances with regulatory oversight provided by the Drug Enforcement Administration (DEA).
- The Medicare Modernization Act of 2003 provides a voluntary drug insurance program to patients eligible for Medicare benefits.
- The Food and Drug Administration (FDA) regulates and enforces investigational and new drug applications to further protect the public.

- OSHA protects the employee from handling hazardous substances.
- State boards of pharmacy have regulations to license pharmacies, pharmacists, and technicians, and they have the power to take administrative actions against those that violate laws, regulations, and standards.
- The legal status of pharmacy technicians and their allowable duties vary from state to state, but in all cases technicians must act under the direct supervision of licensed pharmacists.
- Pharmacy is affected by the potential for tort actions in common law because of negligence or other forms of malpractice.
- Standards for drugs are set by the United States Pharmacopeia (USP) in the *United States Pharmacopeia–National Formulary (USP–NF)*.
- Standards for the practice of pharmacy are set by state boards of pharmacy and by various professional organizations.
- National pharmacy organizations support the advanced training and skills necessary for pharmacy technicians to become certified.

Chapter Review

Checking Your Understanding

Choose the best answer from those provided.

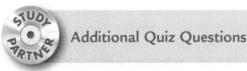 Additional Quiz Questions

1. The Food, Drug, and Cosmetic (FDC) Act of 1938 caused the creation of what agency?
   a. DEA
   b. FDA
   c. NABP
   d. the Joint Commission

2. The Kefauver-Harris Amendment required that all new drugs be proved _____ before being marketed.
   a. safe
   b. affordable
   c. effective
   d. All of the above

3. What organization is responsible for overseeing the policies and procedures in a pharmacy preparing and dispensing hazardous drugs?
   a. OSHA
   b. DEA
   c. FDA
   d. CDC

4. The Omnibus Budget Reconciliation Act of 1990 (OBRA-90) requires the pharmacist to
   a. offer patient counseling regarding medications.
   b. fill prescriptions according to FDA guidelines.
   c. report all prescription drug errors to the FDA.
   d. provide the DEA with information regarding narcotics.

5. What agency is responsible for classifying controlled substances?
   a. Drug Enforcement Agency (DEA)
   b. Food and Drug Administration (FDA)
   c. Medicare
   d. Medicaid

6. The Dietary Supplement Health and Education Act (DSHEA) limited the FDA's authority to regulate
   a. narcotic-prescribing habits of physicians.
   b. the manufacture of orphan drugs.
   c. Medicaid payment for prescriptions.
   d. herbal, vitamin, and nutritional products.

7. Which organization was responsible for the development of the Model State Pharmacy Practice Act (MSPPA)?
   a. Drug Enforcement Agency (DEA)
   b. Food and Drug Administration (FDA)
   c. National Association of Boards of Pharmacy (NABP)
   d. Medicare

8. Who has the authority to remove a pharmacist's or technician's license or registration?
   a. state board of pharmacy
   b. Food and Drug Administration (FDA)
   c. a federal court judge
   d. Drug Enforcement Agency (DEA)

9. If a patient sues a pharmacy, then who has the burden of proof in the case?
   a. pharmacy
   b. pharmacist and technician who filled the prescription
   c. patient
   d. state or local prosecutor

10. A pharmacist may be sued for _____ when he or she fails to meet a minimum standard of care.
    a. libel
    b. slander
    c. negligence
    d. malpractice

Thinking Like a Pharmacy Tech

1. A pharmacy technician accidentally chooses the antidepressant drug Prozac instead of the prescribed medication, the anti-secretory medication Prilosec, used for treatment of heartburn and gastroesophageal reflux disease. The pharmacist fails to check the medication, and the customer experiences no relief of the heartburn and a rare adverse reaction to the Prozac, rendering him temporarily impotent, a condition that causes the patient great psychological distress. The patient decides to sue the pharmacist and the pharmacy technician for negligence. To establish a valid case, what four claims must the patient prove, and to what degree must he prove them? Given the facts as stated, what arguments and/or evidence can the patient put forward to support each of these four claims?

2. In the case of *Baker vs. Arbor Drugs, Inc.,* the plaintiff, Baker, was taking the antidepressant drug tranylcypromine, under a prescription that he regularly filled at Arbor Drugs. The patient went to a physician with a cold, and the physician, despite having records indicating that the patient was taking tranylcypromine, prescribed the decongestant phenylpropanolamine. When Baker came to Arbor Drugs to have his prescription filled, the pharmacy's computer warned a pharmacy technician that a potential interaction existed between the new prescription and Baker's prescription for tranylcypromine that had been filled a few days earlier. The technician overrode the computer warning, and the pharmacist filled the prescription, unaware of the potential drug interaction. As a result of taking the phenylpropanolamine, Baker suffered a stroke. Baker brought suit and on appeal received a judgment against the pharmacy. Discuss this case with other students. Consider the following questions, given the facts as stated:

   a. Were both the pharmacist and the pharmacy technician guilty of negligence? Consider all four criteria for negligence.
   b. In what ways did the physician, the pharmacy technician, and the pharmacist fail to carry out their duties properly?
   c. What requirement, under OBRA-90, did the pharmacist fail to meet? What relevance does this case have to the expanded clinical role of the pharmacist?
   d. Under what legal principle did Baker sue the pharmacy for the actions of its employees—the pharmacist and the technician?
   e. Under what legal principle could Baker not sue the manufacturer of the phenylpropanolamine product, given that the physician and the pharmacy had been warned of the dangerous drug interaction?
   f. What role do computers play, in contemporary pharmacy, in helping pharmacists and technicians to meet the counseling requirements of OBRA-90?
   g. Is this a case in which a court could conceivably make a finding of contributory negligence or comparative negligence? Explain.

3. In the course of her normal duties, a pharmacy technician employed by Hometown Drugs, Inc., discovers from a patient profile that the young man who is dating her daughter is taking a regular prescription for a powerful antipsychotic drug. The technician keeps this information to herself but, in response to the information, attempts to dissuade her daughter from marrying the young man. Has the technician committed a breach of her ethical responsibilities? Explain in writing why you think this is or is not so.

4. Pharmacists with alcohol or substance abuse problems sometimes fail to seek help for fear that a state board of pharmacy might take some disciplinary action should the problem become known. What might professional associations and state boards do, in your opinion, to combat this problem?

5. New legislation or amendments are often passed in response to deficiencies in previous legislation. Give three examples from the text.

Communicating Clearly

1. List three ways to protect patient confidentiality in the community pharmacy.

2. An older patient complains of difficulty opening his medication vial. What procedures can the pharmacy technician take to legally assist this patient?

Researching on the Web

1. Visit the CDER Web site at http://www.fda.gov/cder. Identify two drug approvals for 2007 that were moved from Rx to OTC status. What are the proprietary (or brand) and established (or generic) names of the drugs and what are their indications?

2. Visit a retail pharmacy or go to the state board of pharmacy Web site and try to determine the legal requirements for dispensing insulin and insulin syringes in your state.

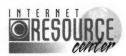

For further study of chapter-related topics, explore the Web links in the Web Center at www.emcp.net/pharmpractice4e.

Pharmacology in Practice

3

Learning Objectives

- Define the term *drug* and distinguish between active and inert ingredients.
- Identify several scientific discoveries of medications that improved our quality and quantity of life.
- Categorize drugs by source as natural, synthetic, synthesized, or semisynthetic.
- Explain the uses of drugs as therapeutic, pharmacodynamic, diagnostic, prophylactic, and destructive agents.
- Explain the parts of a National Drug Code number.
- Identify the function of various commonly used pharmaceutical reference texts.

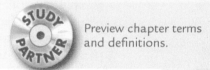 Preview chapter terms and definitions.

In the past five decades technological advances in the synthesis and delivery of pharmaceuticals have transformed everyday lives, providing improved antibiotics, vaccines, and medications to better control chronic diseases such as high blood pressure, high cholesterol, and diabetes. The scientific framework for these medical advances was provided by earlier major research discoveries. The classes, sources, and uses of drugs are covered as well as how drugs and their labeling are approved by the Food and Drug Administration (FDA). This chapter explains the concepts of pharmaceutical and therapeutic equivalence of generic drugs and explores the role of the FDA in monitoring for adverse effects, warning health professionals and consumers, and initiating drug recalls. The chapter also identifies important drug references used by the technician practicing in the community and hospital pharmacy environment.

What Is a Drug?

A **drug** is defined as any substance taken into or applied to the body for the purpose of altering the body's biochemical functions and thus its physiological processes. The active ingredient in a drug exerts a **therapeutic effect** like eradicating bacteria, lowering blood pressure or cholesterol, or controlling heart rate. Pharmacology is the study of how drugs interact with living organisms to produce a change in function.

The term *drugs* typically conjures thoughts of medications prescribed by a physician. The broader definition of *drug* includes not only prescription drugs but also over-the-counter (OTC) drugs, homeopathic remedies, and diet supplements including vitamins, minerals, and herbs. Drugs are available as generic and brand or trade name products; they are available as controlled substances under tight legal and administrative controls and as noncontrolled drugs.

Drugs come from many different sources. In years past, the pharmacist and the physician compounded drugs in a more crude state, often powders, extracts, and tinctures containing herbal remedies from plant sources. Modern science, including our knowledge of DNA and the mapping of human genes, has led to the development of highly researched and standardized medications that are more potent and more toxic than the natural plant herbal remedies of the past.

A drug may contain one or more active ingredients that have many specific therapeutic uses but also contain many other components besides the active ingredient. An **active ingredient** is the biochemically active component of the drug that exerts the desired therapeutic ____ ____ive ingredient is rarely given in pure (i.e., undiluted, uncut) form. Instea____ ____ active ingredients are combined with one or more inert ingredients. ____ ____ent, also called an inactive ingredient, has little or no physiological ____ ____ntain one or more active ingredients commingled, dispersed, ____ ____ion within an inert primary base, or vehicle, that may contai____ ____ antimicrobial preservatives, colorings, and flavorings. The____ ____ed to stabilize the tablet, capsule, or liquid formul____ ____al for many topical creams and ointments, to en____ ____ucts, or to assist in the masking of unpleasant ____ ____atric patients. The role of various inert ingredien____ ____

Drug Discove____ ____neteenth and Twentieth Centuries

As discuss____ ____er 1, during the nineteenth and twentieth centuries the practice of pharmacy____ ____medicine evolved from magic and superstition to a much more scientific basis. Drugs were extracted and purified from various plants and later synthesized in the chemistry lab. The growth of chemistry, biochemistry, pharmacognosy, and pharmacology in both medical and pharmacy education preceded many major drug discoveries.

Many of us take for granted the availability of medications to maintain our health today. What would our lives be like without vaccines, radioactive imaging, insulin, penicillin, or the birth control pill? Significant changes in our quality of life and longevity are due in part to the discoveries discussed here and others in the last 200 years. Pharmacy technicians play an important and integral part in this lifesaving profession.

Smallpox—The First Vaccination

In 1796 Dr. Edward Jenner performed the first experimental vaccination, which was an inoculation of cowpox to treat the dreaded smallpox infection. He had noticed an immunity from smallpox in dairy workers that had previously been exposed to cowpox. Jenner coined the term *vaccination*, which comes from the Latin word *cow*. The cowpox

8522 Kennedy Avenue
Highland, IN 46322

Phone (219) 972-1110
Fax (219) 972-1211

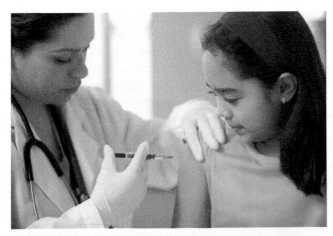

Jenner's experiments with antibodies led to the development of vaccines which today prevent many serious illnesses in children and adults.

exposure produced antibodies that provided cross-immunity with smallpox. An **antibody** is the part of the immune system that neutralizes antigens or foreign substances in the body. Jenner also found that smallpox could be prevented with an inoculation of bacteria from a person with a mild case of smallpox. A **vaccine** is defined as a substance that is introduced into the body in order to produce immunity to disease.

In the late 1700s smallpox was a major cause of premature death much like heart disease and cancer are today. The smallpox vaccine was a success; smallpox was the first disease in history to be eradicated. The use of early vaccinations had a high complication rate due to problems of purity and mass production. It is important for the pharmacy technician to be up to date on his or her (and their family members') vaccination schedule and to reassure the patient that the benefit of vaccine protection outweighs the small risk of adverse reactions.

Radioactive Drugs

At the turn of the century it was rare for a woman to pursue a research career in the sciences, but Madame Marie Curie was the exception. She is most remembered for her pioneering work with *radioactivity*, a term she coined with her physicist husband, Pierre Curie. She was awarded not one but two Nobel prizes—one in physics and the other in chemistry—for her work on the discovery and purification of radioactive chemicals. Madame Curie promoted the use of radium to alleviate the suffering of soldiers during World War I.

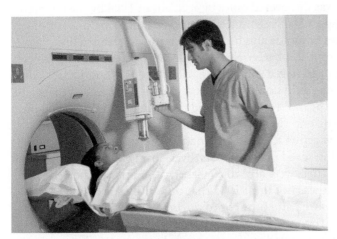

Madame Curie's pioneering study of radioactivity allowed for the development of magnetic resonance imaging (MRI).

Without the discovery of radioactivity there would be no nuclear imaging for diagnosis or treatment of disease. Examples of nuclear imaging include specific organ scans of the thyroid, heart, or bone, as well as total body scans such as a CAT scan and magnetic resonance imaging (MRI). There would be no radiation therapy options for thyroid disease or localized cancers and no specialty of nuclear medicine or nuclear pharmacy without her groundbreaking scientific research.

Insulin—A Lifesaver!

Sir Frederick Banting was a Canadian medical scientist, doctor, and Nobel laureate who with his assistant, Charles Best, discovered insulin in the 1920s while experimenting with beagles. Previous research demonstrated a link between the pancreas and diabetes, which at the time was referred to as "the sugar disease." Dogs with diabetes were kept alive with an extract from the pancreas which they called *isletin*. This extract was later

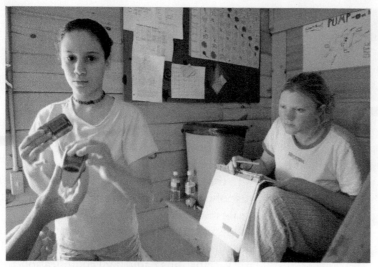

In his later years, Best worked with the American Diabetes Association to provide support groups and educational programs for diabetics, including summer camps for diabetic children.

isolated and purified and named *insulin* after the Latin word *island* (as in the islets of Langerhans, the area of the pancreas secreting insulin).

The discovery of insulin was hailed as one of the most significant advances in medicine at the time. Prior to the discovery of insulin, people with diabetes suffered complications and an early death ("diabetic coma") a short time after the onset of the disorder. This discovery extended the lives of millions of people worldwide who could not be treated and had a very poor prognosis.

Today millions of diabetic patients live near-normal lives while taking one or more types of insulin. Estimates show there are more than 15 million diabetics living today who would have died at a much earlier age without insulin. Pharmacy technicians can assist diabetic patients to lead near-normal lives by helping them select diabetic supplies and stressing the importance of insulin dosing and blood sugar monitoring.

Penicillin—The First Antibiotic

Safety Note

Patients need to complete the full course of any antibiotic treatment in order to avoid developing a resistance to the antibiotic.

An **antibiotic** is a chemical substance that kills or inhibits the growth of bacteria. Penicillin, the first antibiotic, was discovered quite by accident in 1928 by the research scientist Dr. Alexander Fleming and colleagues. Dr. Fleming was the first one to recognize the antibacterial properties of molds and fungi. After returning from a long vacation, Fleming noticed that many of his bacterial culture dishes were contaminated with a fungus. He discarded most but retrieved some and noticed a zone around an invading fungus where the bacteria could not seem to grow. Fleming proceeded to isolate an extract from the mold that prevented the bacteria from growing in the culture dishes. He correctly identified it as being from the *Penicillium* genus and therefore named the agent penicillin.

Penicillin saved many soldiers' lives during World War II. Other researchers were able to concentrate and purify the penicillin, but it was not until 1945 that this antibiotic could be mass-produced and brought to the market.

Today we have many hundreds of synthetic antibiotics, but continued research is needed to overcome bacterial resistance. It is important for the pharmacy technician to communicate to a patient the importance of completing the entire course of therapy for an infection to reduce the incidence of resistance and recurring infection. For example, the required dose of amoxicillin to treat ear infections has doubled in the past 25 years due to drug resistance! With a doubling of dose, there is an increased risk of side effects.

Penicillin is also a drug that causes the most drug allergies. It is important for the technician to be sure to

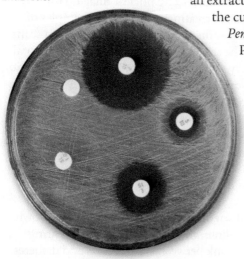

The clear area around the penicillin disk indicates the bacteria's sensitivity to the drug.

check the drug allergy history when receiving a prescription for an antibiotic like penicillin or one of its derivatives. A penicillin allergy may cross-react with other antibiotics. It is also considered good practice to update the drug allergy history, as some patients may become allergic to a drug with later exposure.

The Scourge of Polio

Two American physicians, Jonas Salk and Albert Sabin, independently invented vaccines to prevent polio, which was an infection caused by a virus that attacks the central nervous system. Franklin Delano Roosevelt contracted polio in 1921 before serving as president of the United States from 1932 to 1945. In 1952 more than 21,000 cases of the most serious form of polio—paralytic polio—were reported in the United States alone. Polio sufferers were mainly children who, if they survived, might be paralyzed for life.

Once a patient was infected, there was no cure for polio. The only way to treat severe symptoms was with the use of a noninvasive negative-pressure ventilator, more commonly called an iron lung. The iron lung would artificially maintain respiration during an acute polio infection until the patient could breathe independently. Generally, the treatment lasted about 1 to 2 weeks.

In 1953 Salk created an injectable vaccine from animal cultures that contained the killed viruses of the three kinds of polio that were known at the time. Earlier efforts were unsuccessful because the vaccines covered only one strain of the virus. He developed a process using formalin, which is a chemical that inactivated or killed the whole virus. Mass immunization programs for children were initiated in 1955. In 1955 there were 28,000 reported cases of polio; in 1956, only one year after immunization, there were only 15 cases.

In 1957, in an effort to improve upon the killed Salk vaccine, Albert Sabin began testing a live, oral form of vaccine in which the infectious part of the virus was inactivated (attenuated). Live vaccines contain a small amount of virus that may be contagious to high-risk patients, whereas killed vaccines do not contain live virus. This popular oral vaccine ("sugar cubes") became available for use in 1963. More recent recommendations from the Centers for Disease Control and Prevention (CDC) favor the killed injectable Salk vaccine over the live oral Sabin vaccine. In 1994 polio was declared eradicated in all of the Americas. The polio vaccine is a good example of how a drug discovery has saved thousands of lives.

The Pill

The pill is a common slang name for the birth control pill. Before the birth control pill was developed, there were few contraceptive methods outside of abstinence, the rhythm method, and the use of condoms. Up until the mid-twentieth century some state laws even prohibited teaching about contraceptive methods in medical schools. In the 1920s there were research breakthroughs in the area of reproductive biology. During that decade the female sex hormones estrogen and progesterone were identified and their functions defined. However, it was not until 1954 that Drs. Gregory Pincus and John Rock were able to experiment with the pill in humans.

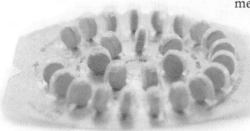

The pill has had a major impact on reproductive rights and helped initiate the women's liberation movement in the 1960s.

Limited trials demonstrated that an oral progesterone pill prevented pregnancy, but larger-scale trials could not be conducted in the United States. Side effects like breakthrough bleeding could be lessened if estrogen was added to the pill. Trials with the new formulation were conducted in Puerto Rico, Haiti, and Mexico. Finally, in 1960, G. D. Searle received FDA approval to market Enovid in low- and high-dose formulations. In 1962 Syntex received FDA approval to market Ortho-Novum from research completed a decade earlier in Mexico by Carl Djerassi. By 1963, 2.3 million American women were using the pill. Today it is estimated that nearly 100 million women worldwide are on the pill.

The early, approved birth control pills contained high doses of both estrogen and progesterone to ensure prevention of a pregnancy. These high doses contributed to a relatively high incidence of side effects including blood clots. With time and additional research, the dosages of the hormones in the pill have steadily decreased, thus reducing the risk of adverse effects. Today there are many different combinations of birth control pills. Some pills have different amounts of estrogen and progesterone during each week of the menstrual cycle. Some pills even decrease the number of menstrual periods. When taken appropriately the pill is 99%+ effective in preventing pregnancy. The pharmacy technician can reinforce the importance of being compliant with the proper administration of birth control pills to ensure their effectiveness.

Drug Classification

Drugs are classified as over-the-counter (OTC), homeopathic, or legend. Vitamins, minerals, and herbs are technically considered diet supplements (not drugs) and are not directly regulated by the FDA. The pharmacy technician must understand the different federal and state laws and regulations regarding the dispensing and retail sale of each of these drug classifications.

Legend or Prescription Drugs

A **legend drug** can be dispensed only upon receipt of a prescription from a healthcare professional licensed to practice in that state. Such drugs are labeled with the legend "Rx only" (Figure 3.1). Prescription drugs were formerly known as *legend drugs*.

A prescription drug may be available as a trade name or branded product (i.e., Norvasc) or it may be available as a generic (i.e., amlodipine). It is important for the

FIGURE 3.1
Legend Drug Labels

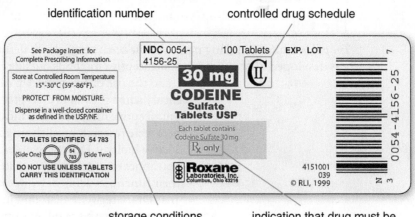

identification number · controlled drug schedule

storage conditions · indication that drug must be dispensed by prescription only

Courtesy of Boehringer Ingelheim Roxane, Inc.
©2008 Boehringer Ingelheim Roxane, Inc. and/or affiliated companies.

pharmacy technician to have a working knowledge of the top 200 trade and generic names of common drugs and their indications (see Appendix A). In most cases insurance will only cover the cost of a generic product if it is available. If a patient does not have drug insurance, he or she will often ask the pharmacy technician if a lower-cost generic product is available.

Legend or prescription drugs are also available as controlled (or scheduled) and noncontrolled medications. Drugs with potential for abuse are classified, under the Comprehensive Drug Abuse Prevention and Control Act of 1970, according to five drug schedules as presented in Chapter 2. Schedule II drugs such as narcotics and amphetamines have the highest potential for abuse, tolerance, and physical or psychological dependence. Misuse of drugs may result in the development of drug tolerance.

Drug tolerance is defined as requiring a higher dose of a controlled substance to exert a similar pharmacological effect with long-term use. For example, many Schedule II or III narcotic medications may not provide the same degree of pain relief if used continuously on a long-term basis. Drug tolerance may lead to psychological and physical dependence or even to drug addiction. **Psychological dependence** is defined as taking a drug on a regular basis because it produces a sense of well-being. Stopping the drug suddenly can lead to anxiety withdrawal symptoms. For example, many medications for sleep may disrupt sleep patterns if used every night, but the patient "feels" a loss of sleep if the medication is not taken every night.

Physical dependence is defined as taking a drug continuously such that when the medication is stopped, physical withdrawal symptoms like restlessness, anxiety, insomnia, diarrhea, vomiting, and "goose bumps" occur. Withdrawal symptoms commonly occur with high doses of Schedule II and III drugs and may occur after 4 weeks of continuous use in some patients. **Addiction** is defined as compulsive and uncontrollable use of controlled substances especially narcotics; addicted patients will do anything to support their drug habit.

If the major role of the profession of pharmacy is to protect the public, it is apparent that closely monitoring prescriptions for controlled drugs is a very important responsibility of the pharmacy technician. The tech must carefully review prescriptions for scheduled drugs for potential forgeries, as well as evaluate requests from patients for early refills on their medications.

OTC Drugs

An **over-the-counter (OTC) drug** is a drug that can be purchased without a prescription. Before an OTC drug is approved for sale, the Food and Drug Administration (FDA) must first recognize it as safe and effective when the patient follows labeled directions on the bottle with regard to dose, frequency, precautions and contraindications, and duration of therapy. The FDA has approved many OTC drugs after the expiration of the manufacturer's patent on the prescription drug. Such examples include Advil (ibuprofen), Aleve (naproxen), Benadryl (diphenhydramine), Claritin (loratadine), Zyrtec (cetirizine), and hydrocortisone. These drugs have been proven relatively safe over the years when appropriately used and sold as OTC medications.

It is very important that OTC drugs have adequate product labeling, written in easily understood terms, to assist the consumer in properly using the product, as there may be no contact with a pharmacist. The FDA requires that labels contain a prominent "Drug Facts" box that lists the active ingredients, purposes, and use of the product, with any warnings and directions including age-appropriate dosing. An expiration date is also required on the label, as well as a list of inactive ingredients for those patients with allergies.

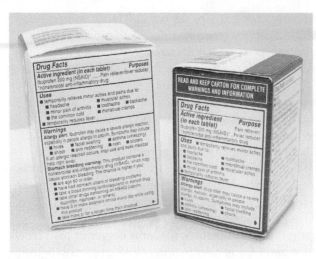

A comparison of the Drug Facts on these two boxes shows that the generic brand (ibuprofen) contains the same ingredients as the brand name drug (Advil).

This standardized labeling allows the consumer to compare active ingredients and assess the benefits and risks for the patient. It also assists the pharmacy technician in identifying a lower-cost generic or store brand OTC medication for the consumer. If a patient is considering the purchase of multiple cold medications, a comparison of active ingredients can identify any overlap or duplication of drugs that may cause adverse effects.

Homeopathic Medications

Another class of drugs under FDA control are called **homeopathic medications**. The term *homeopathy* is derived from the Greek words *homos* (i.e., similar) and *pathos* (i.e., suffering or disease). Homeopathic practice uses subclinical doses of natural extracts or alcohol tinctures. In other words, the active ingredient is diluted from one part per ten (1:10) to more than one part per thousand (1:1000), or even higher. The concept is that these small doses are sufficient to stimulate the body's own immune system to overcome the specifically targeted symptom.

Most homeopathic medications are OTC, but some are prescription only. An OTC homeopathic is one labeled for a self-limiting condition that does not require medical diagnosis or monitoring and is nontoxic. Homeopathy was popular in the United States in the early nineteenth century and remains popular in many areas of Europe today.

Diet Supplements

Most community pharmacies have a large inventory of vitamins, minerals, herbs, and diet supplements. A **diet supplement**, especially an herb, is considered to be a weak drug that can cause side effects, adverse reactions, and drug interactions. Glucosamine is an example of a nonherbal diet supplement that is used in humans and pets to treat mild to moderate arthritis symptoms. As with OTC drugs, diet supplements can be purchased without a prescription. Herbs are further discussed in Chapter 7, *The Business of Community Pharmacy*.

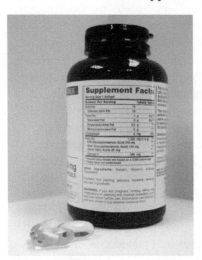

The label on a diet supplement may not contain as much information for the consumer as labels on other OTC drug.

As discussed in Chapter 2, these medications do not have the same stringent controls as legend and OTC medications and are loosely regulated by the Dietary Supplement Health and Education Act (DSHEA) amendments of 1994. The FDA can only regulate when patient safety concerns exist, as in the case of weight loss supplements. The quality of many of these products is suspect when tested by independent consumer laboratories. Diet supplements are considered "food supplements" to maintain health, and a patient should not exceed the recommended daily dose or "serving" without the knowledge of a physician or pharmacist. The pharmacy technician can assist the pharmacist by gathering information on the patient's use of diet supplements and adding this data to the computer profile.

Sources of Drugs

Drugs come from various sources and can be classified as natural, synthetic (created artificially), synthesized (created artificially but in imitation of naturally occurring substances), and semisynthetic (containing both natural and synthetic components). The development of lifesaving and life-altering biogenetically engineered drugs is, and will continue to be, a major source of new drug development in the twenty-first century.

Natural Sources

Some drugs are naturally occurring biological products, made or taken from single-celled organisms, plants, animals, minerals, and humans. Many herbal products come from natural sources. In addition to penicillin and insulin, other examples of modern-day drugs from natural sources are listed:

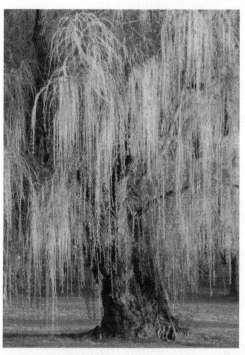

The bark of the willow tree, which contains salicylic acid, has been used for centuries to treat toothaches.

- The antibiotic streptomycin is produced from cultures of the bacterium *Streptomyces griseus*.
- The foxglove plant is a source of digitalis prescribed by doctors to strengthen the heart and regulate its beat.
- Opium, the narcotic, comes from the poppy plant and is a source for both legal drugs such as morphine and illegal drugs such as heroin.
- Quinine, used to treat malaria, and colchicine, used to treat acute gout, both come from the bark of the cinchona tree.
- Acetylsalicylic acid, more commonly known as aspirin, is derived from the bark of the white willow tree (which contains salicylic acid).
- USP thyroid extract is derived from desiccated (dried) thyroid glands, e.g., from pigs.
- The salts of minerals such as iron and potassium, which are commonly found in nature, are used for the treatment of iron deficiency and electrolyte therapy.
- (Milk of) magnesia is a combination of magnesium oxide or hydrated magnesium carbonate and is used as an antacid or a laxative.
- Human growth hormone, or somatropin, comes, as its name suggests, from the human brain.

Synthetic, Synthesized, and Semisynthetic Drugs

Today in the modern era many naturally occurring chemicals have been synthesized. A synthesized drug is a drug created artificially in the laboratory but in imitation of a naturally occurring drug like adrenaline, which is used for heart and asthmatic attacks. A **synthetic drug** exerts a specific pharmacological effect. Barbiturates, sometimes prescribed as a seizure, nerve, or headache medication, are examples of synthetic drugs. A naturally occurring drug like a barbiturate does not exist. A **semisynthetic drug** contains both natural and synthetic molecules like the semisynthetic penicillins, dicloxacillin or nafcillin, which combine artificially created molecules with naturally occurring ones. These new penicillin derivatives are effective against different bacteria or bacteria that have developed resistance to the natural penicillins.

FIGURE 3.2
Modeling DNA

(a) A single nucleotide. (b) A short section of a DNA molecule consisting of two rows of nucleotides connected by weak bonds between the bases adenine (A) and thymine (T) and between the bases guanine (G) and cytosine (C). (c) Long strands of DNA twisted to form a double helix.

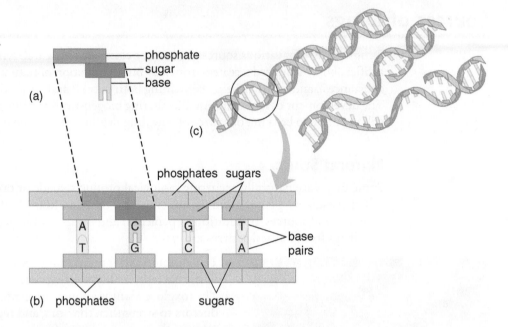

Biogenetically Engineered Drugs

Biotechnology combines the science of biology, chemistry, and immunology to produce synthetic, unique drugs with specific therapeutic effects. These drugs can be created by means of the recombinant deoxyribonucleic acid (recombinant DNA) techniques of genetic engineering. **Deoxyribonucleic acid (DNA)** is the complex, helically shaped molecule that carries the genetic code (Figure 3.2). DNA is made up of four chemical base pairs. These pairs, which are abbreviated as A, T, C, and G, are repeated millions or billions of times throughout a *genome*. A **genome** is the entire DNA in an organism, including its genes. The DNA contains the instructions, or recipe, for creating messenger **ribonucleic acid (RNA)**, which in turn contains the recipe for arranging amino acids into proteins for living organisms. These proteins determine how an organism looks, how well its body metabolizes food or fights infection, and sometimes even how it behaves. A defect in the DNA may increase the risk for developing certain diseases. If you can "unravel" the DNA code, you can more effectively prevent or treat diseases.

Genetic engineering is the process of utilizing DNA biotechnology to create a great variety of drugs, such as insulin for diabetics, clotting factors for treating hemophiliacs, potent anti-inflammatory drugs for rheumatoid arthritis, and drugs for combating viral and bacterial infections, anemia, and some cancers. Such technologies promise to bring many new drugs to the market; almost 200 biogenetically engineered drugs are currently under development.

Biogenetically engineered drugs can treat many serious illnesses. Enbrel is used to treat severe rheumatoid arthritis.

Uses of Drugs

Today medications are being used not just to treat and cure illnesses but also to aid in diagnosis and even prevent illnesses. Several classifications for uses of drugs exist, and most are not mutually exclusive. The following will assist the student in sorting out which classification best describes the various uses of drugs. Some medications may fall into more than one category.

Therapeutic Agents

A **therapeutic agent** is any drug that helps to do the following:

- *Maintain health*—Drugs with this purpose include vitamins and minerals to regulate metabolism and otherwise contribute to the maintenance of normal growth and functioning of the body. A specific example is the use of baby aspirin for patients identified as being at risk for heart attack.
- *Relieve symptoms*—Drugs with this purpose include anti-inflammatory drugs like ibuprofen used to treat fever, pain, or inflammation; narcotics to treat and prevent severe pain in terminally ill patients with cancer; or a diuretic or water pill to control excess fluid or high blood pressure.
- *Combat illness*—Drugs with this purpose include antibiotics to cure pneumonia, strep throat, or a bladder infection. Although antiviral medications do not cure human immunodeficiency virus (HIV) or acquired immunodeficiency syndrome (AIDS), they may allow the immune system to remain sufficiently intact so as to delay disease progression. Drugs for Alzheimer disease will not cure the patient but may delay both disease progression and loss of independence of the patient.
- *Reverse disease processes*—Drugs with this purpose include medications that control depression, blood pressure, cholesterol, or diabetes.

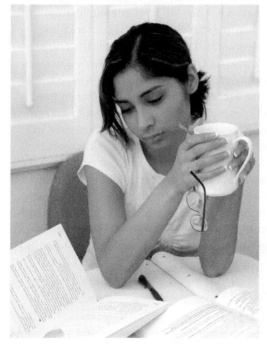

Caffeine is an example of a pharmacodynamic agent that can increase alertness for times such as last minute studying for an exam.

Pharmacodynamic Agents

A **pharmacodynamic agent** alters body functioning in a desired way. Drugs can be used, for example, to stimulate or relax muscles, to dilate or constrict pupils, or to increase or decrease blood sugar. Most of us consume coffee, tea, or a soft drink that contains caffeine to wake us up or keep us more alert. Other examples of pharmacodynamic agents include decongestants for nasal stuffiness, oral contraceptives that depress hormones to prevent pregnancy, expectorants to increase fluid in the respiratory tract, anesthetics to cause numbness or loss of consciousness, glucagon to increase blood sugar in diabetics, and digoxin to increase heart muscle contraction or slow heart conduction in patients with heart disease.

Diagnostic Agents

A chemical containing radioactive isotopes, used diagnostically (and also therapeutically), is known as a **radiopharmaceutical**. Isotopes are forms of an element that contain the same number of protons but differing numbers of neutrons. Unstable, radioactive isotopes give off energy in the form of radiation. These isotopes act as radioactive tracers in the body for diagnosis and treatment.

Nuclear medicine uses radioactive isotopes such as technetium (^{99m}Tc) and iodine (^{131}I) for imaging regional function and biochemistry in the body. Technetium is commonly used for imaging and functional studies of the brain, thyroid, lungs, liver, gallbladder, kidneys, and blood. The radiation exposure is in low doses for short periods of time and not harmful to the patient.

Nuclear pharmacy involves the procuring, storage, compounding, dispensing, and provision of information about radiopharmaceuticals; this is one possible area of specialization for both pharmacists and pharmacy technicians.

Prophylactic Agents

A **prophylactic agent** prevents illness or disease from occurring. Examples of prophylactic agents include the antiseptic and germicidal liquid chemicals used for proper hand hygiene preoperatively for the prevention of infection. Any vaccine is considered a prophylactic agent to prevent diseases such as influenza, pneumonia, shingles, measles, mumps, rubella, chicken pox, smallpox, poliomyelitis, and hepatitis. If you have a history of rheumatic fever, your dentist will most likely prescribe a large one-time dose of an antibiotic taken 1 hour prior to the procedure to prevent the risk of serious bacterial infection. Pharmacists are increasingly becoming involved in the administration of the influenza and pneumonia vaccines to older adults and other high-risk individuals.

Destructive Agents

A **destructive agent** has a *-cidal* action; that is, it kills bacteria, fungi, viruses, or even normal cells or abnormal cancer cells. Many antibiotics, especially given in high doses and intravenous (IV) infusions, are bactericidal (i.e., they kill [rather than just maim] the bacteria if it is sensitive to the drug). Penicillin is an example of a bactericidal drug, though resistance by some bacterial organisms has developed over the years. Another example of a destructive agent is radioactive iodine, which is used to destroy some of the thyroid gland in patients with an overactive thyroid gland.

Another common example of a destructive agent is an **antineoplastic drug** used in cancer chemotherapy to destroy malignant tumors. Cancer is often caused by an unregulated growth of abnormal dysfunctional cells. Different antineoplastics are used in combination to slow the growth of cancer cells at different phases of their growth cycles. Unfortunately, most of these drugs cannot effectively distinguish cancer cells from normal cells, so side effects such as hair loss, further depression of the immune system, and ulcerations of the mouth or gastrointestinal (GI) tract commonly occur.

Agents used in cancer chemotherapy are considered hazardous drugs. These drugs require special storage, preparation, and monitoring (see Chapter 11, *Preparing and Handling Sterile Products and Hazardous Drugs*) in both the community and the hospital pharmacy practice environments.

The Food and Drug Administration (FDA)

The FDA has the very important responsibility to assure the American public that the drugs that are approved are both safe *and* effective. Drugs undergo a fairly lengthy (and expensive) research process before they come to market. In the early 1960s a

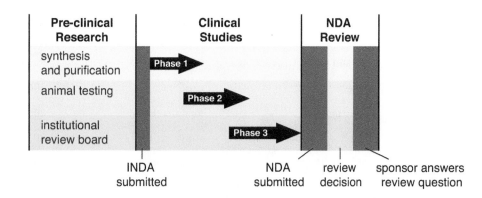

FIGURE 3.3
The Three Phases of the Drug Approval Process

Pre-clinical Research	Clinical Studies	NDA Review
synthesis and purification	Phase 1	
animal testing	Phase 2	
institutional review board	Phase 3	

INDA submitted   NDA submitted   review decision   sponsor answers review question

sedative called thalidomide was approved in Europe but not by the FDA. It was later proven that this drug when taken in pregnancy caused severe congenital birth defects.

Why are drugs so expensive, especially brand name drugs? Are lower-cost generic drugs really as good as the brand name ones? Why doesn't every drug have a generic option available? What is an NDC number and what is its relevance to a pharmacy technician? How does the FDA monitor for side effects of its drugs and vaccines? What is a patient medication guide and why is it important for the tech to be sure to provide it with the drug? How is a drug recalled from the market and what is the role of the pharmacy technician? The answers to these questions will be discovered in this section of the chapter. It is important for the technician to have a basic understanding of these issues, which may be of concern to the consumer. Patient counseling or concerns including discussion of drug side effects, warnings, and recalls should always be referred to the pharmacist.

Drug Approval Process

The FDA has regulations for manufacturers to follow while researching new chemical entities and developing those chemicals into brand or trade name drug products for the market. Scientists conduct three phases of drug testing before the approval process. Before an investigational new drug application (INDA) is reviewed by the FDA or clinical studies are initiated, the pharmaceutical company must do extensive preclinical animal laboratory research; once an investigational new drug (IND) is approved by the FDA and the study has received approval by its institutional review board (IRB), human studies may begin.

Investigational Studies Phase 1 is the initial study or trial of new drugs in humans, usually in a small number of healthy volunteers. The main purpose of this phase is to obtain sufficient information on both the pharmacology and the pharmacokinetics of the drug as well as any side effects. The data obtained are used to design future clinical trials. A Phase 2 study is primarily meant to evaluate the effectiveness as well as the safety of a drug for a given indication or disease state. Phase 2 studies also involve a small number of patients and are well controlled and closely monitored by the FDA. If the results of Phase 1 and Phase 2 studies are promising, Phase 3 studies are conducted in larger clinical trials on patients to better assess the efficacy and safety of the drugs.

New Drug Application (NDA) for Brand Name Drugs If the investigational drug shows promise after Phase 3 studies are completed, the pharmaceutical manufacturer can apply for a new drug application (NDA) to the FDA. In the NDA the applicant must prove the case for both the safety and the effectiveness of the drug before marketing.

Chapter 3 *Pharmacology in Practice*   **67**

TABLE 3.1 Blockbuster Drugs with Patent Expiration Years

Brand Name Drug	Generic Drug Name	Patent Expiration Year
Prevacid	lansoprazole	2009
Topamax	topiramate	2009
Lipitor	atorvastatin	2010
Effexor XR	venlafaxine	2010
Plavix	clopidogrel	2011
Actos	pioglitazone	2011
Zyprexa	olanzapine	2011
Seroquel	quetiapine	2012
Singulair	montelukast	2012

The results of the scientific studies are evaluated by an advisory panel of experts and recommendations are forwarded to the FDA. If the benefits of the drug outweigh the risks, generally the drug is approved. The FDA may request that additional studies be completed. The FDA approval process may take a year or longer in most cases. Occasionally when a medication appears to be very promising early on in the testing, the FDA may opt to fast-track the drug and grant early approval. A recent example includes the quick approval of drugs to control the human immunodeficiency virus (HIV).

Drug development is risky as well as costly. Out of 5,000 to 10,000 screened compounds, only 250 enter preclinical testing, 5 enter human clinical trials, and 1 is approved by the FDA. The cost of developing a new drug today is almost $1 billion, and it can take 10 years or longer to bring a new medicine from the laboratory to the pharmacy shelf.

The patent for a brand name drug like the cholesterol drug Crestor is granted for an extended period of time. This extension allows the manufacturer sufficient time to recover the costs of clinical research. It is important for the pharmacy technician to relay to the patient why there is such a high cost on some unique brand name prescription drugs. If there were no patent protection on new drugs, there would be no financial incentive (plus excessive risk) to develop future breakthrough drug discoveries.

Generic Drugs As discussed in Chapter 2, a **generic drug** contains the same active ingredients as the brand name product and delivers the same amount of medication to the body in the same way and in the same amount of time. Generic drugs are big business in any pharmacy. Over one billion generic prescriptions are dispensed every year. Zocor, for example, is a brand name drug that went "off patent" in 2006; simvastatin is the generic name and is available from several generic manufacturers.

Once the patent has expired on a brand name drug a generic pharmaceutical company may submit an **abbreviated new drug application (aNDA)** to the FDA for drug approval. Generic drug applications are termed "abbreviated" because they are generally not required to include preclinical (animal) and clinical (human) data to establish safety and effectiveness. Instead, generic applicants must scientifically demonstrate that their product is **bioequivalent** (i.e., performs in the same manner as the innovator drug) to an already approved brand name drug.

One way scientists demonstrate bioequivalence between brand name and generic drugs is to measure the time it takes the generic drug to reach the bloodstream in healthy volunteers. This gives scientists the rate of absorption of the generic drug, which they can then compare to that of the innovator (or brand name) drug. The generic version must deliver approximately the same amount of active ingredient into a patient's bloodstream in the same amount of time as the innovator drug.

Pharmaceutically equivalent drug products are formulated to contain the same amount of active ingredient in the same dosage form and to meet the same or *USP–NF* compendial standards (i.e., strength, quality, purity, and identity), but they may differ in characteristics such as shape, scoring configuration, release mechanisms, packaging, excipients (including colors, flavors, preservatives), expiration time, and, within certain limits, labeling. Nearly 80% of all FDA-approved drugs have a pharmaceutically equivalent generic product.

Drug products are considered to be therapeutic equivalents only if they are pharmaceutical equivalents and if they can be expected to have the same clinical effect and safety profile when administered to a patient under the conditions specified in the labeling. Under most circumstances, if a generic drug is both bioequivalent and therapeutically equivalent, it is "substitutable" for the brand name product by the pharmacist without prior approval of the physician. The laws and procedures governing generic substitution in the community pharmacy will be further discussed in Chapter 6.

Pharmaceutical alternative drug products contain the same active therapeutic ingredient but contain different salts (e.g., tetracycline hydrochloride vs. tetracycline phosphate), or may be different dosage forms. Different dosage forms (capsule vs. tablet, immediate-release tablet vs. extended-release tablet) and salts are considered pharmaceutical alternatives and *cannot be substituted* without approval from the physician. Thus, for a prescription written for 100 mg of Wellbutrin SR (sustained release), you cannot substitute 100 mg of generic immediate-release bupropion. Similarly, you cannot substitute 150 mg of Wellbutrin SR for 150 mg of Wellbutrin XL (extended release). Dosage formulations will be discussed further in Chapter 4.

Some drug insurance companies may not allow coverage for a brand name pharmaceutical alternative drug with a unique salt or dosage formulation. If the pharmacy tech observes that insurance will not cover a prescribed drug, or the co-pay is too high for the patient, this observation should be brought to the immediate attention of the pharmacist. Oftentimes once the prescriber is contacted, the prescription may be changed to a generic drug.

Most insurance plans, including the government-sponsored Medicare Part D plans, strongly encourage and provide cost-saving incentives through lower co-pays for the widespread use of generic drugs unless the physician specifies on the prescription the statement *brand name drug necessary*. The pharmacy technician, under the supervision of the pharmacist, may encourage the use of available generic drugs to lower patient out-of-pocket costs.

The dispensing of generic drugs is a major factor in containing the high cost of pharmaceuticals with savings of 30 to 80% compared to the brand name product. In 2006 the average retail price of a generic prescription drug was $32 while the average retail price of a brand name prescription drug was well over $100. Generics save consumers more than $10 billion each year.

There are significant cost savings to patients and pharmacies because generic manufacturers do not have to "front-end" the $1 billion in research cost of the large brand name pharmaceutical houses for each new drug discovery. They do not have to complete the Phase 1–3 studies to prove safety and efficacy, only bioavailability. In addition, once the patent expires, multiple generic companies, including many located outside the United States, manufacture the product, thus fostering competitive pricing.

FIGURE 3.4
NDC Number and Bar Code

For both of these labels for Vistaril, the first four digits of the NDC number (0069) indicate Pfizer Labs. The second four digits indicate the product code. The last two digits of the NDC number define the packaging size and type. (a) The product code (5420) identifies the drug as hydroxyzine pamoate, 50 mg oral capsules. (b) The product code (5440) identifies the drug as hydroxyzine pamoate, 25 mg/5 mL injection.

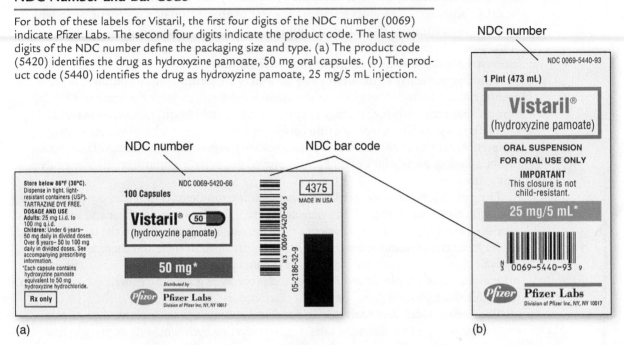

(a)

(b)

National Drug Code (NDC) Number

Under the Drug Listing Act of 1972, discussed in Chapter 2, once a brand name or generic drug receives FDA approval, each one is assigned a unique **National Drug Code (NDC) number** that appears on all drug stock labels as well as on copies of duplicate prescription labels and patient information sheets. The 10- to 11-character NDC number is made up of the following parts:

- a four- or five-digit *labeler code*, identifying the manufacturer or distributor of the drug
- a three- or four-digit *product code*, identifying the drug (active ingredient and its dosage form)
- a two-digit *package code*, identifying the packaging size and type

The NDC number bar code is commonly used by the Food and Drug Administration (FDA) for drug recalls. The NDC code plays a crucial role for the pharmacy technician in the checks and balances of preventing avoidable medication errors during the dispensing process, which is further discussed in Chapters 6 and 12.

Figure 3.4 shows NDC numbers and corresponding bar codes on labels for two different forms of hydroxyzine pamoate.

Drug Information for Health Professionals

The FDA requires that manufacturers provide scientific information to the pharmacist with all prescription drug products. This information is contained in a **product package insert (PPI)** when the stock medication is sent to the pharmacy from the wholesaler. The information on the product package inserts is provided in a specific order as shown in Table 3.2. Of particular interest to the pharmacy technician is the storage information or handling requirements.

TABLE 3.2	Organization of the Information in a Product Package Insert

- description
- clinical pharmacology
- indications and use
- contraindications
- warnings
- precautions ·
- adverse reactions
- drug abuse and dependence
- overdose
- dosage and administration
- how supplied
- date of the most recent revision of the labeling

The PPI is an information resource for the pharmacist and technician, not the patient. If you are not familiar with a new product, the package insert will provide basic information on drug names, doses, indications, side effects, and adverse reactions. Take the opportunity during any "slow time" in the pharmacy to expand your knowledge of new drugs by reading these helpful documents.

Drug Warning Systems

The FDA is increasingly interested in improving its postmarketing surveillance program to detect serious side effects not identified from research studies in the original new drug application or NDA. It is important to remember that all drugs have a risk of toxicity. An **adverse drug reaction (ADR)** is defined as a negative consequence to a patient from taking a particular drug; the ADR may not always be preventable or predictable. Indeed, despite many years of research and clinical studies, some medications will enter the marketplace and place the patient at risk of a serious adverse reaction. Once millions of prescriptions are written (or vaccine doses administered) for patients of all ages, rare adverse effects may suddenly appear in the general population.

It is very important to have a nationwide central reporting mechanism to detect and assess serious adverse effects. The FDA has two such reporting systems for ADR reporting called MedWatch and Vaccine Adverse Event Reporting

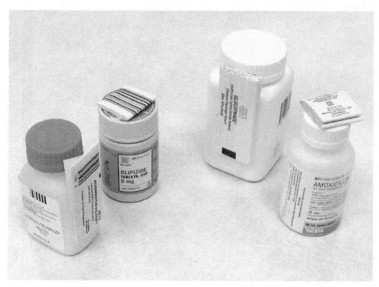

Product package inserts are attached to or placed inside stock bottles. They provide detailed information about the drug for the pharmacist and technician.

System or VAERS. It is also important that the FDA have a mechanism to warn consumers about the risks of selected drugs.

MedWatch The Food and Drug Administration (FDA), working in concert with the Institute of Safe Medication Practices (ISMP), has established a clearinghouse called MedWatch to provide all information on safety alerts for drugs, biologics, diet supplements, and medical devices including drug recalls. It also provides information on all safety-labeling changes to the product package insert (PPI). These changes include contraindications, warnings, boxed warnings, precautions, and adverse reactions.

MedWatch is a voluntary program that allows any healthcare professional to report a serious adverse event that the professional suspects to be associated with the use of an FDA-regulated drug, biological device, or dietary supplement. The FDA uses this information to track unrecognized problems or issues that were not apparent when the medication (or medical device) was initially approved. The occurrence of some side effects may be so rare that it can only be detected in a large population after the drug comes to market.

The recognition of a problem or potential for error does not always mean the product will be removed from the marketplace. Many times, improving prescribing information, educating healthcare professionals or the public, or perhaps simply changing the name or labeling may be all that is necessary to reduce or eliminate a safety risk. The FDA may require the manufacturer to make labeling changes to the patient package insert such as contraindications, warnings, precautions, or adverse reactions.

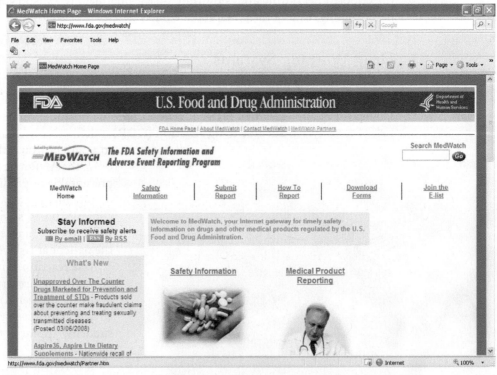

The FDA MedWatch Web site has the latest information on safety information for prescription drugs. The FDA provides an online adverse event reporting 3500 form for the pharmacist to document an adverse drug reaction.

For example, some research studies indicated that the diabetes drug Avandia may increase the risk of heart attack. Rather than recommend withdrawal of Avandia from the market, the FDA recommended labeling changes (see black box warnings in next section) in both the manufacturer information (PPI) to the pharmacist and the required MedGuide to the consumer.

If the adverse reaction is either serious or frequent, the FDA or drug manufacturer will recall the product from the marketplace. For example, the anti-inflammatory drug Vioxx was voluntarily withdrawn from the market by the manufacturer when research studies indicated that it may increase the risk of stroke or heart attack in some patients. Most pharmaceutical companies voluntarily recall products when a problem occurs because it is in their best interest (due to legal liability) to do so.

Beginning in January 2009 the FDA initiated a MedWatch program for consumers to report adverse drug reactions. Medication labeling for all OTC and prescription drugs must include a toll-free number to report adverse effects.

Black Box Warnings If the adverse reaction is a threat to patient safety, the FDA may require the manufacturer to insert a black box warning to health professionals. A **black box warning** (or boxed warning) is a warning statement on the PPI required by the FDA indicating a serious or even life-threatening adverse reaction from a drug. A thick black border surrounds the statement, hence the name. These warnings are also published in the *Physician's Desk Reference* or *PDR*.

Recent black box warning statements were mandated by the FDA for antidepressants like Prozac, Zoloft, and Paxil. The warning on antidepressants was to alert health professionals of the increased risk of suicide in children and adolescents prescribed these drugs.

Patient Medication Guides The FDA communicates black box warnings to the consumer through either a patient package insert—like with all birth control pills—or supplemental printed information called a **MedGuide** or a patient medication guide. The FDA develops the list of drugs requiring these information sheets and approves the information presented on the sheets. Each MedGuide is designed to do the following:

- inform the patient about the drug product
- promote the safe and effective use of prescription drug products by patients
- ensure that patients have the opportunity to be informed of the benefits and risks involved in the use of prescription drug products

The manufacturer of the drug is then responsible for providing the approved information to the pharmacy for sharing with the patient. The information provided on the patient medication guide is designed to further assist the patient in the proper use of the prescribed medication and to minimize the risk of serious adverse drug reactions. The medication guides must also be available in a form using terminology that is understandable to the patient. The medication guide is provided to the patient in addition to the patient information sheet to take home and read.

Common drugs that require an FDA-mandated patient medication guide are listed in Table 3.3. The MedGuides must be used with both brand name and generic drugs. Legally, these medication guides are extensions of the labeling on the drug product, and the laws and regulations involving misbranding or mislabeling apply to them. Thus, it is extremely important that these medication guides be given to the patient at the time of dispensing the medication.

The MedGuide is printed with supplemental medication information sheets at the time of final verification of the prescription, medication, and label by the pharmacist.

TABLE 3.3 Examples of Drugs Requiring a MedGuide

Drug	Risk Factor
Accutane	causes birth defects in women of child-bearing age; women must be on some form of birth control or be advised not to get pregnant while on this medication
Adderall	may cause insomnia, loss of appetite, and changes in pulse and blood pressure; monitor symptoms and vital signs
antidepressants	may be associated with an increase in suicide risk especially in adolescent patients; watch for changes in behavior
birth control pills	cause an increased risk of heart attack or stroke among smokers; the patient taking this type of drug should not smoke
Concerta	is similar to Adderall
Coumadin	reduces blood clotting, so the patient must be careful when working with sharp objects, shaving, and participating in contact sports while taking this drug; interacts with many drugs
NSAIDs	may cause an increase in the risk of stomach ulcers; take with food and no longer than necessary
Ritalin	is similar to Adderall
Serevent	is not effective as a "rescue" drug to reverse acute shortness of breath
Strattera	may interfere with growth and weight in children
Symlin	may cause hypoglycemia in diabetics; eat well-balanced diet

The medication information sheets and medication guides are usually attached to the bag containing the medication(s) when the medications are given to the patient. It is important for the pharmacy technician to confirm that this consumer information is attached to the bag containing the labeled prescription containers. The tech should encourage the consumer to read this information and telephone back with any questions or concerns. If the required MedGuides are not distributed, the pharmacy is subject to heavy fines during an audit.

Vaccine Adverse Event Reporting System (VAERS) A separate reporting system called **Vaccine Adverse Event Reporting System (VAERS)** is a postmarketing national safety surveillance system operated by the FDA and the Centers for Disease Control (CDC) to collect information on adverse events that occur after an immunization.

VAERS collects and analyzes information from reports of adverse events following immunization. The benefits of immunization far outweigh the risks. As with medications, hundreds of thousands of vaccine administrations may be required to detect a potential problem. For example, is there a relationship between vaccine administration and autism? Does the DPT vaccine cause pertussis or whooping cough? Does the polio vaccine cause polio?

Since 1990, VAERS has received over 123,000 reports, most of which describe mild side effects such as fever. Very rarely, people experience serious adverse events following immunization. The CDC and FDA use VAERS information to ensure the safest strategies of vaccine use and to further reduce the rare risks associated with vaccines.

TABLE 3.4   Recall Classes for Drugs

Class	Risk
Class I	A reasonable probability exists that use of the product will cause or lead to serious adverse health events or death. An example of a product that could fall into this category is a label mix-up on a lifesaving drug.
Class II	The probability exists that use of the product will cause adverse health events that are temporary or medically reversible. One example is a drug that is understrength but that is not used to treat life-threatening situations.
Class III	The use of the product will probably not cause an adverse health event. Examples might be a container defect, off taste, or color in a liquid.

In spite of the success of vaccines, even today some parents feel that the risk of adverse effects is greater than the protection that vaccines provide.

A VAERS report can be made online, via an 800 number (1-800-822-7967), or by mail on a downloaded form. Anyone can report a problem with a vaccine. The National Childhood Vaccine Injury Act of 1986 mandates reporting of serious adverse reactions by healthcare professionals.

With pharmacists and their technicians becoming more involved in vaccine administration, especially with the influenza and pneumonia vaccines, it is important to report any adverse effects. The CDC has an online training and continuing education program available at www.vaers.hhs.gov/ce.htm.

Drug Recall Process

Once a drug is approved, FDA oversight continues. A manufacturer is required to report any serious side effects and adverse reactions to the FDA. The FDA has the authority to obtain an injunction from the court and force the manufacturer to recall the drug product if it is contaminated, is poor quality, or causes serious adverse reactions. In some cases where the risk is greater than the perceived benefit, the FDA may issue a **drug recall** and withdraw the drug from the market; in other cases, the manufacturer may voluntarily withdraw the drug due to future liability concerns.

Three classes of recalls exist, and the FDA staff determines which class recall is issued based on reports from the particular manufacturer and from healthcare providers. Table 3.4 describes the three types of recalls.

A pharmacy wholesaler will commonly send a list of drugs with NDC and lot numbers that have been recalled so that the pharmacist or pharmacy technician can remove any such drugs from their inventory "to protect the patient." A Class I recall is serious and requires immediate action by pharmacy personnel. The FDA's role under the guidelines is to monitor company recalls and assess the adequacy of a firm's action. After a recall is completed, the FDA makes sure that the product is destroyed or suitably reconditioned and investigates why the product was defective.

Drug References

The **FDA Online Orange Book** (also called *Approved Drug Products with Therapeutic Equivalence Evaluations*) is available online and provides information on generic substitution of drugs that may have many different brand name or generic manufacturer sources. This online reference lists the drug products that the FDA considers to be (or not to be) therapeutically equivalent to other pharmaceutically equivalent products.

Table 3.5 lists an example from the *Orange Book* of the equivalence of a generic brand with several brand name levothyroxine 25 mcg tablets, a common thyroid medication. Therapeutic equivalence has been established between products that have the same bioequivalence and therapeutic equivalence codes. In the example in Table 3.5, the FDA would allow the pharmacist or pharmacy technician to substitute the generic levothyroxine sodium even if the brand name Unithroid, Levoxyl, or Synthroid is prescribed by the physician. Each state may vary in procedures for dispensing generic or therapeutic equivalents.

Many physicians (and some patients) do not like to substitute brands on their medications even if the medications are considered pharmaceutically and therapeutically equivalent. The prescriber is permitted by law to write "brand medically necessary" on the prescription. On new prescriptions it is important for the pharmacy technician to look for the words "brand medically necessary" on the prescription.

The patient may also request that a brand name product be dispensed even though a higher co-pay from insurance may result. In general, it is not good practice to keep switching among trade or generic products even if they are bioequivalent. For refills, it is important for the pharmacy technician to review the patient profile and see if a brand name or generic product was previously dispensed.

Just as with brand name drugs, not all patients will respond similarly to generic drugs. The technician can, however, reassure the patient that the generic product in stock has received FDA approval. In most cases, the software your pharmacy uses will cross-reference FDA-approved generic equivalents. If in doubt, go online to the FDA Web site or ask the pharmacist before entering information into the computer or filling the prescription.

In addition to the *FDA Online Orange Book*, other references are helpful to the pharmacist and technician working in the community and hospital pharmacy. Two reference works published by the United States Pharmacopeia (USP) establish the official legal standards for drugs in the United States: *United States Pharmacopeia* (which describes drug substances and dosage forms) and the *National Formulary* (which describes pharmaceutical ingredients). Both are revised every 5 years, and supplements are published in the interim between revisions. They are also printed in a combined edition, *United States Pharmacopeia–National Formulary (USP–NF)*. These compendial

TABLE 3.5 Drugs Therapeutically Equivalent to Levothyroxine (25 mcg)

Brand Name	Manufacturer
Unithroid	Jerome Stevens
Levothyroxine Sodium	Mylan
Levoxyl	Jones Pharma
Synthroid	Abbott

standards are utilized by pharmaceutical companies when submitting new drug applications to the FDA.

Several other reference books are also helpful to practitioners:

- *Physician's Desk Reference (PDR)* is published annually with reprints of product package inserts (PPIs) from the pharmaceutical manufacturers of most drugs. It is also useful for identifying unknown drugs by color, shape, and coding. It also will list black box warnings for the pharmacist and pharmacy technician. Pharmacy technicians can learn more about the drugs that they are dispensing by studying the *PDR* and reading package inserts during any free or slow times in the pharmacy. This reference book is also available for consumer purchase in most bookstores.

- *Drug Facts and Comparisons* includes factual information on product availability, indications, administration and dose, pharmacological actions, contraindications, warnings, precautions, adverse reactions, overdose, and patient instructions. It is available as a hardbound copy, as a loose-leaf binder with monthly updates, and as a CD-ROM.

- *DrugPoints*, published by Thomson Healthcare, has replaced the *USP Drug Information*; it features black box warnings, images, and a new toxicology section as well as expanded evidence-based medicine ratings of drug indications.

- *Handbook of Nonprescription Drugs* is published by the American Pharmacists Association and provides a good text reference for OTC drugs.

- *Remington: The Science and Practice of Pharmacy* is an excellent text, especially for use in a compounding pharmacy where determinations of drug stability and compatibility are important.

- *Homeopathic Pharmacopeia of the United States (HPUS)*, now called the *Homœopathic Pharmacopœia Revision Service (HPRS)*, is a compilation of standards for the source, composition, and preparation of homeopathic medications that may be sold in the community pharmacy.

- *American Hospital Formulary Service (AHFS)* is an excellent source of information, especially on parenteral drugs commonly used in the hospital.

- Trissel's *Stability of Compounded Formulations* summarizes specific formulation and stability studies and is an excellent reference for the technician performing sterile compounding in the hospital or specialty compounding pharmacy. The book provides important stability and storage information on compounded drugs in accordance with documented standards.

- *The Lawrence Review of Natural Products* (published by Facts and Comparisons) provides scientific monographs on herbal medications.

Chapter Terms

abbreviated new drug application (aNDA) the process by which applicants must scientifically demonstrate to the FDA that their generic product is bioequivalent to or performs in the same way as the innovator drug

active ingredient the biochemically active component of the drug that exerts a desired therapeutic effect

addiction compulsive and uncontrollable use of controlled substances, especially narcotics

adverse drug reaction (ADR) a negative consequence to a patient from taking a particular drug

antibiotic a chemical substance that is used in the treatment of bacterial infectious diseases and has the ability to either kill or inhibit the growth of certain harmful microorganisms

antibody the part of the immune system that neutralizes antigens or foreign substances in the body

antineoplastic drug a cancer-fighting drug

bioequivalent a generic drug that delivers approximately the same amount of active ingredient into a healthy volunteer's blood-stream in the same amount of time as the innovator or brand name drug

biotechnology the field of study that com-bines the sciences of biology, chemistry, and immunology to produce synthetic, unique drugs with specific therapeutic effects

black box warning a warning statement required by the FDA indicating a serious or even life-threatening adverse reaction from a drug; the warning statement is on the prod-uct package insert (PPI) for the pharmacy staff and in the MedGuide for consumers

deoxyribonucleic acid (DNA) the helix-shaped molecule that carries the genetic code

destructive agent a drug that kills bacteria, fungi, viruses, or even normal or cancer cells

diet supplement a category of nonprescription drugs that includes vitamins, minerals, and herbals that are not regulated by the FDA

drug any substance taken into or applied to the body for the purpose of altering the body's biochemical functions and thus its physiological processes

drug recall the process of withdrawing a drug from the market by the FDA or the drug manufacturer for serious adverse effects or other defects in the product

drug tolerance a situation that occurs when the body requires higher doses of a drug to produce the same therapeutic effect

FDA Online Orange Book an online reference that provides information on the generic and therapeutic equivalence of drugs that may have many different brand names or generic manufacturer sources

generic drug a drug that contains the same active ingredients as the brand name product and delivers the same amount of medication to the body in the same way and in the same amount of time; a drug that is not protected by a patent

genetic engineering process of utilizing DNA biotechnology to create a variety of drugs

genome the entire DNA in an organism, including its genes

homeopathic medications very small dilu-tions of natural drugs claimed to stimulate the immune system

inert ingredient an inactive chemical that has little or no physiological effect that is added to one or more active ingredients to improve drug formulations such as fillers, preserva-tives, colorings, and flavorings; also called inactive ingredient

legend drug a drug that requires a prescrip-tion from a licensed provider for a valid medical purpose

MedGuide written patient information mandated by the Federal Drug Administration (FDA) for select high-risk drugs; also known as a patient medication guide

MedWatch a voluntary program run by the FDA for reporting serious adverse events, product problems, or medication errors; serves as a clearinghouse to provide information on safety alerts for drugs, biologics, diet supplements, and medical devices including drug recalls

National Drug Code (NDC) number a unique number assigned to a brand name, generic, or OTC product to identify the manufacturer, drug, and packaging size

over-the-counter (OTC) drug a drug sold without a prescription

pharmaceutical alternative drug product a drug product that contains the same active therapeutic ingredient but contains different salts or different dosage forms; cannot be substituted without prescriber authorization

pharmaceutically equivalent drug product a drug product that contains the same amount of active ingredient in the same dosage form and meets the same USP–NF compendial standards (i.e., strength, quality, purity, and identity); can be substituted without contacting the prescriber

pharmacodynamic agent a drug that alters body functions in a desired way

physical dependence taking a drug continuously such that physical withdrawal symptoms like restlessness, anxiety, insomnia, diarrhea, vomiting, and "goose bumps" occur if not taken

product package insert (PPI) scientific information supplied to the pharmacist and technician by the manufacturer with all prescription drug products; the information must be approved by the FDA

prophylactic agent a drug used to prevent disease

psychological dependence taking a drug on a regular basis because it produces a sense of well-being; if the drug is stopped suddenly, anxiety withdrawal symptoms can result

radiopharmaceutical a drug containing radioactive ingredients, often used for diagnostic or therapeutic purposes

ribonucleic acid (RNA) an important component of the genetic code that arranges amino acids into proteins

semisynthetic drug a drug that contains both natural and synthetic components

synthetic drug a drug that is artificially created but in imitation of naturally occurring substances

therapeutic agent a drug that prevents, cures, diagnoses, or relieves symptoms of a disease

therapeutic effect the desired pharmacological action of a drug on the body

vaccine a substance introduced into the body in order to produce immunity to disease

Vaccine Adverse Event Reporting System (VAERS) a postmarketing surveillance system operated by the FDA and CDC that collects information on adverse events that occur after immunization

Chapter Summary

- Within the past 200 years several drug discoveries by various scientists have positively impacted the quality and quantity of life.
- Drugs can be classified as over-the-counter (OTC) or legend (prescription drugs) as regulated by the FDA.
- Diet supplements, which include vitamins, minerals, and herbals, are regulated under the DSHEA amendments.
- Drugs are natural, synthetic, synthesized, or semisynthetic substances taken into or applied to the body to alter biochemical functions and achieve a desired pharmacological effect.
- Uses of drug may include one or more of the following: therapeutic, pharmacodynamic, prophylactic, diagnostic, or destructive agents.
- The approval process consists of many different phases of preclinical animal and clinical human studies leading to submission of a new drug application to the FDA.
- For approximately every 10,000 chemicals studied, only one product will be approved by the FDA at a research cost of over $1 billion.

- For FDA approval generic drugs need only show bioequivalence to an innovator product.
- Generic drugs provide a significant cost savings to consumers due to a lower cost of research and more competition in the marketplace.
- In order to substitute for a brand name prescription, a generic drug must show pharmaceutical and therapeutic equivalence.
- The NDC number is specific for each manufacturer, drug product, dose, and package size and is very important to the pharmacy technician to prevent medication errors and in drug recalls.
- The FDA monitors adverse effects of drugs and vaccines through its MedWatch and VAERS postmarketing surveillance programs.
- The FDA communicates serious or life-threatening effects of drugs through black box warnings to health professionals in the PPI and to consumers in MedGuides.
- A multitude of good reference texts and Web sites exist that the practicing pharmacist and pharmacy technician can use to study various pharmaceutical products.

Chapter Review

Checking Your Understanding

Additional Quiz Questions

Choose the best answer from those provided.

1. Which of the following is the most urgent and serious type of drug recall?
   a. Class I
   b. Class II
   c. Class III
   d. Class IV

2. Banting and Best are best known for their discovery of
   a. insulin.
   b. radioactivity.
   c. polio vaccine.
   d. the birth control pill.

3. Which of the following classifications of drugs is not directly under FDA control?
   a. homeopathic medications
   b. legend drugs
   c. diet supplements
   d. OTC drugs

4. The term for a patient requiring higher and higher doses of a narcotic to experience pain relief is
   a. addiction.
   b. tolerance.
   c. psychological dependence.
   d. physical dependence.

5. When a generic manufacturer files an aNDA with the FDA, it must prove
   a. bioequivalence.
   b. safety.
   c. efficacy.
   d. All of the above

6. A radiopharmaceutical used for imaging is an example of a
   a. therapeutic agent.
   b. pharmacodynamic agent.
   c. diagnostic agent.
   d. prophylactic agent.

7. The FDA communicates black box warnings to the consumer on high-risk drugs through which of the following?
   a. product package insert (PPI)
   b. prescription R̥ label
   c. MedGuide
   d. media (TV, radio, newspapers)

8. What should you do if you receive a prescription with the words "brand medically necessary"?
   a. substitute a lower-cost generic drug
   b. check the *FDA Online Orange Book* for acceptable product substitutions
   c. realize that the prescription is written for a Schedule II drug that cannot be refilled
   d. fill the prescription as is with the brand name product

9. A National Drug Code (NDC) number *does not* identify the
   a. product manufacturer.
   b. drug.
   c. packaging size and type.
   d. schedule of the drug.

10. To determine generic equivalency of a brand name product, which reference source would you use?
    a. *Drug Facts and Comparisons*
    b. *FDA Online Orange Book*
    c. *Physician's Desk Reference*
    d. *Homeopathic Pharmacopeia Revision Service* (HPRS)

Thinking Like a Pharmacy Tech

1. Recombinant DNA will, in the future, play a prominent role in gene therapies. Research gene therapy for the treatment of cystic fibrosis, the most common of all fatal genetic diseases. Prepare a brief report explaining how such therapy works.

2. Determine the brand name and primary indication for the following gene therapy or biotechnology-based medications:
   a. epoetin alfa
   b. efavirenz
   c. infliximab
   d. somatropin
   e. trastuzumab
   f. becaplermin
   g. palivizumab

3. Go to a community or retail pharmacy and make a list of five over-the-counter (OTC) products that contain acetaminophen as one of the active ingredients. For each product on your list, give the manufacturer, the brand name, the NDC number, the active and inactive ingredient(s), and the expiration date.

Communicating Clearly

1. Go to the FDA Web site (www.fda.gov) and find a MedGuide for the drug Accutane. What are the serious adverse effects that require a consumer warning?

2. How would you explain to a patient in understandable terms the differences between a brand name product and a generic product? Are both approved by the FDA? Why does the generic drug cost so much less? Why is there not a generic equivalent for each product on the market?

Researching on the Web

1. Go to the Web site of the Association of Natural Medicine Pharmacists (www.anmp.org) and locate the monograph that lists the primary indication, dosage, and clinical efficacy of the following natural medicines:
   a. ginkgo
   b. saw palmetto
   c. ginger

2. Go to www.ornl.gov/sci/techresources/ Human_Genome/home.shtml or search for Human Genome Project and determine how many genes have been identified in the human genome. What is the relationship of this project to treatment for breast cancer?

3. Go to www.fda.gov and find an FDA label warning for Tamiflu issued in March 2008.

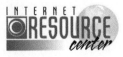 For further study of chapter-related topics, explore the Web links in the Web Center at www.emcp.net/pharmpractice4e.

Dosage Forms and Routes of Administration

4

Learning Objectives

- Define and differentiate between the terms *dosage form* and *route of administration*.

- Enumerate and explain the properties of solid, semisolid, liquid, inhalation, and transdermal dosage forms.

- Identify inactive ingredients and the various coatings of tablets and their functions.

- Differentiate among the various delayed-release dosage formulations.

- Define the emulsion characteristics of topical products such as ointments, creams, and gels.

- Differentiate between a suspension and an emulsion dosage form.

- Explain the advantages of a transdermal dosage form.

- List the major routes of administration and the advantages and disadvantages associated with each route of administration.

- Discuss correct techniques for administration of eye drops, metered-dose inhalers, vaginal medications, and injections.

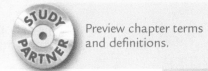

Preview chapter terms and definitions.

I n the modern era, there are many drug formulations and an equally wide variety of ways to get medications into the body. Healthcare providers have numerous agents at their disposal and a wide variety of dosage forms with which to customize patient treatment. A working knowledge of the inherent differences—as well as advantages and disadvantages—of the different dosage forms in use today is primary. The action of a medication cannot be taken into account without considering the dosage form selected.

This chapter discusses the advantages and disadvantages and guidelines for appropriate use for various routes of drug administration. The patient outcome may depend on selecting the most appropriate medication, dosage form, and route of administration to meet the patient's needs. The selection of the most appropriate dosage form and route of administration by the prescriber is based on ease of administration, site of action, onset and duration of action, quantity of drug, and toxicity.

Solid Dosage Forms

A **dosage form** is the physical manifestation of a drug as a solid, liquid, or gas that can be used in a particular way. Currently drugs are administered in a wide variety of dosage forms such as tablets, capsules, creams, ointments, solutions, suspensions, injections, and aerosols. A **drug delivery system** is most commonly a design feature of the dosage form that affects the release of the drug in the body. For example, a drug might have a solid dosage form and be either a tablet or a capsule, but its delivery system may be designed to protect the stomach or delay its release over a 24 hour period of time.

Solid dosage forms are used more frequently than any other formulation. Capsules and tablets are the two most common types and are inexpensive to manufacture. A wide variety of capsule and tablet types and sizes exist. Capsules and tablets generally contain the active ingredient in powders or granules. Such ingredients dissolve in the gastrointestinal (GI) tract and become available for absorption into the bloodstream. Other solid dosage forms, such as implants, lozenges, plasters, powders, and suppositories, though used less frequently, are still very important, for they offer advantages over tablets and capsules and enable physicians and pharmacists to more adequately meet the needs of individual patients.

Tablets

Tablets are available in a wide variety of shapes, sizes, and surface markings. The **tablet** is a solid dosage form produced by compression and contains one or more active ingredients along with inert or inactive ingredients. The common inert ingredients and their uses are listed in Table 4.1. Most tablets are imprinted with a distinctive code and coloring from their manufacturer for drug identification purposes.

TABLE 4.1   Common Tablet Ingredients and Their Uses

Ingredient	Use
diluent	allows for the appropriate concentration of the medication in the tablet
binder	promotes adhesion of the materials in the tablet
lubricating agent	gives the tablet a sheen; aids in the manufacturing process
disintegrant	helps break up the ingredients once the tablet has been consumed
solubilizer	maintains the ingredients in solution; helps the ingredients pass into solution in the body
coloring	differentiates the tablet
coating	assists the patient's swallowing of the tablet; improves the flavor of the tablet; protects the stomach lining from drug side effects; delays the release of the medication once it has been consumed

FIGURE 4.1
**Multiple
Compression
Tablets (MCTs)**

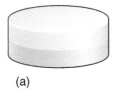

(a)

(a) Two layers or
compression.
(b) Three layers or
compressions.

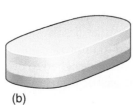

(b)

Punch-and-die machines that compress the ingredients of each tablet in a single stroke create almost all of the tablets produced today. Compression tablets are the most inexpensive and common dosage form used today. A **multiple compression tablet (MCT)** is produced by multiple compressions and is, in effect, either a tablet on top of a tablet or a tablet within a tablet. An MCT may contain a core and one or two outer shells (or two or three different layers, as shown in Figure 4.1), each containing a different medication and colored differently. MCTs are created for a number of reasons: for appearance alone, to combine incompatible substances into a single medication, or to provide for controlled release in successive events or stages.

Some pharmaceutical companies have begun to manufacture an oblong tablet, a hybrid of the capsule and tablet, called the *caplet*. The **caplet** is simply a tablet shaped like a capsule and sometimes coated to look like a capsule. The inside of the caplet is solid, unlike the inside of a capsule, which is often powder or granular material. Caplets are easier to swallow than large tablets and more stable (with a longer shelf life) and tamper-proof than capsules. Caplet formulations on the market include the OTC drug Tylenol and the antibiotic erythromycin.

Most tablets are meant to be swallowed whole and to dissolve in the gastrointestinal (GI) tract, but some tablets are designed to be chewed or dissolved in the mouth.

- A **chewable tablet** contains a base that is flavored and/or colored. The dosage form is designed to be masticated (or chewed). Chewing is preferred for antacids, antiflatulents, commercial vitamins, and tablets designed for children. Single chewable tablets, for example, can be prescribed for small children in lieu of other dosage

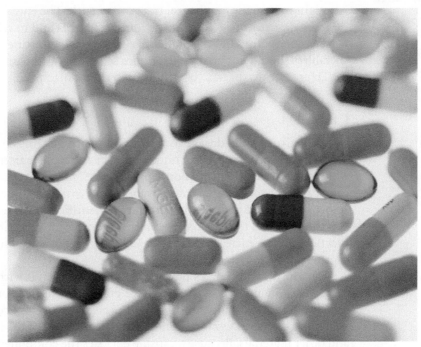

Capsules and tablets are manufactured in a variety of sizes and colors. Distinctive markings help patients identify the drugs.

forms. For example, they can be used to control asthma symptoms or to treat infections. Chewable tablets are absorbed quickly for a faster onset of action.

- An **oral disintegrating tablet (ODT)** is designed to melt in your mouth. ODTs are useful for pediatric and geriatric patients who have difficulty swallowing or for patients with nausea. Examples include Zofran, for treatment of nausea and vomiting, and Maxalt, for the treatment of migraine headaches.

Special Coated Dosage Formulations Most tablets are uncoated, but some tablet dosage forms contain a special outside layer that dissolves or ruptures at the site of application. Coatings on tablets can be used to improve appearance, flavor, or ease of swallowing. A coated drug formulation is often designed to delay absorption of the medication and to resist breakdown by the gastric fluids in the stomach to minimize the risk of causing side effects.

Common tablet coatings include sugar, film, or enteric.

- A **sugar-coated tablet (SCT)** contains an outside layer of sugar that protects the medication and improves both appearance and flavor. Sugar-coating tablets tends to improve taste and increases the chance that the patient will be compliant and take the prescribed medication at the prescribed time. The major disadvantage of a sugar coating is that it makes the tablets much larger and heavier, and thus more difficult to swallow.
- A **film-coated tablet (FCT)** contains a thin outer layer of a polymer (a substance containing very large molecules) that can be either soluble or insoluble in water. Film coatings are thinner, lighter in weight, and cheaper to manufacture than sugar coatings and are colored to provide an attractive appearance. The monthly dosing of Boniva for osteoporosis is an example of the use of an FCT to prevent serious GI side effects.
- An **enteric-coated tablet (ECT)** is used for drugs that are better absorbed by the intestines when they bypass the stomach. ECTs are also used with drugs that might irritate the esophageal tract or stomach. The enteric coating is designed to resist destruction by the gastric fluids' acidic pH and to release the active ingredient once it reaches the higher pH of the small intestine. For this reason, these tablets should not be split. Examples of ECTs are aspirin, potassium chloride, and Trental, drugs that can be irritating to the stomach.

Capsules

The **capsule** is a solid dosage form consisting of a gelatin shell that encloses the drug. Gelatin is a protein substance obtained from vegetable matter and from the skin, white connective tissue, and bones of animals. The gelatin shell of a capsule, which can be hard or soft, may be transparent, semitransparent, or opaque and may be colored or marked with a code to facilitate identification. In commercial manufacturing, the body and the cap may be sealed to protect the integrity of the drug within (a practice that has increased since the 1980s, when highly publicized incidents of capsule tampering occurred).

The capsule will contain powders, granules, or liquids with one or more active ingredients. In most cases these active ingredients will also contain a pharmacologically inert filler substance, or **diluent**. The capsule may also contain disintegrants, solubilizers, *preservatives* (which maintain the integrity of the ingredients), colorings, and other materials. Because a capsule encloses the components, flavorings are not common for this dosage form. Like tablets, capsules can be formulated with delayed-release characteristics to allow less frequent dosing and/or side effects.

Delayed Release Dosage Formulations Most oral tablet and capsule formulations are "immediate-release"; that is, the medication is designed to be activated or released within a short period of time after the drug is taken. In the case of chest pain, or when treating an infection, it is desirable to have a fast onset of action, but in the case of high blood pressure it may not be convenient to take the medication three or four times a day. In fact, most patients will be noncompliant and forget to take a dose or two. Tablet coatings can also be designed to delay drug release.

- A **controlled-release dosage form** is designed not to release the active drug immediately after administration. It is intended to regulate the rate at which a drug is released from the tablet (or capsule) into the body. Such dosage forms may vary the rate of dissolution or the release of the active drug. Common names for controlled-release dosage formulations include the phrases "delayed release," "long acting," and "timed release." Other similar names have specific meanings.
- A **sustained-release (SR) dosage form** allows a frequency of dosing reduced from that of an immediate-release form. For example, the generic bupropion SR (the sustained-release form) should be taken in 2 doses, at least 8 to 12 hours apart. The brand name Wellbutrin XL (the extended-release form), however, should be taken once a day, in the morning.
- An **extended-release (XL) dosage form** allows a frequency of dosing reduced from that of immediate-release and most sustained-release forms. Many medications for blood pressure use this type of dosage form, which allows once-daily dosing and better compliance with a prescribed regimen.

Because of their design, delayed-release dosage forms should not be split. Examples are listed in Table 4.2.

Lozenges, Troches, or Pastilles

A **lozenge**, also known as a *troche* or a *pastille*, is a dosage form containing active ingredients and flavorings, such as sweeteners, that are dissolved in the mouth. Lozenges generally have local therapeutic effects. Compounding pharmacies may prepare these formulations for specific indications in special patients. Commercial OTC lozenges for relief of sore throat are quite common, although many other drugs, including such prescription drugs as nystatin or clotrimazole, are also available in a lozenge form. Some narcotic medications are available in a lollipop-like formulation. Actiq is an example of a solid formulation of fentanyl citrate (a narcotic analgesic) on a plastic stick that dissolves slowly in the mouth.

Powders and Granules

Powders and granules can be used topically or internally. In large-scale commercial manufacturing, as well as in compounding pharmacies (see Chapter 8, *Nonsterile Pharmaceutical Compounding*), **powders** are milled and pulverized by machines. An example of a medication in the powder dosage form is polymyxin B sulfate and bacitracin zinc topical powder, used to prevent infection. Other commonly dispensed powders include antacids, brewer's yeast, laxatives, douche powders, dentifrices and dental adhesives, and powders for external application to the skin. Goody's Headache Powder is a common OTC example.

Granules are larger than powders and are formed by adding very small amounts of liquid to powders; during manufacturing, the mixture is passed through a screen or a granulating device. Tablets are often prepared by compressing granules; capsules are often filled with granules. Granules are generally of irregular shape, have excellent flow characteristics, are more stable than powders, and are generally better suited than powders for use in solutions because they are not as likely to float on the surface of a liquid. They may contain colorings, flavorings, and coatings and may have controlled-release characteristics. Pharmacists and pharmacy technicians often mix granular drug products, such as antibiotic suspensions, with a set volume of distilled water before dispensing.

Effervescent salts are granules or coarse powders containing one or more medicinal agents (such as an analgesic), as well as some combination of sodium bicarbonate with citric acid, tartaric acid, or sodium biphosphate. When dissolved in water, effervescent salts release carbon dioxide gas, causing a distinctive bubbling. Most people are familiar with effervescent tablets such as Alka-Seltzer, used to relieve headaches or hangovers. Domeboro effervescent tablets contain aluminum acetate and are used topically on the skin as a soak or compress for minor skin irritations, such as poison ivy.

Semisolid Dosage Forms

An **emulsion** is a mixture of two immiscible or unblendable substances. One substance (the dispersed phase) is dispersed in the other (the continuous phase). Semisolid dosage forms, such as oil-in-water or water-in-oil, are examples of emulsions. An **oil-in-water (O/W) emulsion** is a formulation that contains a small amount of oil dispersed in water as in a cream or lotion. A **water-in-oil (W/O) emulsion** is a formulation that contains a small amount of water dispersed in oil as in an ointment. If not commercially available, then creams and ointments are commonly prepared in a compounding pharmacy (see Chapter 8). Liquid emulsions will be discussed later in this chapter.

Ointments

An **ointment** is an example of a W/O semisolid dosage form. Many cortisone-like medications and topical antibiotics such as Neosporin are available in an ointment dosage form. Ointments may be medicated or nonmedicated and may contain various kinds of bases.

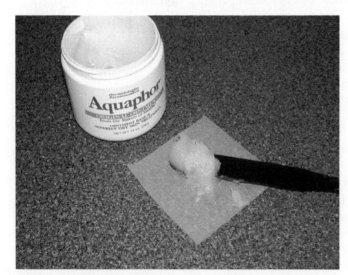

Ointments are referred to as water-in-oil (W/O) preparations. They contain a small amount of water dispersed throughout oil. They will apply smoothly to the skin but will often leave the skin with a greasy feeling. Ointments are often yellowish and opaque.

- oleaginous or greasy bases made from hydrocarbons such as mineral oil or petroleum jelly; a **liniment** meant for rubbing on the skin, such as Ben Gay
- W/O emulsions such as lanolin or cold cream
- O/W emulsions such as hydrophilic ointment containing petrolatum
- water-soluble or greaseless bases such as polyethylene glycol ointment, as in the topical antibiotic Bactroban

A **paste** is like an ointment but contains more solid materials and is thus stiffer and applies more thickly. Examples are zinc oxide paste (an astringent) and triamcinolone acetonide dental paste (an anti-inflammatory preparation). A **plaster** is a solid or semisolid and medicated or nonmedicated preparation that adheres to the body and contains a backing material such as paper, cotton, linen, silk, moleskin, or plastic. An example is the OTC salicylic acid plaster used to remove corns.

Creams

A **cream** is considered an O/W emulsion because it contains a small amount of oil dispersed in water. Most creams are considered "vanishing," which means they are invisible once applied and are thus more cosmetically acceptable to most patients. Many topical prescription products are available in both an ointment and a cream formulation. A **lotion** is also an O/W emulsion for topical application containing insoluble dispersed solids or immiscible liquids. Lotions are easily absorbed and can cover large areas of the skin. Examples include calamine lotion, used for relief of itching, and benzoyl peroxide lotion, used to control acne.

Gels

Much like a suspension, a **gel** contains solid particles in liquid, but the particles are ultrafine, of colloidal dimensions, and sufficient in number (and therefore linked to form a semisolid). Gels are used for both internal and external use. Topically, gels apply evenly and leave a dry coat of the medication in contact with the area. Examples of gels include lidocaine gel and the antacid aluminum hydroxide gel. The following are examples of ultrafine dispersion dosage forms.

- A **jelly** is a gel that contains a higher proportion of water in combination with a drug substance and a thickening agent. Jellies are present in many antiseptics, antifungals, contraceptives, and lubricants. Lubricants are commonly used in pelvic and rectal examinations of body orifices. Lubricants are also used as an aid in sexual intercourse in postmenopausal women having vaginal dryness from an age-related hormone deficiency. Because of their high water content, jellies are subject to contamination and thus usually contain preservatives.
- A **glycerogelatin** is a topical preparation made with gelatin, glycerin, water, and medicinal substances. The hard substance is melted and brushed onto the skin, where it hardens again and is generally covered with a bandage. An example is zinc gelatin (Unna's Boot), used as a pressure bandage to treat varicose ulcers.

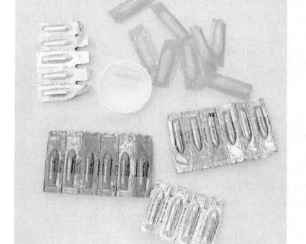

A suppository's site of administration determines the suppository's size and shape.

Suppositories

A **suppository**, another example of a semisolid dosage form, is formulated from a base such as cocoa butter or glycerin to melt in the rectum at body temperature and release an active drug. It is designed for insertion into body orifices such as the rectum or the vagina, or, less commonly, the urethra. Suppositories vary in size and shape, depending on their site of administration and the age and gender of the patient for whom they are designed. Some are meant for local action, as in the treatment of hemorrhoids. Rectal suppositories, however, are often used as vehicles for systemic drugs because the rich supply of blood and lymphatic vessels in the rectum provides for exceptional absorption. Suppositories are often used in children or adults unable to take oral medication for the purpose of controlling symptoms of fever, nausea, or vomiting, as well as to treat those with severe symptoms of inflammatory bowel disease or pain.

Vaginal tablets (or inserts) are designed to be placed into the vagina by means of an applicator; the medication is dissolved and absorbed through the vaginal mucosa. Vaginal tablets may be less messy than equivalent cream formulations, although absorption of the active drug is less predictable. Monistat is an example of an OTC vaginal tablet used to treat yeast infections. Similarly, urethral tablets or inserts may be used in men.

Liquid Dosage Forms

Liquid dosage forms consist of one or more active ingredients in a liquid vehicle such as a solution, suspension, or emulsion. Liquid dosage forms are often less stable than their solid counterparts, and care should be taken to monitor storage conditions, rotate stock, and check expiration dates. Liquid dosage forms also have easier dosage adjustments, especially for pediatric patients. For the patient, taste preference may be either an advantage or disadvantage. For adults this is not usually a concern; however, children's medication is often flavored in the most palatable way possible to improve compliance.

Solutions

A **solution** is a liquid in which the active ingredients are completely dissolved in a liquid vehicle. Solutions may be classified by vehicle as aqueous (water-based), alcoholic (alcohol-based), or hydroalcoholic (water-and-alcohol-based). The vehicle that makes up the greater part of a solution is known as a **solvent**. An ingredient dissolved in a solution is known as a **solute**. Solutions may also be classified by their contents: aromatic waters, elixirs, syrups, extracts, fluidextracts, tinctures, spirits, or irrigating solutions. A low-alcohol or alcohol-free product is preferred for most orally ingested pediatric products.

- An **aromatic water** is a solution of water containing oils or other substances that have a pungent, and usually pleasing, smell and that are volatile (i.e., easily released into the air). Rose water is an example.
- An **elixir** is a clear, sweetened, flavored solution containing water and ethanol (hydroalcoholic). An example of a drug in this dosage form is phenobarbital elixir, containing phenobarbital, orange oil, propylene glycol, alcohol, sorbitol solution, color, and purified water.

- A **syrup** is an aqueous solution thickened with a large amount of sugar—generally sucrose—or a sugar substitute such as sorbitol or propylene glycol. Syrups may contain additional flavorings, colors, or aromatic agents. Syrups may be medicated, such as lithium citrate or ipecac, or nonmedicated, such as cherry syrup or cocoa syrup. Syrups are often the preferred vehicle to mask the taste of pediatric medications, such as cough medicines, because they do not contain alcohol. Syrups are also sometimes used for older patients who cannot easily swallow the commonly available solid forms of certain drugs.
- An **extract** is a potent dosage form derived from animal or plant sources from which most or all the solvent has been evaporated to produce a powder, an oint-

ment-like form, or a solid. Extracts are produced from fluidextracts and are used in the formulation of medications.

- A **fluidextract** is a liquid dosage form prepared by extraction from plant sources and commonly used in the formulation of syrups. Vanilla extract is an example of a fluidextract.
- A **tincture** is an alcoholic or hydroalcoholic solution of extractions from plants. Examples include iodine and belladonna tincture.
- A **spirit** is an alcoholic or hydroalcoholic solution containing volatile, aromatic ingredients. Examples include camphor and peppermint spirit, both of which can be used as medicines or flavorings.
- An **irrigating solution** is any solution for cleansing or bathing an area of the body. Some are used topically in the eye (i.e., normal saline) or ear or for irrigation of tissues exposed by wounds or surgical incisions. Examples of irrigating solutions used in surgical procedures are Neosporin-Polymyxin B and 1% acetic acid. The term *douche* is most commonly used for a cleansing solution, often reconstituted from a powder, administered into the vaginal cavity.

Solutions are sometimes classified by their site or method of administration as topical (local), systemic (throughout the body), epicutaneous (on the skin), percutaneous (through the skin), oral (for or through the mouth), otic (for or through the ear), ophthalmic (for the eye), parenteral (for injection or intravenous [IV] infusion), rectal (for or through the rectum), urethral (for the urethra), or vaginal (for or through the vagina).

An enema is an example of a water-based solution administered rectally for cleansing the bowel before a GI procedure or for delivering an active drug. An evacuation enema, such as Fleet, is administered to clean the bowels in preparation for a colonoscopy. A retention enema, such as Cortenema, is administered to deliver medication locally or systemically in the case of acute inflammatory bowel disease.

A **parenteral solution** is a sterile or microbial-free solution, with or without medication, that is administered by means of a hollow needle or catheter used to place the solution through one or more layers of the skin. Two major delivery systems for parenteral solutions are: (1) infusions and (2) injections. Routes of drug administration include:

- intravenous (IV): into the vein
- intramuscular (IM): into the muscle
- subcutaneous: under the skin
- intradermal (ID): into the skin

Parenteral IV solutions are discussed in greater detail later in this chapter and in Chapter 11, *Preparing and Handling Sterile Products and Hazardous Drugs*.

Dispersions

In a **dispersion**, unlike in a solution, medication is not totally dissolved but simply distributed throughout the vehicle. A **suspension** is the dispersion of an undissolved solid in a liquid, whereas an emulsion is the dispersion of a mixture of two immiscible or unblendable liquids, such as oil-and-vinegar salad dressing; it must be shaken well to mix it evenly before use. In either case, an incomplete mixture of the solid or liquid exists. Dispersions are classified by the size of the dispersed ingredient(s) into suspensions and emulsions, both of which contain relatively large particles, and into magmas, gels, and jellies, which contain fine and ultrafine particles.

Many suspensions are commercially available, but others come in the form of dry powders or granules that are reconstituted with purified water. Suspensions may be

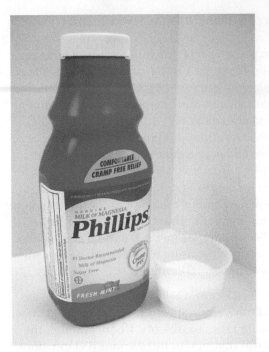
Milk of magnesia is an example of a colloid mixture.

classified by route of administration into oral (taken by mouth) and injection. A well-prepared suspension pours easily and settles slowly but can be redispersed easily by gentle shaking. A suspension may be a preferred method for dispensing a solid to a young or older adult patient who would find it difficult to swallow a solid dosage form. Examples of suspensions include antacids such as the magnesium and aluminum oral suspension sold under the brand name Maalox, antifungal Mycostatin oral suspensions, and NPH (neutral protamine Hagedorn) insulin. Pharmacy technicians should always shake well a stock bottle of an oral suspension before transferring the medication to a smaller, labeled prescription bottle; however, an insulin bottle should be gently agitated rather than shaken well.

Emulsions vary in their viscosity, or rate of flow: from free-flowing liquids, such as lotions, to semisolid dosage preparations, such as ointments and creams (discussed previously). Emulsions contain an emulsifying agent that renders the emulsion stable and less prone to separation. Creomulsion cough and cold products are examples of emulsions available for OTC oral use.

A **colloid** is a mixture having physical properties between those of a solution and a fine suspension. A colloidal dispersion is a heterogeneous mixture in which ultrafine particles of one substance are evenly distributed throughout another substance. Colloidal dispersions can be used internally or externally. A **magma**, or milk, contains colloidal particles in liquid, but the particles remain distinct in a two-phase system. An example is milk of magnesia, containing magnesium hydroxide, used to neutralize gastric acid. Aveeno is made with natural colloidal oatmeal milled into an ultrafine powder. When dispersed in water, this powder forms a soothing milky bath. It moisturizes and relieves dry, itchy, irritated skin caused by rashes, eczema, poison ivy, oak, sumac, and insect bites.

Another type of colloidal dispersion is the microemulsion. A **microemulsion** contains one liquid dispersed in another. Unlike other emulsions, however, it is clear because of the extremely fine size of the droplets of the dispersed phase. An example of a microemulsion is Haley's M-O. Collodion is an example of a vehicle that is a liquid dissolved in a mixture of alcohol and ether, used for a variety of topical purposes. Upon application, the highly volatile alcohol and ether solvent vaporizes, leaving a film coating containing the medication on the skin. The OTC product Compound W Wart Remover consists of acetic acid and salicylic acid in an acetone collodion base used to remove corns or warts.

Inhalation Dosage Forms

Gases, vapors, aerosols, sprays, solutions, and suspensions intended to be inhaled via the nasal or oral respiratory routes are known as inhalations. Many sprays and aerosols are used for topical application to the skin, such as OTC local anesthetics and antiseptics. The patient uses aerosols or sprays administered through the nose or mouth to internally deliver prescription drugs for allergies and asthma.

A **spray** is a dosage form that consists of a container having a valve assembly unit that, when activated, emits a fine dispersion of liquid, solid, or gaseous material. Sprays are often used for nasal decongestants and inhalation aerosols such as an albuterol inhaler for treating the acute symptoms of asthma.

An **aerosol** is a spray in a pressurized container that contains a propellant—an inert liquid or gas under pressure—designed to carry the active ingredient to its location of application. Depending on the formulation of the product and on the design of the valve, an aerosol may commonly emit a fine mist or a coarse liquid spray. Several inhalation products (such as Advair Diskus and Spiriva) are available as breath-activated devices of powders in place of aerosolized propellants.

Many anti-inflammatory medications are available both as a nasal spray for allergies and as an aerosol for inhalation for asthma.

Transdermal Dosage Forms

A **transdermal dosage form** is designed to deliver a drug to the bloodstream via absorption through the skin via a patch or disk. The patch consists of a backing, drug reservoir, control membrane, adhesive layer, and protective strip. The strip is removed, and the adhesive layer is attached to the skin. Chemicals in the patch or disk force the drug across the membranes of the skin and into the layer of skin where optimal absorption into the bloodstream will occur. In some patches, the membrane controls the rate of drug delivery, but in others the skin itself controls it. Although the skin presents a barrier, absorption does occur slowly; therapeutic effects may last for 24 hours up to 1 week. In effect, a transdermal dosage form is similar to a controlled-release tablet or capsule.

Drugs such as nicotine, nitroglycerin, narcotic analgesics, clonidine, scopolamine, estrogen, and testosterone are administered topically for their systemic effects on smoking cessation, chest pain, chronic pain, blood pressure, motion sickness (on cruises), and male and female hormone replacement levels, respectively.

Routes of Administration

Medications can be administered by several routes. A **route of administration** is a way to get a drug into or onto the body. Many drugs, such as nitroglycerin, can be delivered to the body orally (as a tablet or a capsule), sublingually (under the tongue), by inhalation (as a spray), topically (as a patch or ointment), or parenterally (as an IV injection or infusion).

Medication administration for absorption along the gastrointestinal (GI) tract into systemic circulation is referred to as the **oral route of administration**. However, the term *oral* sometimes also refers to applying medication topically to the mouth (as in the local treatment of a cold sore). The abbreviation *po* (from the Latin *per os;* meaning "by mouth") is used to indicate the oral route of medication administration.

Oral medications must proceed through a series of discrete steps such as dissolution in the stomach, absorption in the stomach or small intestine, biotransformation in the liver, and, finally, tissue distribution before they exert their therapeutic effect. This series of steps to get a drug into the bloodstream to exert its effect is called a **systemic effect**. Tablets, capsules, liquids, solutions, suspensions, syrups, and elixirs are all common dosage forms for oral administration of drugs.

- In the **sublingual route of administration** (from *sub*, meaning "under," and *lingua*, meaning "tongue"), the drug is placed under the tongue, where it is rapidly absorbed by the blood vessels under the tongue.
- In the **buccal route of administration**, also called the transmucosal route, the drug is placed between the gums and the inner lining of the cheek, in the so-called buccal pouch, where it is absorbed by the blood vessels in the lining of the mouth.

The **topical route of administration** is typically used to apply a drug directly to the surface of the skin, as in the case of creams, ointments, lotions, gels, and transdermal patches. Drugs given topically for local effects include anesthetics, anti-inflammatories, antifungals, antiseptics, astringents, moisturizers, pediculicides (for killing lice), protectants (e.g., sunscreen), and scabicides (for killing mites).

However, a broader definition of topical includes the administration of drugs to any mucous membrane, such as the lungs, eyes, ears, nose, rectum, vagina, or urethra. Topically administered drugs do not have to be dissolved and absorbed in the stomach to exert their pharmacological effect; most may not need to be absorbed into the bloodstream to work. They are used primarily for localizing their therapeutic effects. Medication that works at a specific body site creates a **local effect**.

- The **intrarespiratory route of administration**, also called inhalation, is defined as the application of a drug through inhalation into the lungs, typically through the mouth. The lungs are designed for the exchange of gases from the tissues into the bloodstream and serve as an excellent site for the absorption of drugs.
- The **ocular route of administration** is the application of a drug to the eye. It may be in a sterile solution or suspension formulation.
- The **conjunctival route of administration** is the application of a drug to the conjunctival mucosa, the lining of the inside of the eyelid.
- The **otic route of administration** is the application of a drug to the ear canal.
- The **nasal route of administration** is the application of a drug into the passages of the nose.
- The **rectal route of administration** is used to deliver drugs into the rectum and includes dosage forms such as suppositories, solutions, ointments, creams, and foams. Rectal solutions or enemas are used for cleansing the bowel, for laxative or cathartic action, or for drug administration in colon disease.
- The **vaginal route of administration** is application of a drug within the vagina; common dosage forms include emulsion foams, inserts, ointments, solutions, sponges, suppositories, and tablets. Generally, this route of administration is for local effects such as cleansing (e.g., douches), contraception, or treatment of common bacterial or yeast infections.
- The **urethral route of administration** is the application of a drug to or within the urethra; common dosage forms include solutions and suppositories. Drugs delivered by this route may be effective in treating incontinence or impotence in men.

Some medications have molecules that are too large to be absorbed or that are broken down so quickly in the stomach or liver that they cannot be taken orally. The **parenteral route of administration** distributes drugs systemically throughout the body by injection or infusion via a needle or catheter inserted into the body. The term *parenteral* comes from the Greek words *para*, meaning "outside," and *enteron*, meaning "the intestine." The derivation of the word indicates that this route of administration bypasses the alimentary canal or GI tract. An **injection** is defined as the administration of a parenteral medication into the bloodstream, muscle, or skin. The parenteral route includes any drug or fluid administered by the intravenous (IV), intramuscular (IM), or subcutaneous routes.

Advantages and Disadvantages of the Oral Route

The oral route of drug administration is convenient, easy to tolerate, safe, and simple to take or self-administer in most instances. A patient can take one tablet, several tablets, or a portion of a tablet, as required. A controlled-release tablet or capsule provides a longer duration of action and/or fewer side effects. An antibiotic liquid or suspension (or a chewable tablet) may be preferable for a young child over a tablet or capsule; a geriatric patient who has swallowing difficulties may also prefer a liquid formulation. Liquid solutions or suspensions work more quickly than oral tablets or capsules, because the medication they contain is more readily available for absorption.

Unlike the dose of a capsule, the dose of a tablet can be altered. Many tablets are *scored* once or twice to facilitate breaking into portions for half (or even quarter) doses. Scoring of a tablet is designed to equally divide the dose in each section. If a tablet is not scored, then it is generally recommended that it should not be broken, because the dose may not be equal in each piece. Due to rising drug costs it is not uncommon for patients, as well as managed-care organizations and Veterans Administration (VA) hospitals, to use a tablet splitter for unscored tablets when treating conditions such as high blood pressure and high cholesterol (providing up to 50% savings). Limited studies suggest that the practice does not appreciably affect the control of the disease state with select medications. Odd-shaped tablets are often difficult to cut—even with a tablet splitter.

The disadvantages of the oral route include the following:

- delayed onset because the tablet and capsule dosage forms must disintegrate in the stomach and small intestines before being absorbed
- destruction of the drug by GI fluids
- delayed absorption of medication because food or drink are present in the stomach

The oral route should not be used in patients who are experiencing nausea or vomiting or who are comatose, sedated, or otherwise unable to swallow. An unpleasant taste is a further disadvantage of some liquid dosage forms and requires that the taste be masked by flavorings to promote compliance. Controlled-release formulations have several disadvantages.

- They cannot be split or crushed (see Table 4.2 on page 96).
- Side effects that occur will take a longer time to subside.
- Many of these medications may be patent-protected, and thus more expensive than generic formulations.

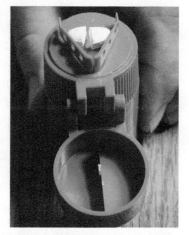

Capsules are a commonly used dosage form, because they are tasteless and easier to swallow than tablets.

A tablet splitter can save money for patients taking high-cost medications.

**TABLE 4.2 Common Delayed Release Tablets and Capsules
That Cannot Be Split**

Adalat CC	Felodipine XR	Pentasa
Adderall XR	Fosamax	pentoxifylline
Aggrenox	Glucophage XR	Plendil XR
Allegra D 12/24	Glucotrol XL	Procardia XL
Avinza	Inderal LA	Propranolol LA
Biaxin XL	indomethacin SR	Ritalin LA
Bupropion SR	Lescol XL	Theophylline XR
Carbidopa/levodopa ER	Metoprolol ER	Toprol XL
Concerta ER	methylphenidate LA	Verapamil XR
Depakote ER	MS contin	Voltaren XR
Diltia XT/diltiazem XL	Niaspan SR	Wellbutrin XL
Ditropan XL	nifedipine XL	
Effexor XR	oxycodone XR	

Safety Note

The oral route is not appropriate for patients who are experiencing nausea or vomiting.

The sublingual administration of medications has a very rapid onset (less than 5 minutes) and is thus appropriate for immediate relief, as in the case of nitroglycerin sublingual tablets for treatment of chest pain. The rapid onset is the result of the medication entering the bloodstream directly without passage through the stomach or breakdown in the liver. A disadvantage of the sublingual tablets is their short duration of action (less than 30 to 60 minutes), making this route of administration inappropriate for the routine delivery of medication. General disadvantages of the buccal route are unpleasant taste and local mouth irritation, as in the case of nicotine gum.

Dispensing and Administering Oral Medications

Patients should be told by the pharmacist what foods to take (and not take) with the medication, as well as what behaviors to avoid while taking the medication (e.g., sun exposure, driving). For most medications, water is preferred to coffee, tea, juices, or carbonated drinks as an aid in swallowing. In fact, taking some antibiotics and osteoporosis medications with milk, coffee, or tea may inactivate the drug. Pharmacists and technicians often add colorful auxiliary labels to the medication container to ensure that the drug is taken in the correct manner.

Patients who can swallow but have difficulty swallowing solids should be instructed to place the dose on the back of the tongue and tilt the head forward. Tilting the head forward stimulates swallowing. Some formulations, such as Theo-Dur, are suitable to be sprinkled on food when swallowing a tablet or capsule proves difficult for a child or adult with asthma. Patients should be reminded not to crush (or split) tablets or open capsules that are intended to be swallowed whole, such as sustained-release, long-acting, and enteric-coated drugs.

The pharmacist or the pharmacy technician under the pharmacist's direction often adds auxiliary labels to the prescription vial or container to further explain proper use to patients and to inform them of certain precautions.

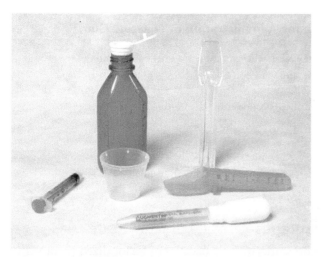

Infants or young children may have less difficulty taking liquid medication when it is administered with one of these devices, which also promote more accurate dosing.

Measuring spoons, cups, oral syringes, and droppers are commonly dispensed in the hospital and community pharmacy setting. It is always important to remind the patient (or parent) that the medication dose in liquid form should be accurately measured in a medication cup or measuring spoon. Common household utensils are often inaccurate measurements of a "teaspoonful" or "tablespoonful." Most manufacturers provide a measuring cup for OTC liquids for use in treating fever, cough, cold, and the like.

An **oral syringe** is used to deliver oral liquid medications to pediatric patients. It is an example of a calibrated device consisting of a plunger and a cannula, or barrel, used without a needle for administration of precisely measured amounts of medication by mouth. An oral syringe may be used to slowly administer an oral liquid medication to patients who cannot open their mouths or for infants and small children. Most pharmacies will provide a measuring spoon, oral syringe, or dropper when dispensing oral liquids and suspensions, including antibiotics.

Droppers are critically important for delivering the correct dosage of medication to infants. A **dropper** contains a small, squeezable bulb at one end and a hollow glass or plastic tube with a tapering point. Squeezing the bulb creates a vacuum for drawing up a liquid. The dropper may be incorporated into the cap of a vial or other container. The abbreviation *gtt* is used as a unit of pharmaceutical measurement for droppers and IV infusions to indicate *drops*. Because of the differing viscosities (the thicknesses and flow characteristics) of differing fluids, the size of a drop varies considerably from medication to medication—especially between suspensions and solutions. Some medication droppers that are packaged with the medication can only be used to measure the specific medication they accompany.

The pharmacy technician should remind the patient of proper storage conditions for medications. If the liquid medication is a suspension, then patients should be reminded to store it properly and shake the bottle before dosing. The expiration date for most pediatric antibiotic suspensions reconstituted or mixed with water is 7 days at room temperature and 14 days if stored in the refrigerator. Some antibiotics are best stored at room temperature, rather than refrigerated, after reconstitution.

Pharmacy technicians should also reinforce instructions on the proper storage of nitroglycerin. Sublingual nitroglycerin tablets should be stored in their original container (brown bottle) with the lid screwed on tightly to prevent sunlight and air from causing a loss of potency. The use of pillboxes is not recommended for these tablets. Physicians usually advise patients to refill their nitroglycerin with a fresh bottle every 3 to 6 months.

For buccally administered medication it is important that the patient understand the difference between the technique for chewing regular gum and taking nicotine gum medication. If the nicotine gum is chewed vigorously like chewing gum, then too much nicotine will be released, causing unpleasant side effects. Proper administration allows the gum to release the nicotine slowly, decreasing cravings. Counseling on the proper technique for administration of the nicotine gum is provided in Table 4.3.

TABLE 4.3 Proper Technique for Administration of Nicotine Gum

1. Chew the gum slowly and stop chewing when you notice a tingling sensation in the mouth.
2. Park the gum between the cheek and gum and leave it there until the taste or tingling sensation is almost gone.
3. Resume slowly chewing a few more times until the taste or sensation returns.
4. Park the gum again in a different place in the mouth.
5. Continue this chewing and parking process until the taste or tingle no longer returns when the gum is chewed (usually 30 minutes).
6. Do not eat or drink for 15 minutes before or while using the gum.

Advantages and Disadvantages of the Topical Route

The topical route of administration works quickly because of its localized therapeutic effects. Most drugs applied topically are not designed to be well absorbed into the deeper layers of the skin or mucous membrane. For example, most mild cases of poison ivy may be treated with an OTC product such as hydrocortisone cream; if the equivalent dose of tablets were administered, then the risk of side effects would be much greater. Alternatively, an asthmatic may have faster relief and fewer side effects with an inhaled metered dose medication rather than a tablet or capsule.

Compared to creams and gels, ointments are sticky and will leave the area feeling greasy. An ointment is especially good for extremely dry areas where moisture needs to be retained, as well as for areas prone to friction from clothing or other body parts. Ointments generally have a longer contact time with the skin and thus a longer duration of action. Creams and gels apply smoothly to the skin and leave a very thin film; they are more readily absorbed and are more cosmetically acceptable for most patients. Lotions are best applied to hairy areas of the body.

The transdermal route offers a method of administering medications that will provide a slow-release, steady level of drug in the system. Patient convenience and compliance are improved with the use of transdermal patches. The main disadvantages of the patch are cost and occasional skin irritation at the site.

The ocular, conjunctival, nasal, and otic routes of administration are almost always prescribed for their local effects, to treat conditions of the eye, the nose or sinuses, or the ear. Sprays for inhalation through the nose, however, may be used for either local or systemic effects. Some ophthalmic and nasal medications have systemic side effects, and precautions are advised if the patient has certain medical conditions. If the OTC medication label instructions are not clear, the patient should consult the pharmacist for appropriate and safe use of the selected product.

The usual dosage form for the inhalation route of administration is an aerosol. Entry into the bloodstream is extremely rapid—second only to the IV route of drug administration. This route is primarily used to deliver bronchodilators and anti-inflammatory drugs to asthma sufferers. An example is the "rescue" medication albuterol, commonly prescribed for asthmatics with acute onset of shortness of breath.

Medicated inhalations intended for the lung are often administered via devices such as metered-dose

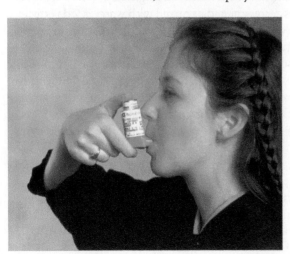

A metered-dose inhaler (MDI) is a common device used to administer a drug through inhalation into the lungs.

inhalers or nebulizers. A **metered-dose inhaler (MDI)** is a handheld, propellant-driven inhaler commonly used for patients with asthma or chronic lung disease. The metered-dose inhaler (MDI) provides medication with compressed gas. The MDI will deliver a specific, measured amount of medication each time the device is activated.

Beginning in 2009, "environmentally friendly" hydrofluroalkane (HFA) propellants are required by the government to replace all chlorofluorocarbon (CFC) propellants because of concerns about their adverse effect on earth's ozone layer. Some manufacturers use a **diskus** or a nonaerosolized, breath-activated powder for inhalation to avoid the propellants. This newer dosage form administers a higher concentration of drug as a micronized powder into the lungs. The result may be a controlled release of active ingredients for prevention of recurring symptoms, with potentially fewer side effects.

The major disadvantage of all MDIs is poor inhalation technique by the patient, thus decreasing the amount of drug that reaches into the pulmonary circulation. Proper technique and use of spacer devices are addressed later in the chapter.

A **nebulizer** is an atomizing machine that delivers a sterile solution of medication as a mist that is more effective in penetrating into the lungs. Common vehicles for inhalation solutions include sterile water for injection (SWI) and sodium chloride, also called *normal saline (NS)*. The solution is placed in a device that will aerosolize both the medication and the vehicle. An example of a medication delivered by inhalation is albuterol for relief of bronchial spasms and wheezing, commonly used in children. A "nebulized" mist of medication is more effective than an "aerosolized" spray in delivering more medication into deeper areas of the lungs in infants and young children.

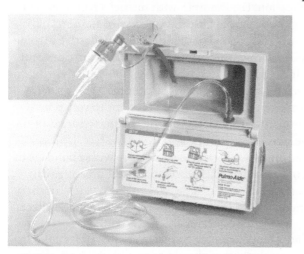

Nebulizers, also called atomizing machines, are effective for delivering mists or micronized powders to the lungs.

Vaporizers and humidifiers are other mechanical devices commonly used to deliver moisture to the air for relief of cold symptoms. Volatile medications can be used with some vaporizers. A good example of a volatile medication is Vicks Vaposteam.

An advantage of vaginal and urethral topical medications is the ability to treat an infection "locally" rather than "systemically" through tablets or capsules; this provides a higher concentration of the medication at the site while minimizing exposure to side effects. The major disadvantage of vaginally administered medications is the inconvenience and messiness of the creams and ointments. Inconvenience and localized pain and discomfort are disadvantages of the urethral inserts.

Rectal administration may be a preferred method of delivery for systemic drugs in four situations:

- when an oral drug might be destroyed or diluted by acidic fluids in the stomach
- when an oral drug might be too readily metabolized by the liver and eliminated from the body
- when the patient is unconscious and needs medication
- when the patient may be unable to take oral drugs because of nausea and vomiting or because of severe acute illness in the GI tract

Rectal doses do not transverse the digestive system for absorption and can be used in both young children and adults. For example, a young child with a high fever who will not (or cannot) take an oral formulation may need an acetaminophen suppository.

An adult with severe nausea and vomiting from a bad case of the flu, or perhaps from chemotherapy, may require a suppository to treat the acute symptoms and prevent dehydration. A major disadvantage of the rectal route of administration is its inconvenience, including discomfort and sometimes premature expulsion. Another disadvantage is erratic and irregular drug absorption.

Dispensing and Administering Topical Medications

Topical administration of drugs can provide a desirable therapeutic effect while minimizing side effects and adverse reactions that may be more prevalent when a drug is systemically absorbed in the body. It is important for the patient to fully understand the appropriate use and administration of each topical drug at the time of dispensing. Improper technique or overuse of topical drugs can increase the risk of side effects or alter drug efficacy.

Ointments, Creams, Lotions, and Gels Some topical products require special precautions and counseling for proper application. For example, with nitroglycerin ointment the patient or caregiver should wear gloves to avoid absorbing excessive amounts of drug, which could cause headaches. An OTC cream containing capsaicin (active ingredient is hot chili peppers) must be applied with gloves because severe irritation can occur if the cream is inadvertently rubbed into the eyes. Capsaicin is available in both regular and high potency formulas and is used for treating arthritis symptoms.

Many topical corticosteroids exist, from mild OTC hydrocortisone to very potent prescription agents. Most of these drugs are applied "sparingly" to affected areas of the body for short periods of time; some steroids cannot be applied to the face. Unless directed by the physician, the affected area should not be covered up with a bandage or other dressing (or, in the case of an infant, a diaper), because occlusive dressings can significantly increase drug absorption and the risk of side effects. The overuse, or inappropriate use, of potent topical corticosteroids can lead to serious systemic side effects.

Transdermal Patches The site of administration for transdermal patches should be relatively hair-free (usually the upper arm); patches should not be placed over a large area of scar tissue, which may decrease the release of the drug. Some patches are replaced every day, but others maintain their therapeutic effect for 3 to 7 days. The site of application should be rotated to minimize localized skin reactions.

A Lidoderm and nitroglycerin patch provides 24 hours of relief from a 12 hour application. Most physicians advise their patients to remove the nitroglycerin patch at bedtime to prevent the development of drug tolerance. As defined in Chapter 3, a drug tolerance occurs when the body requires higher doses of drug to produce the same therapeutic effect. Patients should be advised to carefully discard their used patches; the nicotine patch, for example, could cause serious side effects if ingested by children or pets.

Another transdermal patch delivers fentanyl, a potent Schedule II opiate analgesic. This drug is slowly absorbed through the skin into the blood-

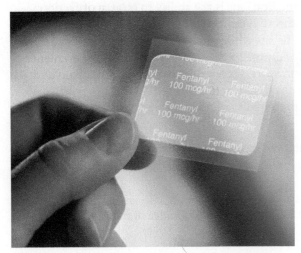

A transdermal patch offers a convenient delivery system for many medications. Transdermal patches should not be placed on skin that is overly hairy or on scar tissue.

stream and can relieve chronic pain for up to 3 days upon a single patch application. Sun exposure should be avoided, and heating pads, electric blankets, heat lamps, saunas, hot tubs, or heated water beds cannot be used with this drug. Localized heat speeds up the movement of fentanyl from the patch into the body. If the patch is damaged, then increased absorption of the active drug can occur. Both situations will create a higher risk for a serious drug overdose.

Ophthalmic Medications Ophthalmics must be at or near room temperature or body temperature before application into the eye. All medications should be stored according to the package insert to reduce bacterial growth and to ensure drug stability. Only medications with preservatives can be used repeatedly.

Before application, patients should be advised to wash their hands to prevent contamination of the application site or of the medication. The opening of the container (i.e., tube or dropper) should not touch the application site, to avoid contaminating the medication. The eye is prone to infection, so only sterile ophthalmic solutions or suspensions should be used. For example, a nonsterile otic medication for the ear cannot be dispensed as an ophthalmic medication even if it contains the same dose and drugs and concentration.

Previously applied medications should be cleaned away, as should any drainage from the eye. Cotton balls work well for this purpose. The intended location is usually the conjunctiva, the outer surface of the eye. Poorly administered eye drops could result in loss of medication through the tear duct; poorly placed eye ointments may be distributed over the eyelids and lashes.

To apply either drops or ointment, the patient's head should be tilted back. Once the medication is administered, it is important for the patient to place a finger in the corner of the eye, next to the nose, to gently close the duct, thus preventing loss of medication through the tear duct. The patient should also keep the eye closed for 1 or 2 minutes after application. Figure 4.2 shows the application of both ophthalmic drops and ointment.

When multiple drops of more than one medication are to be administered, the patient should be advised to wait 5 minutes between different medications lest the first drop be washed away. If an ointment and a drop are to be used together, then the drop is used first; the patient should then wait 10 minutes before applying the ointment. Ointments are generally applied at night; they are the drug form of choice when extended contact with the medication is desired, because tears wash them out less easily. The patient should be reminded that he or she might experience some temporary blurring of vision after application.

Safety Note

Unused medication should be discarded 30 days after the container is opened. Manufacturer expirations do not apply once a patient has opened the medication.

Safety Note

Eardrops can never be used in the eye, but eyedrops can be used in the ear.

FIGURE 4.2
Administering Ophthalmic Medication

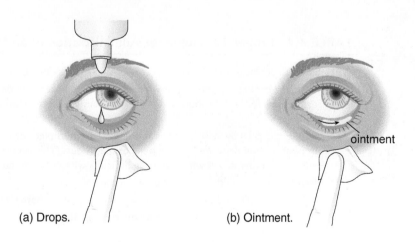

(a) Drops.

(b) Ointment.

ointment

FIGURE 4.3
**Administering
Otic Medications**

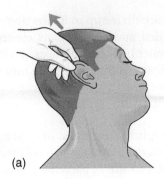
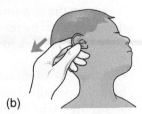

(a) Children over 3 years of age and adults should have the lobe pulled up and back when otic medications are administered.
(b) Children under 3 years old should have the lobe pulled down and back.

Otic Medications Like ophthalmics, otics must be stored at room temperature or body temperature. Heated drops may cause rupturing of the eardrum. Cold drops can cause vertigo and discomfort. Alcohol causes pain and burning sensation and therefore should not be used if the patient has a ruptured tympanic membrane (eardrum). If eardrum damage is suspected, then a low-alcohol content otic solution or suspension should be used.

The head is tilted to the side with the ear facing up (Figure 4.3). Anyone 3 years of age or older should have the lobes pulled up and back. Children under 3 years of age should have their ear lobes pulled down and back. The head should remain tilted for 2 to 5 minutes. Cotton plugs placed in the ear after administration of drops will prevent excess medication from dripping out of the ear. The plugs will not reduce the amount of drug that is absorbed.

Nasal Medications Nasal medications are applied by drops (instillation), sprays, or aerosols (i.e., spray under pressure). Application may be for relief of nasal congestion or allergy symptoms. The patient should be instructed to tilt the head back, insert the dropper, spray, or aerosol tip into the nostril, point it toward the eyes, and apply the prescribed number of drops or sprays (repeating the process in the other nostril if indicated). Breathing should be through the mouth to avoid sniffing the medication into the sinuses. It is very important that the patient not overuse OTC nasal decongestants (not more than three days) and that the patient carefully follow label instructions.

Inhaled Medications Proper administration of aerosolized medications is extremely important to ensure that medication reaches the lungs to control or relieve symptoms. Table 4.4 lists steps patients should follow when administering MDIs.

TABLE 4.4 Proper Technique for Administration of an MDI

1. Shake the canister well (or else only the propellant may be administered).
2. Prime the canister by pressing down and activating a practice dose. (Check priming instructions for each product as they vary depending on the manufacturer and active ingredient.)
3. Prepare the MDI by inserting the canister into a mouthpiece or spacer to reduce the amount of drug deposited on the back of the throat. (This is especially helpful for young children or older adults who may have difficulty with eye-hand coordination.)
4. Breathe out and hold the spacer between the lips, making a seal.
5. Activate the MDI and take a deep, slow inhalation at the same time.
6. Hold the breath briefly and slowly exhale through the nose.

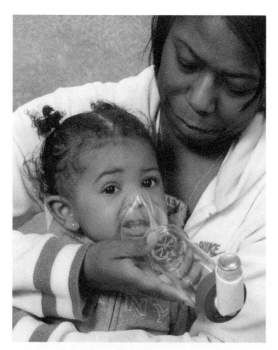

A spacer device improves the delivery of inhaled medications, especially in children and older adults.

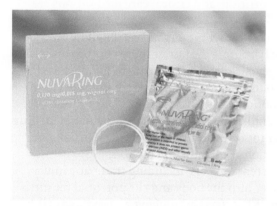

The NuvaRing offers an innovative system to deliver hormones in a vaginal ring to prevent conception.

If the MDI (metered-dose inhaler) contains a cortisone-like drug, then the patient should rinse the mouth thoroughly after receiving a dose to prevent a fungal infection in the mouth. The MDI device should be washed with soap and water at least weekly.

Spacer devices are used to improve the rate of drug delivery to the lungs, especially in children and in older patients with chronic lung diseases. Spacer devices may be packaged with the medication or dispensed separately. Eye and hand coordination and timing of inhalation is critical with an MDI. With a spacer device the medication is released into a "storage chamber" where it can be more easily inhaled by the patient. A higher concentration of medication is inhaled, thus improving symptoms.

Vaginal Medications The vaginal route is generally indicated for bacterial or fungal infection or for hormone replacement therapy. The patient is instructed to use the medication for the prescribed period to ensure effective treatment. Many vaginal creams and ointments are delivered to the site with the use of an applicator tube. If the medication is to be applied with an applicator, then the application should follow the steps outlined in Table 4.5.

For contraception a ring may be inserted into the vagina to surround the cervix. The ring contains hormones similar to birth control pills and provides nearly the same contraceptive protection. These hormones are released on contact and are slowly absorbed and distributed into the bloodstream. NuvaRing is an example of this type of delivery system. This steady, consistent release of medication may result in fewer hormonal ups and downs than when using other birth control methods. Occasionally, the patient will experience side effects or discomfort or have difficulty with proper insertion.

An **intrauterine device** is a way to deliver medication to prevent conception or to treat cancer within the uterus.

TABLE 4.5   Proper Technique for Administration of Vaginal Medications

1. Empty the bladder and wash hands.
2. Open the container and place the dose in the applicator.
3. Lubricate the applicator with a water-soluble lubricant if it is not prelubricated.
4. Lie down, spread the legs, and open the labia with one hand. With the other hand, insert the applicator about 2 inches into the vagina. (An alternative application is to insert the applicator and medication by standing with one foot on the edge of a bathtub.)
5. Release the labia; use the free hand to push the applicator plunger, releasing the medication.
6. Withdraw the applicator and wash hands. Wash applicator and dry it if being reused.

Rectal Medications The patient or caregiver should be instructed to be sure that the suppository is unwrapped and removed from its package. The suppository should then be inserted, small tapered end first, into the rectum with the index finger for the full length of the finger. The suppository may need to be lubricated with a water-soluble gel such as Vaseline to ease insertion. Another rectal route of drug administration is the enema, which is an application of a solution to evacuate the bowels for diagnostic procedures involving the lower GI tract.

Rectal enemas and suppositories should be used after a bowel movement. The patient should be instructed to lie on his or her left side with the left knee bent toward the chest. Shake the enema, and then unwrap it and gently insert the nozzle into the rectum. Firmly squeeze the bottle to release the entire drug. The whole bottle should be used unless otherwise directed. The patient should continue to lay on the left side. The patient should try to keep the medicine in the rectum as long as possible before having a bowel movement.

Safety Note

The patient must
remove the foil
packaging before
inserting the
suppository!

Advantages and Disadvantages of the Parenteral Route

Parenteral administration deserves special attention because of its complexity, widespread use, and potential for both therapeutic benefit and danger. The most common parenteral route of administration is the IV route—that is, directly into a vein. An **intravenous (IV) infusion** is a method for delivering a large amount of fluid and/or a high concentration of medication directly into the bloodstream over a prolonged period of time and at a slow, steady rate. In the hospital and in many home healthcare pharmacies, antibiotics, chemotherapy, nutrition, and critical care medications are administered via this route.

IV medications act rapidly to control and treat symptoms and can be administered to almost any organ or part of the body. The IV route is the fastest route of drug administration and is the preferred route in an emergency situation. Drugs can be administered by IV bolus or push, or by infusion. With a bolus injection, the drug is administered all at once, whereas an IV infusion provides a continuous amount of needed medication over a given period of time. The advantage of an infusion is that there is less fluctuation in drug blood levels than is experienced with other routes of administration; the infusion rate can be adjusted to provide more or less medication as the situation dictates.

The IV route does have associated inherent dangers, including traumatic injury from the insertion of the needle or catheter into the body and the potential for introducing toxic agents, microbes, or **pyrogens** (i.e., fever-producing by-products of microbial metabolism). To minimize infection from any type of injection, the site needs to be carefully "prepped" with an alcohol wipe, and the correct syringe, needle, and technique must be used. IV products are prepared in isolated rooms using special equipment to ensure sterility. Germ theory and the importance of aseptic technique are covered in more detail in Chapter 10, *Infection Control*.

IV injections and infusions must also be free of air bubbles and particulate matter. The introduction of air or particles might cause an embolism, or blockage, in a vessel or a severe painful reaction at the injection site. Another potential disadvantage of IV drug administration is that it is impossible to retrieve the drug if an adverse or allergic reaction occurs.

Safety Note

Do not use the
abbreviations
"SQ" or "SC."
Instead, write out
subcutaneous to
minimize potential
medication errors.

The intramuscular (IM) and subcutaneous routes of administration offer a more convenient way to deliver medications. Although the onset of response to the medication is slower than with the IV route, the duration of action is much longer, making it more practical for use outside the hospital. The absorption of the drug by the IM route is often unpredictable in a patient who is unconscious or in a shocklike state so the IM route is not recommended for these patients. The most commonly used medication that is administered subcutaneously is insulin; its proper administration will be discussed later in this chapter.

The major use of the intradermal (ID) route of administration is for diagnostic and allergy skin testing. If the patient is allergic or has been exposed to an allergen similar to tuberculosis (TB), then the patient may experience a severe local reaction.

Dispensing and Administering Parenteral Medications

The body is primarily an aqueous, or water-containing, vehicle. Because of this, most parenteral preparations introduced into the body are made up of ingredients placed in a sterile-water medium. Parenteral preparations are most commonly solutions in which ingredients are dissolved with water, normal saline, or other sterile solutions.

A basic understanding of various syringe and needle sizes by the technician will allow him or her to better assist the patient. Assisting the diabetic patient will be discussed further in Chapter 7, *The Business of Community Pharmacy*. Only trained professionals and healthcare providers should give injections. In recent years patients have been taught how to self-administer injections or infusions at home by the home health nurse or pharmacist. Many pharmacists are becoming increasingly involved in vaccine administration programs after completion of training and certification. Pharmacy technicians will not give injections unless they have received specialized training and certification and their state regulations allow the practice.

A **syringe** is a calibrated device used to accurately draw up, measure, and deliver medication to a patient through a needle. All injections, whether IV, IM, subcutaneous, or other, must be sterile, because they introduce medication directly into the body. Two types of syringes are commonly used for injections: (1) glass and (2) plastic. Glass syringes are fairly expensive and must be carefully sterilized between uses. Plastic syringes are easy to handle, disposable, and come from the manufacturer in sterile packaging. Plastic is clearly preferred and used both in and out of the hospital setting.

The larger hypodermic syringes have cannulas or barrels ranging from 3 to 60 mL of liquid. The **cannula** is the bore area inside the syringe that correlates with the volume of solution. Common types of syringes (Figure 4.4) include the insulin syringe (which measures from 30 to 100 units) and the tuberculin syringe (with cannulas ranging from 0.1 to 1 mL [used for skin tests and for drawing up very small volumes of solution]). The syringe and needle will be explained in more detail in Chapter 11.

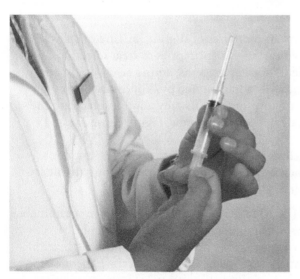

Disposable syringes and needles are used to administer drugs by injection. Different sizes are available depending on the type of medication and injection needed.

An injectable may be reconstituted and filled at the time of injection from a single-use vial or an ampule (no preservatives) or a multidose vial with preservatives. An injectable may also be available in a prefilled syringe. An example of a medication in a prefilled syringe drug delivery system is an insulin penfill (Figure 4.5). Short-, intermediate-, and long-acting insulins and mixtures are available with this delivery system. The patient simply "dials up" the correct units on the syringe and injects. The penfills commonly use short, fine, or ultrafine disposable needles to help make injecting less painful.

FIGURE 4.4
Typical Syringes

(a) Insulin syringes in 100 unit and 50 unit sizes.
(b) Hypodermic syringes in 6 mL and 3 mL sizes.
(c) Tuberculin syringes marked with metric measures.

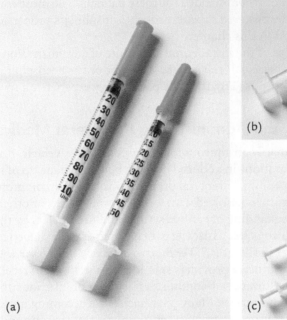

(a)

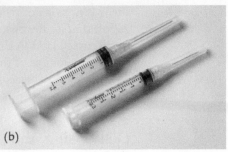

(b)

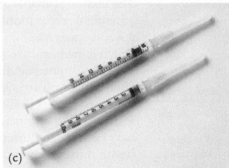

(c)

Safety Note

The syringes in Figure 4.4b are marked with the abbreviation *cc* (cubic centimeters). Because *cc* is considered a dangerous abbreviation, healthcare professionals, including the pharmacy technician, are encouraged to use the abbreviation for milliliters (mL) instead.

Different states have different regulations on the sale of syringes because of their potential diversion for the injection of illegal drugs; some states (or insurance companies) may require a prescription or the placement of syringes behind the prescription counter to control access to their sales. The proper disposal of plastic syringes and needles is both a health and environmental concern.

Intravenous Injections or Infusions Typical uses of IV infusions are to deliver pain-killing or bloodclot-busting medications, or antibiotics to treat infections. Blood, water, electrolytes, and nutrients such as proteins, amino acids, lipids, and sugars, as well as drugs, are also commonly administered by IV infusion. Although other sites are also used, injections and infusions are usually administered into the superficial veins of the arm on the side opposite the elbow. Figure 4.6 shows an IV injection.

Infusion pumps continuously deliver medication 24/7 to regulate the amount, rate, and/or timing of injections. They are used in both hospital and outpatient settings. Examples of infusion pumps include:

Safety Note

Only the patient should control the PCA pump button.

- a **patient-controlled analgesia (PCA) infusion device**, which is a programmable machine that delivers small doses of painkillers upon patient demand
- a jet injector, which uses pressure rather than a needle to deliver the medication
- an ambulatory injection device, such as an insulin pump, that the patient can wear while moving about

FIGURE 4.5
Insulin Penfill

The insulin penfill is easy to learn, simple to use, and convenient to carry, especially while traveling.

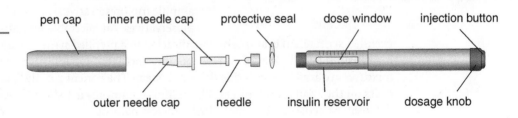

pen cap   inner needle cap   protective seal   dose window   injection button

outer needle cap   needle   insulin reservoir   dosage knob

106   **Unit 1** *Principles of Pharmacy Practice*

FIGURE 4.6
Intravenous Injection

Intravenous (IV) injections are administered at a 15 to 20 degree angle.

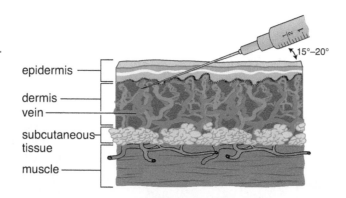

epidermis
dermis
vein
subcutaneous tissue
muscle

15°–20°

FIGURE 4.7
Intramuscular Injection

Intramuscular (IM) injections are administered at a 90 degree angle.

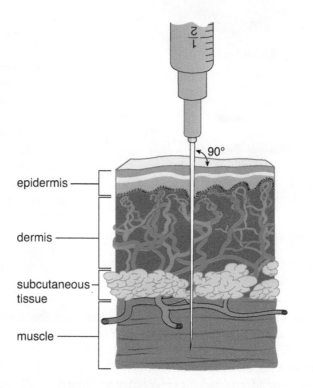

90°

epidermis

dermis

subcutaneous tissue

muscle

Intramuscular Injections The IM route is used to administer antibiotics, narcotics, pain medications for migraine headaches, vitamins, iron, and several vaccines. The volume of injection is limited to less than 2 or 3 mL. Care must be taken during deep IM injections to avoid hitting a vein, artery, or nerve. In adults, IM injections are generally given into the upper, outer portion of the gluteus maximus, the large muscle on either side of the buttocks. Another common site, especially for children, is the deltoid muscles of the shoulders. The typical needle used for IM injections is commonly a 22 to 25 gauge, ½ to 1 inch needle. The needle must be sufficiently long to inject the drug into the muscle. Figure 4.7 shows the needle angle and injection depth for an IM injection.

Subcutaneous Injections Subcutaneous injections administer parenteral medications below the skin into the subcutaneous tissue. Subcutaneous injections are given just beneath the skin with the syringe held at a 45 degree angle (Figure 4.8), usually on the outside of the upper arm, the top of the thigh, or the lower portion of each side of the abdomen. In lean older patients with less tissue, and in obese patients with more tissue, the syringe should be held nearer to a 90 degree angle.

The needle used is normally a 25 or 26 gauge needle that is ⅜ to ⅝ inch in length. The correct length of the needle is determined by a skin pinch in the injection area. The proper needle length will be one half the thickness of the pinch. Subcutaneous injections should not be made into grossly adipose, hardened, inflamed, or swollen tissue. To avoid pressure on sensory nerves causing pain and discomfort, no more than 1.5 mL should be injected into the site. Usually less than 1 mL is used.

Insulin, the most common type of subcutaneous injection, is given using 28 to 31 gauge short, fine, or ultrafine needles in a special syringe that measures the drug in units. The patient should carefully administer the insulin while following a plan for site rotation. (The site of insulin administration must be rotated to avoid or minimize

FIGURE 4.8

Subcutaneous Injection

Subcutaneous injections usually are administered just below the skin at a 45 degree angle.

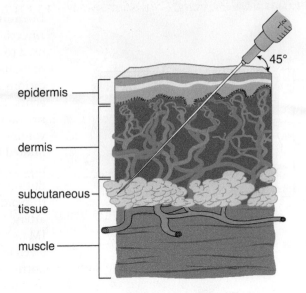

FIGURE 4.9

Intradermal Injection

Intradermal (ID) injections pierce the skin at a 10 to 15 degree angle. A small amount of medication (0.1 mL) is injected slowly into the dermal layer to form a wheal.

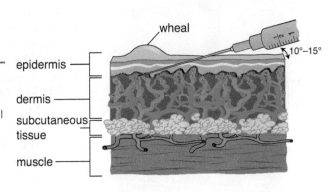

Safety Note

The patient should be instructed to agitate but not shake the insulin vial.

local skin reactions.) The absorption of insulin may vary depending on the site of administration and the activity level of the patient.

Patients should be instructed to keep insulin refrigerated and to check expiration dates frequently. Opened vials should generally be discarded after 1 month, because the insulin can lose a portion of its potency even if stored under ideal conditions. A vial of insulin is agitated and warmed by rolling between the hands and should never be shaken. The rubber stopper should be cleaned with an alcohol wipe. An amount of air should be injected into the vial approximately equal to the amount of insulin to be withdrawn. To remove air bubbles from the syringe, the patient should hold the syringe needle up and tap it lightly. Then gently push the air from the syringe with the plunger. The patient should be cautioned about planning meals, exercise, and insulin administration to gain the best advantage of the medication and avoid the chances of creating hypoglycemia or low blood sugar.

In addition to insulin, other common medications administered subcutaneously include epinephrine (or adrenaline) for emergency asthmatic attacks or allergic reactions, heparin or low-molecular-weight heparins such as Lovenox to prevent blood clots, sumatriptan or Imitrex for migraines, and many vaccines.

Intradermal Injections ID injections, given into the more capillary-rich layer just below the epidermis (Figure 4.9), are given for local anesthesia and for various diagnostic tests and immunizations. A common ID injection is a skin test for tuberculosis (TB); the typical site is the upper forearm, below the area where IV injections are given. Another example of ID injections is allergy skin testing in which small amounts of various allergens are administered (usually on the surface of the back) to detect allergies before beginning desensitization allergy shots.

Chapter Terms

aerosol a pressurized container with propellant used to administer a drug through oral inhalation into the lungs

aromatic water a solution of water containing oils or other substances that have a pungent, and usually pleasing, smell and are easily released into the air

buccal route of administration oral administration in which a drug is placed between the gum and the inner lining of the cheek; also called transmucosal route of administration

cannula the barrel of a syringe or bore area inside the syringe that correlates with the volume of solution

caplet a hybrid solid dosage formulation sharing characteristics of both a tablet and a capsule

capsule the dosage form containing powder, liquid, or granules in a gelatin covering

chewable tablet a solid oral dosage form meant to be chewed that is readily absorbed; commonly prescribed for school-age children

colloid the dispersion of ultrafine particles in a liquid formulation

conjunctival route of administration the placement of sterile ophthalmic medications in the conjunctival sac of the eye(s)

controlled-release dosage form the dosage form that is formulated to release medication over a long duration of time; also called delayed release

cream a cosmetically acceptable oil-in-water (O/W) emulsion for topical use on the skin

diluent an inactive ingredient that allows for the appropriate concentration of the medication in the tablet or capsule; also used to reconstitute parenteral products

diskus a nonaerosolized powder that is used for inhalation

dispersion a liquid dosage form in which undissolved ingredients are mixed throughout a liquid vehicle

dosage form the physical manifestation of a drug (e.g., capsule, tablet)

dropper a measuring device used to accurately dose medication for infants

drug delivery system a design feature of the dosage form that affects the delivery of the drug; such a system may protect the stomach or delay the release of the active drug

effervescent salts granular salts that release gas and dispense active ingredients into solution when placed in water

elixir a clear, sweetened, flavored solution containing water and ethanol

emulsion the dispersion of a liquid in another liquid varying in viscosity

enteric-coated tablet (ECT) a tablet coated in a way designed to resist destruction by the acidic pH of the gastric fluids and to delay the release of the active ingredient

extended-release (XL) dosage form a tablet or capsule designed to reduce frequency of dosing compared with immediate-release and most sustained-release forms

extract a potent dosage form derived from animal or plant sources from which most or all the solvent has been evaporated to produce a powder, an ointment-like form, or a solid

film-coated tablet (FCT) a tablet coated with a thin outer layer that prevents serious GI side effects

fluidextract a liquid dosage form prepared by extraction from plant sources and commonly used in the formulation of syrups

gel a dispersion containing fine particles for topical use on the skin

glycerogelatin a topical preparation made with gelatin, glycerin, water, and medicinal substances

granules a dosage form larger than powders that are formed by adding very small amounts of liquid to powders

injection the administration of a parenteral medication into the bloodstream, muscle, or skin

intrarespiratory route of administration the administration of a drug by inhalation into the lungs; also called inhalation

intrauterine device a device to deliver medication to prevent conception or to treat cancer within the uterus

intravenous (IV) infusion the process of injecting fluid or medication into the veins, usually over a prolonged period of time

irrigating solution any solution used for cleansing or bathing an area of the body, such as the eyes or ears

jelly a gel that contains a higher proportion of water in combination with a drug substance, as well as a thickening agent

liniment a medicated topical preparation for application to the skin, such as Ben Gay

local effect the site-specific application of a drug

lotion a liquid for topical application that contains insoluble dispersed solids or immiscible liquids

lozenge a medication in a sweet-tasting formulation that is absorbed in the mouth

magma a milklike liquid colloidal dispersion in which particles remain distinct, in a two-phase system; for example, milk of magnesia

metered-dose inhaler (MDI) a device used to administer a drug in the form of compressed gas through the mouth into the lungs

microemulsion a clear formulation that contains one liquid of extremely fine size droplets dispersed in another liquid; for example Haley's M-O

multiple compression tablet (MCT) a tablet formulation on top of a tablet or a tablet within a tablet, produced by multiple compressions in manufacturing

nasal route of administration the placement of sprays or solutions into the nose

nebulizer a device used to deliver medication in a fine-mist form to the lungs; often used in treating asthma

ocular route of administration the placement of ophthalmic medications into the eye

oil-in-water (O/W) emulsion an emulsion containing a small amount of oil dispersed in water, as in a cream

ointment a semisolid emulsion for topical use on the skin

oral disintegrating tablet (ODT) a solid oral dosage form designed to dissolve quickly on the tongue for oral absorption and ease of administration without water

oral route of administration the administration of medication through swallowing for absorption along the GI tract into systemic circulation

oral syringe a needleless device for administering medication to pediatric or older adult patients unable to swallow tablets or capsules

otic route of administration the placement of solutions or suspensions into the ear

parenteral route of administration the injection or infusion of fluids and/or medications into the body, bypassing the GI tract

parenteral solution a product that is prepared in a sterile environment for administration by injection

paste a water-in-oil (W/O) emulsion containing more solid material than an ointment

patient-controlled analgesia (PCA) infusion device a device used by a patient to deliver small doses of medication to the patient for chronic pain relief

plaster a solid or semisolid, medicated or nonmedicated preparation that adheres to the skin

powders fine particles of medication used in tablets and capsules

pyrogen a fever-producing by-product of microbial metabolism

rectal route of administration the delivery of medication via the rectum

route of administration a way of getting a drug onto or into the body, such as orally, topically, or parenterally

solute an ingredient dissolved in a solution or dispersed in a suspension

solution a liquid dosage form in which the active ingredients are completely dissolved in a liquid vehicle

solvent the vehicle that makes up the greater part of a solution

spirit an alcoholic or hydroalcoholic solution containing volatile, aromatic ingredients

spray the dosage form that consists of a container with a valve assembly that, when activated, emits a fine dispersion of liquid, solid, or gaseous material

sublingual route of administration oral administration in which a drug is placed under the tongue and is rapidly absorbed into the bloodstream

sugar-coated tablet (SCT) a tablet coated with an outside layer of sugar that protects the medication and improves both appearance and flavor

suppository a solid formulation containing a drug for rectal or vaginal administration

suspension the dispersion of a solid in a liquid

sustained-release (SR) dosage form a delayed-release dosage form that allows less frequent dosing than an immediate-release dosage form

syringe a device used to inject a parenteral solution into the bloodstream, muscle, or under the skin

syrup an aqueous solution thickened with a large amount of sugar (generally sucrose) or a sugar substitute such as sorbitol or propylene glycol

systemic effect the distribution of a drug throughout the body by absorption into the bloodstream

tablet the solid dosage form produced by compression and containing one or more active and inactive ingredients

tincture an alcoholic or hydroalcoholic solution of extractions from plants

topical route of administration the administration of a drug on the skin or any mucous membrane such as the eyes, nose, ears, lungs, vagina, urethra, or rectum; usually administered directly to the surface of the skin

transdermal dosage form a formulation designed to deliver a continuous supply of drug into the bloodstream by absorption through the skin via a patch or disk

urethral route of administration the administration of a drug by insertion into the urethra

vaginal route of administration the administration of a drug by application of a cream or insertion of a tablet into the vagina

water-in-oil (W/O) emulsion an emulsion containing a small amount of water dispersed in an oil, such as an ointment

Chapter Summary

- Drugs are administered in many dosage forms. The choice of dosage form is based on dose, route of administration, onset, and duration of desired therapeutic effect.
- Solid dosage forms commonly include tablets and capsules. Tablets may be coated, chewable, controlled release, effervescent, and/or specially formulated for buccal, sublingual, vaginal, or rectal use.

- Liquid dosage forms include a wide variety of solutions, as well as suspensions and emulsions.
- Measuring spoons, oral syringes, and droppers are critical for accurate dosing of liquid medication in infant and pediatric patients.
- Topical dosage forms include creams and ointments, which are special emulsions for application to the skin.

- Factors influencing the decision on route of administration include ease of administration; site, onset, and duration of action; quantity to be administered; drug metabolism by the liver or excretion by the kidney; and drug toxicity.
- Major routes of medication administration are oral, topical, and parenteral.
- The oral route of drug administration offers many advantages over other routes and is the one most commonly used.
- Topical administration includes not only medication applied to the skin but also ophthalmic, nasal, otic, inhaled, vaginal, urethral, and rectal formulations.

- Topical agents often require additional counseling by the pharmacist in technique for proper administration.
- Parenteral administration commonly includes IV, IM, subcutaneous, and ID injections, as well as IV infusions.
- Infusions are given for a variety of purposes, including the delivery of fluids and electrolytes, nutrients, and drugs.
- IV injections and infusions are injected directly into the bloodstream, and special precautions must be taken in their preparation and administration to maintain sterility and to prevent air embolisms.

Chapter Review

Checking Your Understanding

Choose the best answer from those provided.

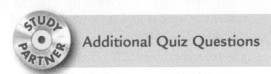
Additional Quiz Questions

1. The most common drug dosage form is a(n)
   a. tablet.
   b. capsule.
   c. cream.
   d. aerosol.

2. Administration of a medication under the tongue is called
   a. topical.
   b. sublingual.
   c. intradermal (ID).
   d. buccal.

3. Drugs with an enteric coating primarily release the active drug in the
   a. stomach.
   b. intestines.
   c. pancreas.
   d. liver.

4. Some examples of dispersions are
   a. suspensions and emulsions.
   b. tinctures, fluidextracts, and extracts.
   c. aromatic waters.
   d. elixirs and syrups.

5. Dosage forms that are often or always sweetened include
   a. parenteral solutions.
   b. medicated syrups and elixirs.
   c. collodions.
   d. liniments.

6. A transdermal formulation makes use of which organ of the body for its site of absorption?
   a. skin
   b. eyes
   c. ears
   d. lungs

7. The route of administration with the fastest onset of action is
   a. sublingual.
   b. subcutaneous.
   c. intramuscular (IM).
   d. intravenous (IV).

8. In a patient with severe nausea and vomiting, the most appropriate dosage form would be a
   a. liquid suspension.
   b. caplet.
   c. suppository.
   d. magma.

9. The word *parenteral* means, literally, *outside the*
   a. *stomach.*
   b. *intestine.*
   c. *mouth.*
   d. *liver.*

10. Insulin needles for subcutaneous administration are usually
    a. 28 gauge.
    b. 22 gauge.
    c. 18 gauge.
    d. 15 gauge.

Thinking Like a Pharmacy Tech

1. Nitroglycerin is an example of a drug that comes in a wide variety of dosage forms appropriate for a wide variety of routes of administration. Research the different routes of administration used for nitroglycerin. Refer to Internet sites or reference works, as well as to healthcare professionals. Pose the following questions: What are the various dosage forms of nitroglycerin? What routes of administration are used? Why do people choose one route of administration over another? Use the table below to list the advantages and disadvantages of each dosage form.

2. In a small group, discuss the advantages and disadvantages of the various routes of administration. Which is the most convenient? Safest? Fastest in onset? Longest in duration? Which poses the most compliance problems? Present your group's opinions to the class.

Dosage Form	Advantages	Disadvantages
a. tablet sustained release		
b. capsule sustained release		
c. sublingual tablet		
d. buccal tablet		
e. aerosol spray		
f. transdermal patch		
g. ointment		
h. IV		

3. Create a chart with a schematic diagram of the human body illustrating the various routes of administration described in this lesson. To visualize administration techniques, if you have access in your classroom to a syringe, then use IM, subcutaneous, and ID techniques to inject an orange with water or normal saline.

4. Check the *Physician's Desk Reference (PDR)* for the following information on reconstituted antibiotic suspensions for these drugs: amoxicillin, azithromycin, and Omnicef. How should each of these medications be stored? What expiration date is recommended after reconstitution? What auxiliary labels are needed for each?

Communicating Clearly

1. A prescription has been brought in for a steroid cream (0.25%) to be applied to an infant's eczema on the cheeks. The mother states that she has a similar drug at home in an ointment (1%) and wants to know whether she can use what she has at home because the drug is expensive. Creams and ointments are very different, and in this case the strength (and maybe the drug) is different as well. How should the pharmacy tech respond to this question? What will the pharmacist tell this mother about the differences between the two products?

2. A young man has come in to pick up some prescriptions for his asthma. His physician has just changed his prescription from oral prednisone to an inhaled steroid to control an exacerbation of his asthma. The physician told the patient that the inhaled product would be safer for him in the long run. Why? What are the advantages of the inhaled product over the oral tablets?

3. An older man has just picked up two prescriptions for nitroglycerin. One is for sublingual tablets and the other is for transdermal patches. Why is the patient using two different forms of the same drug? What are the advantages and disadvantages of each?

4. A patient has come in to pick up some prescriptions for fertility drugs. Some of the medications are given subcutaneously and others IM. The pharmacist has selected the appropriate syringes for them.

   a. Which of the following syringes is for the IM injection, and which is for the subcutaneous injection?

   > **22G1½**
   > Needle
   >
   > Do not reshield used needles.
   > Discard after single use. STERILE.

   > **27G ½**
   > Needle
   >
   > Do not reshield used needles.
   > Discard after single use. STERILE.

   b. Prepare a brief statement for the patient explaining which syringe is used for each type of injection, as well as the technique and location used for each injection.

Researching on the Web

1. Visit a drug information site, such as www.drugs.com or www.Rxlist.com, and research the following drugs. For each drug identify the various dosage forms available and the route by which each dosage form is administered. (Each drug is available in at least two dosage forms.)
   a. Imitrex
   b. promethazine
   c. Valium
   d. morphine
   e. triamcinolone
   f. Proventil

2. Visit the following site and provide information on the proper use of the Duragesic transdermal patch: www.fda.gov/cder/drug/infopage/fentanyl/DuragesicPPI.pdf. In your report, include directions for correct physical application of the patch and the appropriate sites to be used.

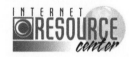 For further study of chapter-related topics, explore the Web links in the Web Center at www.emcp.net/pharmpractice4e.

Pharmaceutical Measurements and Calculations

5

Learning Objectives

- Describe four systems of measurement commonly used in pharmacy and convert units from one system to another.

- Explain the meanings of the prefixes most commonly used in metric measurement.

- Convert from one metric unit to another (e.g., grams to milligrams).

- Convert Roman numerals to Arabic numerals.

- Convert time to 24 hour military time.

- Convert temperatures to and from the Fahrenheit and Celsius scales.

- Round decimals up and down.

- Perform basic operations with proportions, including identifying equivalent ratios and finding an unknown quantity in a proportion.

- Convert percentages to and from fractions, ratios, and decimals.

- Perform fundamental dosage calculations and conversions.

- Solve problems involving powder solutions and dilutions.

- Use the alligation method to prepare solutions.

- Calculate the specific gravity of a liquid.

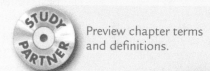 Preview chapter terms and definitions.

The daily activities of pharmacists and pharmacy technicians require making precise measurements. When pharmacy personnel measure liquids for reconstituted solutions (mixing water to a powder to make a solution), compound drugs, and prepare parenteral infusions, the amounts or quantities and calculations must always be precise. A mistake in a calculation can have severe consequences, such as drug toxicity. Therefore, it is essential for the practicing pharmacy technician to understand the basic measurement systems and mathematical techniques used in the field, as discussed in this chapter.

Systems of Pharmaceutical Measurement

Systems of measurement are widely accepted standards used to determine such quantities as area, distance (or length), temperature, time, volume, and weight. Of these, temperature, distance, volume, and weight are the most important to the pharmacy profession.

- Quantities of temperature and weight are the simplest and most familiar measurements.
- Distance is a measurement of extension in space in one dimension.
- Volume, the least intuitive of these quantities, is a measurement of extension in space in three dimensions (i.e., cubic volume).

The Metric System

The **metric system** is the legal standard of measure for pharmaceutical measurements and calculations in the United States. Developed in France in the 1700s, the metric system became the legal standard of measure in the United States in 1893.

The metric system has several distinct advantages over other measurement systems:

- The metric system is based on decimal notation, in which units are described as multiples of ten (0.001, 0.01, 0.1, 1, 10, 100, 1000). This decimal notation makes calculation easier.
- The metric system contains clear correlations among the units of measurement of length, volume, and weight, again simplifying calculation. For example, the standard metric unit for volume, the liter, is almost exactly equivalent to 1000 cubic centimeters. (A centimeter is a metric unit of length.)
- With slight variations in notation, the metric system is used worldwide, especially in scientific measurement, and so, like music, is a "universal language."

The modern metric system makes use of the standardized units of the Système International (SI), adopted by agreement by governments worldwide in 1960. Three basic units in this system are the (1) meter, (2) liter, and (3) gram. The **meter** is the unit for measuring distance, length, and area and has limited use in pharmacy. Figure 5.1 shows an application of the metric system in measuring distance, area, and volume. Prefixes—syllables placed at the beginnings of words—can be added to these basic metric units to specify a particular measure. Because SI is a decimal system, the prefixes denote powers of 10. Table 5.1 lists the prefixes in the SI language.

The major metric units used most commonly in pharmacy are the gram and the liter. The **gram,** the unit for measuring weight, is used for measuring the amount of medication in solid form and for indicating the amount of solid medication in a solution. The gram is the weight of 1 cubic centimeter of water at 4 °C. The **liter** is the unit for measuring the volume of liquid medications and also liquids for solutions.

The metric units most commonly used in pharmacy practice, along with their abbreviations, are listed in Table 5.2. Note that the same abbreviations are used for both single and plural measurements (e.g., 1 g, 3 g).

In prescriptions using the metric system, numbers are expressed as decimals rather than as fractions. Weights are generally given in grams, and volumes in milliliters.

For numbers less than 1, a 0 is placed before the decimal point to prevent misreading, as in ℞ digoxin 0.25 mg. Note that an error of a single decimal place is an error by a factor of 10. It is therefore extremely important that decimals be written properly.

Safety Note

An error of a single decimal place is an error of a factor of 10.

FIGURE 5.1
Measurements in the Metric System

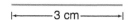

(a) Distance (length) = 3 cm.

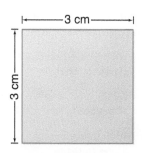

(b) Area = 9 cm² or
3 cm × 3 cm.

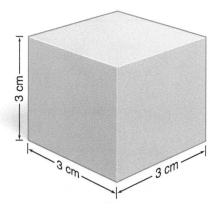

(c) Volume = 27 mL or 3 cm³ or
3 cm × 3 cm × 3 cm.

TABLE 5.1 Système International Prefixes

Prefix	Symbol	Meaning
micro-	mc	one millionth (basic unit × 10⁻⁶, or unit × 0.000001)
milli-	m	one thousandth (basic unit × 10⁻³, or unit × 0.001)
centi-	c	one hundredth (basic unit × 10⁻², or unit × 0.01)
deci-	d	one tenth (basic unit × 10⁻¹, or unit × 0.1)
hecto-	h	one hundred times (basic unit × 10², or unit × 100)
kilo-	k	one thousand times (basic unit × 10³, or unit × 1000)

TABLE 5.2 Common Metric Units

Measurement Unit	Equivalent
Length: Meter	
1 meter (m)	100 centimeters (cm)
1 centimeter (cm)	0.01 m; 10 millimeters (mm)
1 millimeter (mm)	0.001 m; 1000 micrometers, or microns (mcm)
Volume: Liter	
1 liter (L)	1000 milliliters (mL)
1 milliliter (mL)	0.001 L; 1000 microliters (mcL)
Weight: Gram	
1 gram (g)	1000 milligrams (mg)
1 milligram (mg)	1000 micrograms (mcg); one thousandth of a gram (g)
1 kilogram (kg)	1000 grams (g)

TABLE 5.3   Common Metric Conversions

Conversion	Instruction	Example
kilograms (kg) to grams (g)	multiply by 1000 (move decimal point three places to the right)	6.25 kg = 6250 g
grams (g) to milligrams (mg)	multiply by 1000 (move decimal point three places to the right)	3.56 g = 3560 mg
milligrams (mg) to grams (g)	multiply by 0.001 (move decimal point three places to the left)	120 mg = 0.120 g
liters (L) to milliliters (mL)	multiply by 1000 (move decimal point three places to the right)	2.5 L = 2500 mL
milliliters (mL) to liters (L)	multiply by 0.001 (move decimal point three places to the left)	238 mL = 0.238 L

To convert from one metric unit to another, simply move the decimal point. Move the decimal point to the left to convert to larger units. Move the decimal point to the right to convert to smaller units. The most common metric calculations in pharmacy involve conversions to and from milliliters and liters and to and from grams, milligrams, and kilograms. Table 5.3 shows how to do these conversions.

Common Measures

Like languages, measurement systems tend to evolve by folk processes. Thus a foot was originally a length approximately equal to that of the average person's foot. By its nature, common measure is approximate. Many households still use these common systems of measure, and U.S. pharmacies often use the common measure systems when dispensing medications.

Three types of common measures encountered in pharmacy are (1) apothecary, (2) avoirdupois, and (3) household. Table 5.4 provides a key to the symbols used in the apothecary system. Tables 5.5, 5.6, and 5.7 provide conversion equivalents for common units in these systems and compare them to the metric system.

When the household system was formed, 1 fluidram became synonymous with 1 teaspoonful or 5 mL. Therefore, Table 5.5 states that there are 6 fluidrams per 1 fluid ounce, and that 1 fluidram equals 5 mL. When converting from fluid ounces to

TABLE 5.4   Apothecary Symbols

Volume		Weight	
Unit of Measure	Symbol	Unit of Measure	Symbol
minim	♏	grain	gr
fluidram	f℥	scruple	Ꝫ
fluidounce	f℥	dram	ℨ
pint	pt	ounce	℥
quart	qt	pound	℔ or #
gallon	gal		

TABLE 5.5 Apothecary System

Measurement Unit	Equivalent within System	Metric Equivalent
Volume		
1 ♏ (minim)	–	0.06 mL
16.23 ♏	–	1 mL
1 f𝔷 (fluidram)	60 ♏	5 mL (3.75 mL)*
1 f℥ (fluid ounce)	6 f𝔷	30 mL (29.57 mL)†
1 pt (pint)	16 f℥	480 mL
1 qt (quart)	2 pt or 32 f℥	960 mL
1 gal (gallon)	4 qt or 8 pt	3840 mL
Weight		
1 gr (grain)	–	65 mg††
15.432 gr	–	1 g
1 ℈ (scruple)	20 gr	1.3 g
1 𝔷 (dram)	3 ℈ or 60 gr	3.9 g
1 ℥ (ounce)	8 𝔷 or 480 gr	30 g (31.1 g)
1 # (pound)	12 ℥ or 5760 gr	373.2 g

*In reality, 1 f℥ contains 3.75 mL; however, that number is usually rounded up to 5 mL or 1 tsp.
†In reality, 1 f℥ contains 29.57 mL; however, that number is usually rounded up to 30 mL.
††Many manufacturers use 60 mg instead of 65 mg as the equivalent for 1 gr (grain).

TABLE 5.6 Avoirdupois System

Measurement Unit	Equivalent within System	Metric Equivalent
1 gr (grain)	–	65 mg
1 oz (ounce)	437.5 gr	30 g (28.35 g)*
1 lb (pound)	16 oz or 7000 gr	454 g

*An avoirdupois ounce actually contains 28.34952 g; however, we often round up to 30 g. It is common practice to use 454 g as the equivalent for a pound (28.35 g × 16 oz/lb = 453.6 g/lb, rounded to 454 g/lb).

Safety Note

For safety reasons, the use of the apothecary system is discouraged. Use the metric system.

milliliters in pharmacy calculations, it is common practice to round up: for example, 29.57 mL up to 30 mL. In this chapter, use 30 mL when converting from apothecary, avoirdupois, or household measure fluid ounces.

Another calculation performed on a frequent basis is a conversion from ounces to grams. An apothecary ounce is 31.1 g, and the avoirdupois ounce is 28.35 g. In both cases it is common practice to round to 30 g. Many physicians are accustomed to writing prescription orders in ounces of medication, in both liquid and solid forms; however, the metric system is considered more accurate and is becoming the system of choice in the United States. In addition, many pharmacy computer systems are programmed to accept only amounts given in metric units.

TABLE 5.7 Household Measures

Measurement Unit	Equivalent within System	Metric Equivalent
Volume		
1 tsp (teaspoonful)	–	5 mL
1 tbsp (tablespoonful)	3 tsp	15 mL
1 fl oz (fluid ounce)	2 tbsp	30 mL (29.57 mL)*
1 cup	8 fl oz	240 mL
1 pt (pint)	2 cups	480 mL†
1 qt (quart)	2 pt	960 mL
1 gal (gallon)	4 qt	3840 mL
Weight		
1 oz (ounce)	–	30 g
1 lb (pound)	–	454 g
2.2 lb	–	1 kg

*In reality, 1 fl oz (household measure) contains less than 30 mL; however, 30 mL is usually used.
†When packaging a pint, companies will typically present 473 mL, rather than the full 480 mL, thus saving money over time.

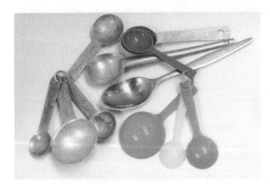

The volume held by a household teaspoon may vary, but a true teaspoon equals 5 mL.

As stated earlier, it is common practice to round a household fluid ounce (29.57 mL) up to 30 mL. When measuring this amount, it is often appropriate to make this estimation, because the volume differs by such a small amount. However, the discrepancy becomes far more apparent when measuring multiple fluid ounces that have been rounded up to the 30 mL equivalent. For example, if asked to measure a household pint (16 fl oz), one would measure roughly 480 mL. This becomes problematic, because 29.57 mL multiplied by 16 is equal to only 473.12 mL, not 480 mL. Products in most stock bottles will be labeled 473 mL, yet pharmacies will bill according to the estimation of 480 mL and measure out fluid ounces in 30 mL increments. For the purposes of this chapter, use the rounded 30 mL and 480 mL values.

Note that the only equivalent unit in both the apothecary and avoirdupois systems is the unit of dry measure known as the *grain*. This is the most commonly encountered nonmetric unit in pharmacy practice. Phenobarbitol and thyroid medications are often prescribed in grains. Pharmacists sometimes make use of apothecaries' weights for extemporaneous compoundings that come in 5 grain, 4 grain, 3 grain, 2 grain, 1 grain, and ½ grain units. In Table 5.5, the grain is equal to 65 mg, but many other references use 60 mg instead. Most pharmacists use the 65 mg conversion.

Safety Note

Always carefully check and double-check all calculations.

Numeric Systems

Two types of numbers are used in pharmaceutical calculations: Roman and Arabic. The Arabic system uses numbers, fractions (such as ³/₅), and decimals. In the

TABLE 5.8 Comparison of Roman and Arabic Numerals

Roman	Arabic	Roman	Arabic
s̅s̅	0.5 or ½	L or l	50
I or i or ī	1	C or c	100
V or v	5	D or d	500
X or x	10	M or m	1000

Safety Note

New safety guidelines discourage use of Roman numerals.

Roman system, numerals are expressed in either lowercase letters or as capital letters. The most frequently used numerals are the upper case I, V, and X, which represent the Arabic numbers 1, 5, and 10, respectively. A prescription using an apothecary measure is commonly written in lowercase Roman numerals that follow rather than precede the unit of measurement. Thus "aspirin gr vi" means "six grains of aspirin." Roman numerals are also sometimes used to express other quantities, as in tablets (C = 100 tablets) or volume (tbsp iii = 3 tablespoonsful). The lowercase Roman numerals i, ii, and iii are often written with a line above to prevent errors in interpretation (for example: ī, īī, īīī). Table 5.8 summarizes the Roman numeral system and gives equivalents in Arabic numerals.

Roman numerals are equal or smaller when reading left to right; the total value equals the sum of their individual values. Thus iii = 3, and xi = 10 + 1 = 11. Otherwise, first subtract the value of each smaller numeral from the value of the larger numeral that it precedes, and then add the individual values. Thus iv = 5 − 1 = 4, and xxiv = 10 + 10 + (5 − 1) = 10 + 10 + 4 = 24.

Time

Safety Note

Military time reduces errors.

In the hospital setting, medication orders are commonly time-stamped with military time (also referred to as international time). Dosage administration schedules for unit dose and IV admixtures also use this method. **Military time** is based on a 24 hour clock, with midnight being considered time 0000. The first two digits are the time in hours, and the second two digits are the time in minutes.

0000	Midnight
0600	6 AM
1200	Noon
1800	6 PM

No AM or PM are used, thus causing less confusion—and fewer medication errors. Military time eliminates the potential to confuse between 4 AM or 4 PM.

Example 1

At 0125, you receive an order for gentamicin 80 mg IV every 8 hours. The order is due to be administered at 0200, 1000, and 1800. When was the order received, and when should doses be prepared and sent to the patient care unit?

The order was received at 1:25 AM. The first dose is to be immediately prepared and sent to the patient care unit in order to be given at 2:00 AM. Follow-up doses are scheduled at 10:00 AM and 6:00 PM.

Temperature

The United States is one of the few countries in the world that commonly uses Fahrenheit as its temperature scale. The **Fahrenheit temperature scale** uses 32 °F as the temperature when ice freezes and 212 °F as the temperature when water boils; the difference between these two extremes is 180 °F.

In the 1700s a Swedish scientist with the last name of Celsius suggested a thermometer with a difference of 100 degrees between freezing and boiling. He used zero degrees (0 °C) as the freezing point and 100 °C as the boiling point. The **Celsius temperature scale** is commonly used in Europe and globally in science. Celsius is often the scale used in healthcare settings, including the pharmacy.

Storing unstable drugs under proper refrigeration and maintaining refrigerated equipment at the appropriate temperature are important responsibilities for the pharmacy technician. Most often the temperature requirements in the drug package inserts or in the policy and procedure manual will be given in Celsius. Most refrigerators in the pharmacy need to maintain a temperature of 5 °C to 10 °C. Pharmacy technicians will need to know how to convert between the Celsius scale and the Fahrenheit scale.

Every 5 °C change in temperature is equivalent to a 9 °F change (as indicated in Table 5.9). In addition to using this chart, here are several mathematical methods of converting from Fahrenheit to Celsius and vice versa. One method uses the following equations:

Pharmacy technicians may be asked to help patients convert between temperature readings in degrees Celsius and Fahrenheit. As with all conversions, this calculation must be done accurately.

$$°F = (1.8 \times °C) + 32°$$

$$°C = (°F - 32°) \div 1.8$$

An alternative method uses the following algebraic equation:

$$5 °F = 9 °C + 160$$

When calculating the conversion, the final temperature is usually rounded up to the closest whole number. The use of these equations is demonstrated in the following examples.

Example 2

Convert 75 °F to degrees Celsius.

$$°C = (°F - 32°) \div 1.8$$
$$°C = (75° - 32°) \div 1.8$$
$$°C = 43° \div 1.8$$
$$°C = 23.888°, \text{ rounded to } 24°$$

Example 3

Convert 75 °C to degrees Fahrenheit.

$$°F = (1.8 \times °C) + 32°$$
$$°F = (1.8 \times 75°) + 32°$$
$$°F = 135° + 32°$$
$$°F = 167°$$

TABLE 5.9 Temperature Equivalencies between Celsius and Fahrenheit

Celsius	Fahrenheit
0 °C	32 °F
5 °C	41 °F
10 °C	50 °F
15 °C	59 °F
20 °C	68 °F

Example 4

According to the package insert, the manufacturer requires that a vial of reconstituted antibiotic be stored at a temperature from 2 to 8 °C. What should the range of the Fahrenheit temperature setting be on the thermostat in the refrigerator?

First, convert the degrees Celsius at the low end of the range.

$$°F = (1.8 \times °C) + 32°$$
$$°F = (1.8 \times 2°) + 32°$$
$$°F = 3.6° + 32°$$
$$°F = 35.6°, \text{ rounded to } 36°$$

Second, convert the degrees Celsius at the high end of the range.

$$°F = (1.8 \times °C) + 32°$$
$$°F = (1.8 \times 8°) + 32°$$
$$°F = 14.4° + 32°$$
$$°F = 46.4°, \text{ rounded to } 46°$$

The technician should be sure the thermostat setting is between 36 and 46 °F, inclusively.

Example 5

An anxious mother telephones the pharmacy on a Saturday night. Her 6 month old child has a fever. The only thermometer she has records a temperature of 38.3 °C. Her pediatrician told her to call if the child's temperature reached 101 °F. What is the child's temperature in degrees Fahrenheit? Should the mother call the pediatrician?

$$°F = (1.8 \times °C) + 32°$$
$$°F = (1.8 \times 38.3°) + 32°$$
$$°F = 68.94° + 32°$$
$$°F = 100.94°, \text{ rounded to } 101°$$

The parent should call the child's pediatrician.

Basic Calculations Used in Pharmacy Practice

Many tasks in pharmacy—determining dosages, compounding medications, and preparing solutions—use calculations involving the units of measure given in the preceding section. Pharmacy work often requires performing fundamental operations involving fractions, rounding numbers, ratios and proportions, and percentages.

Fractions

The technician needs to be comfortable with adding, subtracting, multiplying, and dividing fractions. For a review of these skills, check out the tutorial in the Study Hall at www.emcp.net/pharmpractice4e.

When something is divided into parts, each part is considered a **fraction** of the whole. For example, a pie might be divided into eight slices, each one of which is a fraction, or ⅛, of the whole pie. In this example, 1 is a piece of the pie and 8 is the number of slices in the whole pie. A simple fraction consists of two numbers: a **numerator** (the number on the top) and a **denominator** (the number on the bottom).

$$\frac{1}{2} \quad \begin{matrix} \longleftarrow \text{numerator} \\ \longleftarrow \text{denominator} \end{matrix}$$

A fraction is simply a convenient way of representing an operation, the division of the numerator by the denominator. Thus the fraction 6/3 equals 6 divided by 3, which equals 2. The fraction ⅞ is 7 divided by 8, which equals the decimal value 0.875. Thus, the number obtained upon dividing the numerator by the denominator is the value of the fraction.

Decimals

An understanding of decimals is crucial to dosage calculations because most medication orders are written using decimals. An example would be:

℞ **Synthroid 0.75 mg #30**
Take 1 tablet every morning for thyroid.

A **decimal** is any number that can be written in decimal notation using the integers 0, 1, 2, 3, 4, 5, 6, 7, 8, and 9 and a point (.) to divide the "ones" place from the "tenths" place. Figure 5.2 illustrates the relative value of each decimal unit and provides the names of the place values. Numbers to the left of the decimal point are whole numbers; numbers to the right of the decimal point are decimal fractions (parts of the whole).

$$0.131313 \qquad 2.09 \qquad 43.09$$

Safety Note

For a decimal value less than 1, use a leading zero to prevent errors.

Notice that in the decimal expression of a fraction, a zero (0) is placed before the decimal point if the number is less than 1. This zero is called a **leading zero;** using this zero helps to prevent potential medication errors when reading decimals.

A fraction can be expressed as a decimal by dividing the numerator by the denominator.

$$\frac{1}{2} = 1 \div 2 = 0.5$$

$$\frac{1}{3} = 1 \div 3 = 0.33333\ldots$$

$$\frac{438}{64} = 438 \div 64 = 6.84375$$

FIGURE 5.2
Decimal Units and Values

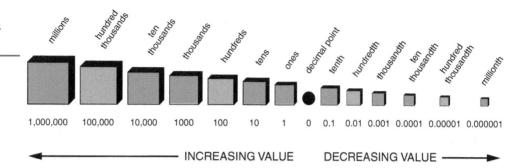

millions	hundred thousands	ten thousands	thousands	hundreds	tens	ones	decimal point	tenth	hundredth	thousandth	ten thousandth	hundred thousandth	millionth
1,000,000	100,000	10,000	1000	100	10	1	0	0.1	0.01	0.001	0.0001	0.00001	0.000001

◄——————— INCREASING VALUE   DECREASING VALUE ———————►

Converting Decimals to Fractions The metric system generally uses numbers in decimal form. Any decimal number can be expressed as a decimal fraction that has a power of 10 as its denominator. The decimal-fraction equivalents shown in Table 5.10 correspond to the decimal place names previously presented in Figure 5.2.

To express a decimal number as a fraction, remove the decimal point and use the resulting number as the numerator. To obtain the denominator, count the number of places to the right of the decimal point. Use Table 5.10 to find the corresponding power of ten to put in the denominator.

$$2.33 = \frac{233}{100} \qquad 0.1234 = \frac{1234}{10,000} \qquad 0.00367 = \frac{367}{100,000}$$

Once a decimal number is expressed as a fraction, the fraction can be simplified by dividing it by a fraction equivalent to 1.

$$0.84 = \frac{84}{100} = \frac{84}{100} \div \frac{4}{4} = \frac{21}{25}$$

$$0.1234 = \frac{1234}{10,000} = \frac{1234}{10,000} \div \frac{2}{2} = \frac{617}{5,000}$$

Rounding Decimals To round off an answer to the nearest tenth, carry the division out two places, to the hundredths place. If the number in the hundredths place is 5 or greater, add 1 to the tenths-place number. If the number in the hundredths place is less than 5, round the number down by omitting the digit in the hundredths place.

5.65 becomes 5.7   4.24 becomes 4.2

TABLE 5.10   Decimals and Equivalent Decimal Fractions

$1 = \frac{1}{1}$	$0.01 = \frac{1}{100}$	$0.0001 = \frac{1}{10,000}$
$0.1 = \frac{1}{10}$	$0.001 = \frac{1}{1000}$	$0.00001 = \frac{1}{100,000}$

The same procedure may be used when rounding to the nearest hundredths place or thousandths place.

$$3.8421 = 3.84 \text{ (hundredths)}$$
$$41.2674 = 41.27 \text{ (hundredths)}$$
$$0.3928 = 0.393 \text{ (thousandths)}$$
$$4.1111 = 4.111 \text{ (thousandths)}$$

Safety Note

When rounding calculations of IV fluid drops per minute (gtt/min), round partial drops down. So, if a calculation indicates 28.6 gtt/min, the answer is rounded down to 28 gtt/min, not 29 gtt/min. Calculations involving drops are discussed in Chapter 11.

When rounding numbers used in pharmacy calculations, it is common to round off to the nearest tenth. However, sometimes a dose is very small (as when prescribed for a child or an infant) and rounding to the nearest hundredth or thousandth may be more appropriate. Check with the pharmacist to confirm proper rounding practices on a case-by-case basis.

The exact dose calculated is 0.08752 g

Rounded to nearest tenth: 0.1 g

Rounded to nearest hundredth: 0.09 g

Rounded to nearest thousandth: 0.088 g

Ratios and Proportions

A **ratio** is a comparison of two like quantities and can be expressed in a fraction or in ratio notation (using a colon). For example, if a beaker contains two parts water and three parts alcohol, then the ratio of water to alcohol in the beaker can be expressed as the fraction ⅔ or as the ratio 2:3. The ratio is read not as a value (2 divided by 3) but as the expression "a ratio of 2 to 3."

One common use of ratios is as follows: the numerator is the number of parts of one substance contained in a known number of parts of another substance, which is the denominator. For example, suppose that 60 mL of sterile solution contains 3 mL of tetrahydrozoline hydrochloride. This can be expressed as the ratio ³⁄₆₀ or ¹⁄₂₀. In other words, the ratio of the active ingredient to the sterile solution is 1 to 20, or 1 part in 20 parts.

Two ratios that have the same value, such as ½ and ²⁄₄, are said to be equivalent ratios. When ratios are equivalent, the product of the numerator of the first ratio and the denominator of the second ratio is equal to the product of the numerator of the second ratio and denominator of the first ratio.

Therefore if $2{:}3 = 6{:}9,$ then $\dfrac{2}{3} = \dfrac{6}{9};$ thus $2 \times 9 = 3 \times 6 = 18$

The same thing is true of the reciprocals.

Therefore if $3{:}2 = 9{:}6,$ then $\dfrac{3}{2} = \dfrac{9}{6};$ thus $3 \times 6 = 2 \times 9 = 18$

Two equivalent ratios are said to be in the same proportion. Equivalent, or proportional, ratios can be expressed in three different ways.

$$\frac{a}{b} = \frac{c}{d} \qquad \text{example: } \frac{1}{2} = \frac{2}{4}$$

$$a{:}b = c{:}d \qquad \text{example: } 1{:}2 = 2{:}4$$

$$a{:}b :: c{:}d \qquad \text{example: } 1{:}2 :: 2{:}4$$

Pairs of equivalent ratios are called a **proportion.** The first and fourth, or outside, numbers are called the extremes, and the second and third, or inside, numbers are called the means.

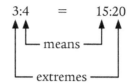

A very useful fact about proportions was illustrated in the previous examples: the product of the extremes equals the product of the means. If the proportion is expressed as a relationship between fractions, then the numerator of the first fraction times the denominator of the second is equal to the denominator of the first fraction times the numerator of the second. This can be stated as a rule:

$$\text{If} \quad \frac{a}{b} = \frac{c}{d} \quad \text{then} \quad a \times d = b \times c$$

This equation proves extremely valuable because it can be used to calculate an unknown quantity in a proportion when the other three variables are known. In mathematics, it is common to express unknown quantities using letters from the lower end of the alphabet, especially x, y, and z.

When setting up ratios in the proportion, it is important that the numbers remain in the correct ratio and that the numbers have the correct units of measurement in both the numerator and denominator. Table 5.11 lists the rules for solving proportions. Table 5.12 lists the steps for solving for an unknown quantity, which we usually label x, using the ratio-proportion method. Example 6 will demonstrate the basic steps for solving for x using the ratio-proportion method.

TABLE 5.11   Rules for Solving Proportions

- Three of the four amounts must be known.
- The numerators must have the same unit of measurement.
- The denominators must have the same unit of measurement.

TABLE 5.12   Steps for Solving for an Unknown x Using the Ratio-Proportion Method

Step 1.   Create the proportion by placing the ratios in fraction form so that the x is in the upper-left corner.

Step 2.   Verify that the unit of measurement in the numerators is the same and that the unit of measurement in the denominators is the same.

Step 3.   Solve for x by multiplying both sides of the proportion by the denominator of the ratio containing the unknown, and cancel.

Step 4.   Check your answer by verifying that the product of the means equals the product of the extremes.

Example 6   **Solve for x.**

$$\frac{x}{35} = \frac{2}{7}$$

By the proportion rule,

$$x \times 7 = 35 \times 2$$

$$7x = 70$$

Then, dividing both sides by 7,

$$\frac{7x}{7} = \frac{70}{7}$$

$$x = 10$$

The ratio-proportion method is commonly used in the hospital pharmacy. It can be used to convert within or between different measurement systems, such as translating from household measure to the preferred metric system. The ratio-proportion method is also used to calculate specific dosages.

Converting Quantities between the Metric and Common Measure Systems Many situations in pharmacy practice call for conversion of quantities within one measurement system or between different measurement systems. When possible, convert to the metric system, because it is the preferred system. To convert between metric measurements and apothecary units, it is necessary to know the equivalent measures shown in Table 5.5. The following examples will demonstrate some common pharmacy conversions using the ratio-proportion method.

Example 7   **How many milliliters are there in 1 gal, 12 fl oz?**

According to the values in Table 5.7, 3840 mL are found in 1 gal. In addition, because 1 fl oz contains 30 mL, you can use the ratio-proportion method to calculate the amount of milliliters in 12 fl oz as follows:

$$\frac{x \text{ mL}}{12 \text{ fl oz}} = \frac{30 \text{ mL}}{1 \text{ fl oz}}$$

$$\frac{(12 \text{ fl oz}) \, x \text{ mL}}{12 \text{ fl oz}} = \frac{(12 \text{ fl oz}) \, 30 \text{ mL}}{1 \text{ fl oz}}$$

$$x \text{ mL} = 360 \text{ mL}$$

Add the two values:

$$3840 \text{ mL} + 360 \text{ mL} = 4200 \text{ mL}$$

Example 8   A solution is to be used to fill hypodermic syringes, each containing 60 mL. There is 3 L of the solution available. How many hypodermic syringes can be filled with the available solution?

From Table 5.2, 1 L is 1000 mL. The available supply of solution is therefore

$$3 \times 1000 \text{ mL} = 3000 \text{ mL}$$

Determine the number of syringes by using the ratio-proportion method:

$$\frac{x \text{ syringes}}{3000 \text{ mL}} = \frac{1 \text{ syringe}}{60 \text{ mL}}$$

$$\frac{(3000 \text{ mL}) \, x \text{ syringes}}{3000 \text{ mL}} = \frac{(3000 \text{ mL}) \, 1 \text{ syringe}}{60 \text{ mL}}$$

$$x \text{ syringes} = 50 \text{ syringes}$$

Therefore 50 hypodermic syringes can be filled.

Example 9   You are to dispense 300 mL of a liquid preparation. If the medication amount (the dose) is 2 tsp, how many doses will there be in the final preparation?

Begin solving this problem by converting to a common unit of measure using conversion values in Table 5.7.

$$1 \text{ dose} = 2 \text{ tsp} = 2 \times 5 \text{ mL} = 10 \text{ mL}$$

Using these converted measurements, the solution can be determined using the ratio-proportion method.

$$\frac{x \text{ doses}}{300 \text{ mL}} = \frac{1 \text{ dose}}{10 \text{ mL}}$$

$$\frac{(300 \text{ mL}) \, x \text{ doses}}{300 \text{ mL}} = \frac{(300 \text{ mL}) \, 1 \text{ dose}}{10 \text{ mL}}$$

$$x \text{ doses} = 30 \text{ doses}$$

Example 10

A prescription calls for acetaminophen 400 mg. How many grains of acetaminophen should be used in the prescription?

Solve this problem by using the ratio-proportion method. The unknown number of grains and the requested number of milligrams go on the left side, and the ratio of 1 gr = 65 mg goes on the right side, per Table 5.5.

$$\frac{x \text{ gr}}{400 \text{ mg}} = \frac{1 \text{ gr}}{65 \text{ mg}}$$

$$\frac{(400 \text{ mg}) \, x \text{ gr}}{400 \text{ mg}} = \frac{(400 \text{ mg}) \, 1 \text{ gr}}{65 \text{ mg}}$$

$$x \text{ gr} = 6.1538 \text{ gr, rounded to } 6 \text{ gr}$$

Rounding down, 6 gr should be used in the prescription.

Example 11

A physician wants a patient to be given 0.8 mg of nitroglycerin. On hand are tablets containing nitroglycerin 1/150 gr. How many tablets should the patient be given?

Begin solving this problem by determining the number of grains in a dose by setting up a proportion and solving for the unknown. The unknown number of grains and the requested number of milligrams go on the left side, and the ratio of 1 gr = 65 mg goes on the right side, per Table 5.5.

$$\frac{x \text{ gr}}{0.8 \text{ mg}} = \frac{1 \text{ gr}}{65 \text{ mg}}$$

$$\frac{(0.8 \text{ mg}) \, x \text{ gr}}{0.8 \text{ mg}} = \frac{(0.8 \text{ mg}) \, 1 \text{ gr}}{65 \text{ mg}}$$

$$x \text{ gr} = 0.0123076 \text{ gr, rounded to } 0.012 \text{ gr}$$

Determine the number of tablets that the patient should receive by first converting the fraction value to a decimal value:

$$1/150 \text{ gr} = 0.00666 \ldots \text{ gr, rounded to } 0.0067 \text{ gr}$$

Then, set up another proportion and solve for the unknown:

$$\frac{x \text{ tablets}}{0.012 \text{ gr}} = \frac{1 \text{ tablet}}{0.0067 \text{ gr}}$$

$$\frac{(0.012 \text{ gr}) \, x \text{ tablets}}{0.012 \text{ gr}} = \frac{(0.012 \text{ gr}) \, 1 \text{ tablet}}{0.0067 \text{ gr}}$$

$$x \text{ tablets} = 1.79 \text{ tablets, rounded to } 2 \text{ tablets}$$

The dose of medications is often based on body weight in kilograms, and sometimes the pharmacy technician will need to convert a patient's weight from pounds to kilograms. The following example will show this conversion using the ratio-proportion method.

Example 12

A patient says she weighs 135 lb. What is her weight in kilograms?

Remember

2.2 lb = 1 kg

Because 1 kg equals 2.2 lb, using the ratio-proportion method,

$$\frac{x \text{ kg}}{135 \text{ lb}} = \frac{1 \text{ kg}}{2.2 \text{ lb}}$$

$$\frac{(135 \text{ lb}) \, x \text{ kg}}{135 \text{ lb}} = \frac{(135 \text{ lb}) \, 1 \text{ kg}}{2.2 \text{ lb}}$$

$$x \text{ kg} = 61.3636 \text{ kg, rounded to } 61.4 \text{ kg}$$

Calculating Dosages One of the most common calculations in pharmacy practice is that of dosages. The available supply is usually labeled as a ratio of an active ingredient to a solution.

$$\frac{\text{active ingredient (available)}}{\text{solution (available)}}$$

The prescription received in the pharmacy gives the amount of the active ingredient to be administered. The unknown quantity to be calculated is the amount of solution needed to achieve the desired dose of the active ingredient. This yields another ratio.

$$\frac{\text{active ingredient (to be administered)}}{\text{solution (needed)}}$$

The amount of solution needed can be determined by setting the two ratios into a proportion.

$$\frac{\text{active ingredient (to be administered)}}{\text{solution (needed)}} = \frac{\text{active ingredient (available)}}{\text{solution (available)}}$$

Safety Note

Always double-check the units in a proportion and double-check your calculations.

When solving medication-dosing problems, use ratios to describe the amount of drug in a dosage form (tablet, capsule, or volume of solution). It is important to remember that the numerators and denominators of both ratios must be in the same units. For example, in oral medications, the active ingredient is usually expressed in milligrams and the solution is expressed in milliliters. Similarly, the pharmacy stock will most likely be a milligram per milliliter solution. Because it is so easy to confuse units, setting up proportions with the units clearly shown is the safest way to solve these types of calculations.

Example 13

You have a stock solution that contains 10 mg of active ingredient per 5 mL of solution. The physician orders a dosage of 4 mg. How many milliliters of the stock solution will have to be administered?

Using the information provided, set up a proportion, but flip the ratios so that the unknown variable is in the upper left corner of the proportion.

$$\frac{\text{solution (needed)}}{\text{active ingredient (to be administered)}} = \frac{\text{solution (available)}}{\text{active ingredient (available)}}$$

$$\frac{x \text{ mL}}{4 \text{ mg}} = \frac{5 \text{ mL}}{10 \text{ mg}}$$

$$\frac{(4 \text{ mg}) \, x \text{ mL}}{4 \text{ mg}} = \frac{(4 \text{ mg}) \, 5 \text{ mL}}{10 \text{ mg}}$$

$$x \text{ mL} = 2 \text{ mL}$$

Thus 2 mL of solution are needed to provide the 4 mg dose.

Example 14

An order calls for Demerol 75 mg IM q4 h prn pain. The supply available is in Demerol 100 mg/mL syringes. How many milliliters will the nurse give for one injection?

This order is calling for an intramuscular (IM) injection of 75 mg every 4 hours as needed for pain. Determine the number of milliliters in an injection by setting up a proportion:

$$\frac{\text{solution (needed)}}{\text{active ingredient (to be administered)}} = \frac{\text{solution (available)}}{\text{active ingredient (available)}}$$

$$\frac{x \text{ mL}}{75 \text{ mg}} = \frac{1 \text{ mL}}{100 \text{ mg}}$$

$$\frac{(75 \text{ mg}) \, x \text{ mL}}{75 \text{ mg}} = \frac{(75 \text{ mg}) \, 1 \text{ mL}}{100 \text{ mg}}$$

$$x \text{ mL} = 0.75 \text{ mL}$$

Notice that 0.75 mL is three quarters of a syringe.

Proportions can be used to solve other types of dosage calculations, such as converting an adult dose, based on body surface area (BSA), to an appropriate child's dose. **Body surface area (BSA)** is an expression of a patient's weight and height, used to calculate patient-specific dosages. Many medications have a wide dosage range, and the patient's response and adverse reactions can vary widely, even in adults. For this reason, many physicians prefer to prescribe to children only those medications that have a known pediatric-suggested dose. As you will see in Example 15, the calculated pediatric dose is rounded down, rather than up, for safety reasons.

Example 15

An average adult has a BSA of 1.72 m² and requires an adult dose of 12 mg of a given medication. The same medication is to be given to a child in a pediatric dose. The child has a BSA of 0.60 m², and the proper dose for pediatric and adult patients is a linear function of the BSA (in other words, think of the child as a small adult). What is the proper pediatric dose? Round off the final answer.

The assumptions regarding the calculation of pediatric doses make it possible to use a proportion to answer this question.

$$\frac{\text{child's dose}}{\text{child's BSA}} = \frac{\text{adult dose}}{\text{adult BSA}}$$

$$\frac{x \text{ mg}}{0.6 \text{ m}^2} = \frac{12 \text{ mg}}{1.72 \text{ m}^2}$$

$$\frac{(0.6 \text{ m}^2) \, x \text{ mg}}{0.6 \text{ m}^2} = \frac{(0.6 \text{ m}^2) 12 \text{ mg}}{1.72 \text{ m}^2}$$

$$x \text{ mg} = 4.186 \text{ mg, rounded to 4 mg}$$

Because this dose is for a child, it is customary to round the dosage down to 4 mg rather than up to 4.2 mg.

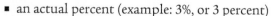

Percents

The word *percent* comes from the Latin phrase *per centum,* meaning "in one hundred." A **percent** is a given part or amount in a hundred. Percents can be expressed in many ways, and all of the following expressions are equivalent.

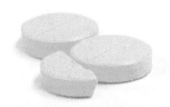

A pharmacy technician will need to be able to describe the piece of tablet as a ratio (1:2), a fraction (½), and a percentage (50%).

- an actual percent (example: 3%, or 3 percent)
- a fraction with 100 as the denominator (example: ³⁄₁₀₀)
- as a ratio (example 3:100)
- as a decimal (example: 0.03)

Percent conversions from both ratios and decimals are often calculated by the pharmacy technician. Accuracy when calculating these conversions is critical to minimizing medication errors.

Converting Ratios and Percents To express a ratio as a percent, designate the first number of the ratio as the numerator and the second number as the denominator. Multiply the fraction by 100 and add a percent sign after the product.

$$5:1 = \frac{5}{1} \times 100 = 5 \times 100 = 500\%$$

$$1:5 = \frac{1}{5} \times 100 = \frac{100}{5} = 20\%$$

$$1:2 = \frac{1}{2} \times 100 = \frac{100}{2} = 50\%$$

To convert a percent to a ratio, first change it to a fraction by dividing it by 100 and then reduce the fraction to its lowest terms. Express this as a ratio by making the numerator the first number of the ratio and the denominator the second number.

$$2\% = 2 \div 100 = \frac{2}{100} = \frac{1}{50} = 1:50$$

$$10\% = 10 \div 100 = \frac{10}{100} = \frac{1}{10} = 1:10$$

$$75\% = 75 \div 100 = \frac{75}{100} = \frac{3}{4} = 3:4$$

$$\frac{1}{2}\% = \frac{1}{2} \div 100 = \frac{\frac{1}{2}}{100} = \frac{1}{2} \times \frac{1}{100} = \frac{1}{200} = 1:200$$

Converting Percents and Decimals To convert a percent to a decimal, drop the percent symbol and divide the number by 100. Dividing a number by 100 is equivalent to moving the decimal two places to the left and inserting zeros if necessary.

$$0.75\% = 0.75 \div 100 = 0.0075$$

$$4\% = 4 \div 100 = 0.04$$

$$200\% = 200 \div 100 = 2$$

To change a decimal to a percent, multiply by 100 or move the decimal point two places to the right and add a percent symbol.

$$0.25 = 0.25 \times 100 = 25\%$$

$$1.35 = 1.35 \times 100 = 135\%$$

$$0.015 = 0.015 \times 100 = 1.5\%$$

Advanced Calculations Used in Pharmacy Practice

The pharmacy technician will need to calculate the amount of ingredients required to create prescribed solutions. For example, parenteral products are often reconstituted by adding a diluent to a lyophilized or freeze-dried powder to prepare a solution for intravenous administration. The product is commercially manufactured in powder form because of the instability of the drug in solution over a long period of time. In addition, the pharmacy technician may be asked to create solutions of a specific concentration by combining measured amounts of solutions of more and less concentrated ingredients. This section will present these types of calculations.

Preparing Solutions Using Powders

In preparing solutions, although the active ingredient is discussed in terms of weight, it also occupies a certain amount of space. When working with dry pharmaceuticals, this space is referred to as **powder volume (pv).** It is equal to the difference between the final volume (fv) and the volume of the diluting ingredient, or the diluent volume (dv), as expressed in the following equation:

$$powder\ volume = final\ volume - diluent\ volume$$

or

$$pv = fv - dv$$

Example 16

A dry powder antibiotic must be reconstituted for use. The label states that the dry powder occupies 0.5 mL. Using the formula for solving for powder volume, determine the diluent volume (the amount of solvent added). You are given the final volume for three different examples with the same powder volume.

Final Volume	Powder Volume
(1) 2 mL	0.5 mL
(2) 5 mL	0.5 mL
(3) 10 mL	0.5 mL

$$dv = fv - pv$$

$$(1)\ dv = 2\ mL - 0.5\ mL = 1.5\ mL$$

$$(2)\ dv = 5\ mL - 0.5\ mL = 4.5\ mL$$

$$(3)\ dv = 10\ mL - 0.5\ mL = 9.5\ mL$$

Example 17

You are to reconstitute 1 g of dry powder. The label states that you are to add 9.3 mL of diluent to make a final solution of 100 mg/mL. What is the powder volume?

Step 1. Calculate the final volume. The strength of the final solution will be 100 mg/mL. Since you start with 1 g = 1000 mg of powder, for a final volume x of the solution, it will have strength 1000 mg/x mL. Using the ratio-proportion method,

$$\frac{x\ mL}{1000\ mg} = \frac{1\ mL}{100\ mg}$$

$$x\ mL = \frac{(1000\ mg) \times 1\ mL}{100\ mg} = 10\ mL$$

Step 2. Using the calculated final volume and the given diluent volume, calculate the powder volume.

$$pv = fv - dv$$

$$pv = 10 \text{ mL} - 9.3 \text{ mL} = 0.7 \text{ mL}$$

Working with Dilutions

Medications may be diluted for several reasons. They are sometimes diluted prior to administration to children, infants, and older adults to meet the dosage requirements of those patients. Medications may also be diluted so that they can be measured more accurately and easily. For example, volumes less than 0.1 mL are usually considered too small to measure accurately. Therefore they must be diluted further. Many pharmacies have a policy as to how much an injection can be diluted. A rule of thumb is for the required dose to have a volume greater than 0.1 mL and less than 1 mL.

The following example will demonstrate the method for solving typical dilution problems. The first step is to use the ratio-proportion method to solve for the volume of the final product by using a ratio of diluted solution to desired concentration. The second step is to determine the amount of diluent simply by subtracting the concentrate from the total volume. Both of these volumes are approximate because they depend on the calibration and accuracy of the measuring devices used.

Although the second step is used to determine the amount of diluent added, the amount will actually be determined by adding "up to" the desired total quantity. The abbreviation QS for "sufficient quantity" is used to describe the process of adding enough of the last ingredient in a compound to reach the desired volume. It is helpful to calculate the necessary amount beforehand so that an adequate supply of medication is available.

Example 18

Dexamethasone is available as a 4 mg/mL preparation; an infant is to receive 0.35 mg. The volume needed would be a miniscule 0.08 mL, which is very difficult to accurately measure.

Prepare a dilution so that the final concentration is 1 mg/mL. How much diluent will you need if the original product is in a 1 mL vial and you dilute the entire vial? What is the volume of final dose to be measured?

Step 1. Determine the volume (in milliliters) of the final product. Because the strength of the dexamethasone is 4 mg/mL, a 1 mL vial will contain 4 mg of the active ingredient. Then, for a final volume x of solution, you will have a concentration of 4 mg/x mL.

Diluted solution	Desired concentration

$$\frac{x \text{ mL}}{4 \text{ mg}} = \frac{1 \text{ mL}}{1 \text{ mg}}$$

$$x \text{ mL} = \frac{(4 \text{ mg} \times 1 \text{ mL})}{1 \text{ mg}} = 4 \text{ mL final product}$$

Step 2. Subtract the volume of the concentrate from the total volume to determine the volume of diluent needed.

$$4 \text{ mL total volume} - 1 \text{ mL concentrate} = 3 \text{ mL diluent needed}$$

Therefore an additional 3 mL of diluent are needed to dilute the original 1 mL of preparation to arrive at a final concentration of 1 mg/mL.

Step 3. Set up a ratio and proportion to determine the volume of medication to be prepared from the diluted medication.

$$\frac{x \text{ mL}}{0.35 \text{ mg}} = \frac{1 \text{ mL}}{1 \text{ mg}}$$

$$x \text{ mL} = 0.35 \text{ mL}$$

This volume is much more accurately measured in a syringe.

Using Alligation to Prepare Compounded Products

Physicians often prescribe concentrations of medications that are not commercially available, and these prescriptions must be compounded (added together) at the pharmacy. When an ordered concentration is not commercially available, it may be necessary to combine two different solutions with the same active ingredient in differing strengths. The resulting concentration will be greater than the weaker strength, but less than the stronger strength. For example, 1% and 5% hydrocortisone ointments may be combined to provide a 3% ointment. This is called **alligation.** An alligation is used when the two quantities needed to prepare the desired concentration are both relatively large.

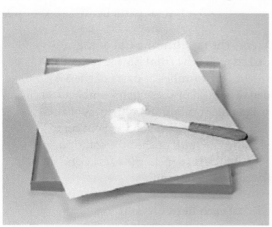

When the desired concentration of a cream is not available, the pharmacy technician will use an alligation to calculate how much cream of the lesser concentration, and how much of a greater concentration, should be mixed together.

The amount of each stock product to be added together is calculated by using the alligation alternate method. This is the calculation used to determine the proportions of available products needed to prepare the desired concentration. The alligation alternate method requires changing the percentages to parts of a proportion and then using the proportion to obtain the amounts of the two ingredients. The answer can then be checked using the following formula.

$$\text{milliliters} \times \text{percent (expressed as a decimal)} = \text{grams}$$

It is important to note that this formula works for any strength solution.

The following examples will demonstrate the application of the alligation alternate method.

Example 19

Prepare 250 mL of dextrose 7.5% weight in volume (w/v) using dextrose 5% (D$_5$W) w/v and dextrose 50% (D$_{50}$W) w/v. How many milliliters of each will be needed?

Step 1. Set up a box arrangement and at the upper left corner write the percent of the highest concentration (50%) as a whole number. At the lower left corner, write the percent of the lowest concentration (5%) as a whole number, and in the center, write the desired concentration.

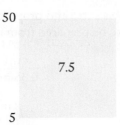

Step 2. Subtract the center number from the upper left number (i.e., the smaller from the larger) and put it at the lower-right corner. Now subtract the lower left number from the center number (i.e., the smaller from the larger), and put it at the upper right corner.

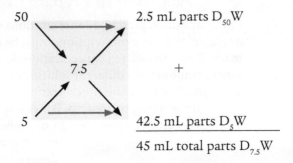

The number 2.5 mL represents the number of parts of the 50% solution that will be needed to make the final 7.5% solution, and the number 42.5 mL represents the number of parts of the 5% solution that will be needed. The sum of these two numbers, 2.5 mL + 42.5 mL = 45 mL, is the total number of parts of the 7.5% solution. In terms of ratios, the ratio of the 5% solution to the 7.5% solution is 42.5:45, and the ratio of the 50% solution to the 7.5% solution is 2.5:45. Much less of the 50% solution (2.5 mL) is needed to make the 7.5% solution.

Step 3. Calculate the volume needed of each dextrose solution.

50% Dextrose

$$\frac{x \text{ mL of } 50\%}{250 \text{ mL}} = \frac{2.5 \text{ mL parts D}_{50}\text{W}}{45 \text{ mL total parts D}_{7.5}\text{W}}$$

$$x \text{ mL} = \frac{(250 \text{ mL}) \times 2.5 \text{ mL parts}}{45 \text{ mL total parts}}$$

$$x \text{ mL} = 13.8888 \text{ mL D}_{50}\text{W, rounded to } 13.9 \text{ mL}$$

5% Dextrose

$$\frac{x \text{ mL of } 5\%}{250 \text{ mL}} = \frac{42.5 \text{ mL parts D}_5\text{W}}{45 \text{ mL total parts D}_{7.5}\text{W}}$$

$$x \text{ mL} = \frac{(250 \text{ mL}) \times 42.5 \text{ mL parts}}{45 \text{ mL total parts}}$$

$$x \text{ mL} = 236.11 \text{ mL D}_5\text{W, rounded to } 236.1 \text{ mL}$$

Step 4. Add the volumes of the two solutions together. The sum should equal the required volume of dextrose 7.5%.

$$\begin{array}{r} 236.1 \text{ mL} \\ + \ 13.9 \text{ mL} \\ \hline 250.0 \text{ mL} \end{array}$$

Step 5. Check your answer by calculating the amount of solute (dextrose) in all three solutions. The number of grams of solute should equal the sum of the grams of solutes from the 50% solution and the 5% solution, using the following formula.

$$\text{mL} \times \% \text{ (as a decimal)} = g$$

$$250 \text{ mL} \times 0.075 = 18.75 \text{ g}$$

$$13.9 \text{ mL D}_{50}\text{W} \times 0.5 = 6.95 \text{ g}$$

$$236.1 \text{ mL D}_5\text{W} \times 0.05 = 11.805 \text{ g, rounded to } 11.8 \text{ g}$$

$$\begin{array}{r} 11.805 \text{ g} \\ + \ 6.945 \text{ g} \\ \hline 18.750 \text{ g} \end{array}$$

The amounts measured to prepare this prescription will be rounded to the nearest milliliter: 14 mL D$_{50}$W and 236 mL D$_5$W.

Example 20

You are instructed to make 454 g of 3% zinc oxide cream. You have in stock 10% and 1% zinc oxide cream. How much of each percent will you use?

Step 1.

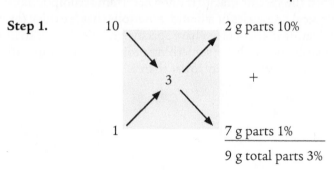

Step 2.

10% zinc oxide cream

$$\frac{x \text{ g of } 10\%}{454 \text{ g}} = \frac{2 \text{ g parts } 10\%}{9 \text{ g total parts } 3\%}$$

$$x \text{ g of } 10\% = 101 \text{ g of } 10\% \text{ zinc oxide cream}$$

1% zinc oxide cream

$$\frac{x \text{ g of } 1\%}{454 \text{ g}} = \frac{7 \text{ g parts } 1\%}{9 \text{ g total parts } 3\%}$$

$$x \text{ g of } 1\% = 353 \text{ g of } 1\% \text{ zinc oxide cream}$$

Step 3. Check your work.

$$353 \text{ g} + 101 \text{ g} = 454 \text{ g}$$

Calculating Specific Gravity

Calculating specific gravity is an example of a ratio and proportion application. **Specific gravity** is the ratio of the weight of a substance to the weight of an equal volume of water, the standard, when both are at the same temperature. Final weight can be measured in grams, because 1 mL of water weighs 1 g.

> **1 mL, volume of water = 1 g, weight of water**
> **specific gravity of water = 1**

The specific gravity represents the weight of 1 mL of the substance and has no units of measure. The ratio called specific gravity is in essence a comparison of the weight of a liquid to the weight of water when exactly 1 mL of each is measured out. Water is the standard that is used, and the specific gravity assigned to it is 1. The formula for determining specific gravity is as follows:

$$\text{specific gravity} = \frac{\text{weight of a substance}}{\text{weight of an equal volume of water}}$$

When the specific gravity is known, certain assumptions can be made regarding the physical properties of a liquid. Solutions that are thick (or viscous) or have particles floating in them often have specific gravities higher than 1. Solutions that contain volatile chemicals (or something prone to quick evaporation), such as alcohol, often have a specific gravity lower than 1.

Example 21   If the weight of 100 mL of dextrose solution is 117 g, what is the specific gravity of the dextrose solution?

$$\text{specific gravity} = \frac{\text{weight of a substance}}{\text{weight of an equal volume of water}}$$

$$= \frac{117 \text{ g}}{100 \text{ g}}$$

$$= 1.17$$

If the specific gravity is known, you can determine the weight of a volume of a liquid.

Example 22   If a liquid has a specific gravity of 0.85, how much does 125 mL of it weigh?

Because the specific gravity of the liquid is 0.85,

$$\text{specific gravity} = \frac{\text{weight of a substance}}{\text{weight of an equal volume of water}}$$

$$0.85 = \frac{85 \text{ g (weight of 100 mL of the liquid)}}{100 \text{ g (weight of 100 mL of water)}}$$

Now, use the ratio-proportion method to find the weight of 125 mL.

$$\frac{x \text{ g}}{125 \text{ mL}} = \frac{85 \text{ g}}{100 \text{ mL}}$$

$$\frac{(125 \text{ mL}) x \text{ g}}{125 \text{ mL}} = \frac{(125 \text{ mL}) 85 \text{ g}}{100 \text{ mL}}$$

$$x \text{ g} = \frac{10{,}625 \text{ g}}{100}$$

$$x \text{ g} = 106.25 \text{ g}$$

Math skills do not come easily to everyone. However, knowledge of the basic fundamentals of math, especially in the metric system, is critical to minimizing medication errors involving dosage, flow rates, and concentrations. Be sure to double-check your calculations as well as the calculations done by the pharmacist. The end-of-chapter exercises should assist you in gaining both confidence and competence in mathematical skills. Additional math skills are covered in Chapter 7, *The Business of Community Pharmacy,* as well in Chapter 11, *Preparing and Handling Sterile Products and Hazardous Drugs.*

Chapter Terms

alligation the compounding of two or more products to obtain a desired concentration

body surface area (BSA) a measurement related to a patient's weight and height, expressed in meters squared (m^2), and used to calculate patient-specific dosages of medications

Celsius temperature scale the temperature scale that uses zero degrees (i.e., 0 °C) as the temperature at which water freezes at sea level and 100 °C as the temperature at which it boils

decimal any number that can be written in decimal notation using the integers 0 through 9 and a point (.) to divide the "ones" place from the "tenths" place (e.g., 10.25 is equal to 10¼)

denominator the number on the bottom part of a fraction that represents the whole

Fahrenheit temperature scale the temperature scale that uses 32 °F as the temperature at which water freezes at sea level and 212 °F as the temperature at which it boils

fraction a portion of a whole that is represented as a ratio

gram the metric system's base unit for measuring weight

leading zero a zero that is placed in the ones place in a number less than zero that is being represented by a decimal value

liter the metric system's base unit for measuring volume

meter the metric system's base unit for measuring length

metric system a measurement system based on subdivisions and multiples of 10; made up of three basic units: meter, gram, and liter

military time a measure of time based on a 24 hour clock in which midnight is 0000, noon is 1200, and the minute before midnight is 2359; also referred to as international time

numerator the number on the upper part of a fraction that represents the part of the whole

percent the number or ratio per 100

powder volume (pv) the amount of space occupied by a freeze-dried medication in a sterile vial, used for reconstitution; equal to the difference between the final volume (fv) and the volume of the diluting ingredient, or the diluent volume (dv)

proportion a comparison of equal ratios; the product of the means equals the product of the extremes

ratio a comparison of numeric values

specific gravity the ratio of the weight of a substance compared to an equal volume of water when both have the same temperature

Chapter Summary

- The metric system is preferred worldwide for making accurate, standard measurements.
- The metric system of measurement makes use of decimal units, including the basic units of the gram (for weight) and the liter (for volume). Pharmacy professionals should be able to convert between different systems such as metric, avoirdupois, apothecary, and household measures.
- The most widely used units of measure in pharmacy include milligrams, grams, kilograms, milliliters, liters, and grains.
- Pharmacy technicians working in hospital pharmacies must be comfortable reading military time (also called international time).
- In the pharmacy, technicians must be able to convert temperatures from Fahrenheit to Celsius.

- Pharmacists and pharmacy technicians should be familiar with the standard prefixes for abbreviating metric quantities and with the basic mathematical principles used to calculate and convert doses and prepare reconstituted solutions from powdered drug products.
- Those working in the pharmaceutical profession should be able to find an unknown quantity in a proportion when three elements of the proportion are known; they should also be able to use the alligation method to compound a product from products having different concentrations.

Chapter Review

Checking Your Understanding

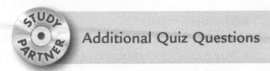

Additional Quiz Questions

Choose the best answer from those provided.

1. The modern metric system makes use of the standardized units of the
   a. avoirdupois system.
   b. Système International (SI).
   c. household measurement system.
   d. apothecary system.

2. The metric prefix that indicates one millionth is
   a. nano-.
   b. micro-.
   c. milli-.
   d. deci-.

3. A gram is equal to
   a. 1000 micrograms.
   b. 1000 milligrams.
   c. 1000 centigrams.
   d. 1000 nanograms.

4. In the metric system the liter is a standard measurement of
   a. distance.
   b. area.
   c. volume.
   d. weight.

5. The Varicella (chicken pox/shingles) vaccine requires a storage temperature of –15 °C or colder. What is the equivalent temperature in degrees Fahrenheit?
   a. 0 °F
   b. 5 °F
   c. 10 °F
   d. 32 °F

6. A decimal fraction has as its denominator a power of
   a. 2.
   b. 5.
   c. 10.
   d. 25.

7. 58% means 58 out of one
   a. hundred.
   b. thousand.
   c. million.
   d. billion.

8. What is the specific gravity of 250 mL of water?
   a. 0.25
   b. 0.5
   c. 1.0
   d. 1.25

9. The only unit of measure that is the same in the apothecary and avoirdupois system is the
   a. grain.
   b. gram.
   c. liter.
   d. ounce.

10. Which measurement is commonly used to convert an adult dose to an appropriate child's dose?
    a. height
    b. age
    c. body surface area (BSA)
    d. body mass index (BMI)

Thinking Like a Pharmacy Tech

1. Convert the following:
   a. 34.6 g = _____ mg
   b. 735 mg = _____ g
   c. 3400 mL = _____ L
   d. 1.2 L = _____ mL
   e. 7.48 kg = _____ g
   f. 473 mL = _____ L

2. Convert the following:
   a. 24 fl oz = _____ pt
   b. 40 gr (apothecary) =
      _____ Э (apothecary)
   c. 6 ʒ (apothecary) =
      _____ # (apothecary)
   d. 6.25 tbsp = _____ tsp
   e. 8 qt = _____ gal
   f. viii = _____ (Arabic numeral)
   g. C = _____ (Arabic numeral)

3. Solve the following conversion problems:
   a. You have 2 L of solution in stock. The solution is to be used to fill vials that hold 40 mL each. How many vials can you fill with the 2 L of solution?
   b. The patient has received a bottle containing 200 mL of a liquid medication. The patient is to take 3 tsp of the medication per day. How many days will the bottle last?
   c. A prescription calls for codeine sulfate 40 mg. How many grains of codeine sulfate should be used in the prescription? (Assume 65 mg = 1 gr)
   d. A patient takes two 1/150 gr nitroglycerin tablets per day. How many milligrams of nitroglycerin does the patient receive each day?

4. Solve the following problems:
   a. In stock you have a solution that contains 8 mg of active ingredient per 10 mL of solution. A customer has a prescription calling for a quantity of 4 doses of 6 mg each of the active ingredient. How many milliliters of the solution should the customer be given?
   b. A medication order calls for phenobarbital 60 mg. The supply available is phenobarbital 100 mg/mL of solution. How many milliliters of the solution will the patient be given?
   c. If the adult dose of a medication is 30 mg and the average adult body surface area (BSA) is 1.72 m², what would be the appropriate pediatric dose for a child with a BSA of 0.50 m²?

5. Solve the following solution preparation problems:
   a. You have been asked to prepare a solution containing a powder with a volume of 0.7 mL. The total volume of the solution that you are to prepare should be 30 mL. How much diluent will you use in the solution, and what will be the percentage, by volume, of powder in the solution?
   b. You are instructed to make 240 mL of a 0.45% w/v solution. You have a 3% concentrate in stock. How much of the full-strength solution will you use, and how much diluent will be needed?
   c. You must prepare 300 mL of a solution containing 42.5% dextrose. In stock you have solutions containing 5% dextrose (solution 1) and 50% dextrose (solution 2). How many milliliters of each stock solution must you use in the solution that you prepare?

Communicating Clearly

1. Interview a hospital and community pharmacy technician or pharmacist regarding their experience with calculations in their practice setting. Discuss your findings with the class.

2. Visit a Web site or interview a lawyer to learn past litigation involving calculation errors in health care that may have led to serious disability or death. Report your findings to the class.

3. Get one 1cc oral syringe (without needle) from a local pharmacy for an experiment. Measure 0.09 mL of water and 0.35 mL of water. Which is easier and more accurate? (See Example 18.)

Researching on the Web

1. Visit ismp.org and search file under "fluorouracil" and "heparin." Look for discussions of medication errors. What were the patient outcomes?

2. Investigate the markings on an aspirin 5 gr bottle and ferrous sulfate 5 gr bottle by different manufacturers to see what "mg" they say is in each table. Check rxlist.com and see how many milligrams of codeine are in Tylenol #3, which contains ½ grain of codeine.

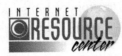

For further study of chapter-related topics, explore the Web links in the Web Center at www.emcp.net/pharmpractice4e.

Unit

2

Community Pharmacy

Dispensing Medications in the Community Pharmacy

6

Learning Objectives

- Discuss overall community pharmacy operations including restricted area, hours of operation, drive-through options, and general responsibilities of the pharmacy technician with regard to dispensing prescription drugs.

- Identify the parts of a patient profile, detail the steps required to select a patient from the database, and discuss the importance of including up-to-date allergy and adverse drug reaction information.

- Describe the parts of a prescription and identify the most commonly used abbreviations for amounts, dosage forms, times of administration, and sites of administration.

- Describe controls necessary for reviewing prescriptions of scheduled drugs, including the identification of possible forgeries.

- Explain the typical procedures for processing new and refill prescription orders.

- Identify the parts of a prescription stock label and know the importance of comparing NDC numbers in medication selection and filling.

- Describe the parts of a typical medication container label.

- Contrast the purposes of the patient medication information sheet and leaflet with those of the medication guide.

- Discuss the importance of a final check and verification by the pharmacist prior to dispensing to the patient.

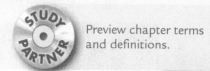

Preview chapter terms and definitions.

The primary role of the pharmacist is to dispense medications safely, accurately, and in accordance with state and federal laws upon receipt of valid medication orders from prescribers. Prescribers are most often physicians but may also include dentists, veterinarians, nurse practitioners, or physician's assistants. The technician plays a critical role assisting in customer service, updating patient demographics and insurance information, and accurately filling prescription orders. By supporting the pharmacist, the pharmacy technician frees the pharmacist to spend more time resolving medication-related problems and counseling patients about their medications.

Almost 75% of all pharmacy technician positions are in community pharmacy settings. This chapter will outline in detail the major responsibilities of both the pharmacist and the pharmacy technician in dispensing new and refill prescriptions in a typical community pharmacy. The exact procedures outlined in this chapter may vary within a specific community pharmacy, but the basic components are similar and must be learned by the aspiring pharmacy technician. Chapter 7, *The Business of Community Pharmacy*, will focus on the role of the technician in the business operations of a community pharmacy, including the sale of nonprescription products and supplies.

An Overview of the Operations of a Community Pharmacy

The community pharmacy is a business designed to serve the needs of its customers. The hours of operation of a community pharmacy may vary from 40 to 168 hours weekly. After-hours availability is convenient for working families and shift workers, as well as for patients recently discharged from emergency rooms and hospitals. To increase the convenience of the pharmacy to its customers, many pharmacies include a drive-through area for prescription drop-off and pick-up.

Almost 4 billion prescriptions are dispensed annually in the pharmacies of the United States. With an increasingly older population and the expansion of Medicare Part D and other prescription drug insurance programs, major growth is expected for the foreseeable future in all community pharmacies. A majority of prescriptions today are filled in a chain or independent community pharmacy. If a local need exists, then some community pharmacies will also prepare and deliver prescriptions to nontraditional healthcare sites such as nursing homes, personal care homes, and prisons.

Customer service and convenience provided by the community pharmacy is important, because patients can also choose to send their prescription orders to large, less expensive, out-of-state, mail-order pharmacy warehouses. Mail-order pharmacies can charge less for their prescriptions because they use automation and centralized, round-the-clock filling operations. In addition to reducing costs, automation assists mail-order pharmacies to make fewer dispensing errors. The Veterans Administration (VA), with its regional centralized warehouses, operates this type of drug distribution system. These operations differ from a local community pharmacy primarily by their sheer workload volume and lack of direct access to patients.

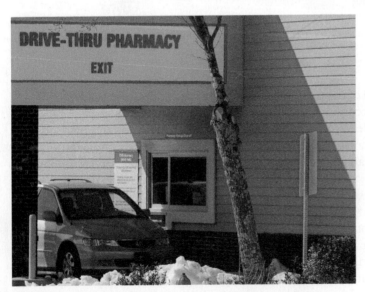

Parents with children, as well as older patients and patients with disabilities, often prefer the convenience of a pharmacy with a drive-through.

Some prescription insurance programs encourage patients to use mail-order pharmacies by offering lower co-payments on a 90 day supply of a medication. The potential cost savings of mail-order may be partially offset by delays in the receipt of a needed medication (to the potential detriment of health), drug wastage if a patient's medication or dosage is changed, and minimal counseling offered to the patient. For example, patient information on prescribed medications provided by mail-order pharmacies is usually limited to preprinted typed sheets or toll-free 800 numbers. On the other hand, patients receiving prescription medications from a community pharmacy will have direct access to the on-duty pharmacist at any time.

Defining the Pharmacy Technician's Role in the Community Pharmacy

In the community pharmacy, a technician needs to do many near-simultaneous tasks with focused care and attention to detail. The technician greets customers on the phone, in the store, and at the drive-through. The pharmacy technician plays an important role in reducing patient waiting time by efficiently and correctly scanning or entering information into a patient database. The technician also assists with the filling of prescriptions by doing such things as retrieving drug stock bottles and labeling medications to be dispensed to patients. A pharmacy technician may also be involved in resolving insurance issues. Often the technician's role changes during the day, and because the technician may be involved in all these responsibilities at the same time, good multitasking skills are necessary.

The duties the pharmacy technician may be asked to carry out in relation to the dispensing of prescription drugs in the community pharmacy are listed in Table 6.1. Use this list only as a general reference; each pharmacy will differ in its own policies and procedures. A pharmacy's approved policies and procedures are generally explained as a central part of an on-the-job training program for new pharmacy technicians or, in some cases, in a written policy and procedure manual. The training program (or manual) not only reflects the requirements of the relevant state laws and regulations but also defines those guidelines for the safe and effective operation that have been established within the pharmacy itself. It is important for the pharmacy technician to understand these policies and procedures and to follow them carefully.

A pharmacy technician working in the community pharmacy is involved in selling medications and healthcare-related products to customers. The sale of prescription medications, called legend drugs, is regulated and carefully monitored. Customers

TABLE 6.1 Key Pharmacy Technician Duties in the Community Pharmacy

- greeting customers and receiving written prescriptions
- answering the telephone and referring call-in prescriptions to the pharmacist
- initiating refills requested by patients in person or by telephone
- resolving questions about the prescription (name, directions, and so on) with the physician's office
- updating the patient's patient profile, including patient demographics, allergies, and health conditions
- entering or updating billing information for third-party reimbursement
- entering new prescriptions (or refill requests) into the patient profile
- preparing medication container labels for prescriptions, including partial fills and out-of-stock medications
- submitting prescription claims online to insurance providers
- contacting insurance companies to resolve eligibility or prescription processing issues
- retrieving drug products from storage in the restricted prescription area
- counting, reconstituting, packaging, and repackaging products
- returning stock bottles to the proper storage location
- distributing labeled medications to the patient after final verification by the pharmacist
- offering a medication counseling opportunity for the patient
- accepting payments, including co-payments
- storing completed prescriptions for patient pickup
- retrieving medications for patient pickup once patient verification is completed

FIGURE 6.1

The Rx Only Designation

The "Rx only" on this medication label designates that this medication can only be dispensed according to a prescription.

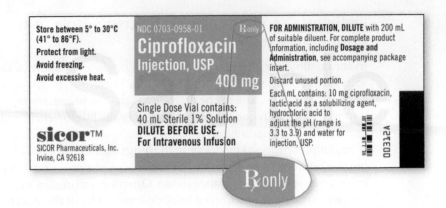

Store between 5° to 30°C (41° to 86°F).
Protect from light.
Avoid freezing.
Avoid excessive heat.

NDC 0703-0958-01   Rₓonly
Ciprofloxacin
Injection, USP
400 mg

Single Dose Vial contains:
40 mL Sterile 1% Solution
DILUTE BEFORE USE.
For Intravenous Infusion

sicor™
SICOR Pharmaceuticals, Inc.
Irvine, CA 92618

FOR ADMINISTRATION, DILUTE with 200 mL of suitable diluent. For complete product information, including **Dosage and Administration**, see accompanying package insert.
Discard unused portion.
Each mL contains: 10 mg ciprofloxacin, lactic acid as a solubilizing agent, hydrochloric acid to adjust the pH (range is 3.3 to 3.9) and water for injection, USP.

Rₓonly

cannot buy these drugs without an appropriate prescription from a healthcare provider. Legend drugs are identified on their stock bottle with the label "Rx only" (Figure 6.1).

Identification of potential medication errors is a dual responsibility of both the pharmacist and the pharmacy technician. It is of utmost importance to clarify the legal responsibility of the pharmacy technician in contrast to that of the pharmacist in the dispensing process, something that may vary from state to state.

Controlling Access to Prescription Drug Inventory

To limit the access to prescription medications, the area of the pharmacy where the prescription medications are stored and prepared for sale is usually secured by code or key and is off-limits to the public. The secured area where the prescription drugs are stored may be entered only by authorized employees, such as the pharmacist and the pharmacy technician. If there is no pharmacist on duty, as when the pharmacist is out for lunch or has gone home for the day, then this area of the pharmacy must be locked and closed to the public or secured as per state law.

Filling a Prescription

A **prescription** is defined as an order of medication for a patient, ordered by a physician or a qualified licensed practitioner for a valid medical condition, to be filled by a pharmacist. Table 6.2 reviews the path a single new prescription follows once it crosses the threshold of a community pharmacy. Although a patient may bring in multiple prescriptions, each prescription more or less follows the same critical path. Each step in the critical path is discussed in the following sections of this chapter.

The prescription filling process that begins with the receipt and review of the prescription for completeness and ends with dispensing to the patient takes about 5 to 10 minutes per prescription (without interruptions, such as phone calls,

To limit access to legend drugs, only authorized employees can enter the ℞ area of the pharmacy.

TABLE 6.2 The Critical Path of a New Prescription

1. After the patient drops off the prescription, the pharmacy technician checks the prescription to make certain it is complete and authentic.

2. The pharmacy technician verifies that the patient information is contained in the pharmacy database. If the patient is not in the pharmacy database, then the technician obtains necessary demographic, insurance, allergy, and health information from the patient and enters the information into the computer.

3. The pharmacy technician enters (or scans) the prescription into the computer database, billing the insurance company or calculating the cost to the patient.

4. The pharmacist verifies the accuracy of the technician's computerized entry against the original prescription (or a photocopied image) and generates the medication container label.

5. The pharmacy technician asks the pharmacist to check the drug utilization review (DUR) or drug interaction warning screen when required.

6. The pharmacy technician selects the appropriate medication and verifies the National Drug Code (NDC) number on the drug stock bottle against the computer-generated medication container label. In some pharmacies the bar codes on the stock bottle and medication container label are compared for accuracy.

7. The pharmacy technician prepares the medication (the prescribed number of tablets or capsules are counted or the prescribed amount of liquid measured). Controlled drugs are often double-counted and initialed.

8. The pharmacy technician packages the medication in the appropriate container.

9. The pharmacy technician labels the prescription container with the computer-generated medication container label. In some states the law requires the pharmacist to affix the label to the container.

10. The pharmacy technician prepares the filled prescription (including original prescription, drug stock bottle, medication container label, and medication container) for the pharmacist to check.

11. The pharmacist checks the prescription and may initial the label and prescription.

12. The pharmacist or pharmacy technician bags the approved prescription for patient sale and attaches an information sheet about the prescription, including indications, interactions, and possible side effects.

13 The pharmacy technician returns the drug stock bottle to the shelf. If the bottle is opened, then the bottle is so marked or labeled for inventory ordering.

14. The pharmacy technician delivers the packaged prescription to the cash register area for patient pickup (or storage) and pharmacist counseling. The pharmacy technician verifies that the correct patient is receiving the prescription by asking for address or birth date verification. If someone other than the patient is picking up a controlled drug prescription, then a photo ID may be required.

15. If payment is due, then the patient pays by cash, credit card, or check. Most insurance providers require the patient to sign a form verifying that the prescription was picked up.

Safety Note

Steps 6, 7, 10, 11, 13, and 14 in Table 6.2 should include verification that the proper product has been selected.

---

patients dropping off prescriptions, and so on). The pharmacy technician should ask the patient whether he or she prefers to wait for the prescription to be filled and, based on workload and staffing, should provide a good estimate for the waiting time should the patient elect to shop or run errands.

Safety Note

100% accuracy is expected with all prescriptions.

Although speed is important, 100% accuracy is paramount. If prescriptions filled in a given day were 99% correct, then the average pharmacy filling 200 prescriptions daily would have filled two prescriptions incorrectly. This is unacceptable. In order to strive to eliminate errors, the prescription and product selection are checked several times for accuracy during the fill process by both the pharmacist and the pharmacy technician. The prescription should be mentally checked again before the original prescription is filed or stock bottle is returned to the shelf. Medication safety is discussed in more detail in Chapter 12, *Medication Safety*.

The Patient Profile

A **patient profile** contains all prescriptions that have been dispensed in the past at the pharmacy for a patient. It also documents other relevant demographic information about the patient. This profile is maintained as part of a confidential database used by the pharmacy to track all prescriptions dispensed by the pharmacy. Every patient who presents a prescription to the pharmacy must have a current updated profile. The profile must be updated with each prescription presented to the pharmacy for filling. A major part of the pharmacy technician's job is maintaining a profile for each patient receiving prescription medications from the pharmacy. The patient profile will generally contain the information listed in Table 6.3.

Some chain pharmacies, such as Walgreens, use a common database, allowing prescription information in the patient profile to be shared among all their pharma-

TABLE 6.3   Components of the Patient Profile

Component	Content
identifying information	Patient's full name (including middle initial), street address, telephone number, birth date, and gender. Increasingly, some programs are entering e-mail addresses so that refill notifications and other communications can be made.
insurance and billing information	Information necessary for billing. More information on insurance billing is contained in Chapter 7.
medical and allergy history	Information concerning existing conditions (e.g., diabetes, heart disease) and known allergies and adverse drug reactions the patient has experienced. (The pharmacy software reviews the profile's medical history for the pharmacist to make sure that the prescription is safe to fill for a given patient.)
medication and prescription history	Most databases allow the listing of any prescriptions filled at this pharmacy location; some software may allow listing of OTC medications. The new prescription will be compared to previously filled prescriptions in the database. (The pharmacy software reviews this information for the pharmacist to make sure that the prescription will not cause adverse drug interactions [i.e., negative consequences] because of the combined effects of drugs and/or drugs and foods.)
prescription preferences	Patient preferences as they apply to prescriptions (e.g., child-resistant or non–child-resistant containers, generic substitutions, large print labels, foreign language preference, and so on).
HIPAA confidentiality	Each new patient is required by law to receive a statement on patient confidentiality of information on the patient profile, which must be documented. (This statement is for the protection of the pharmacy.)

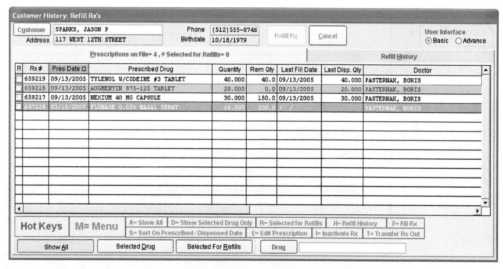

A computerized profile is maintained for each patient receiving a prescription from the pharmacy. This profile is part of a confidential database that helps the pharmacist and technician confirm that medications are dispensed safely.

cies nationally. A new prescription (or refill request) may be entered into a central database and be accessed at a pharmacy other than the one where the prescription was originally received. The patient may pick up the prescription at the receiving pharmacy rather than the originating pharmacy. This is extremely helpful for patients with medication needs who travel frequently or share residencies in two or more states.

If a patient profile already exists for a patient, then it is important for the pharmacy technician to verify that the correct one is selected. A patient identifier, in addition to the patient's name is used to verify that the correct patient is selected. A second patient identifier may be an address, telephone number, or date of birth. Failure to do so may result in a medication error—a prescription entered and filled for the wrong patient. It is also important for the technician to update the information on the profile, especially the patient's contact information and any changes in prescription drug insurance.

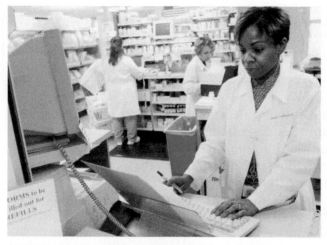

An important responsibility of the technician is keeping records such as the patient profile up to date.

Creating a New Patient Profile

Prescriptions cannot be filled for patients who do not have a current patient profile on record in the pharmacy. If a patient is a new customer to the pharmacy, then a new profile will have to be created, either at the time the prescription is submitted to the pharmacy or, in the case of phoned-in prescriptions, prior to dispensing the medication(s) to the patient. Figure 6.2 is an example of a patient profile form used to obtain information from the patient for the profile.

Creating a patient profile might require asking questions related to each of the items indicated in Table 6.3. If a patient profile is not complete, then the technician may need

FIGURE 6.2
**Patient Profile
Form**

PATIENT PROFILE

Patient Name

Last	First	Middle Initial

Street or PO Box

City	State	ZIP

Phone (__)__ __	Date of Birth Month Day Year	Social Security No. __ __ __
	□ Male □ Female	

□ Yes, I would like medication dispensed in a child-resistant container.
□ No, I do not want medication dispensed in a child-resistant container.

Medication Insurance   Card Holder Name _____
□ Yes   □ Card Holder   □ Child   □ Disabled Dependent
□ No   □ Spouse   □ Dependent Parent □ Full Time Student

MEDICAL HISTORY

HEALTH		ALLERGIES AND DRUG REACTIONS
□ Angina	□ Epilepsy	□ No known drug allergies or reactions
□ Anemia	□ Glaucoma	□ Aspirin
□ Arthritis	□ Heart condition	□ Cephalosporins
□ Asthma	□ Kidney disease	□ Codeine
□ Blood clotting disorders	□ Liver disease	□ Erythromycin
□ High blood pressure	□ Lung disease	□ Penicillin
□ Breast feeding	□ Parkinson disease	□ Sulfa drugs
□ Cancer	□ Pregnancy	□ Tetracyclines
□ Diabetes	□ Ulcers	□ Xanthines
Other conditions _____		□ Other allergies/reactions _____

Prescription Medication(s) Being Taken   OTC Medication(s) Currently Being Taken

Would you like generic medication when possible? □ Yes □ No

Comments

Health information changes periodically. Please notify the pharmacy of any new medications, allergies, drug reactions, or health conditions.

_____ Signature _____ Date   □ I do not wish to provide this information.

to interview the patient (or the parent or patient representative) to obtain the necessary information. In some pharmacies, the customer may complete a hard-copy form with medical and allergy information. Any time the technician notices a patient having difficulty with filling out or reading and understanding the form, the pharmacy technicians should offer assistance to the patient.

The information provided on the form is then typed into the patient profile by the pharmacy technician. At the time of an initial visit, the patient will likely be given a copy of the store's confidentiality policy. It is extremely important that confidentiality of patient medical information be maintained at all times (see Chapter 13, *Human Relations and Communications*).

Documenting Medication Allergies and Adverse Drug Reactions

When creating and maintaining the patient profile and when receiving a new prescription, it is extremely important for the pharmacy technician to ask the patient about allergies to medications, as well as about past adverse drug reactions. An **allergy** is a hypersensitivity to a specific substance that may be manifested as a rash, shortness of breath, runny nose, watery eyes, etc. Common allergic reactions include sweating, rashes, swelling, and difficulty in breathing. In extreme cases, allergic reactions can lead to shock, coma, or death. An adverse drug reaction (ADR) is any unexpected negative consequence from taking a particular drug.

If the patient indicates that he or she does not have any allergies, then the notation NKA (or NKMA), for *no known allergies* (or *no known medication allergies*), should be recorded on the back of the prescription form and in the computerized patient profile. If the patient indicates that he or she does have an allergy, then that allergy must be documented and entered into the patient profile.

Many community pharmacies will require the pharmacy technician to ask patients at each visit about changes in allergies, medical conditions, or new medications, including OTC drugs and diet supplements, in order to keep the patient profile current. This information may assist the pharmacist in reviewing the prescription for potential medication-related problems.

Inquiring about allergies every time a patient comes to the pharmacy with a prescription for an antibiotic is a good practice. Antibiotics, especially penicillin and sulfa drugs, are the most common types of medication allergies and allergies can begin at any age. A patient could have safely taken an antibiotic several times in the past and become allergic to it on a subsequent occasion.

Patients can be allergic to any medication or ingredient. Other common medications that can cause allergic reactions include aspirin, NSAIDs (such as ibuprofen), codeine, and anesthetics. Some patients who report stomach upset or nausea may be experiencing an allergic reaction. However, these are more likely expected side effects of the prescribed medication, not a true allergy. Therefore the technician should ask the patient to describe the symptoms before documenting the allergy into the patient profile.

Once a patient profile contains allergy-related information, the computer software will alert the pharmacist that a potential allergy or that a hypersensitivity reaction may occur if a prescription is filled for that drug. For example, if hydrocodone, a codeine derivative, is being prescribed to a patient whose profile indicates that he or she may be allergic to codeine, then the pharmacist will receive a precautionary message on the computer screen. The pharmacist then has the option to call the physician, counsel the patient, or review the profile. The pharmacist may ask the patient whether he or she remembers taking hydrocodone in the past without an allergic reaction. In such instances, it is important that the action taken by the pharmacist be documented. In addition to potentially causing patient harm, a missed drug allergy could trigger a major negligence law suit. More discussion on this topic appears in the *Pharmacist Verification and Drug Utilization Review (DUR) Evaluation* section, later in this chapter.

Components of a Prescription

The reason many people go to a community pharmacy is to fill a prescription. The prescription will usually be on a preprinted form bearing the name, address, and telephone (and fax) number of the prescriber. Table 6.4 lists the parts of a prescription. Prescriptions may also be called into the pharmacy from the medical office or transferred from another pharmacy. The use of hard-copy prescriptions is slowly diminish-

TABLE 6.4 Parts of a Prescription

Part	Description
prescriber information	name, address, telephone number, and other information identifying the prescriber, including state license and DEA number
date	date on which the prescription was written; this may not be the same day as the prescription is received
patient information	full name, address, telephone number, and date of birth of the patient
℞	symbol ℞, for the Latin word *recipe*, meaning *take*
inscription	medication prescribed, including generic or brand name, strength, and amount
subscription	instructions to the pharmacist on dispensing the medication
signa	directions for the patient to follow (commonly called the sig)
additional instructions	any additional instructions that the prescriber deems necessary
signature	the signature of the prescriber

ing each year as new technologies develop. For example, more and more the pharmacy is receiving prescriptions via fax or other electronic transmission.

With the increased use of personal digital assistants (PDAs) by physicians, and at the encouragement of the federal government, all states now approve e-prescribing. **E-prescribing** is the transmission of electronic prescriptions to the pharmacy. The advantages of electronic submission of prescriptions to the pharmacy are speed, accuracy, improved billing, and decreased potential for forgeries and medication errors. Prescriptions for Schedule II–controlled substances must remain as hard-copy or print documents. It is important that pharmacy technicians be aware of state laws regarding patient confidentiality of prescription faxing and the transferring of prescriptions electronically or via a database.

Reviewing the Prescription for Completeness

One of the responsibilities of the pharmacy technician will be to check to make sure that each prescription received in the pharmacy is complete and that the information about the medication order is documented accurately. Figure 6.3 shows an example of a complete prescription. The pharmacy technician will do this work under the supervision of the pharmacist. The following are some general guidelines for the pharmacy technician when reviewing a prescription for completeness:

Safety Note

Amounts on prescriptions should be written out to prevent alterations.

- The **DEA number** is issued to a physician authorizing him or her to prescribe controlled substances. This number (and often the state license number) is required on prescriptions to file any third-party insurance claims, even for noncontrolled prescriptions. In most cases, for security reasons, the DEA number of the prescribing physician is handwritten rather than preprinted on the prescription form.
- Patient name should be given in full, including at least the full first and last names. Initials alone are not acceptable. If the writing is illegible, then the technician should rewrite the patient's name in full above the name on the prescription and verify the spelling of the patient's name.

- Patient address and telephone number are needed for patient records. Requesting the telephone number is often helpful in identifying the patient and minimizing dispensing errors. A secondary phone (cell or business) is often helpful to contact the patient for additional information. If this information is missing, then the pharmacy technician should request it from the patient and add it to the prescription.

- Preprinted prescriptions often contain a space for the patient's birth date. If this space is not filled in, then the technician should request this information. The patient birth date is helpful for third-party billing and for distinguishing among patients having the same name. Knowing the patient's age also helps the pharmacist evaluate the appropriateness of the drug, its quantity, and the dosage form prescribed, thus minimizing medication errors.

- The date the physician wrote the prescription should be provided. For pharmacy records, the date when the prescription is received should be written on the prescription as well, if different from the current date. If no date is written on the prescription, then the date the prescription is brought into the pharmacy should be recorded and noted as such. If the undated prescription is for an antibiotic, then the pharmacist may wish to verify that the patient is under the current care of a physician. The date on a prescription holds special importance for controlled substances (see *Receiving a Controlled-Drug Prescription*, later in this chapter).

- The **inscription** is the part of the prescription that lists the medication prescribed, including the strength and amount. A medication may be listed on a prescription using a brand or generic name. As discussed in Chapter 3, a given drug (i.e., one with a particular generic name) may be marketed under various brand names. For example, Prinivil and Zestril are two brand names under which the generic drug lisinopril is marketed by pharmaceutical companies. Generic drugs are often

FIGURE 6.3
A Complete Prescription

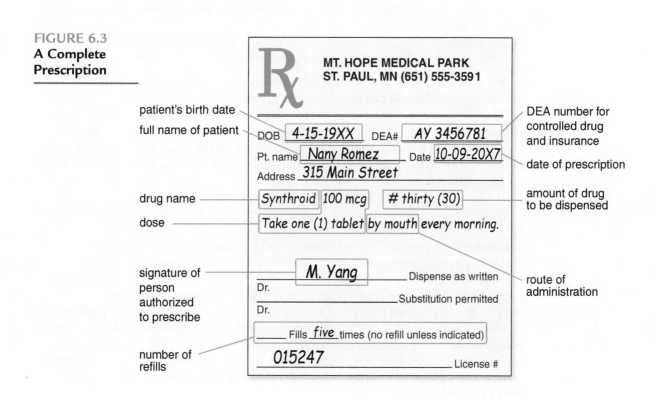

less expensive than brand name drugs and are often automatically substituted by pharmacy software, under regulations now existing in every state, for brand name drugs. A patient may request a brand name product, but his or her insurance may not cover the additional cost. If the prescription for a brand name drug is filled with a generic equivalent, then the name, strength, and manufacturer of the generic substitution must be included on the dispensed medication container label.

- The **subscription** is the part of the prescription that lists the instructions to the pharmacist about dispensing the medication, including compounding instructions, labeling instructions, refill information, and information about the appropriateness of dispensing drug equivalents.

- A **refill** is an approval by the prescriber to dispense the medication again without requiring a new order. If the refill section on the prescription is left blank, then the prescription cannot be refilled. The words *no refill* (sometime abbreviated NR) will appear on the medication container label, and *no refill* will be entered into the patient's record. Even if the refill blank on the prescription indicates *as needed*, or *prn*, unlimited duration is not allowed. Most pharmacies and state laws require at least yearly updates on prn, or as needed, prescriptions and medical supplies.

- Regulations in a given state may require two signature lines at the bottom of the prescription: one reading *dispense as written* and the other reading *substitution permitted*. If the **dispense as written (DAW)** line is signed, then substitution of a generic equivalent is not permitted. Other states may require only one signature line; **brand name medically necessary**, which is sometimes shortened to "brand necessary," must be designated on the prescription if a prescriber wishes that only the brand name product be dispensed. At times a patient may request a brand name to be dispensed in lieu of a generic drug (called DAW2); this will often result in a higher patient co-pay.

- The **signa** (or "**sig**" for short) is the part of the prescription that communicates the directions for use. This information is transferred onto the label that is placed on the medication container.

- The signature of each local physician should be recognizable by both the pharmacy technician and pharmacist to detect possible forged prescriptions.

If there are any doubts about the authenticity or completeness of a prescription, then this should be called to the immediate attention of the pharmacist. A telephone call from the pharmacy technician or the pharmacist to the prescriber's office might be necessary to clarify an order. The technician is allowed to clarify a prescription in some states, but all changes should be documented on the prescription (and/or in the patient profile) with the technician's initials and the name of the nurse who clarified the prescription.

Reading the Prescription

It is extremely important for the pharmacy technician to accurately transcribe the physician's prescription order into the patient profile. Many drugs have similar names, and the incorrect drug can be easily chosen from the computer database (see Appendix B). After a prescription has been received and reviewed, the trained pharmacy technician is given the task of recording the new prescription in the profile to provide such information as the prescription number, drug prescribed, dosage form, quantity, number of refills authorized (if any), and patient cost for the prescription. The medication container label's instructions should read exactly as indicated on the prescription's signa. In addition, any signa comments written on the prescription must be included on the label.

FIGURE 6.4
**Hard-to-Read
Prescription**

This prescription is for a Z-PAK (azithromycin) and directs the patient to take "as directed for sinus infection."

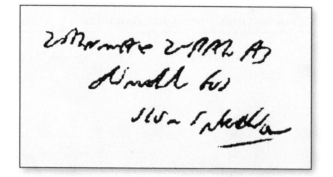

The subscription and the sig may be written by the prescriber using abbreviations. If the prescription is handwritten by the prescriber, then the combination of the use of abbreviations and the handwriting style might make the prescription difficult to read. Figure 6.4 shows an example of a hard-to-read prescription.

In order to read and interpret a physician's medication order, the technician must become familiar with the approved abbreviations for physician use on prescriptions. If any part of the prescription is unclear or undecipherable, then the technician must check with the pharmacist prior to beginning the prescription-filling process. A list of common prescription abbreviations is given in Table 6.5. A more complete listing of abbreviations is available in the Pharmacy Library section of the Internet Resource Center for this book at www.emcp.net/pharmpractice4e.

Misinterpretation of the abbreviations on a prescription could result in a serious medication error—wrong drug or wrong dose or wrong directions to, perhaps, the wrong patient. The importance to the filling process of each of the components of a prescription is detailed throughout this chapter.

Other Types of Prescriptions Received in the Community Pharmacy

In addition to newly written or e-prescribed prescriptions, the community pharmacy will receive requests for other types of prescriptions, including refill requests from the patient, called-in prescriptions from the prescriber's office, transfer prescriptions *to* or *from* another pharmacy, and prescriptions for controlled substances. These types of prescriptions require special attention.

Prescription Refill Requests

Pharmacy technicians often receive a telephone call or personal request from a patient at the pharmacy counter to refill a medication. If the patient has the prescription container with label information, then the processing of the request is much easier. In this case the prescription information has already been previously entered (and verified) into the computerized patient profile. The role of the technician is to verify that refills do indeed exist for the requested medication and to forward the request for pharmacist review and approval if they do. Most pharmacies and insurance plans will allow medications to be refilled up to a week prior to the next refill date; if the request for refill is too early, then it will be rejected by third-party insurance.

For example, suppose a patient requests a refill of Motrin 600 mg #90 with the sig: 1 tab tid prn; this prescription represents a 30 day supply of this drug. The patient's profile indicates the prescription was filled on April 1. Because this is a 30 day supply, the refill is due May 1 and the technician can initiate the refill request on or after April 23. Each pharmacy will have a policy defining the procedure for handling early refills.

TABLE 6.5 Common Prescription Abbreviations

Category	Abbreviation	Meaning
amount	cc *	cubic centimeter (mL)
	g	gram
	gr	grain
	gtt	drop
	mg	milligram
	mL	milliliter
	qs	a sufficient quantity
	tbsp	tablespoonful
	tsp	teaspoonful
dosage form	cap	capsule
	MDI	metered-dose inhaler
	sol	solution
	supp	suppository
	susp	suspension
	tab	tablet
	ung	ointment
time of administration	ac	before meals
	am	morning, before noon
	bid	twice a day
	hs *	at bedtime
	pc	after meals
	pm	evening, after noon
	prn	as needed
	q6 h	every 6 hours
	qid	four times a day
	tid	three times a day
	tiw	three times a week
site of administration	ad *	right ear
	as *	left ear
	au *	each ear
	od *	right eye
	os *	left eye
	ou *	each eye
	po	oral, by mouth
	pr	per rectum
	sl	sublingual (under the tongue)
	top	topical (skin)
	vag	vaginally

*Do not use these abbreviations. Although commonly used, they are easily misread; the Institute for Safe Medication Practices (IMSP) lists these as dangerous abbreviations.

In some circumstances (e.g., when a customer is leaving on vacation), an early refill for a medication might be appropriate. Insurance companies often will not pay for these early refills automatically; the pharmacy technician may offer to call the insurance and get approval for a "one time" early refill. Often the patient may need to pay for the prescription and send in the receipt for possible reimbursement at a later date.

Some prescriptions written in the emergency department, such as antibiotics or other medications, are commonly prescribed with no refills. In some cases, patients with chronic disease medications for conditions such as high cholesterol and high blood pressure are written with limited refills so that patients will be required to follow up with their primary care physicians for repeat office visits or needed blood tests. In other cases, the refills will be fully used and a call (or fax) to the physician will be necessary to authorize additional refills. If the patient has not been seen recently, then the physician's office may deny the refills until the patient makes an appointment.

Most states allow pharmacists to use their best professional judgment to provide a short-term emergency supply (usually 2–3 days) of needed chronic medication such as for high blood pressure, high cholesterol, or epilepsy. This is often the case at night or on weekends, when contacting the physician for refill authorization is not feasible.

There are circumstances where refills are not permitted despite refills being listed on the medication container label, such as the following:

- A prescription that is more than 12 months old
- A prescription for a controlled drug (Schedules III–IV) that was written more than 6 months ago or refilled 5 times
- A prescription that has been previously transferred to another pharmacy

It is important for the pharmacy technician to communicate to the patient why refills are not available, when "too early" refills will be allowed, and when additional refills might be authorized by the physician (usually 24–48 hours after the request, excluding weekends).

New Telephone Orders

When a new telephone prescription from a prescriber's office is received by the technician, it needs to be referred to the pharmacist. These prescriptions may be telephoned into the pharmacy or left on a message line for later transcription. Once the pharmacist submits a prescription to writing and verifies its accuracy, the technician can enter the information into the patient profile, as with a new prescription.

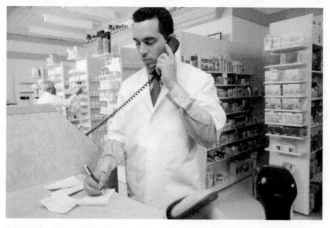

In most states, only the pharmacist may take verbal prescriptions over the telephone.

Transfer Prescriptions

At the patient's request, a pharmacy may call the pharmacy that originally filled a prescription to transfer or copy the remaining refills on that prescription. The information is documented on the original prescription on file; if the patient has the medication vial with the prescription number, then the transfer is easier, but it can also be done with the patient name and birth date and the name of the medication to be transferred. Figure 6.5 shows the form used to document the information that must be received for each transfer prescription.

FIGURE 6.5
Information
Needed for
a Transfer
Prescription

The Corner Drug Store　　**Transferred Rx**　　Open/Copy from Competitor

Patient Name _____　Date _____

Address _____

Phone Number _____　Birth Date _____

Allergies/Health Conditions _____　Hold ☐　　DAW ☐

Pharmacy Phone # _____　Pharmacy _____

RPh _____

Rx # _____

First Fill _____

Last Fill _____

Original Date _____

Original Qty _____

Original Refills _____

Remaining Refills _____

Prescriber _____

Prescriber Address _____

Prescriber Phone # _____

MD DEA _____　Pharmacist initials _____

Pharmacy DEA (if controlled substance) _____

Pharmacies provide transfer service to patients, but careful documentation is required. Common reasons for a transfer may be cost and service issues, including hours of operation or location. The processing of transfer prescriptions will require additional time to make a telephone call, initiate a hard-copy prescription after talking to a pharmacist, and enter the prescription into the patient profile. If the prescription is for a new patient, then more time is needed to get demographic and insurance information to complete the patient profile.

In most states, by law only a licensed pharmacist can transfer or copy a prescription from (or to) another pharmacy. In states that do not allow pharmacy technicians to receive these orders, the pharmacist must talk to a pharmacist at the originating pharmacy.

Once the prescription information is transcribed to an order by the pharmacist, that order is usually sent to the pharmacy technician for entry into the computerized patient profile. The technician should resolve any difficulty reading or interpreting the pharmacist's transcribing prior to entry into the patient profile to minimize medication errors. If a transfer prescription has no remaining refills (or the date is beyond one year), then the physician's office must be called or faxed to request a new prescription before it can be filled by the pharmacy.

Some prescriptions are transferred to another pharmacy. Some states only allow the transfer of one refill while others require you to transfer all the remaining refills and it cannot be transferred again. Once transferred, the prescription is "closed" at the originating pharmacy. In most states no additional refills can be authorized without a new prescription once transferred. Some states have limitations on the number of transfers, especially with controlled drugs.

Prescriptions Not Yet Due

Often a patient may present a written prescription that does not have to be filled until a future date. The patient may have insufficient medication at home, especially if the dose was changed, or may have insufficient cash-on-hand to pay for all prescribed medications. Although procedures will differ by pharmacy, the prescription is commonly held or stored in an alphabetized file box or in the computerized patient profile for easy retrieval at a later date. In most states, prescriptions for Schedule II drugs cannot be stored or held in the pharmacy.

Controlled-Drug Prescriptions

As discussed earlier, a prescription for a controlled drug (Schedule II–V) requires additional care because of the potential for a patient to intentionally or unintentionally abuse the drug. Many of these drugs have a high likelihood of tolerance or physical or psychological dependence, as discussed in Chapter 3. Many of these drugs are addicting if used inappropriately or for a long duration of time.

Federal law requires a physical address (not a post office box) in the patient profile on all prescriptions (or in the patient profile) for Schedule II substances. A controlled drug can only be dispensed upon receipt of a valid prescription written for a valid medical condition. The prescription must be carefully reviewed by both the pharmacy technician and the pharmacist for authenticity, because these drugs are the most likely to be the subject of forged or altered prescriptions.

The date of the original prescription on all controlled drugs should be entered into the profile, rather than the date the prescription was filled. State laws or regulations may control the time period for initially filling a Schedule II prescription. In some states, a Schedule II prescription must be filled within 7 days of issue; in other states, it must be filled within 72 hours. Prescriptions for Schedule II controlled substances should be handwritten or typed; Schedule II prescriptions cannot be faxed or phoned in to the pharmacy. Most states do not allow a nurse, nurse practitioner, or physician's assistant to write a prescription for a Schedule II medication, even if the physician signs it. Signatures on all Schedule II prescriptions should be handwritten, not stamped.

The drug, dose, and quantity of a prescription for a Schedule II drug cannot be altered in any way by the physician, nurse, pharmacist, or technician and can never be refilled. A new prescription is required each time it is dispensed. There may also be limits on the quantity of a controlled drug that may be dispensed; in some states the limit may be 120 units (tablets or capsules) or a 30 day supply, whichever is less. Insurance company policies often also limit the supply. If insurance has limited the quantity the patient is allowed, then the patient may purchase the remainder of the prescription.

Emergency Dispensing of Controlled Substances A Schedule II medication is rarely dispensed without an authorized prescription except under exceptional circumstances. Occasions may arise in which the usual and customary procedures for filling and dispensing a Schedule II drug will result in the delay of an urgent medication needed for a patient. Pursuant to a valid medical reason, an emergency supply of a drug can be provided to a patient in most states. The prescriber may provide an oral or facsimile prescription. Again the stricter of state versus federal regulations apply. An emergency procedure is described as follows:

- A controlled substance administration is to be immediate if the patient is to receive proper treatment.
- The pharmacist immediately converts an oral order into writing.
- The pharmacist documents the need for the emergency dispensing of the Schedule II prescription.
- If the pharmacist does not know the prescriber, then good faith efforts are made by the pharmacy to verify that the prescriber is authentic.

- Within 7 days (72 hours in some states), the prescriber must deliver a written version of the emergency oral order to the pharmacy that includes "authorization for emergency dispensing" written on its face.

Authentication of Controlled-Substance Prescriptions The legitimacy of the prescription for all scheduled drugs, especially Schedule II drugs, must be carefully assessed by both the pharmacy technician and the pharmacist. Forgeries may be written on stolen or preprinted facsimiles of prescriptions. Those with access to blank prescription blanks (and controlled substances) include all health professionals, including pharmacy technicians and clerical personnel. Prescription pads in physicians' offices should be kept by prescribers only or in locked drawers in the examining rooms.

Some physicians have their DEA number preprinted on their prescriptions, but others write it on the prescription when writing out a prescription order for a controlled substance medication. Some states and insurers require all such prescriptions to be written on authorized **safety paper**, which is tamper-resistant. Most pharmacies have a computerized physician database containing DEA, state license number, and contact information. All insurance plans require a pharmacy to have a physician's DEA number (and state license number) on file to be reimbursed for prescriptions, even when the drug is for a nonscheduled medication. Pharmacy personnel can also check for a falsified DEA number by following the procedure listed in Table 6.6.

Forgeries are often difficult to recognize, especially during a typically busy pharmacy workload. Any discrepancies must be resolved by the pharmacist by talking directly to the prescribing physician. However, many tell-tale signs of potential forgeries or prescriptions exist. Pharmacy technicians should be alert to the indicators listed in Table 6.7. Physicians should be encouraged to use Roman numerals and should write out quantities so that #12 tablets of a narcotic cannot be altered by adding a zero, thus creating #120. Also, it is important to learn to recognize the signatures of the legal prescribers who send prescriptions to the pharmacy.

Pharmacy technicians should also take care when another person (other than the patient or a family member) attempts to call in a refill or to pick up medication. When in doubt, the pharmacy technician should call the patient to verify the authenticity of the prescription or the validity of the refill request. Some pharmacies request a photo ID in order to confirm information written on a received prescription.

A **drug seeker** is a patient who may receive prescriptions for the same or similar controlled drugs from several physicians or who constantly requests "early refills." A drug seeker may be tolerant or addicted to the medication or may be illegally selling the drugs. Many drug-seeking patients pay with cash to minimize computerized tracking and use more than one pharmacy and physician or dentist. Most pharmacies and physicians' offices (including emergency rooms) require that all prescribed medications must be dispensed when a controlled-substance prescription is submitted. Because the role of the pharmacy profession is to safeguard the public health, the

---

TABLE 6.6 Steps for Checking a DEA Number

1. Add the first, third, and fifth digits of the DEA number.
2. Add the second, fourth, and sixth digits of the number and multiply the sum by two.
3. Add the results of steps 1 and 2. The last digit of this sum should be the same as the last digit of the DEA number.
4. The second letter of the DEA number should be the same as the first letter of the physician's last name.

TABLE 6.7   Indicators of a Potentially Forged Prescription

- The prescription is altered (for example, a change in quantity).
- There are misspellings on the prescription.
- A refill is indicated for a Schedule II drug.
- A prescription from the emergency department is written for more than a 7 day supply.
- A prescription is cut and pasted from a preprinted, signed prescription.
- A second or third prescription is added to a legal prescription written by a physician. More than one handwriting style is used.
- A patient presents a prescription containing several medications but only wants the pharmacy to fill the narcotic prescription.
- The prescription is signed with different handwriting or in different ink, or not signed by the physician.
- The DEA number is missing or is incorrect.
- The prescription is written by an out-of-state physician or a physician practicing in an area far from the pharmacy. This can be especially questionable if the prescription is received at night or on the weekend, when it will be difficult to confirm the prescription.
- Someone other than the patient drops off the prescription.

technician and the pharmacist must carefully review and monitor all new and refill controlled-drug medications.

If a forgery is suspected, then the prescription should be retained for evidence, the "patient" detained if possible, and the police notified. The pharmacist or technician can detain the person presenting the prescription by saying, "This may take some time to fill. Can you come back in one hour?"

The Right to Refuse a Controlled-Substance Prescription A pharmacist has the right to refuse to fill a controlled-substance prescription. For example, it may not make sense to have a narcotic prescription for severe pain filled three months after the date it was written! If a legitimate concern exists that a prescription was not written in good faith, then the pharmacist's duty is to determine the reason for issuing the prescription from the prescriber.

Safety Note

A pharmacist has the right to refuse to fill a prescription for a controlled substance.

If there is concern that the patient is abusing a legal prescription or receiving controlled substances from more than one prescriber, then the pharmacist should contact the prescriber. Even if the prescriber approves the order, the pharmacist can exercise the option to not fill the prescription. For example, if the prescriber prescribes an excessive amount of narcotic that could do harm to the patient, then the pharmacist may elect not to fill the prescription. However, if a diagnosis of cancer is known, or the patient is under care of a hospice team or oncologist (cancer physician), then use of high-dose narcotics for comfort and pain relief is understandable.

Refilling Controlled-Substance Prescriptions The safeguard of not allowing the refill of Schedule II drugs frequently causes an inconvenience to a parent whose child may be treated with a Schedule II drug for attention-deficit hyperactivity disorder (ADHD). In some states a prescriber is permitted to write two additional future dated prescriptions for such medications for a patient, or the patient's representative, to hold until needed. It is illegal in most states for pharmacies to store or "hold" future prescriptions of Schedule II drugs.

A prescription for a Schedule III or IV drug may be refilled up to five times if allowed by the physician, but these refills must occur within a 6 month period, after which time a new prescription is required. *The 6 month time frame starts with the date the prescription was written, not with the date it was filled.* The five refills include both completely and partially filled prescriptions. If you are not sure whether a prescription (or refill) is for a controlled drug, then check the medication stock bottles on the shelf (or the medication container label) for a C-III or C-IV designation.

Early refill requests by patients for Schedule III–IV drugs must be carefully monitored by the pharmacy technician. If refills are indicated for a controlled drug, then prescriptions are refilled no sooner than 1 or 2 days before the customer's supply will run out (although this is not a hard-and-fast rule). If the request for refill is too early for a controlled medication such as pain or nerve medications, then it may be rejected by the pharmacist. Each pharmacy has a policy defining the procedure for handling early refills of Schedule III–IV controlled substances.

A prescription for a Schedule V controlled substance (required in some states) may be refilled only if authorized by a prescribing physician; some states allow patients to purchase a limited supply of a Schedule V medication (see Chapter 7 for further discussion). Most Schedule V medications contain codeine in a cough syrup formulation.

Generally, by state law, refills for prescriptions of controlled medications can only be transferred to another pharmacy one time. Careful attention must be given to the transfer and documentation of Schedule III–IV prescriptions. If a controlled substance is transferred between pharmacies, then the DEA numbers of both the originating and receiving pharmacies must be exchanged and reduced to writing on the prescription form or in the computerized pharmacy database.

If a Schedule III or IV prescription was filled and in "storage" at the originating pharmacy, then the technician may be directed by the pharmacist to "reverse" (or credit to insurance) via online billing (if covered by insurance) and to place the unused medication back into inventory. This prevents patients from transferring narcotics to one pharmacy but returning to the original pharmacy to pick up the original prescription before the drug is taken out of storage.

Documenting Insurance Information

Once the demographic and prescription information is reviewed and entered into the correct patient profile, the pharmacy technician often submits an online claim to an insurance plan. If there is a problem with insurance eligibility (incorrect ID or group number or date of birth) or drug coverage (drug not covered), then the pharmacy technician must try to resolve the issue. It is not uncommon for insurance to only cover a 30 day supply of medication even if the prescriber approved a higher quantity. For example, a prescriber may write a 90 day supply of verapamil for blood pressure, but insurance may only cover a 30 day supply. Again, suppose a prescription is received for Ambien CR 12.5 mg #30 for sleep. Insurance may only cover 18 tablets per 30 days; however, the patient does have the option to purchase the other 12 tablets personally.

If the drug on the prescription is not covered by insurance (usually expensive drugs), or if it is not included on a preferred drug formulary list, then a prior authorization may be required. A **prior authorization (PA)** requires the pharmacy technician or pharmacist to call or fax the prescriber's office so that the prescriber can explain the justification for the use of the drug with the patient's insurer. This often delays filling the prescription for 72 hours or longer. An alternative drug may be prescribed. The patient always has the option to pay for the medication personally instead of waiting for the outcome of the PA. If insurance approves the PA, then the technician can process the prescription claim online and fill the prescription. Chapter 7 will provide more details about online billing and insurance claims.

Pharmacist Verification and Drug Utilization Review (DUR) Evaluation

It is nearly impossible for any pharmacist (or physician) to remember doses, adverse effects, and drug interactions for all medications, especially while juggling a typically busy pharmacy workload. In addition, because patients may go to more than one pharmacy or more than one physician specialist, a complete medication profile may not exist. Pharmacy software will compare a prescription with others the patient has received to determine whether a drug utilization review is necessary. A **drug utilization review (DUR)** requires a closer review of the patient profile and an override by the pharmacist indicating that the prescription is safe to dispense. This software is specifically designed for pharmacies and insurance companies to provide an additional level of protection with which to detect a potentially serious medication error.

A DUR may be needed for a prescribed medication if the prescribed drug may:

- Interact with existing or past medications on the patient's profile (i.e., blood thinners such as warfarin)
- Be contraindicated because of the patient's allergy or medical history (penicillin allergy, diabetes, or asthma)
- Be a duplicate of a similar drug prescribed in the past (i.e., two different migraine headache drugs, both narcotics)
- Have been prescribed in doses too low (sub-therapeutic) or too high (toxic) for this patient
- Not be indicated in certain patients or used with caution (i.e., in pregnancy, pediatrics, or with older adults)

Most DUR notifications will be categorized by their potential severity, for instance as mild, moderate, or severe. The pharmacist must use his or her professional judgment to determine what type of action is necessary before dispensing the drug. These options include:

- Reviewing the patient profile
- Contacting the prescribing physician
- Counseling the patient on potential issues prior to dispensing
- Overriding the DUR and filling the prescription

In most pharmacies, the action taken on severe DURs must be documented. The pharmacist will use his or her training and experience to review the patient profile and assess the significance of any potential interaction or adverse effect.

The pharmacy technician will not be able to fill or dispense the prescription to the patient until the verification is complete and the DUR, if any, is resolved by the pharmacist. It is important for the technician to alert the pharmacist that a DUR exists and effectively communicate to the patient that a potential problem exists with the prescribed medication that must be resolved prior to dispensing. Often the pharmacist will write a reminder note to counsel the patient at the time of prescription pick-up to increase awareness of a potential side effect or adverse reaction. Once the DUR is resolved by the pharmacist, the technician can then continue the process of filling the prescription order.

Medication Selection and Preparation

In order to efficiently and accurately select medications from the pharmacy stock to fill the prescriptions received, the technician must become familiar with the precise location of drug inventory. Drugs are usually stocked by brand or generic drug name. High-volume pharmacies may have an additional section of the pharmacy dedicated to fast-moving Top 200 drugs, enhancing dispensing efficiency. Antibiotic powders for reconstitution are usually stocked in a separate area (as are all solutions, syrups, and suspensions). Some pharmacies may also have a separate shelving section for birth control pills, topical creams, ointments and gels, nasal and lung sprays and inhalers, and otic (ear) and ophthalmic (eye) medications.

Schedule II drugs can be dispersed throughout the stock or can be stored in a locked cabinet. In most pharmacies access to these medications is limited to the pharmacist. This requires the pharmacist to unlock the cabinet, select the appropriate stock bottle, compare the NDC number with the medication container label, and count out the medication. Other controlled Schedule III–V substances may be distributed throughout the drug stock. Be sure to know the policy and procedure for filling controlled substance prescription orders in your pharmacy.

The pharmacy technician fills a medication order based on a printed medication container label or a patient-specific medication information sheet after computer entry from the original prescription has been reviewed and approved by the pharmacist. The printout often indicates whether the medication order is for a new or refill prescription. In addition to patient information, the printout contains the generic or brand drug name, dose, quantity, and NDC number.

Figure 6.6 identifies the standard parts of a pharmacy stock drug label. The drug name, strength, package size, and NDC number should always be checked immediately and compared with the printout before the technician counts out and places the medication in a container. On the unit stock bottle the brand name is often in bolder print, and the generic name is in smaller print under or beside the brand name. The dosage form is also indicated in this area. The dose or strength per unit is prominently displayed near the drug name. The package size is commonly a drug stock bottle of 30, 60, 90, 100, or 500 tablets or capsules.

Safety Note

The expiration date should always be checked by the pharmacy technician before filling, especially on infrequently used medications.

Safety Note

Use the medication's NDC number to confirm that the correct medication has been pulled from stock.

FIGURE 6.6
Parts of a Stock Drug Label

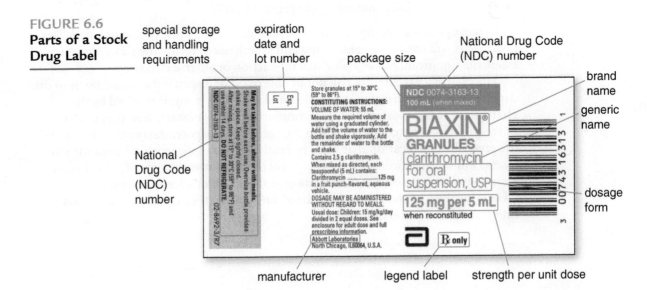

special storage and handling requirements · expiration date and lot number · package size · National Drug Code (NDC) number · brand name · generic name · dosage form · National Drug Code (NDC) number · manufacturer · legend label · strength per unit dose

Safety Note

Check each drug at least three times to confirm that the correct drug is dispensed.

Safety Note

Review Appendix B for a listing of common sound-alike medications and recommendations by the ISMP.

The NDC number is used by many pharmacists and technicians to aid in identifying the exact drug, dose, and package size for the preparation of the prescription. It is very important that the technician compare the NDC number of the stock bottle with the printout. Automation in some pharmacies allows the comparison of the bar code of the printout and the drug stock bottle, minimizing the chance of human error.

Pharmacy technicians are often in a better position to identify potential sources of error related to filling the prescription order. Often, in the pharmacy, drugs are arranged alphabetically, with drugs of similar spelling and strength or similar generic manufacturer nearby. Packaging of the same drug in various doses, dosage forms, strengths, or concentrations may be similar. To minimize dispensing errors, some drugs may be purposely stocked slightly out of order to get the attention of pharmacy personnel.

A common error is the selection of the wrong drug stock bottle or dose or package size because two products look alike (similar labeling) or have names that sound alike (see Appendix B). Good work habits are to read each stock drug label three times and to avoid basing product identification on size, color, package shape, or label design. The technician should develop the habit of making three checks to ensure that the correct drug was selected: (1) when the product is initially being pulled from the inventory shelf, (2) at the time of preparation, and (3) when the product is returned to the shelf. Medication error prevention is more thoroughly discussed in Chapter 12.

It is important that the pharmacy technician select the correct drug from stock. The NDC number will confirm that the appropriate drug was selected.

Occasionally, the NDC number of the prescription order will not match the drug stock bottle. The pharmacy (or wholesaler) may have changed the generic source of a drug product because of a more favorable price. Thus, a patient may receive a different shaped or colored tablet upon refill of a pain medication because of this "change of manufacturer." A new printout of the medication order will reflect the new NDC number of the drug product. It is important that the technician notify the patient at the time of pickup that the appearance of the medication may have changed; otherwise, the patient may think that an error was made in the filling process.

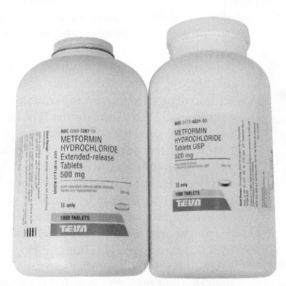

It is important that the pharmacy technician carefully check the drug's name, strength, and formulation when selecting the drug from stock. In this case, both drugs are metformin 500 mg, but one bottle is immediate-release and the other is extended-release. Selecting the wrong formulation would result in a serious medication error.

FIGURE 6.7 Counting Tablets

(a) Tablets should be counted by fives and moved to the trough with a spatula. (b) The unneeded tablets should be returned to the stock container by pouring them from the spout. (c) The counted tablets should then be poured into the appropriately sized medication vial.

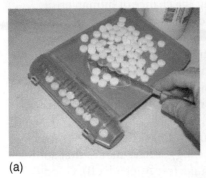

(a)

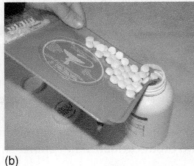

(b)

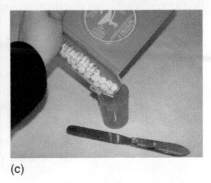

(c)

Preparing Oral Dosage Forms

Oral drug products are available in many different dosage forms, each of which has its own dispensing requirements. The most commonly used form is the oral tablet or capsule. Tablets and capsules must be counted out and placed in the appropriately sized vial or medication container.

Figure 6.7 shows the equipment and procedure for counting tablets and capsules. A special counting tray is used that has a trough on one side to hold counted tablets or capsules and a spout on the opposite side to pour unused medication back into the stock bottle. The technician should minimize any direct finger contact with the medication, because germs and oils from the skin could contaminate the medication. The tablets and capsules should always be counted with a clean spatula and picked up with forceps if they are dropped on the counter. The spatula, tray, and forceps should be cleaned often throughout the workday with 70% isopropyl alcohol. Because of the frequency of severe patient allergies, this equipment should be cleaned immediately after counting sulfa, penicillin, or aspirin products, as well as any product leaving visible powder residue on surfaces.

Safety Note

Equipment should be cleaned after counting sulfa, penicillin, or aspirin products.

Some higher volume pharmacies may use bar-code scanners and automated counting machines to minimize the chance of human error in drug selection and to facilitate the counting of tablets and capsules. The bar scanners are also used for refills, comparing the NDC numbers of drug stock bottles with the prescription order (patient information leaflet) and final verification of the medication container label with a drug identification screen.

The counting machines take into account the weight per unit of an individual tablet or capsule based on its NDC number. However, the machine is not 100% accurate and should not be used to count prescription orders for controlled drugs. The counting machine must be calibrated and documented daily by the pharmacy technician; a known weight (e.g., 200 g) is placed on the balance and the device is recalibrated.

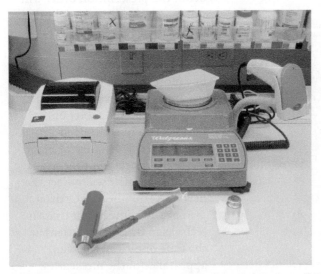

Top, from left: a label printer, an automatic counting machine with calibrated weight, and a bar-code scanner used to verify the prescription with the bar code on the stock bottle. Bottom, at left: a counting tray and spatula.

Most pharmacies allow the pharmacy technician to fill Schedule III–IV drugs (those usually not contained in a locked cabinet). Many pharmacies' procedures may require a manual double-count of all controlled substances (Schedule II–IV) and the pharmacist or pharmacy technician initialing the medication container label. This prevents potential abusing or drug-seeking patients from returning to the pharmacy to complain that the pharmacist or technician shorted the count on their prescription.

Liquid products, such as pediatric cough and cold syrups and suspensions, are sometimes dispensed in their original packaging. They are also commonly poured from a stock bottle directly into an appropriately sized dispensing bottle (from 2 fl oz to 16 fl oz). The pharmacy technician should present the original stock bottle to the pharmacist for final check along with the original prescription, the patient information leaflet, and the medication in the labeled container.

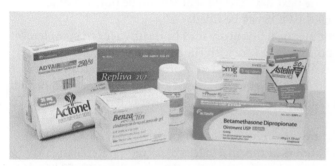

Unit-of-use packaging for commonly prescribed drugs saves time and reduces medication preparation errors.

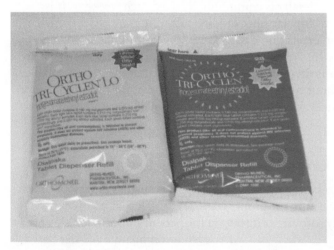

Birth control pills are prepackaged for dispensing.

Dispensing Prepackaged Drugs

Filling a prescription often involves simply retrieving from stock a drug with the correct name, manufacturer, quantity, and strength. Counting out the medication may not be necessary. A drug may be commercially available in a prepackaged, unit-of-use form. A **unit of use** is a fixed number of dosage units in a drug stock container. Many drugs are prescribed as one dose daily, and many insurance companies reimburse for only a 1 month supply of medication. Unit-of-use packaging consists of a month's supply, which is often 30 tablets or capsules.

Other examples of prepackaged drugs are birth control pills, topical ointments or creams, and eye and ear drops. Filling the prescription with medications in unit-of-use packaging thus amounts to little more than locating the correct drug, in the correct strength, in storage, verifying the NDC number, and affixing the correct medication container label.

Sometimes filling a prescription involves retrieving a multiple-dose container of a premixed drug, measuring out the prescribed quantity, and placing it into a container with a label. Because antibiotic powders are available in multiple strengths and volumes, checking the drug label (and NDC number) carefully is critical to minimizing mistakes. Pediatric antibiotic suspensions must be reconstituted with a given amount of distilled water before being dispensed to the parent.

Even with prepackaged drug formulations, the pharmacist must verify the quality of the technician's work, ensuring that the proper drug, dosage form, and amount were chosen and placed in the proper container, as well as that a proper label was prepared and the correct amount of distilled water added, for medications needing reconstitution.

Safety Note

The pharmacist must check all drugs prepared by the pharmacy technician.

Dealing with Out-of-Stock and Partially Filled Medications

Most pharmacies maintain a limited drug inventory to remain profitable, so it is not uncommon to be either out of a prescribed medication or unable to completely fill a prescription order. A medication can go **out of stock (OOS)** if an uncommon specialty medication is ordered or if there has been a higher than normal demand for such a prescription, such as during the allergy season. In the case of an OOS, options include:

- Allowing the patient to take the prescription to another pharmacy
- Borrowing the medication from another pharmacy
- Ordering the medication from the wholesaler

Unless the prescription is received on the weekend (or late at night), the medication can usually be received by the next day. The patient should be notified of an expected "promised time" when the OOS can be filled.

Even when a drug is not out of stock, inventory may be insufficient to completely fill the prescription. Though policies may vary with the pharmacy, the pharmacy may provide the patient with a partial fill. A **partial fill** may provide a 2 day to 5 day supply of medication, which should be sufficient until the new drug inventory is received. The medication container label and patient information leaflet will indicate that a partial fill was dispensed.

Partial fills on Schedule II drugs are only allowed on an emergency basis if the remainder can be supplied in 72 hours at the pharmacist's discretion. Receiving new inventory for a Schedule II drug may, depending on the pharmacy, take 48–72 hours because of required federal and state recordkeeping and paper trails. Many pharmacies have adopted a secure online ordering process to expedite orders for Schedule II drugs.

Inventory from the drug wholesaler is commonly received each weekday. It is important that the pharmacy technician check in or "post" the drug order (which usually includes NDC number, expiration dating, and drug cost updates) and then initiate the prescription filling for any OOS or partial-fill prescriptions from the day before. The prescription order is then processed and filled so that it can be available for the patient to pick up without further delay. The inventory implications of filling out of stock and partial fill medications and ordering controlled substances is discussed in Chapter 7.

Choosing Medication Containers

A wide variety of plastic vial sizes are available for tablets and capsules in various dram sizes (from 10 to 60 drams). Selecting the proper vial size is a skill that becomes easy with experience. The pharmacy software printout on the patient information sheet may even recommend a vial size based on the count and weight of the specific drug product. Most containers in the pharmacy are amber colored to prevent ultraviolet (UV) light exposure and subsequent degradation of the medication.

Other containers common to the retail pharmacy include amber liquid containers and solid white ointment jars for creams or ointments. Cardboard boxes may be

Amber-colored containers protect medications from UV light exposure.

available as well for products such as suppositories, unit-of-use packages, or injectable syringes. Many products, such as metered-dose inhalers (MDIs) and oral contraceptives, are available in a manufacturer-provided container; the prescription label is attached directly to the product or the box.

Some pharmacists prefer to apply prescription labels for topical products directly to the tube or jar, but others prefer to have the label placed on the box in which the product is packaged. A disadvantage of the latter method is that if the box is lost or discarded, then the physician's directions to the patient will not be available. If the packaging of an ointment tube or bottle of an ophthalmic or otic medication is too small for a label, then the medication is often placed in an appropriately sized, child-resistant prescription vial and labeled.

All medications should be dispensed in child-resistant containers that are designed to be difficult for children to open. Pediatric medications should always be dispensed with an appropriate measuring device. The Poison Prevention Packaging Act of 1970 requires (with some exceptions, such as nitroglycerin sublingual tablets) that all prescription drugs be packaged in child-resistant containers but states that a non–child-resistant container may be used if the prescriber prescribing the drug or the patient receiving it makes a request for such a container. This information should be added to the patient profile for future reference. Many older patients, especially those with arthritis, may have difficulty opening child-resistant containers and may request an exemption from child-resistant containers.

The regulations of a given state may require the patient to initiate a special request for dispensing a prescription in a non–child-resistant container. Some state laws allow pharmacy patients to complete a blanket request form for non–child-resistant containers. Others require patients to sign such a request for each prescription. Often pharmacies make use of a stamp on the back of the prescription for this purpose. Some unit dosed prepackaged tablets or capsules may need to be dispensed in a zip-locked plastic bag; unit dosed medication is considered child-resistant packaging. Some OTC drugs that are potentially toxic to children, such as aspirin and iron, require the manufacturer to use child-resistant containers.

Medication Information for the Patient

It is important to provide each patient with sufficient information to correctly take the prescribed medication. Written information is delivered through the medication container labels. Additional written drug information is given to the patient to take home and review for each new and refill medication. Although the pharmacy technician is not allowed to counsel the patients, by law the pharmacy technician is legally bound to offer the patient verbal counseling to be provided by the pharmacist.

Drug labeling will summarize and reinforce the dosing instructions in most cases. However some prescription labels will read "take as directed." The pharmacy technician should verify that the physician did indeed give the patient specific directions or request that the pharmacist counsel the patient on the appropriate use.

Written medication information, such as patient information sheets and MedGuides, will be generated by the pharmacy software and is strictly regulated by the FDA. The pharmacy technician will assist the pharmacist in assuring that these resources are available to the patient or to a family member picking up the medication on his or her behalf.

Creating the Medication Container Label

A **medication container label** is a label containing the dosage directions from the prescriber and is affixed to the container of the dispensed medication. This label is usually generated by the computer after verification by the pharmacist but before the preparation or "filling" of the prescription. In some pharmacies, this label is generated only after the bar code of the patient medication sheet is compared to the bar code of the drug stock bottle. This provides additional protection from selecting the wrong drug or dose.

The information required on a medication container label depends on the laws and regulations of a given state. As indicated previously, manufacturers' labels for prescription medications must carry the legend "℞ only." Some states require veterinary labels to carry the name and address of the animal owner and the species of the animal. Typical information required on a medication container label prepared by a pharmacy includes the information in Table 6.8.

Once the prescribed medication is in the appropriate container, the medication container label is affixed directly to the container by the person generating the label or may be kept separate for review by the pharmacist before being affixed, depending on state laws and regulations. Figure 6.8 compares a prescription and a medication container label.

From a legal point of view, a medication should be accompanied by information to help a patient understand the appropriate use and common side effects of the dispensed medication. The medication container label contains the information provided on the prescription written by the prescriber. Further information is included: patient medication sheets, FDA-mandated MedGuides, and auxiliary labels. These additional sources of information will be discussed in more detail in the following sections of this chapter.

Medication container labels for Schedule II–V drugs must contain the transfer warning "Caution: Federal law prohibits the transfer of this drug to any person other than the patient for whom it was prescribed." It is common practice for this statement to be placed in small print on all medication container labels.

TABLE 6.8 Medication Container Label Information

- date when prescription filled
- prescription serial number
- pharmacy name and address
- patient name
- prescriber name
- all directions for use given on the prescription
- all necessary auxiliary labels, containing patient precautions
- medication name, whether generic or brand
- medication strength
- drug manufacturer name
- drug quantity
- drug expiration date or date after which drug should not be used because of possible loss of potency or efficacy
- initials of the licensed pharmacist
- number of refills allowed, or the phrase "No Refills"

FIGURE 6.8
**Prescription
and Label
Comparison**

(a) The original
prescription contains
the information that
should be included
on the label.
(b) The medication
container label trans-
lates the instructions
for the patient.

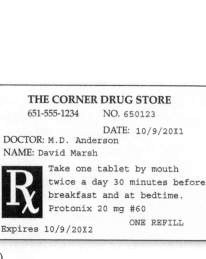

(a)

THE CORNER DRUG STORE
651-555-1234   NO. 650123
                 DATE: 10/9/20X1
DOCTOR: M.D. Anderson
NAME: David Marsh

℞ Take one tablet by mouth
   twice a day 30 minutes before
   breakfast and at bedtime.
   Protonix 20 mg #60
                  ONE REFILL
Expires 10/9/20X2

(b)

Applying Auxiliary Labels

In addition to medication container labels typed with prescriber directions, a medication may be labeled with an auxiliary label. An **auxiliary label** is a small, colorful label that is added to a dispensed medication. An auxiliary label supplements the directions on the medication container label. The application of these auxiliary labels requires a thorough knowledge and understanding of the drug and is thus usually restricted to the professional judgment of the pharmacist. Some pharmacy software may automatically print auxiliary labels when the medication container label is printed. Auxiliary labels may include warnings such as to avoid exposure to sunlight, take with food, take on an empty stomach, and avoid alcohol. With experience, the pharmacist may allow the technician to add auxiliary labeling; if in doubt, be sure to ask the pharmacist for the appropriate labels.

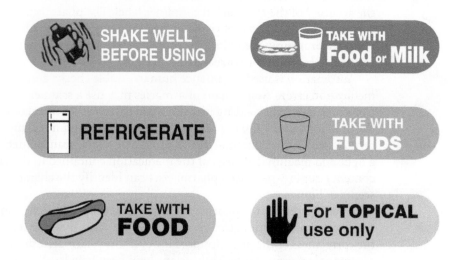

Auxiliary labels are affixed to the medication container by the pharmacist or the pharmacy technician under his or her direct supervision. These labels aid the patient in taking the medication in the safest and most appropriate manner.

Patient Information Sheets

Written information in easily understood terms is available to a patient for each prescription medication. In addition to pharmacists' providing verbal consultation, all pharmacies will print out a take-home patient information sheet or leaflet for the patient. A **patient information sheet** provides details on how to safely use the prescribed medication and is provided to the patient after the prescription is verified by the pharmacist, and after any drug utilization reviews are resolved. Although the information sheet does not replace the counseling provided by the pharmacist or prescriber, the patient may not remember the counseling details if only verbal instructions are given. The written information will provide more detailed information that the patient can review at home when actually taking the medication.

Patient Medication Guides

As discussed in Chapter 3, a patient medication guide, or MedGuide, must be provided to patients receiving a select number of high-risk drugs. The MedGuide is basically a "black box" warning advising consumers of a potential adverse reaction or of the proper use of a medication with a special dosage formulation, such as the inhaled pulmonary drugs Advair or Serevent.

The Final Check of the Prescription

It is extremely important—and required by law—that the pharmacist check every prescription before it is dispensed to the patient to verify its correctness. Typically, the pharmacy technician will present the original prescription, the patient information sheet, and the labeled medication container for final check to the pharmacist. Often the unit stock bottles of tablets, capsules, or liquids will be provided to check the source (and NDC number) of the medication.

The pharmacist reviews the original prescription order, compares it with the patient profile, confirms that the patient information sheet has been printed, verifies that the drug selected by the technician (from the stock bottle) is correct, and checks the accuracy of the medication container label. The pharmacist will often open the vial and perform a physical visual inspection to verify the medication. Additionally, the price or insurance eligibility is often checked to see whether the prescribed drug is covered or billed to the correct insurance plan.

Automation is used to enhance human double checks and minimize the chance of medication errors. Some chain pharmacies may use a scanner to evaluate the medication container label via drug identification software. The bar code may suggest that the prescription for 250 mg of cephalexin should contain red and gray capsules with certain markings. A pharmacist will often do a visual scan (sometimes with the help of a light and magnifying glass) of the medication contained in the vial to verify the contents; some experienced pharmacists can identify the characteristic smells and scents of liquids.

After this review, the pharmacist may initial the medication container label and/or the original prescription. In doing so, the pharmacist assumes legal responsibility for the correctness of the prescription. However, the pharmacist does not necessarily assume sole responsibility. Technicians have been held legally responsible for dispensing and labeling mistakes, especially in situations in which the dispensing error was the result of negligence on their part (e.g., improperly overriding a computerized adverse interaction warning or medication allergy without checking with the pharmacist).

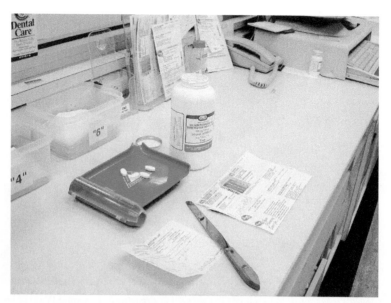

The pharmacy technician must have all prepared prescriptions checked by the supervising pharmacist.

A duplicate of the computer generated copy of the medication container label is usually affixed to the back of the original new prescription by the pharmacist or pharmacy technician. This provides a paper trail of exactly which product (drug, dose, quantity, directions, and NDC number) was used in filling the prescription. It is not uncommon for the filling technician and the verifying pharmacist to initial this copy, especially in the case of a controlled substance.

Once the prescription has completed the final check and the copy of the label has been affixed, the original prescription is filed numerically. Prescription records must be stored and readily retrievable for potential review. Before filing a prescription for a controlled Schedule II substance, the pharmacist must, by law, sign the front or back of the prescription. Some pharmacies require the pharmacist to maintain a perpetual inventory (exact unit count) of these drugs. If the technician records this information, then it must be cosigned by the pharmacist. Even minor discrepancies must be reported to state and federal authorities.

Delivering the Filled Prescription to the Patient

After the final verification and filing of the original prescription, the medication is available for immediate or future distribution to the patient. If the prescription is a "partial fill" or "change of manufacturer," then the pharmacy technician should be sure to relay this information to the patient; in case of a partial fill, the technician should provide the patient with a promised time when the remainder of the prescription can be filled.

Most medications are stored in alphabetical or numeric storage bins. Some medications, such as all insulins, many injections, and suppositories, should be stored in the refrigerator once the final verification by the pharmacist is completed. Other medications, such as antibiotic suspensions, must be mixed just before dispensing. Suitable measuring devices should be provided on all pediatric suspensions and liquids. If "half-tablets" are prescribed, then the pharmacist should recommend that the customer purchase a **tablet splitter** to divide the tablets, especially if the tablets are scored.

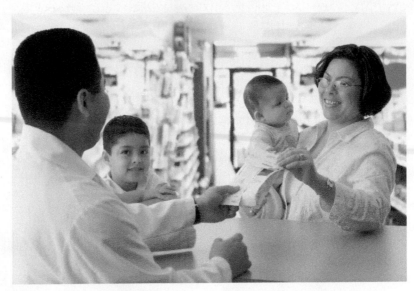

When a patient receives a prescription, the medication will be provided with written information as well as the opportunity to discuss any questions about the medication with the pharmacist.

Medications may be picked up at the pharmacy window (inside the store) or, in some cases, a pharmacy drive-through window. It is very important for the pharmacy technician to verify that the correct patient is receiving the dispensed medication, especially if someone else (i.e., a family member or a friend) picks up the prescription. It is common practice to verify patient address and/or birth date before ringing up the prescription. In the case of controlled substances, a photo ID may be required and documented—a good practice.

The patient information sheet is usually attached to the bag containing the labeled medication and any necessary FDA-mandated MedGuides. Manufacturers of birth control pills provide their own patient labeling. Most pharmacists try to make every effort to counsel every patient on a new prescription and to be available for counseling for any questions on refill medications. The pharmacist may initiate a request to counsel a patient if a questionable allergy, duplicate therapy, potential side effect, or drug–drug interaction warning appeared during the prescription filling process. A private or semiprivate area should be available for medication counseling. The acceptance or decline of counseling by the patient is often documented by the pharmacy technician in the pharmacy software.

Safety Note

By law, the technician must offer the patient (or the patient's representative) the opportunity for verbal counseling by the pharmacist.

Chapter Terms

allergy a hypersensitivity to a specific substance, manifested in a physiological disorder

auxiliary label a supplementary label added to a medication container at the discretion of the pharmacist that provides additional directions

brand name medically necessary a designation on the prescription by the physician indicating that a generic substitution by the pharmacist is not allowed; commonly seen on prescriptions for thyroid medication; often abbreviated as "brand necessary"

DEA number an identification number assigned by the Drug Enforcement Administration (DEA) to identify someone authorized to handle or prescribe controlled substances within the United States

dispense as written (DAW) a notation indicating on a prescription that a brand name drug is necessary or that a generic substitution is not allowed; DAW2 is often used to indicate patient preference for a brand name drug

drug seeker a customer who requests early refills on medications or gets prescriptions from multiple physicians for controlled substances in order to obtain more than the normally prescribed amount of medication

drug utilization review (DUR) a procedure built into pharmacy software designed to help pharmacists check for potential medication errors in dosage, drug interactions, allergies, and so on

e-prescribing the transmission of a prescription via electronic means

inscription the part of the prescription listing the medication or medications prescribed, including the drug names, strengths, and amounts

medication container label a label containing the dosage directions from the physician, affixed to the container of the dispensed medication; the technician may use this hard copy to select the correct stock bottle and to fill the prescription

out of stock (OOS) a medication not in stock in the pharmacy; a drug that must be specially ordered from a drug wholesaler

partial fill a supply dispensed to hold the patient until a new supply is received from the wholesaler because insufficient inventory in the pharmacy prevents completely filling the prescription

patient information sheet a leaflet printed from the prescription software and provided to patients on each medication dispensed; the tech may use this hard copy to select the correct drug stock bottle and fill the prescription

patient profile a record kept by the pharmacy listing a patient's identifying information, insurance information, medical and prescription history, and prescription preferences

prescription an order written by a qualified, licensed practitioner for a medication to be filled by a pharmacist for a patient in order to treat a qualified medical condition

prior authorization (PA) approval for coverage of a high-cost medication or a medication not on the insurer's approved formulary, obtained after a prescriber calls the insurer to justify the use of the drug; must be obtained before the drug is dispensed by the pharmacy in order to be covered by insurance

refill an approval by the prescriber to dispense the prescribed medication again without the need for a new prescription order

safety paper a special tamper-proof paper required in many states for C-II prescriptions to minimize forgeries

signa ("sig") the part of the prescription that indicates the directions for the patient to follow when taking the medication

subscription the part of the prescription that lists instructions to the pharmacist about dispensing the medication, including information about compounding or packaging instructions, labeling instructions, refill information, and information about the appropriateness of dispensing drug equivalencies

tablet splitter a device used to manually split or score tablets

unit of use a fixed number of dose units in a drug stock container, usually consisting of a month's supply, or 30 tablets or capsules

Chapter Summary

- In the community pharmacy, a pharmacy technician assumes a number of responsibilities related to legend drugs; these depend on federal and state laws and regulations.
- The technician assists in the filling of prescriptions, which commonly involves retrieving stock bottles of drugs, counting the prescribed quantity of medications, filling the appropriate containers, and affixing medication container labels.
- A technician can legally take written prescriptions from walk-in customers but cannot take new or transfer prescriptions by telephone and transcribe them.
- The parts of a prescription include prescriber information, the date, patient information, the symbol ℞, the inscription (i.e., the medication or medications prescribed and their amounts), the subscription (i.e., instructions to the pharmacist), the signa (i.e., directions to the patient), additional instructions, and the signature.
- The pharmacy technician is often responsible for entering the new prescription order and creating or updating the computerized patient profile, including identifying information, medical history, medication/prescription history, drug allergy information, insurance/billing information, and prescription preferences.
- The pharmacy technician must become familiar with common abbreviations that are needed to interpret prescriptions and enter information into the patient profile database.

- Both technicians and pharmacists must be able to identify possible forged prescriptions for controlled drugs.
- Prescriptions for controlled substances require special recordkeeping procedures. Pharmacy technicians should be sure to follow any labeling requirements given under state and federal law.
- The patient receives medication information by way of drug and auxiliary labeling on the medication container, patient information sheet, MedGuide, and counseling by the pharmacist.
- Medication container labels must contain a unique prescription number, the name of the patient, the date of the prescription, directions for use, the name and strength of the medication, the manufacturer of the medication, the quantity of the drug, the expiration date or beyond-use date, the initials of the pharmacist, and the number of refills. Auxiliary labels may also be affixed to the container at the discretion of the pharmacist.
- The pharmacist is responsible for the final check of the original prescription and for reviewing the patient profile, the accuracy of the drug and quantity used, and the medication container label.

Chapter Review

Checking Your Understanding

Choose the best answer from those provided.

Additional Quiz Questions

1. The technician's duties with regard to C-II drugs include all the following *except*
   a. receiving the prescription from the patient.
   b. entering the prescription information into the computer patient profile.
   c. retrieving the drug from the secured storage area.
   d. dispensing the drug to the patient.

2. In a prescription, the signa is the
   a. signature of the prescriber.
   b. initials of the pharmacist.
   c. directions for the patient to follow.
   d. instructions to the pharmacist on dispensing the medication.

3. The symbol ℞ stands for the Latin word *recipe* and means
   a. *give.*
   b. *take.*
   c. *prepare.*
   d. *mix.*

4. A signature on a prescription for a Schedule II controlled substance
   a. may be stamped.
   b. must be handwritten.
   c. is not necessary if the prescription is faxed directly from the physician's office.
   d. may be that of the prescriber's agent, such as a nurse, physician assistant, or nurse practitioner.

5. In most states, a generic drug may be substituted for a brand name or proprietary drug provided the generic drug
   a. is the same color and shape of the brand name drug.
   b. has undergone clinical efficacy trials.
   c. is bioequivalent to the brand name or proprietary drug.
   d. is nontoxic.

6. Pharmacy personnel can check to see whether a DEA number has been falsified by
   a. looking up the number in the *FDA Online Orange Book.*
   b. performing a mathematic calculation.
   c. checking the number in *Drug Facts and Comparisons.*
   d. using a code to translate the number into an alphabetic form, which is the name of the prescriber.

7. Refills are commonly dispensed for a 1 month supply of a Schedule III drug
   a. whenever the patient requests it.
   b. when approved by online claims processing to an insurer.
   c. no sooner than 21 days after the last refill.
   d. no sooner than 28 days after the last refill.

8. A pharmacy technician may
   a. receive a new prescription from a patient.
   b. take a new prescription over the phone and immediately transcribe it.
   c. counsel patients on medications when the pharmacist is busy.
   d. check another technician's work before dispensing the drug to the patient.

9. A Schedule III prescription may be refilled a maximum of
   a. once.
   b. twice.
   c. five times, or within 6 months.
   d. twelve times, or within 1 year.

10. For select high-risk drugs, the FDA requires
   a. auxiliary labels.
   b. a patient information sheet.
   c. a medication container label.
   d. a MedGuide.

Thinking Like a Pharmacy Tech

1. For each of the prescriptions below, answer the following questions.
   a. Is any essential item missing from the prescription? If so, then what is this item?
   b. What medication has been prescribed? In what strength? In what amount?
   c. What special instructions, if any, are provided in the subscription?
   d. What directions are given for the patient to follow?

MT. HOPE MEDICAL PARK
MY TOWN, USA 555-3591

\# _127352_   DEA \# _____

PT. NAME _Fred Figule_   DATE _____

ADDRESS _____   DOB _____

_____

Rx   Prednisone   5 mg tabs #12
     Take AM   5 tabs day 1
                   3   "   2
                   2   "   3
                   1 tab " 4 and 5

REFILLS _0_ TIMES

_____ M.D. _A Demomis_ _____ M.D.
DISPENSE AS WRITTEN   SUBSTITUTE PERMITTED

MT. HOPE MEDICAL PARK
MY TOWN, USA 555-3591

\# _42573_   DEA \# _____

PT. NAME _H.R. Rubbins_   DATE _11-24-20XX_

ADDRESS _____   DOB _____

_____

Rx   Tylenol/Codeine No.4
     Take 1 prn pain q4-6 h

                    #30

REFILLS _0_ TIMES

_____ M.D. _J. Jutten_ _____ M.D.
DISPENSE AS WRITTEN   SUBSTITUTE PERMITTED

MT. HOPE MEDICAL PARK
MY TOWN, USA 555-3591

\# _____   DEA \# _____

PT. NAME _Abby Gee_   DATE _9-10-20XX_

ADDRESS _____   DOB _____

_____

Rx   Nexium 40 mg
     Take 1 cap before eating daily

                    #30

REFILLS _0_ TIMES

C. Janew _____ M.D. _____ M.D.
DISPENSE AS WRITTEN   SUBSTITUTE PERMITTED

---

2. Prepare a medication container label for each of the prescriptions shown in the previous question.

a.

Paragon Pharmacy   AP 1111111
670 Main Street   220-555-3245
Anytown, USA

Patient: _____   Prescriber: _____

Drug: _____

Date: _____   Refills: _____

b.

Paragon Pharmacy   AP 1111111
670 Main Street   220-555-3245
Anytown, USA

Patient: _____   Prescriber: _____

Drug: _____

Date: _____   Refills: _____

c.

Paragon Pharmacy   AP 1111111
670 Main Street   220-555-3245
Anytown, USA

Patient: _____   Prescriber: _____

Drug: _____

Date: _____   Refills: _____

3. Review the patient profile below and then answer the following questions.
   a. What essential information is missing from this patient profile?
   b. What allergies and drug reactions does the patient have?
   c. What known medical conditions does the patient have?
   d. What prescriptions and OTC medications is the patient currently taking?
   e. Should the customer's prescription be filled in a child-resistant container? Explain why or why not.
   f. Does the customer have prescription insurance? If so, then in whose name is this insurance held?

PATIENT PROFILE

Patient Name

Frames   *Ted*   *R.*
Last   First   Middle Initial

111 Black Road
Street or PO Box
Guston   *SC*   *29052*
City   State   ZIP

Phone   Date of Birth   Social Security No.
(803) 555 7989   ☐ Male   ___ __ ___
                   Month   Day   Year   ☐ Female

☒ Yes, I would like medication dispensed in a child-resistant container.
☐ No, I do not want medication dispensed in a child-resistant container.

Medication Insurance   Card Holder Name *Ted Frames*
☒ Yes   ☒ Card Holder   ☐ Child   ☐ Disabled Dependent
☐ No   ☐ Spouse   ☐ Dependent Parent   ☐ Full Time Student

MEDICAL HISTORY

HEALTH		ALLERGIES AND DRUG REACTIONS
☐ Angina	☐ Epilepsy	☐ No known drug allergies or reactions
☐ Anemia	☐ Glaucoma	☒ Aspirin
☒ Arthritis	☒ Heart condition	☐ Cephalosporins
☐ Asthma	☐ Kidney disease	☐ Codeine
☐ Blood clotting disorders	☐ Liver disease	☐ Erythromycin
☐ High blood pressure	☐ Lung disease	☐ Penicillin
☐ Breast feeding	☐ Parkinson disease	☒ Sulfa drugs
☐ Cancer	☐ Pregnancy	☐ Tetracyclines
☐ Diabetes	☐ Ulcers	☐ Xanthines
Other conditions ____		☐ Other allergies/reactions ____

Prescription Medication(s) Being Taken   OTC Medication(s) Currently Being Taken
Feldene   20 mg   *Nasalcrom*
Isoptin   80 mg

Would you like generic medication when possible? ☒ Yes ☐ No

Comments

Health information changes periodically. Please notify the pharmacy of any new medications, allergies, drug reactions, or health conditions.

Ted Frames _____ Signature *9-9-XX* Date ☐ I do not wish to provide this information.

4. Determine which of the following is a valid
   DEA number:
   AY 1234563
   AY 2749122

Communicating Clearly

1. Sometimes customers have difficulty identifying the pharmacist and do not understand the different roles of the pharmacist and the pharmacy technician. This can be frustrating for a customer seeking assistance. What types of things could you do, as a pharmacy technician, to help customers identify the pharmacist and his or her capacity?

2. Discuss how you would handle a prescription for a controlled substance that you suspected to be forged.

3. How would you communicate to a patient the following information?
   a. Our pharmacy does not have that medication in stock.
   b. We did not have a sufficient amount of medication to fill your prescription, so we dispensed only a partial fill.
   c. We could not fill your prescription as written; a PA was required.
   d. We could not fill your prescription as written because a serious interaction may occur.

Researching on the Web

1. Visit Walgreens.com.
   a. Find the closest store to your zip code.
   b. Look under Pharmacy: how much does it cost to flavor Prelone syrup?
   c. Again under Pharmacy, find common uses and side effects for Valtrex 500 mg caplets?
   d. Calculate your body mass index in the Health Library.

2. Visit www.dea.gov.
   a. What are the "Facts and Stats" of drug abuse for your state (look under Law Enforcement)?
   b. Under "For Young Adults," check for information concerning drug abuse involving common cough syrups sold in the pharmacy.

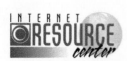

For further study of chapter-related topics, explore the Web links in the Web Center at www.emcp.net/pharmpractice4e.

The Business of Community Pharmacy

7

Learning Objectives

- Understand the roles, responsibilities, and limitations of the technician in the sale of over-the-counter (OTC) drugs, dietary supplements, and medical supplies, especially in the case of a patient who is diabetic.

- Accurately process special OTC sales, such as Schedule V cough syrups, decongestants containing pseudoephedrine, and the Plan B contraceptive.

- Understand the importance of necessary cash register management functions.

- Identify procedures for inventory management, including the purchasing, receiving, and storage of prescription drugs, including controlled substances.

- Discuss drug insurance coverage for private, Medicaid, Tricare, and Medicare plans.

- Define and explain the terms prescription benefits manager (PBM), tiered co-pay, and prior authorization.

- Know how to process a workers' compensation insurance claim.

- Identify the necessary insurance information needed to process online claims for prescription drugs.

- Calculate days supply of medication for online billing.

- Resolve problems with online claims processing.

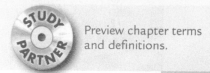

Preview chapter terms and definitions.

The chapter provides an overview of the business functions that are critical to the success of any community pharmacy operation. The pharmacy technician performs an important role in assisting in the sale of OTC medications, herbals, diet supplements, vitamins, and medical supplies. Cash register management is an important skill to learn for all sales. The technician also assists the pharmacist in inventory management—the purchasing, receiving, and stocking of all pharmaceuticals. A key responsibility for the technician is the online billing of third-party insurance. This chapter discusses how to correctly identify, enter, and verify prescription insurance plans for private and government insurance plans. The pharmacy technician must possess a basic understanding of computer and mathematical skills in order to be an invaluable asset in the business operations of a community pharmacy.

Nonprescription Sales

Community pharmacies are generally organized into two areas, a front area and an ℞ area. In the ℞ area, medications requiring a prescription and related items, such as syringes and restricted nonprescription drugs, are stored. In the front area, medications that can be purchased without a prescription, medical supplies, and other merchandise are available for sale. Nonprescription products are commonly stocked by drug class or by indication, such as pain, fever, allergy, first aid, antacid, laxative, foot care, and so on. Condoms or contraceptive jellies for pregnancy protection are also available in this area. The pharmacy technician has a major role in assisting customers in locating necessary OTC drugs, diet supplements, and medical supplies.

Over-the-Counter Drugs

An **over-the-counter (OTC) drug** is one that is approved for sale without a prescription. The FDA approves and regulates OTC drugs only after the drug and dosage are generally recognized as *safe and effective* for the approved indication when taken according to labeled directions. A broad definition of nonprescription products includes not only OTC drugs but also vitamins, minerals, herbal medications, and other products that are sometimes classified as diet supplements.

Many OTC drugs of today, such as hydrocortisone, loperamide (Imodium), and ibuprofen (Advil, Motrin IB) once required a prescription. Although OTC medications may be purchased without a prescription, the active ingredients are often the same as those found in higher-strength prescription formulations. For example, ibuprofen is available in an OTC strength of 200 mg, whereas the prescription strengths are 400 mg, 600 mg, and 800 mg.

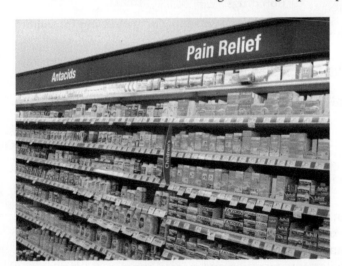

OTC medications are commonly stocked by symptom, such as pain relief, antacids, and so on.

Customers are purchasing OTC products for self-administration at an ever-increasing rate. The increase in the use of OTC drugs is related to a number of factors, including the increased cost and inconvenience (that is to say, taking time off work) of physician visits, the rising cost of prescription medications, and lack of health or drug insurance coverage. With OTC products, patients can obtain medications to treat everyday symptoms of illness or to maintain health.

OTC drugs can be purchased in nearly any retail outlet, not just the pharmacy. This, in addition to the fact that the consumer often self-selects and self-medicates with an OTC drug, demonstrates the importance of product labeling. The manufacturer must include all information on the OTC product label that is necessary for the safe and effective use of the product by the consumer. The language on the product label must be both understandable and readable. Such information should include dosage and frequency of administration for different age groups, as well as precautions, warnings, and expiration dates.

Consumers using OTC drugs need to remember that OTC drugs should be used for a limited duration of time (usually less than 7 days) for self-limiting indications such as a cold or cough, unless directed by a physician. For example, a physician may direct an adult patient to take a baby aspirin on a long-term daily basis in order to lower a patient's risk of heart disease. If the pharmacist cannot determine the source of a self-limited problem, or if the patient has self-medicated with an OTC drug for 7 or more days, the patient should be referred to the appropriate healthcare professional.

The technician and the consumer must also remember that no drug, even an OTC, is completely safe and without side effects or adverse reactions. Even OTC cough medicines could potentially be misused if the dosage recommended by the manufacturer is exceeded. In fact, for OTC products that contain the cough suppressant dextromethorphan (DM), the technician must confirm that the age of the customer is greater than 18 years before the sale can be completed. The use of OTC cough and cold products for children under the age of six years is strongly discouraged by the FDA because the risk of adverse reactions is greater than the benefit.

Customers often seek the counsel of the pharmacist to verify the assessment of their symptoms. For example, a pharmacist may need to identify and select a sugar-free cough syrup for a young patient who is diabetic, a laxative for a pregnant patient who is taking a prenatal vitamin and iron, or an appropriate nasal decongestant for a patient with high blood pressure. A pharmacy technician's support allows the pharmacist the necessary time from prescription-filling duties to assess a self-limited problem, make an appropriate drug product selection, and counsel the patient.

OTC drugs are becoming an increasingly important part of the technician's responsibilities. Technicians often carry out such functions as selling and stocking of the OTC products, ordering or rearranging inventory, and removing stock when the shelf life has expired. However, questions about drug product selection, indications, dosage and administration, expected therapeutic effect, side effects, contraindications, and interactions should always be referred to the pharmacist.

Schedule V Drugs A **Schedule V drug** is a medication with a low potential for abuse and a limited potential for creating physical or psychological dependence. A common example of a Schedule V medication is a cough medication containing codeine. Although federal law allows the dispensing of Schedule V medications without a prescription, there are restrictions and requirements for the sale. For example:

- The drugs must be stored behind the counter, in the prescription area.
- The amount of cough syrups sold to a single customer is generally limited to a specific volume (such as 120 fl oz or 4 fl oz) within a 48 hour period.
- Only a pharmacist (or the pharmacy technician under direct supervision) can make the sale.
- The purchaser must be 18 years of age and have proof of identity.

A state may have more stringent laws for Schedule V drugs than the federal government. For example, some states require a signed prescription from a licensed healthcare professional for Schedule V drugs, so be sure to check the laws in your state. To discourage potential drug abuse, many pharmacies have instituted a policy of dispensing no Schedule V drugs (even if legally allowed) without a prescription from a physician.

If the sale of an OTC drug that is also a Schedule V drug is allowed, then the pharmacy technician or the pharmacist must record all sales in a record book. This record must include the following information:

- Name and address of the purchaser
- Date of birth of the purchaser
- Date of purchase
- Name and quantity of the Schedule V drug sold
- Name and initials of the pharmacist handling or approving the sale

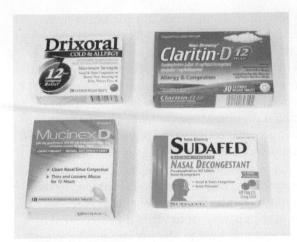

OTC products that contain pseudoephedrine must be stored in the prescription area and certain conditions must be met before a sale is completed.

Drugs That Contain Pseudoephedrine The federal government and many states have passed legislation restricting the access and sale of OTC products that contain pseudoephedrine (and ephedra). These restrictions have been put in place because the common ingredients of OTC cold and sinus medications have been used as raw products in the illegal manufacture of methamphetamine. Mandated limits determine how many "units" of these drugs can be legally purchased at one time at one location. These products must be stocked behind the prescription counter and sold to the patient directly by the pharmacist or the pharmacy technician. The purchaser must be 18 years old or older.

The sale of pseudoephedrine requires a written (or computerized) record similar to that for Schedule V drugs (see Figure 7.1). The information required prior to the sale of these products includes:

- A validated and current photo ID, which is usually a driver's license
- A driver's license number or a personal identification card number
- Proof that the customer is 18 years old or older
- The street address, state, and ZIP code of the customer
- The customer's signature

Plan B "Prescription" Plan B is an emergency contraceptive drug that can be dispensed in most states without a prescription. However, federal and state laws require that the patient (or the patient's representative) be over the age of 18 years (17 years in some states) in order to be allowed to purchase the drug. All patients purchasing Plan B should be counseled by the pharmacist on the appropriate use and expected side effects of this drug.

Diet Supplements

A **diet supplement** can be a vitamin, mineral, or an herbal product. Diet supplements are sold in retail outlets and in nutrition and wellness stores, as well as in pharmacies. Most consumers do not realize that diet supplements are not regulated by the FDA in the same stringent manner as are OTC drugs, and scientific studies on the efficacy of these products are usually quite limited.

FIGURE 7.1
Form for Recording Sales of Restricted Products Containing Pseudoephedrine

Pseudoephedrine (PSE) Products Dispensing Record							
Purchaser's Name	Driver's License Number	Purchaser's Address	Date of Purchase	Product Name	Quantity Purchased	Dispensed by (Initials)	Purchaser's Signature

TABLE 7.1   Indications for Common Diet Supplements

Diet Supplement	Indications
calcium and vitamin D	osteoporosis
echinacea	boosts immune system
garlic	antibacterial and antiviral action; maintains healthy cholesterol
ginger	nausea, motion sickness
gingko	memory
glucosamine/chondroitin	osteoarthritis
melatonin	insomnia, especially in shift workers or time zone travelers
Policosanol	maintains healthy cholesterol
omega-3 fatty acids (fish oil)	lowers triglycerides
saw palmetto	benign prostatic hypertrophy or BPH
St. John's wort	mild depression
vitamin C	common cold
zinc	boosts immune system, common cold

As you learned in Chapter 2, diet supplements are primarily regulated by DSHEA. The FDA does not approve diet supplements; however, they must be *safe and accurately labeled*. If a diet supplement is deemed dangerous or if the marketing claims or labels include disease indications, then the FDA can act to remove the drug from the market. This has occurred with "diet pills" in the past. Another example of unregulated diet supplement use is the misuse of androgenic hormones by professional and high school athletes to enhance their athletic performance.

The dosage of a dietary supplement is usually indicated as a daily serving size rather than dose; the label can make no "disease" claim (without prior approval by the FDA), and information to the patient on the label is quite limited compared to that for an OTC drug. The amount of active ingredient in the product may not always match the labeled amount because of inconsistencies in quality control or product contamination.

In addition to vitamins and minerals, diet supplements may include natural herbals, such as ginger, garlic, saw palmetto, or other products such as glucosamine and soy. Indications for some common diet supplements are listed in Table 7.1. As with the use of other OTC medications, it is important that the pharmacy technician not counsel customers in regard to the appropriate use of diet supplements unless directed to do so by the pharmacist.

Medical Supplies

A community pharmacy is a source of multiple disposable and durable medical supplies that may be needed by a customer or a member of the customer's family. Some community pharmacies specialize in the sale or rental of **durable medical equipment (DME)**. DME includes hospital beds, wheelchairs, canes, walkers, crutches, ostomy supplies, and so on.

Some pharmacies are licensed as medical suppliers, with the ability to provide direct Medicare Part B insurance coverage for many medical supplies and drugs for those patients over the age of 65 years. In addition to DME equipment, diabetic supplies, and nebulizer drugs, the pharmacy may also cover enteral nutrition and expensive injectable drugs for anemia or for nausea and vomiting caused by cancer chemotherapy.

Supplies to Manage Diabetes Customers with diabetes will require specific medical supplies to monitor and manage their blood sugar levels. For example, they need insulin syringes, a glucometer, diabetic test strips, lancets to pierce the skin for blood, and alcohol wipes for use before and after using the lancet and needle sticks. These supplies are often purchased in the community pharmacy. The pharmacy technician can assist the customer in locating the requested products and medical supplies in the pharmacy.

Patients who are diabetic require insulin syringes to self-administer their daily insulin shots. The policy for the sale of insulin syringes in a community pharmacy may vary by state in order to prevent diversion to potential illegal drug administration. Many pharmacies have a policy that no insulin syringes can be sold unless the patient is a proven diabetic or known customer of the pharmacy.

Insulin syringes and needles come in different sizes. Syringes are generally available in 0.3 mL, 0.5 mL, and 1 mL sizes depending on the dosage of the insulin prescribed. Instead of being marked in milliliters, the insulin syringe is marked in units in order to make the insulin administration more accurate. Most needles are "short"—either ½ inch or ⁵⁄₁₆ inch or ¼ inch—for easier and less painful injection under the skin rather than muscle. The needle width is commonly between 29 and 31 gauge; the higher the gauge number, the smaller the width of the needle, with potentially less pain at the injection site.

The proper disposal of insulin syringes is important to minimize the transmission of communicable diseases such as hepatitis or human immunodeficiency virus (HIV). A patient should purchase a sharps container to dispose of insulin syringes safely; alternatively, many pharmacies may offer to dispose of used insulin syringes properly.

Glucometers are devices that measure blood sugar for patients who are diabetic. Glucometers are available in different sizes and with different features, such as the amount of blood needed to make a reading, the amount of time to provide the results of a reading, memory capacity, and the ability to interface with a computer. These products often can be purchased with a generous rebate that negates a majority of the original purchase price. Companies frequently upgrade their glucometers, so it is important for both the pharmacist and the technician to keep abreast of product changes.

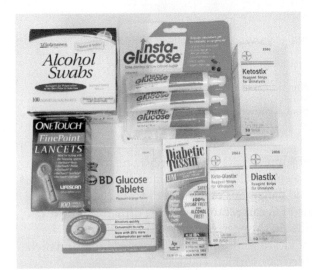

A patient who is diabetic is a frequent customer in the community pharmacy, with needs for glucose tablets and gel, lancets, alcohol wipes, and other supplies.

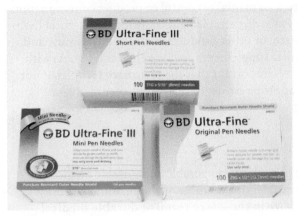

The technician can assist the patient who is diabetic in selecting the correct size and gauge of insulin needles.

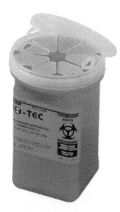

The proper disposal of insulin syringes in a sharps container is important to minimize the transmission of infectious diseases, even in the home.

Disposable test strips are needed with the glucometer to test the blood sugar. A test strip is the piece of paper on which the patient puts a drop of blood after piercing his or her finger with a lancet device. The test strip is then put into the glucometer for a blood sugar reading. Test strips are machine-specific and must be matched for the type of glucometer that the patient is using. Some test strips come with a computer chip (lot number) that must be inserted in the glucometer. Failure to replace this chip with a new bottle (different lot number) of test strips will lead to an error in the blood glucose readings. Test strips may be used from one time daily up to six times daily. Test strips can be expensive if the patient does not have insurance coverage. The expiration date of the strips should be checked carefully by the technician prior to sale.

Insulin syringes and other diabetic supplies are sometimes covered by drug insurance or Medicare Part B if a prescription is written by the physician. If a patient is going to apply insurance coverage to the purchase of diabetic medical supplies, then it is important that the patient have a prescription from the prescriber indicating the ICD-9 diagnosis code and frequency of daily insulin injections and blood glucose testing. A **certificate of medical necessity** for diabetic supplies for each patient may need to be completed and signed by the prescriber (see Figure 7.2).

The proper use of diabetic supplies is important in monitoring the patient's diabetes. A level of blood sugar, maintained in an acceptable range, delays or minimizes the development of long-term complications of diabetes and improves both the quality of

FIGURE 7.2
Certificate of Medical Necessity

If a physician writes a prescription and completes a certificate of medical necessity, then the cost of diabetic supplies may be partially covered by Medicare Part B or prescription insurance for some patients.

Patient Demographics			
Select Type of Diabetes ☐ Type 1 IDDM, Insulin Dependent ☐ Type 2 NIDDM, Non Insulin Dependent ☐ Type 2 NIDDMIR, Requires Insulin		**Indicates Diabetes Diagnosis** ICD-9 _ _ _ . _ _ ICD-9 _ _ _ . _ _ Type 1 Diabetic, ICD-9 must end in odd number. Type 2 Diabetic, ICD-9 must end in even number.	

	Required Supplies		
Number of Tests/Day	**Number of Test Strips**	**Number of Lancets**	**Healthcare Orders**
☐ 1			
☐ 2			
☐ 3			_____ test strips
☐ 4			_____ lancets
☐ 5			_____ glucometer(s)
☐ 6			_____ lancet skin piercing device(s)
☐ 7			_____ bottle(s) of control solution
☐ 8			
☐ 9			
☐ 10			
☐ 11			
☐ 12			
Provider Demographics with Date and Signature			

life and life expectancy. Matching the specific needs of the patient with the proper equipment and supplies is an important responsibility for the pharmacist. Many pharmacists acquire specialty training and certifications in this area. Experienced pharmacy technicians can now complete training, pass an examination, and become certified in patient education for diabetic patients. Such skills are considered valuable within the pharmacy and may enhance hourly pay.

Test Kits In addition to testing for blood sugar, patients come to the pharmacy to purchase any number of test kits to help them monitor their health conditions. Women may be interested in purchasing pregnancy or ovulation test kits. There are test kits to measure cholesterol level in the blood. Urine test kits measure the amount of sugar or ketones in the urine of a patient who is diabetic and test for bladder infections. Kits are also available to test for various illegal drugs. Occasionally, the pharmacy may need to special order a test kit product from a wholesaler for a customer. The pharmacy technician can be helpful in the identification, selection, and sale of a needed test kit and can help the patient understand the kit's instructions.

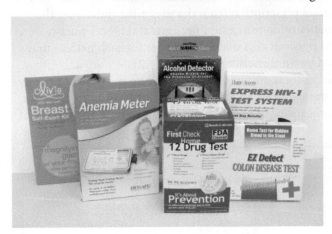

A typical community pharmacy sells many kinds of test kits. The pharmacy technician can assist the customer in selecting the best product to meet his or her needs.

General Medical Supplies Customers purchase several types of general medical supplies from a community pharmacy, and the pharmacy technician also assists with these transactions. Parents may need to purchase thermometers to check for fever in their kids. Patients with high blood pressure may need to purchase a measuring device for home use; the results can be recorded and brought to the physician's office on the next visit. Patients with asthma may need a spacer device to deliver inhaled medication more accurately or a peak flow meter to measure their expirations and assess severity of symptoms or benefit of therapy. Others may need wrist splints, back braces, bathroom accessories, nebulizer tubing and masks, and so on. Customers also need bandages, gauze pads, adhesive tape, hydrogen peroxide, or isopropyl or rubbing alcohol to attend to their first-aid needs.

Computer Systems in the Pharmacy

A computer is a critical tool needed for the safe and efficient dispensing of prescriptions and online billing in the community pharmacy. A **computer** is simply an electronic device used for inputting, storing, processing, and/or outputting information. Because of the complexity of overall pharmacy operations , the computer is an absolutely essential tool in the community pharmacy.

The aspiring pharmacy technician needs to have a working knowledge of computer hardware; the software is often pharmacy-specific and must be learned on-the-job. Competency at basic keyboarding (in other words, typing), with a minimum proficiency of 30 words per minute, is essential.

In most small, independent pharmacies, the computer is a **smart terminal** that contains its own storage and processing capabilities. In larger pharmacies, including most drug chains, the technician or pharmacist may work at a **dumb terminal**, a computer device that contains a keyboard and a monitor but does not contain its own storage and processing capabilities. The terminal is connected to a **remote computer**—often a mini-computer or a mainframe at the company headquarters or home office—that stores and processes data such as patient information, prescription history, and insurance coverage.

The software is designed to help the pharmacy technician process the prescription with both speed and accuracy. Pharmacy software varies widely from pharmacy to pharmacy, but most pharmacies use a software program application that allows one to enter, retrieve, and query patient records. This type of software is referred to as a **database management system (DBMS)**. Examples of DBMS include the patient profile, physician database, and pharmacy drug inventory. Often the software is menu-driven (or Windows-based), allowing the technician to choose fields or functions easily from a menu of options on the screen by typing a single number, letter, or function key on the keyboard.

The patient profile discussed in Chapter 6 is created and managed through a DBMS. The software stores demographic, insurance, and prescription information on every patient. The software allows the technician to retrieve patient profiles on-screen and to enter new prescription information. Care must be taken to identify the correct patient, not only by name but by date of birth or telephone number. The database software contains many fields of information that can be sorted (or queried) to meet the needs of that pharmacy or drug chain. Fields of information may include the patient's name, address, phone number, and date of birth; the prescription's number, drug name, and NDC number, dosage and quantity of drug, and number of refills; and the prescriber's name, address, phone, and DEA number.

Contemporary pharmacy computer systems have evolved into complex systems offering a wide range of functions, such as checking for possible allergies and drug

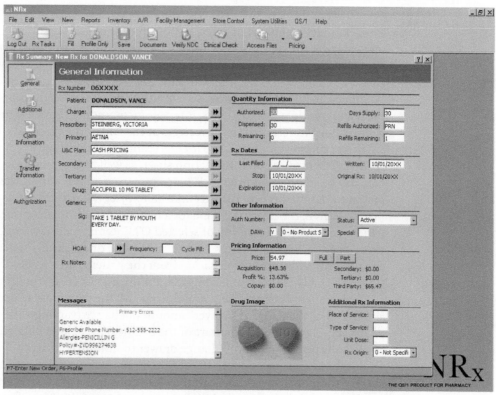

On-screen entry of patient and prescription data via a database management system (DBMS) is a valuable tool used by the pharmacy technician to easily and accurately process prescriptions.

interactions or printing medication container labels and patient information sheets. As discussed in Chapter 6, most pharmacy computer systems contain automatic warnings about possible allergic or other adverse reactions as part of the drug utilization review (DUR). These automatically generated warnings provide the pharmacist with an opportunity to review the prescriptions and the profile to minimize medication errors.

The pharmacy software accesses insurance plans via telecommunications (in other words, connecting to the remote computer via telephone lines, digital subscriber line [DSL], cable, or wireless connections) to perform immediate online billing. Wireless communications involve the transmission of data or voice signals through the air via transmitters, receivers, and, often, satellites. Wireless communications are critical for determining patient eligibility and online processing of prescription claims (discussed later in this chapter). Links to online insurance plans may also warn of potential errors with prescriptions previously dispensed at another pharmacy.

Some specially designed computer systems are capable of controlling automatic or robotic dispensing and compounding devices, tracking expenses and inventory reports, generating reports concerning controlled substances or patient insurance, performing special dosing calculations, or retrieving medical and pharmacy literature. Other systems may provide a picture or description of the medication for a final visual check by the pharmacist, in order to minimize medication errors.

Computers occasionally break down and are susceptible to such problems as power failures and surges. Therefore copies, or backups, of all data should be made at regular intervals. A pharmacy may use a CD, magnetic tape backup devices, or remote storage to back up its prescription records, usually on a daily basis.

Cash Register Management

The pharmacy technician is often responsible for collecting money that the patient owes to cover the cost of prescriptions and OTC drugs, vitamins, herbs, diet supplements, medical supplies, and other store merchandise. Payment may be with cash, check, or credit card. The procedures for cash register management differ with each pharmacy. In larger pharmacies with multiple pharmacy technicians (and pharmacists) and multiple cash registers, it is not uncommon to have a sign-on and password code to assist in reconciling the receipts at the end of the day or shift.

Larger pharmacies may use bar-code scanning technology in concert with the cash register. The medication information sheet, as well as any nonprescription merchandise, can be scanned for pricing. When a prescription is scanned, the computer system may automatically prompt the technician to offer the patient counseling by the pharmacist. (Often, the pharmacist makes a note on the information sheet to initiate patient counseling.) Scanning of selected OTC items, such as pseudoephedrine products, Schedule V cough syrups, and contraceptive drugs (as discussed earlier), prompts a request for additional information from the patient, such as proof of age and identification. Finally, if the item is nonprescription, a sales tax is usually added.

Cash transactions are fairly straightforward: the cash register usually calculates the amount of change needed. A given amount of change (varying with the size of the pharmacy) is provided at the start of the business day. Large bills, such as $50 or $100, are usually placed under the change drawer to minimize mix-ups.

Some patients may elect to pay for their pharmacy purchases with a personal check. Procedures may differ with the pharmacy. If the patient is not recognized as a regular customer, then the technician may need to ask for identification, such as a

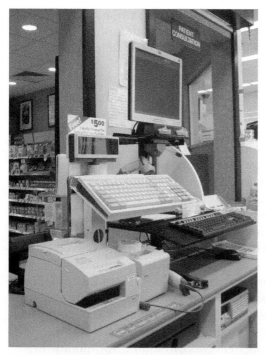

The workstation of the pharmacy technician often consists of a bar-code scanner, cash register, computer, and telephone.

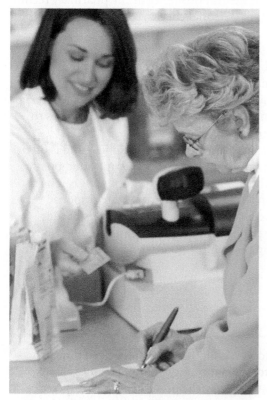

An important part of the pharmacy technician's role is to accept payment for pharmacy purchases in cash, check, or credit card from a customer.

driver's license, and to transfer that information to the check. The amount of the check and the signature should always be verified. In a nonautomated system, it is possible for the pharmacy to receive a check with insufficient funds to cover the bill. Most pharmacies have a policy on the additional cost of rebilling bad checks; in most cases, this higher cost acts as a deterrent. In some cases, the pharmacy may keep a list of customer names from whom the technician is not allowed to accept checks.

Larger pharmacies may have a check reader connected to the cash register. The signed check is fed into the reader and the bank account is immediately accessed; in some cases, the check reader prints the entire check, ready for customer signature. If the account shows insufficient funds for the check, then a prompt alerts the technician not to accept the check and to seek an alternate source of payment.

In addition to cash and check transactions, payments may be made by a credit, debit, Flex, or even a store gift card. Scanning technology is usually available for the patient or the technician to swipe any type of card and follow the prompts. A **credit card** doesn't deduct the money directly but is a type of loan that is either paid off at the end of the month or accrues a finance charge. Depending on the policy of the pharmacy, patients may or may not need to sign a credit card expense of less than $50. Some chain pharmacies have express pay options such that the credit card is automatically billed at the time of prescription filling.

A **debit card** is also a form of online cash payment; unlike a credit card, a debit card instantly deducts the cost of the purchase from the customer's bank account. A debit card purchase requires the customer to enter a confidential PIN number for account activation. A debit card can be used as a credit card if it is inconvenient for the customer to enter a PIN number, such as picking up prescriptions at the drive-through pharmacy. The amount of the purchase should be verified prior to processing. Generally these cards do not require a signature because the money is immediately transferred from the bank account. Credit and debit cards allow the option of the customer to request cash back after the claim is processed.

A **Flex card** is a medical credit card for prescription co-pays and select IRS-approved OTC items. The Flex card is cross-referenced with the bar code of the product so that coverage is known immediately. The Flex card option is available to customers with high deductible medical insurance plans. An individual contributes to a medical fund for out-of-pocket costs for medical and pharmacy co-pays as well as OTC drugs. The Flex card minimizes the need for submission of receipts and prevents delays in reimbursement. In addition there are tax advantages when individuals file their income taxes at year end if a Flex card account is used.

Gift cards are handled similarly to credit, debit, and Flex cards, with the amount embedded in the bar code. With product or store coupons, as well as drug rebate forms, the technician must carefully review the requirements and expiration date before scanning. All credit card receipts (and coupons) are placed under the change drawer or in a separate secure location for later reconciliation.

Some small independent pharmacies allow their best customers to run a charge account and settle with the pharmacy at the end of the month. Personal charge accounts usually add to the overhead of the pharmacy because billing statements may need to be mailed out each month. If discretion is not used, then the pharmacy may have a lot of unpaid bills that cannot be collected, especially if ownership is being transferred.

Regardless of form of payment, the technician should always present a receipt at the conclusion of the purchase. A **receipt** is a proof-of-purchase printout.

Occasionally sales of prescription or nonprescription items are voided—drugs may not be covered by insurance, the co-pay may be too high, or the merchandise may not be available at the same price as the customer assumed. In such cases, the sale must be voided and some record of the event must be recorded by the technician. Often the cash register also can verify the price of store items, and, in some cases, modify the price of prescription or nonprescription items. If the patient is due a refund from a prior purchase, then it may be necessary to get administrative approval from either the pharmacist or the store manager.

At the end of the business day, it is often the responsibility of the pharmacy technician to reconcile the cash, credit card receipts, personal checks, coupons, rebates, voided sales, and patient charges (if allowed) with the tape printout from the cash register. It is common to be off a few cents or dollars once in a while, but frequent or large discrepancies must be immediately brought to the attention of the pharmacist. In a chain pharmacy, the store manager may be responsible for reconciling the cash register, but technicians must be accountable for all customer receipts. The technician needs to understand that surveillance cameras are available in many pharmacies to protect the pharmacy from money loss or drug diversion.

The pharmacy technician is the one most accessible to the customer—and is often the final contact with the customer at the time of prescription pickup. Good public relation skills are required. Dealing with the public for an eight hour shift can be difficult and tiring. It is not uncommon in larger pharmacies to rotate responsibilities so that every two to four hours the technician may have different responsibilities— collecting payments and dealing with the public, entering new prescriptions and refill requests, resolving insurance claims, filling prescriptions, ordering medications, and so on.

Inventory Management

The entire stock of pharmaceutical products on hand for sale at any given time in a community pharmacy is known as **inventory**. Community pharmacies must stock, or have ready access to, all drugs that may be written by the prescribers in their practice area. Unlike some businesses, however, a pharmacy may need to keep some very slow-moving drugs in stock as a service to a few customers. If the inventory is too tight, then

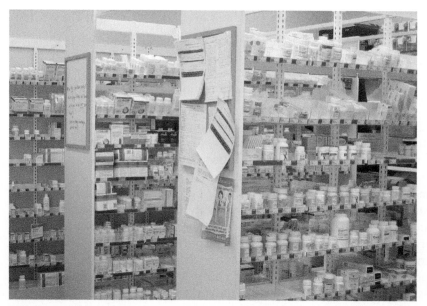

The pharmacy inventory must be carefully maintained to have an adequate but not excessive stock of drugs.

the pharmacy frequently runs out of needed medication, causing either a loss of sale or an inconvenience to the patient, who must make another trip to the pharmacy when the inventory has been replenished.

Inventory value is defined as the total value of the drugs and merchandise in stock on a given day. In addition to prescription drugs, inventory includes OTC drugs, diet supplements, medical supplies, and front-end merchandise. Inventory management should be designed so that medications arrive shortly before they are dispensed and sold, to minimize shelf space needed and maximize cash flow. The primary purposes of inventory management are the timely purchase and receipt of pharmaceuticals and establishing and maintaining appropriate levels of materials in stock.

Several important issues with regard to inventory management include the following: how much inventory should be maintained, when inventory levels should be adjusted, and where inventory should be stored. Factors that bear on decisions regarding these issues include turnover of products, floor space allocation, design and arrangement of shelves, and demands on available refrigerator or freezer space.

Managing inventory is an important responsibility of the pharmacy technician. Restocking drug inventory, doing proper shelf labeling, locating stock, setting inventory reorder levels, rotating stock, and checking expiration dates are all important roles in the pharmacy. Checking for expired vitamins and herbs is especially important, because they can lose their labeled potency quickly. Pharmacy technicians should remove all expired products from stock and return them for credit.

Purchasing, receiving, and inventory processes should be as uncomplicated as possible so as not to disrupt or interfere with the other activities of the pharmacy. Pharmacies must maintain a record of drugs and other supplies and merchandise purchased and sold in order to know when to reorder and when to adjust inventory levels of each item. The purchase and receipt of controlled drugs require additional procedures and documentation.

Purchasing

Purchasing is defined as the ordering of products for use or sale by the pharmacy and is usually carried out by either an independent or group process. In independent purchasing, the pharmacist deals directly with a drug wholesaler regarding matters such as price and contractual terms. In group purchasing, a number of independent pharmacies work together to negotiate a discount for high-volume purchases and more favorable contract terms. The state pharmacy association may act as a facilitator for group purchasing, contracting for its members as a benefit.

The following three primary purchasing methods or systems are used in pharmacies:

- **Wholesaler purchasing** enables the community pharmacy to use a single source to purchase and receive numerous products from multiple manufacturers of brand and generic name pharmaceuticals. Some pharmacies use more than one wholesaler. Advantages of wholesaler purchasing include reduced turnaround time for orders, lower inventory and lower associated costs, and reduced commitment of time and staff. Disadvantages include higher purchase cost, occasional supply shortages (called back orders), and unavailability of some pharmaceuticals. The turnaround time for receipt of drug orders is usually the next day, with the possible exception of weekends and Schedule II drugs.

- **Just-in-time (JIT) purchasing** involves frequent purchasing in quantities that just meet supply needs until the next ordering time. JIT reduces the quantity of each product on the shelves and thus reduces the amount of money committed to inventory. However, such a system can be used only when supplies are readily available and pharmaceutical needs can be accurately predicted. Automation can enhance the accuracy of replacing needed inventory levels of drugs. In large chain pharmacies, a regional or centralized warehouse may provide JIT purchasing.

- **Prime vendor purchasing** involves an exclusive agreement made by a pharmacy for a specified percentage or dollar volume of purchases. Prime vendor purchasing offers the advantages of lower acquisition costs, competitive service fees, electronic order entry, and emergency delivery services. This type of purchasing is more common in hospital pharmacies.

The pharmacy technician plays a critical role in the purchasing of pharmaceuticals. Today a variety of methods may be used for inventory management to determine when a product needs to be reordered A small independent pharmacy may use a "want book" to record inventory that needs to be replaced; after a time, the technician has a good sense of how fast drug products move off the shelves and when they need to be reordered. Manual or automated inventory records based on usage and seasonal patterns may be used. For example more antibiotics and cough and cold products may be purchased during the winter season. For fast movers, the purchase decision is often based on the most economic order quantity or best value (in other words, ordering capsules in a 1000 count size rather than 100 count size, or buying a case of antacid liquid rather than one or two bottles).

Other pharmacies have software to automate the drug ordering process, which can automatically generate purchase orders under predetermined conditions. An important goal of computerized inventory control is to reduce the time and staff required for inventory management, as well as to maintain an appropriate balance of adequate stock with adequate inventory turnover. Each time that drugs are purchased from the wholesaler, the product, quantity, and price are entered into the computer database. As each prescription is dispensed or as a customer purchases a nonprescription product, the computer system automatically adjusts the inventory record. Pharmacies usually establish an inventory range for each item (in other words, a maximum and a minimum number of units to have on hand). When the inventory drops to the minimum level, the item is purchased to restock the supply. This predetermined order point and the order quantity are based on the historical use of each drug. The following is an example of a calculation used to make inventory management decisions.

Example 1	The maximum inventory level for amoxicillin 500 mg capsules is 2000 capsules. At the end of the day, the computer prints a list of items to be reordered; the list indicates an inventory level of 975 amoxicillin capsules, the minimum quantity—and the point to reorder automatically is 1000 capsules. Has the automatic reorder level been reached? How many capsules should be ordered?

$$\text{maximum inventory} - \text{present inventory} = \text{amount sold}$$

$$2000 \text{ capsules} - 975 \text{ capsules} = 1025 \text{ capsules}$$

Because 1025 capsules sold is more than the minimum number needed to reorder automatically, the automatic reorder level has been reached. One bottle of 1000 capsules (or two bottles of 500 capsules) is ordered.

As discussed in Chapter 6, the technician also needs to consider special onetime orders for a specific patient, partial-fill prescriptions, and out-of-stock (OOS) requests that occur during the day when placing an order. Most drug ordering occurs online, but telephoning a wholesaler may be needed for special or late-in-the-day orders. Special orders for seldom stocked injectable products may require additional delivery time if they are not in the wholesaler's inventory.

Occasionally a pharmaceutical product is temporarily or permanently unavailable from a supplier. The reason should be determined—back ordered by warehouse, drug recalled by the manufacturer, drug discontinued, and so on. An alternate source or product may need to be identified, or the drug may need to be borrowed from another pharmacy if a patient is waiting for a certain medication. A policy and procedure for control and accountability for loaned or borrowed products are necessary. If a pharmacy does not have a certain medication, then it is common to check with a local competing pharmacy and transfer the prescription if such a pharmacy has the product in stock.

The pharmacy technician also has other inventorying responsibilities that are important to making the business of a community pharmacy successful. The technician is responsible for ordering and stocking necessary prescription supplies (various sizes of vials and bottles, medication and auxiliary labels, information sheets, measuring devices, paper). These supplies may or may not be available from the wholesaler and may require several days to receive if ordered directly from a manufacturer, so an adequate inventory must be kept on hand.

Receiving and Posting

The physical delivery of an order of products from a wholesaler, warehouse, or other pharmacy initiates a series of procedures known as **receiving**. As part of the receiving process, the pharmaceutical products must be carefully checked against the purchase order or requisition. The pharmacist or technician usually signs an invoice from a delivery representative, verifying the receipt of the number of totes or boxes delivered from the wholesaler. A separate invoice is required for the receipt of controlled substances.

The contents of any shipment should be verified for name of product, manufacturer, quantity received versus ordered, product strength, and package size. As discussed in Chapter 3, the NDC, a number assigned to every drug product, consists of three parts

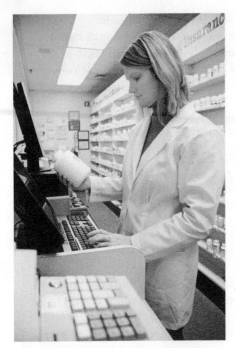

Pharmaceuticals in a shipment should be carefully checked by the pharmacy technician for NDC numbers, price updates, and expiration dates and then entered into the computer database.

separated by dashes: the first part represents the number assigned to the manufacturer of the drug product, the second represents the drug entity (generic name and strength), and the third indicates the package size of the drug. A drug ordered but not received should immediately be brought to the attention of the pharmacist, who can initiate the appropriate action.

Posting is the process of reconciling the invoice and updating inventory in the pharmacy product database. Any large price increases should be brought to the attention of the pharmacist for verification. As part of the posting process, the pharmacy technician affixes stickers to the received unit stock bottles. These stickers document the wholesaler's item number and pricing information.

Each pharmacy has a policy for an acceptable range of product expiration dates. A typical requirement might be that products have expiration dates of at least six months from the date of receipt. After products are received and checked, they are placed in a proper storage location and under proper storage conditions (in other words, refrigeration). New products may require new shelf labeling. An accepted method for stocking pharmaceuticals is to position the units of product with the shortest expiration dates where they will be the first units selected for use.

Once the wholesaler order is received and posted as part of the inventory, all partial-fill and out-of-stock (OOS) prescriptions from the day before should be filled, and the patient should be notified that the prescription is now ready.

Drug Returns and Credits

Product shortages or products that are damaged in shipment or improperly shipped or stored must be reported to the pharmacist and vendor immediately. Stringent laws regulate the return of pharmaceuticals to manufacturers, especially controlled substances. In the case of a damaged or incorrect shipment, the wholesaler should be notified immediately and authorization should be secured for the return of the defective shipment as soon as possible.

The pharmacy technician is often responsible for handling drug returns to the wholesaler for credits of both prescription and nonprescription drugs. These returns may be because of drug overstocks, expired drugs, drug recalls by the drug manufacturer or FDA, reformulated drugs, drugs in new packaging, or drugs that are no longer manufactured. This process often involves a lot of paperwork and is time-consuming; however, it is an important part of inventory management and maintaining a profitable business.

Prescription medication vials returned by the patient—even if unopened—cannot, by law, be returned to stock once they have left the pharmacy. This law exists to protect patients from product tampering. In the case of a drug recall, the patient can return the drug for credit or for a refund provided by the manufacturer. Depending on the policy of the pharmacy, the cost of returned drugs may or may not allow a reimbursement to the patient. The pharmacy or store manager must generally approve any such refund. The returned drug should be disposed of per the pharmacy's policy and defined procedure.

Requirements for Controlled Substances

The purchasing, receipt, and inventory of controlled-drug substances requires special procedures and recordkeeping requirements. The Controlled Substances Act (CSA) defines procedures for purchasing and receiving and requirements for inventory and recordkeeping. Each pharmacy must register with the Drug Enforcement Administration (DEA) to purchase controlled substances.

How can a new pharmacy technician tell whether or not a medication is a controlled substance? As you may recall from Chapter 2, the FDA requires that all controlled-substance containers be clearly marked with their *schedule* on the product label. This mark is an uppercase Roman numeral with or without a *C* symbol.

II or C-II

III or C-III

IV or C-IV

V or C-V

The symbol *C* and/or the Roman numeral must be at least twice the size of the largest letters printed on the label. When a bottle is too small to receive the symbol or numerals, then the box and package insert must contain them. Symbols and/or numerals are not required on the containers of dispensed medications.

Schedule III, IV, V Drugs   In most pharmacies, the technician can order Schedule III–V medications. The pharmacist must, however, verify the receipt of these drugs. Receipt includes comparing the invoice with the drug name, dosage, and quantity of physical inventory. Once the receipt is verified by the pharmacist, these drugs may be stored by the technician among the drug stock, usually alphabetically by drug name. All Schedule III, IV, and V prescriptions and records, including purchasing invoices, are commonly kept separate from other records and must also be kept in a readily retrievable form. Prescription records for nonscheduled drugs are often filed separately.

Schedule II Drugs   All Schedule II drugs should be received in a special tote with an unbroken seal. If the seal is broken, then the tote should not be accepted at delivery and the wholesaler should be notified immediately. The pharmacist must break the seal on the tote and verify the contents with the invoice. After verification, the invoice is signed and dated, and the information, such as NDC number, price, and expiration date, is entered into the pharmacy database.

The pharmacist usually is responsible for the receipt and secure storage of all controlled drugs, but especially Schedule II drugs. Many community pharmacies use a perpetual inventory to maintain close control of the Schedule II drug stock. A **perpetual inventory record** is a method of maintaining ongoing accountability for Schedule II medications on a tablet-by-tablet (or other dosage form) basis. Figure 7.3 shows an example of a perpetual inventory record. A perpetual inventory record documents each and every dosage of Schedule II drugs received and dispensed. This record includes product, dosage, quantity, date received or dispensed, prescription number, remaining inventory, and signature or initials of the pharmacist.

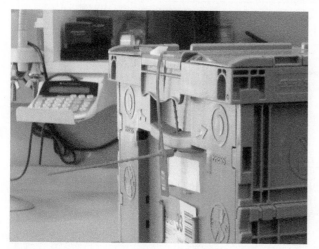

The seal on totes for controlled substances can only be broken by the pharmacist.

FIGURE 7.3
**Perpetual
Inventory Record**

A perpetual inven-
tory record accounts
for each unit of a
Schedule II drug
dispensed or
received.

Drug and Dose	Oxycodone 5mg/325 mg APAP
Record Starting Date	01/02/20XX
Record Starting Quantity	500

Prescription Number	Dispensing Date	Quantity Dispensed	Cumulative Total	RPh Initials
246734	01/03/20XX	40	460	RJA
247981	01/06/20XX	16	444	RJA
248103	01/07/20XX	120	324	RJA
DEA 001234988	01/10/20XX	+500	824	RJA
249008	01/12/20XX	60	764	RJA

If allowed by the policy and procedures of the pharmacy, the technician will make entries on new inventory or prescription dispensing into this notebook. All entries should be co-initialed by the pharmacist. The correct drug, dosage, and quantity must be documented. Any discrepancies should be reported to the pharmacist; if the discrepancy cannot be resolved, then the pharmacist must contact the state drug inspector and the DEA.

Documentation The purchase of Schedule II controlled substances must be authorized by a pharmacist and executed on a DEA 222 form (Figure 7.4). This form provides the record of any Schedule II substances sold or delivered to another DEA-registered dispenser. Ordering such drugs from a wholesaler may involve a wait of 48 or 72 hours because of the paperwork and special handling. Online ordering of

FIGURE 7.4
DEA 222 Form

This form must
be completed
and signed by the
pharmacist for the
ordering of
all Schedule II
controlled
substances.

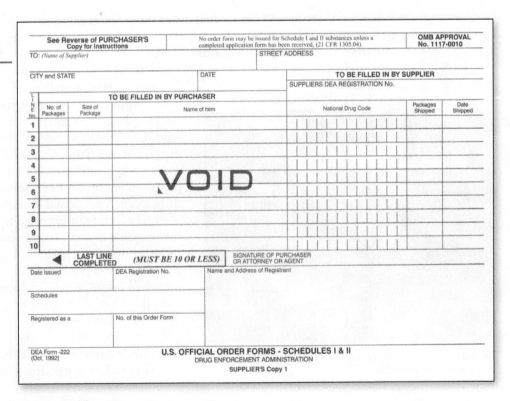

Schedule II drugs is available to most community pharmacies, but it requires registration, user name, and password protection for each pharmacist. Online access to ordering allows next-day delivery in most cases. The pharmacist—not the technician—is legally responsible for the ordering of all Schedule II controlled substances, whether by submitting a DEA 222 form or ordering online.

The pharmacy must maintain complete and accurate records of all controlled substances. Receiving records include the DEA order form, with the DEA number of the supplier, as well as all receipts. The order form must contain medication name, dosage form, strength or concentration per dosage unit, and amount of dosage units per commercial container. The invoice must be signed and dated by the pharmacist. If Schedule II drugs are received, then the amount and date received, as well as the NDC numbers, should be completed on the DEA 222 form.

The DEA requires that a complete paper trail of records be maintained for each Schedule II drug as the drug travels from manufacturer to the community pharmacy to the patient. The DEA 222 form documents the request from the manufacturer, the shipment receipt documents the delivery to the pharmacy, and the prescription documents the dispensing of the drug to the patient. The signed invoice and DEA 222 form must be filed together and be readily retrievable in case of an audit. All Schedule II prescription records must be kept separate from other prescription records and also be readily retrievable.

Estimating Drug Inventory

Often today's pharmacies have $150,000 to $300,000 or more in inventory on the shelves as drug products. If a chain has ten stores in the region, then the amount of money in goods on the shelf adds up very quickly.

To minimize the cost of doing business, inventory levels must be adequate but not excessive, with a rapid turnover of drug stock on the shelf. Keeping medications on the shelf is a cost to a pharmacy, and an excessive inventory can hinder cash flow. Keeping excess inventory in stock has a number of associated costs, including the capital that is tied up in the inventory, wastage because of product expiration, and increased likelihood of theft.

Although all of the transactions of drugs and products coming in and out of the pharmacy are carefully documented, the technician should occasionally take a physical count of the pharmacy's inventory. A counting of the items in stock is usually taken once or more each year, and the task is often assigned to a senior pharmacy technician or else it is outsourced to complete the project. An inventory value is used to determine average inventory and turnover rate and to make any necessary adjustments in stock levels. Whenever a pharmacy is in the process of being sold, an inventory is required and included in the purchase price.

When the inventory is counted, unopened bottles receive full credit. All opened bottles are assumed to be half-full for inventory purposes. When filling a prescription, the technician should make a note (usually an "X") on the drug stock bottle (or affix an "Open Bottle" sticker) to indicate that the bottle has been opened. Similarly, drug stock bottles should not be overfilled. For example, the

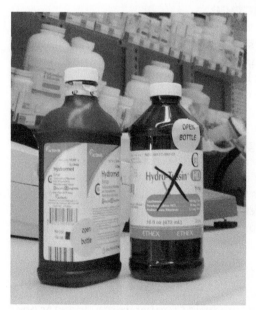

It is a common procedure to mark stock bottles with an "X" or to affix an "Open Bottle" label once the bottles have been opened. When the technician is counting inventory, an opened bottle is assumed to be half-full.

technician should not add 100 tablets of cyclobenzaprine to a stock bottle of 500 tablets; on inspection, the bottle would be counted as half-full (250 tablets) and the inventory would be understated by 350 tablets. For most expensive drugs, this practice could understate inventory costs and negatively impact the purchase price of the pharmacy.

There is a special policy and procedure for counting the inventory of controlled drug substances. The DEA requires that a complete inventory of all controlled substances must be taken every two years. Some states have even more stringent requirements, such as a yearly inventory. An exact unit count (number of tablets, capsules, patches, or milliliters) is required for all Schedule II drugs. For Schedules III, IV, and V, an estimated count and/or measure is permitted unless a container holds more than 1000 capsules or tablets. If the container has been opened, then an exact count is required.

The date of the taking of an actual inventory should not vary by more than four days from the biennial inventory date. The complete inventory record must contain the following information for each controlled substance:

- name of the drug
- dosage form and strength
- number of dosage units or volume in each container
- number of containers

Prescription records for all controlled substances must be maintained for a minimum of two years. Some states require holding records for five years. For legal purposes, most pharmacies keep all prescription records indefinitely. Any disposal of a controlled drug must be recorded, witnessed, and signed by the pharmacist. In most cases, expired or defective formulations (broken tablets) of Schedule II drugs are saved for destruction on the next visit of the state drug inspector or returned to an authorized destruction depot.

Business Math Used in Pharmacy Practice

A community pharmacy operates under the same principles as any other business: it deals with expenses and receipts. In addition, like any other business, the pharmacy must make a **profit** (in other words, it must have more receipts than expenses to continue to provide customer services). One of the responsibilities of the pharmacy technician is to help ensure that inventory turns over and that the insurance reimbursements and receipts are greater than the expenses.

The technician often takes care of pricing in the pharmacy by billing online insurance, marking products up by a certain percentage over the cost, and marking products down by a percentage discount at other times. The successful pharmacy technician needs to master basic mathematic skills used in markup, discount, and average wholesale price (AWP). Understanding the terminology and mathematics used in community pharmacy is an important part of the pharmacy technician's job and can directly affect the profitability of the business.

Markup

Like all businesses, pharmacies purchase their products (in other words, drugs) at one price and sell them at a higher price. This difference is called the **markup**, but it is sometimes referred to as the **gross profit**. Prescription pricing is subject to governmental laws and regulations, as well as competition within the marketplace. Markup plays an important part in the pricing system. The markup is computed as follows:

$$\text{selling price} - \text{purchase price} = \text{markup}$$

The markup rate is expressed as a percentage and is calculated as follows:

$$\text{markup} \div \text{cost} \times 100 = \text{markup rate}$$

Example 2

A 30 day supply of insulin sells for \$75 and costs the pharmacy \$50. What is the markup and what is the markup rate?

The markup is computed as follows:

$$\text{selling price} - \text{purchase price} = \text{markup}$$

$$\$75 - \$50.00 = \$25.00 = \text{markup}$$

$$\$25.00 = \text{markup}$$

The markup rate is computed as follows:

$$\text{markup} \div \text{cost} \times 100 = \text{markup rate}$$

$$\$25.00 \div \$50.00 \times 100 = \text{markup rate}$$

$$50\% = \text{markup rate}$$

Discount

Sometimes a wholesaler offers an item to a pharmacy at a lower price. This reduced price is a **discount**. Often this discount may be passed on to the consumer, or it may help offset expenses and low reimbursements from insurance. The pharmacy may offer the consumer a discount, or a deduction from what is normally charged, as an incentive to purchase an item, especially on a nonprescription product or store merchandise. Discount and discounted price are calculated with the following formulas:

$$\text{purchase price} \times \text{discount rate} = \text{discount}$$

$$\text{purchase price} - \text{discount} = \text{discounted price}$$

Example 3

Assume that the pharmacy purchases five cases of hydrocortisone cream at \$100.00 per case. If the account is paid in full within fifteen days, then the supplier (wholesaler) offers a 15% discount on the purchase. What is the total discounted purchase price?

Begin by calculating the total purchase price.

$$\text{quantity of product} \times \text{cost per unit} = \text{total purchase price}$$

$$5 \text{ cases} \times \$100.00/\text{case} = \$500.00$$

Next calculate the discount for payment within fifteen days.

$$\text{total purchase price} \times \text{discount rate} = \text{discount}$$

$$\$500.00 \times 0.15 = \$75.00$$

Finally, to obtain the discounted price, subtract the discount from the original price.

$$\text{total purchase price} - \text{discount} = \text{discounted purchase price}$$

$$\$500.00 - \$75.00 = \$425.00$$

Average Wholesale Price Applications

A pharmacy may potentially receive payment for the drug product and its services from several sources. Historically, patients have been responsible for paying for their own medications, but this situation is much less common than in the past. More recently, health maintenance organizations (HMOs) and health insurance companies (or PBMs) have become major players in determining the cost of health care, including patient medications. The very survival of a pharmacy depends on its ability to contain drug costs.

The **average wholesale price (AWP)** of a drug is an *average* price that wholesalers charge the pharmacy. Usually, third parties reimburse a pharmacy based on the AWP less a discount that has been agreed on. Therefore the pharmacy has an incentive to purchase a drug at a price that is as far below its AWP as possible. Drugs are sold below AWP in some situations (that is to say, via group purchasing, volume discounts, contract situations, rebates from manufacturers). The AWP is used to calculate a prescription reimbursement with the following formula:

$$\text{prescription reimbursement} = \text{AWP} + \text{percentage} + \text{dispensing fee}$$

Example 4

Plavix comes in a quantity of 90 tablets and has an AWP of $150.00. The pharmacy has an agreement with the supplier to purchase the drug at the AWP minus 15%. The insurer is willing to pay the AWP plus 5% plus a $3.00 dispensing fee. A patient on this insurer's plan purchases 30 tablets for $55.50. How much profit does the pharmacy make on this prescription?

Begin by calculating the amount of the discount.

$$\$150 \times 0.15 = \$22.50$$

Use the discount to calculate the purchase price of the drug.

$$\$150.00 - \$22.50 = \$127.50$$

Therefore, the pharmacy can purchase 90 tablets for $127.50.

The insurance company pays the pharmacy AWP plus 5%. (Note that 5% = 0.05.)

$$\$150.00 + (\$150.00 \times 0.05) = \$150.00 + \$7.50 = \$157.50$$

Using the insurance reimbursement of $157.50 for 90 tablets, calculate the reinbursement for 30 tablets.

$$(\$157.50 \div 3) + \$3 \text{ (dispensing fee)} = \$52.50 + \$3.00 = \$55.50$$

Compare this to the pharmacy's cost of 30 tablets.

$$\$127.50 \div 3 = \$42.50$$

Therefore, the pharmacy's profit on 30 tablets is:

$$\$55.50 - \$42.50 = \$13.00$$

Health Insurance

Health insurance is coverage of incurred medical costs such as physician visits, laboratory costs, and hospitalization. In the past, this medical coverage was primarily limited to hospitalizations and emergency room visits. A patient had to pay cash for each physician visit and at the time of picking up a prescription. Today most patients have health and prescription drug insurance coverage from a private insurance company through their employer or from the state (in other words, Medicaid) or federal government (in other words, Medicare, Tricare). Many Medicare patients may have additional supplemental insurance to cover medical and/or prescription expenses.

Unfortunately, the cost of health care and health insurance is far outpacing the rate of inflation. In many industries, the competitiveness of the United States with global markets is threatened by the escalating cost of healthcare benefits for employees and retirees. Health costs are nearly 20% of the gross domestic product (GDP), nearly double the costs only 20 years ago. Without major changes, the solvency of the Medicare insurance program after the year 2018 is questionable.

Medicaid and Medicare offer medical and drug benefit coverage, with limitations and restrictions on age, income, and disability. Many small employers elect not to provide health insurance coverage. For individuals who are unemployed, work part-time, or are underinsured by their employers, the cost of private health insurance is prohibitive. There are more than 47 million adults and children in the United States, or 16% of the population, who do not have any type of health or drug insurance. Many states are experimenting with providing basic health insurance to all of their citizens. Healthcare policy will continue to be debated in each political election for years to come.

Prescription Insurance Plans

Many insurance companies including Blue Cross/Blue Shield, Aetna, United Health, some Medicaid, and all Medicare Part D plans elect to outsource (or contract outside the insurance company) for the administrative processing of drug claims to a PBM. A **prescription benefits manager (PBM)** is a company that provides such service by administering the prescription drug benefits and pharmacy reimbursements for many insurance companies. Common examples of PBMs who agree to process drug claims for insurance companies include Express Scripts International (ESI), PAID, and Medco.

With the exception of Medicaid (low income, disabled) and Tricare (military), most patients with prescription insurance pay a monthly premium for prescription drug coverage that may or may not be subsidized by their employer. Private health insurance usually includes some combination of individual and family deductible, co-payment per visit or per prescription, and limits on total or lifetime benefits. A wide variety of private insurance is available, ranging from premium to more basic plans based on cost.

Several important terms for the pharmacy technician to understand are related to prescription insurance plans. The **deductible** is an amount that must be paid by the insured before the insurance company will consider paying its portion of the medical and medication cost. This annual deductible is commonly $500 to $1000 and usually starts with the first of the calendar year. A **co-payment (co-pay)** is the flat amount that the patient is to pay for each prescription; co-pays vary by both drug and insurance company. **Co-insurance** is a percentage-based plan, whereby the patient must pay a certain percentage of the prescription price, which is not as common as deductible and co-pay insurance arrangements. The deductible, co-pay, or co-insurance are all methods by which an insurance company tries to control healthcare costs. The higher-cost premium plans may have no deductible or lower deductibles and co-pays.

In some cases, a patient may have a dual co-pay—one co-pay for brand names and a lower one for generics (that is to say, $30.00 for brand names; $5.00 for generics). Co-pays are for each drug; most insurance plans only cover a 30 day supply of medication in a community pharmacy (but a 90 day supply if a mail-order pharmacy is used) regardless of how the prescription was written. A more common drug insurance plan of today is the use of a tiered co-pay. The **tiered co-pay** has an escalating cost for a generic, a preferred brand, and a nonpreferred brand. For preferred medications, the patient pays a lower co-pay than for a nonpreferred drug that has a higher co-pay or is not covered at all.

Patients are often provided with the insurance company's list of preferred drugs and are encouraged to share them with their physicians so that these medications may be selected whenever possible. Often, prescribers do not know or do not remember which drug is on which PBM formulary, so the patient, or the pharmacist acting as the patient advocate, may need to discuss therapy options with the prescriber, especially if drug affordability is an issue. To complicate matters, these formulary listings for each PBM are constantly changing. For example, a PBM may elect to cover the generic drug simvastatin for the treatment of high cholesterol: the co-pay for simvastatin may be $10, the co-pay for Lipitor (the preferred brand name drug) may be $30, and the co-pay for Crestor (the *nonpreferred* brand name drug) may be $50.

Online adjudication is defined as using wireless communications to process prescription claims. It usually takes less than 30 seconds during the prescription-filling process and can save the pharmacy a great deal of time and paperwork when it is performed properly. When the prescription is billed to a PBM, the pharmacy is immediately notified as to what amount it should charge the patient and what amount the pharmacy will be reimbursed; if the cost is not covered, the patient may need to meet a deductible first, or the drug may simply not be covered under the insurance plan. It is common for many plans to list the amount saved by insurance coverage on the medication information sheet that accompanies the dispensed medication.

Even with drug insurance coverage, a patient commonly pays five or six co-pays at the time of each refill with medications for high blood pressure, diabetes, and high cholesterol. Depending on the insurance plan and formulary status of the medications, the patient may need to pay $100 to $250 per person per month out-of-pocket in addition to monthly insurance premium expenses.

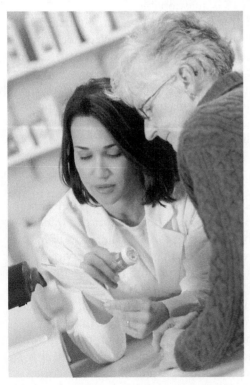

Pharmacy technicians may discuss insurance coverage with patients to help them understand their medication expenses.

Medicaid **Medicaid** subsidizes the cost of health care, including drugs, for indigent and disabled citizens of its state who meet age and income eligibility requirements. Each state has its own policies, procedures, and regulations on the reimbursement of prescription drugs for patients who are eligible for Medicaid. Eligibility for Medicaid is frequently renewed by the state and checked online by the pharmacy each time that a prescription is processed.

Most community pharmacies sign a contract to agree to provide prescription benefits to this disadvantaged population according to the terms of that state. With very few exceptions, OTC drugs are not covered by Medicaid. Some states may have a formulary of acceptable drugs that they cover. Other states provide a maximum number of prescriptions (usually five) that can be covered in any single month. Most states have instituted a minimal co-pay on some prescriptions (usually less than $5.00 per prescription) to discourage misuse.

The state reimbursement rate to pharmacies is generally *usual and customary charges*. This means that the pharmacy cannot charge the state more for the same prescription dispensed to a patient with private or commercial insurance. Thus the pharmacy must avoid agreeing to nonprofitable contracts with PBMs, because patients eligible for Medicaid add more financial loss to the balance sheet.

Many states are outsourcing their drug coverage to PBMs because of the rising nature of drug costs and shrinking state tax revenues. In Georgia, for example, an eligible patient may be covered by Medicaid, AmeriGroup, Peach Care, or Wellpoint. Each of these plans has different requirements. Insurance coverage frequently changes once or twice during the year to another PBM without notice to the patient or issuance of a new insurance card. During the process of online drug claims, the new insurance coverage information may be provided and identified by the experienced technician.

Some community pharmacies elect not to accept Medicaid coverage because of low reimbursement, delays or errors in receipt of payment, and challenges on legitimate drug claims from accounting audits. The pharmacy can receive stiff financial and civil penalties for intentional or unintentional errors in billing.

Tricare **Tricare** is a federal health and prescription drug insurance plan that is available to active and inactive members of the military and their families. The program has generous coverage of drug costs. The prescription insurance coverage has relatively low co-pays for generic and brand name drugs and usually covers a 90 day supply of medication from any community pharmacy.

Medicare The Medicare Prescription Drug, Improvement, and Modernization Act (MMA) of 2003, also called **Medicare Part D**, offers eligible patients the option to add drug insurance to their existing health coverage. Starting in January 2006, patients who qualified for Medicare coverage were eligible to add drug benefit coverage for an additional monthly charge to their current premium. In addition to patients over the age of sixty-five years, patients with chronic kidney disease and those who are "dual eligible" for Medicare and Medicaid are covered under the plan. More than 40 million patients who are eligible for Medicare have taken advantage of this insurance program. If eligible patients opt not to join when eligible, then the monthly cost may be higher if they decide to join in the future.

In this voluntary program, a patient may elect to continue current drug coverage through his or her existing supplemental health insurance or employer or to select an insurer participating in the Medicare Part D program in his or her state. The plan has special provisions for low-income seniors who would likely benefit most from this program. This Medicare plan provides catastrophic coverage for all patients who develop serious medical conditions requiring expensive drug treatments.

Medicare Part D is complex, with many choices for coverage, but each patient can expect to save an average of 25 to 30% from annual out-of-pocket cost of prescriptions. For example, in some plans a $100 or $250 deductible must be paid before the patient is eligible for benefits. After the deductible is met, patients pay an average of 25% of the cost for their new and refilled prescriptions until the total drug costs (from out-of-pocket and insurance) reach approximately $3000. From $3000 to approximately $5500, patients are responsible for 100% of the cost of their medications. This gap in coverage is what patients and the media refer to as the **doughnut hole**. Once approximately $5500 in drug costs has been reached in the calendar year, the patient only pays 5% of the cost of the medications. The premium, as well the annual drug costs, is adjusted annually with inflation.

Older adults can choose from several insurance plans that are available in each region of the country. Patients are often frustrated and confused, and they continue to have many questions about Medicare Part D insurance coverage. Patients are often shocked by the reality of drug costs when in the doughnut hole. By becoming more knowledgeable, the pharmacy technician can better serve the needs of the patient.

Each plan has its advantages and disadvantages, and each has a different list of lower-cost, *preferred* drugs. Most plans cover all or most of the cost for generic drugs. Preferred and nonpreferred formulary drugs are subject to a tiered co-pay. If a patient has a brand name product with a high co-pay, then the technician should alert the pharmacist, who could suggest a lower-cost alternative; if financial hardship exists, many physicians are willing to change to a less costly product.

Although far from perfect, Medicare Part D addresses the important issue of partial and catastrophic insurance coverage for prescription drugs. The pharmacy technician can provide a valuable service by educating patients on drug insurance coverage for their individual drug regimens. Patients should research their options on the Internet or get assistance from a family member or the pharmacist in selecting the drug insurance program that best fits their needs.

Workers' Compensation   In addition to PBMs representing commercial insurers, Medicare, Tricare, and Medicaid, some patients may present prescriptions which are to be billed to **workers' compensation** (or workers' comp). Workers' comp provides insurance to cover medical care and compensation for employees who are injured in the course of employment or from an accident, in exchange for a waiver of the employee's right to sue his or her employer. Drug coverage is usually limited to specific classes of drugs that are needed to treat the injury. For example, if back pain is the primary symptom, analgesic and back spasm medication may be covered, but antibiotics for a sinus infection would not be covered.

The pharmacy must have a contract with the third-party PBM that is providing reimbursement to the pharmacy for the workers' comp claim. The patient must present certain information to the pharmacy technician so that it can be entered in the patient profile; in addition to PBM information, the social security number, date of injury, and the name of the business compensating the patient must be entered. The initial data entry may take additional time and require a telephone call to verify information and drug coverage.

A workers' comp claim is generally entered as a secondary insurer (assuming that the patient has other drug insurance coverage); the coverage is usually time limited, from three to twelve months, based on the extent and severity of the injury. For covered drugs, the patient pays no co-pay. Depending on the pharmacy, there may be contracts for one or more workers' comp PBMs.

The pharmacy technician should become familiar with the policy and procedure for handling workers' comp claims. The patient may have multiple claims to process; some drugs may be billed to the primary insurer and selected approved claims sent to the workers' comp PBM.

Coordinating Drug Benefits Another common scenario involves a patient who has a primary and a secondary drug insurance plan. The claim is processed to the primary insurer; if the drug is not covered, or a co-pay exists, then the technician must bill the secondary insurer. This process is called **coordination of benefits (COB)**, and its successful resolution differs according to the pharmacy software. Having the technician learn about the various insurance plans and their interface with the pharmacy's software package is an ongoing daily process and an asset to any pharmacy operation.

Receiving and Entering Insurance Information

For the pharmacy technician, learning the ins and outs of various insurance plans is a most challenging skill, second only to learning all of those generic and trade names. The experienced pharmacy technician can greatly assist the pharmacist and the patient by making the drug insurance claim process a success. The procedures to bill online PBMs are similar—but not identical—whether the billing is to private insurance, the federal government (Medicare, Tricare), or state government plans.

If the customer has drug insurance, then he or she should carry a prescription insurance card containing information such as the following: the name of the primary insured person, the insurance carrier, a group number, a nine digit cardholder identification number, information on coverage of dependents, an expiration date, and, sometimes, the amount of the co-pay for prescriptions (see Figure 7.5). The technician must request this information and enter it into the patient profile for every new patient or for new changes in insurance coverage. Unfortunately, the information on these cards is not standardized or always accurate, making the job of online billing for the technician very challenging.

The technician must carefully review the information contained on the prescription insurance card. Customers often have both a medical (including Medicare) card as well as a drug insurance card. The technician should identify the correct insurance card because many customers are confused by the various cards for healthcare coverage.

There are thousands of drug insurance plans. For example, Blue Cross and Blue Shield may have hundreds of PBMs that process their prescription claims. Most pharmacies have contracts with most plans, but some plans, especially those out-of-state, may not be covered.

FIGURE 7.5
Parts of an Insurance Identification Card

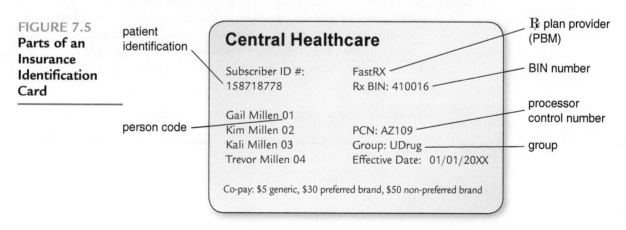

Calculating Medication Amount and Days Supply

Preparing a drug claim for online billing includes filling in specific information about each prescription filled, including the medication amount and days supply of medication. A **days supply** is the time that a given amount of medication dispensed lasts. If the information submitted is incorrect, then the claim may be denied, or, if audited, the pharmacy may not be reimbursed for the medication. Thus, calculating days supply of medication accurately is an important skill.

The following examples show how to calculate medication amounts and days supply for actual prescriptions.

Example 5

A prescription is received for Ciprofloxacin 500 mg and the sig "take one tablet twice daily Quantity: 28." What is the medication amount and the days supply?

$$\text{days supply} = 28 \text{ tablets} \div 2 \text{ tablets/day} = 14 \text{ days}$$

Example 6

A prescription is received for Augmentin 600 mg/5 mL with the sig "give ¾ teaspoonful twice daily for 10 days." Augmentin is available as a generic in 75 mL, 100 mL, and 150 mL. What is the days supply? What size bottle should be used? How much dispensed product will be unused?

Step 1. Calculate volume taken in each dose by converting ¾ teaspoonful to milliliters (abbreviated as mL). Because 1 tsp = 5 mL,

$$\frac{3}{4} \text{ tsp/dose} \times 5 \text{ mL/1 tsp} = 3.75 \text{ mL/dose}$$

Step 2. Calculate the amount of drug prescribed per day.

$$2 \text{ doses/day} \times 3.75 \text{ mL/dose} = 7.5 \text{ mL/day}$$

Step 3. Determine the number of days the prescription should last. According to the prescription, the days supply is 10 days.

Step 4. Calculate total volume needed.

$$7.5 \text{ mL/day} \times 10 \text{ days} = 75 \text{ mL}$$

Step 5. Select the bottle size from the available stock and determine how much product will remain after the patient takes the prescribed amount. Because Augmentin comes in 75 mL, 100 mL, and 150 mL bottles, the 75 mL bottle will be selected. Because the bottle amount equals the prescribed amount, none of the drug will be left over.

$$75 \text{ mL/dispensed amount} - 75 \text{ mL/prescribed amount} = 0 \text{ mL}$$

Example 7

The pharmacy receives a prescription for Augmentin 400 mg/5 mL. It reads "Give 1 tsp tid for 7 days." Medicaid insurance does not cover this strength, but will cover Augmentin 600 mg/5 mL. If the substitution to the insured strength is made, what will the new sig be? Augmentin suspensions are available in 50 mL, 75 mL, and 100 mL sizes. Which bottle will be dispensed and how much should remain after 7 days?

Step 1. Calculate the volume of Augmentin 600 mg/5 mL needed to provide the prescribed dose of 400 mg tid. Set up a ratio comparing the prescribed dose to the insured product.

$$\frac{x \text{ mL}}{400 \text{ mg}} = \frac{5 \text{ mL}}{600 \text{ mg}}$$

$$\frac{(400 \text{ mg}) \, x \text{ mL}}{400 \text{ mg}} = \frac{(400 \text{ mg}) \, 5 \text{ mL}}{600 \text{ mg}}$$

$$x \text{ mL} = 3.333 \text{ mL, rounded to } 3.33 \text{ mL}$$

The sig must be changed to read "Take 3.33 mL 3 times daily for 7 days."

Step 2. Calculate volume needed per day.

$$3.33 \text{ mL} \times 3 \text{ doses/day} = 9.99 \text{ mL/day, rounded to } 10 \text{ mL}$$

Step 3. Calculate the total volume needed for the days supply.

$$7 \text{ days} \times 10 \text{ mL/day} = 70 \text{ mL}$$

Step 4. Use the 75 mL volume of the 600 mg/5 mL Augmentin. Approximately 5 mL will remain after 7 days and should be discarded. Because of the "3.33 mL dose," a measuring device should be included with the prescription. If you incorrectly chose the 100 mL size, then more product would be wasted and the claim would not be processed.

Example 8

A prescription is written for Hydrocodone/APAP in a strength of 500 mg/500 mg #90 with the sig "take 1–2 tablets every 4 to 6 hours prn pain" with one refill. How many days will the dispensed medication last?

Step 1. Calculate the maximum number of tablets taken each day. If the patient takes 2 tablets every 4 hours, 12 tablets could be taken in a day. However, (as you learn with experience) the maximum safe amount for this drug is 8 tablets per day.

Step 2. Assuming the patient takes 8 tablets per day, calculate the days of supply for the 90 tablets dispensed.

$$90 \text{ tablets} \div 8 \text{ tablets/day} = 11.25 \text{ days, or } 11 \text{ days}$$

This means that the prescription cannot be refilled—or the claim processed—prior to 11 days from the date of initial dispensing.

Example 9

A prescription is written for Cortisporin Otic suspension with the sig "place 4 gtt AS qid for 5 days." This product is available as a generic in sizes of 5 mL and 10 mL. Assuming there are 16 gtt in 1 mL, how much medication is dispensed to fill the prescription?

Step 1. Because the available stock is in milliliters (mL), convert the prescribed units of measure, drops, which is abbreviated as gtt, to milliliters (mL).

$$4 \text{ gtt/dose} \times 1 \text{ mL/16 gtt} = 0.25 \text{ mL/dose}$$

Step 2. Calculate the amount of drug used per day.

$$0.25 \text{ mL/dose} \times 4 \text{ doses/day} = 1 \text{ mL/day}$$

Step 3. Calculate the amount of drug needed to complete the prescribed therapy.

$$1 \text{ mL/day} \times 5 \text{ days/therapy} = 5 \text{ mL/therapy}$$

Because the product is available as a 5 mL size, which meets the needs of the prescription, the 5 mL size should be dispensed. If the 10 mL size were dispensed, then the insurance claim would not be accepted.

Example 10

A prescription is written for 30 g of Lotrisone Cream with the sig "apply to affected area tid" with one refill. How many days will the prescribed medication last?

Estimate may be 7 or 10 days; after this time, the medication can be refilled and billed online to insurance.

Example 11

A prescription is received for #2 vials of Novolin N with the sig "inject 40 units under the skin in the morning and 25 units in the evening" with prn refills. Insulin is available in 10 mL vials (or 1000 units per 10 mL). How many days will the prescribed medication last?

Step 1. Calculate the total daily dose of insulin.

$$40 \text{ units/morning} + 25 \text{ units/evening} = 65 \text{ units/day}$$

Step 2. Calculate the number of days supply that 2 vials will satisfy. Each vial contains 1000 unit vials of insulin.

$$2 \text{ vials} \times 1000 \text{ units/vial} = 2000 \text{ units}$$

$$2000 \text{ units} \div 65 \text{ units/day} = 30.769 \text{ days, or 30 days supply}$$

If you arbitrarily put 60 days (30 days for each vial) supply, then the initial claim will be processed; however, the patient will not be able to get a needed refill after 30 days without calling the insurance provider to change the original claim.

Example 12

A prescription is received for Cialis 20 mg, #30 with no refills and the sig "take as directed 1 hour prior to sexual intercourse." What is medication amount and days supply?

Your first impression is that the ℞ is written for 30 tablets, so it must be a 30 days supply. Much to your dismay, the insurance claim is denied. Although each PBM may differ, insurance may cover only 5 tablets for 30 days.

Step 1. Update your prescription entry in the computer with 5 tablets and 30 days supply and resubmit to insurance; this time it worked!

Step 2. Explain to the patient that insurance only covers 5 tablets dispensed for a $30 co-pay. He or she has the option of purchasing the remaining #25 for $250 cash. Explain that he or she actually can get 5 refills of 5 tablets each month, because the total quantity written on the prescription was #30 tablets!

Learning the subtleties of insurance and its interface with a specific pharmacy software package is one of the biggest challenges to working as a pharmacy technician in a community pharmacy. Such expertise can only come with dedicated study and experience.

Processing Prescription Drug Claims

The prescription drug insurance information allows online billing from the pharmacy to a third-party PBM as the new prescription (or refill) is being processed. The pharmacy receives immediate feedback to determine patient or dependent eligibility, whether or not the drug is covered, and the amount of co-pay, if any, that must be collected from the patient at the time of dispensing.

If the patient has prescription insurance, then the technician should identify the name of the insurer and the PBM servicing that plan. In addition to patient ID number, user number or person code, and group number of the plan, the technician should locate the BIN and processor control number (PCN) on the insurance card. The BIN and PCN allow the technician to identify the correct PBM. Finding the needle in the haystack is a primary job of the technician.

The patient's relationship to the cardholder (spouse, child, and so on) is often required for processing the online claim. Some patients have more than one insurer, in which case the primary and secondary insurer should be designated. If the cardholder's employment status has changed recently, then the drug insurance may have expired. Figure 7.5 (on page 217) demonstrates an example of what a drug insurance card may look like.

The technician should be aware of several potential errors when processing a prescription claim. The customer name in the database should exactly match the name on the card; for example, "Rick Smith" may be in the insurance database as "Charles R. Smith." If a technician tries to process a drug claim under Rick Smith, then it will be denied with the error message "unmatched recipient." This is important to remember for all insurance, but especially for Tricare, which covers military retirees and their dependents.

Another common processing error on insurance is date of birth. If either the pharmacy or the insurance company has the incorrect date of birth, then the claim will not be processed. Even if the pharmacy has the correct date of birth, if the date does not match the one in the PBM database, the claim will not be approved. To correct this error, the technician must call the PBM, verify the birth date, and enter the incorrect date in the patient profile in order to process the claim. The patient (or parent) must then call the insurance company to correct the dates and advise the pharmacy on his or her next visit to update the birth date in the patient profile.

If the drug claim is not processing (in other words, causing an error message), then take another look at the ID numbers. Many plans may use letters preceding the ID number, such as XYZ1199A2883; some insurance plans require the letters, but some do not. Letters in the middle of the ID number are required. Tricare uses the social security number as the ID number for both retired military personnel and their dependents. To make matters more complicated, the group number on the prescription card may be missing or incorrect; some plans do not require a group number!

Some insurance plans (or pharmacy software) require a user number or person code to follow the ID number, but some do not. For example, the husband may be there to pick up a prescription, but his wife is the primary insured under the plan; his ID number may be 119922883-02 (or 002), whereas his wife may have the same ID number but a different user number of 01 (or 001). Dependent children may be 03, 04, 05, and so on. Most Medicare Part D (see the following discussion) and Medicaid programs have a patient-specific ID number without a user number. Does it sound confusing? It is!

The notation "refill too soon" may be one reason that a claim cannot be processed. Most insurance plans allow refills to be processed if the request is within 7 days of the patient's running out of medication, but some plans are more restrictive. If the refill involves a controlled substance, then the pharmacist may not allow early refills, depending on the policy at the community pharmacy.

Another claim processing error may be because the pharmacy technician entered the incorrect days supply of medication into the patient profile. The prescription may have been written for a 90 day supply of Lipitor but only 30 days are covered. Or a prescription is received for 10 mL of an ophthalmic solution with the sig "place 2 drops in the right eye qid." The technician must know that 20 drops of solution is equal to 1 mL, so 10 mL would be equal to 200 drops. See Table 7.2 for some common and useful volume equivalences. If the patient is taking 8 drops of medication daily, then the days supply would be 25 days (8 drops/day × 25 days = 200 drops); if the technician entered 10 days, then the claim may be rejected.

Calculating days supply of creams, ointments, and gels is difficult, but it can be estimated—depending on the size of the tube (usually 15 g, 30 g, 45 g, or 60 g) and the application site (face, arm, body, and so on). For some prescriptions, dispensing the exact days supply is not practical. For example, a prescription is written for Omnicef antibiotic suspension with a sig "give 1 teaspoonful daily for 10 days." The total volume is 50 mL (5 mL/day × 10 days), but the smallest bottle of Omnicef suspension is

TABLE 7.2   Medication Volume Equivalences

Medication	Equivalences	
otic/ophthalmic solution	1 mL	20 drops
otic/ophthalmic suspension	1 mL	16 drops
MDI asthma	1 bottle	200 inhalations
nasal sprays for allergies	1 bottle	120 doses
insulin (Novolog, Humulin, Lantus, and so on)	10 mL vial	100 units/mL or 1000 units/vial

60 mL. Insurance plans recognize that there will be 10 mL of wastage and approve the claim. In this circumstance, the technician should add the statement "discard remainder after 10 days" to the medication container label.

The customer should know that his or her co-pay and drug coverage are determined by the insurance plan, not by the pharmacy. The process of online billing is similar among all pharmacies, and the co-pays are identical, regardless of where the prescription is filled. With drug insurance, a patient may go to any pharmacy to get his or her prescriptions filled; the only differences are location, hours of operation, and quality of service.

Billing Prescription Drug Claims

Billing policies and procedures differ from pharmacy to pharmacy and from customer to customer. In a majority of cases, billing involves direct online billing by the pharmacy to the customer's insurance plan. A claim is processed, and the patient cost of the prescription is determined if the patient is eligible. Billing is accomplished by wireless communications, phone modem, or, rarely, by a written universal claim form (UCF).

Some patients use a drug discount card or present a coupon from their physician to partially cover or discount the cost of the medication. The conditions for the discount card or coupon (including expiration date, amount of drug allowed, and so on) must be carefully reviewed by the pharmacy technician. Coupons may require rebates to be made directly to the customer rather than online billing by the pharmacy. If they are billed to the pharmacy, then the technician enters the BIN, ID, and group number into the patient profile as for any other insurance plan. Some discount cards or coupons can only be used if no additional insurance claim is processed or if no government insurance (Medicaid, Medicare, Tricare) is available.

When a medication is not covered by drug insurance, or when the physician decides that the patient must have a medication that is not on the PBM's formulary, the physician may have to call the PBM in order to obtain **prior authorization (PA)** for the prescription to be covered properly. For example, in the preceding example, if the patient's cholesterol could not be controlled with lovastatin (a generic cholesterol drug) and the patient suffered an adverse reaction to the Lipitor (the preferred brand cholesterol drug), then the PBM would, in most cases, approve drug coverage and a lower co-pay for Crestor ($30 as opposed to $50 in this example). The pharmacy sends a PA request to the physician, whose representative contacts the insurance company to determine whether coverage will be approved (and for how long) or alternative drug prescribed. Pending legislation in some states would allow the pharmacist to act on the physician and patient's behalf in resolving PAs.

Cases exist in which the medication selected by the physician and needed by the patient is not covered by the insurance under any circumstances. This lack of coverage applies to newly marketed innovative drugs that are extremely expensive; drugs in certain classes, such as weight loss and those for sleep or nerves; as well as drugs that have less costly alternatives or that are available as OTC drugs. If a question about coverage arises, then having a photocopy of the patient's insurance card on file, with the appropriate (toll-free) contact phone numbers, is helpful.

If a claim cannot be resolved, then the technician should telephone the toll-free number on the back of the insurance card, but this may take 10 to 15 minutes or more to resolve. The pharmacy technician often has to be empathetic to a patient who does not fully understand why his or her medications are so expensive but not covered—or only partially covered—by the insurance company. Clearly, much can go wrong when the technician is processing a drug claim. The technician should have a personal notebook to make entries for future reference, including helpful tips and shortcuts, on the various insurance plans.

Chapter Terms

average wholesale price (AWP) the average price that wholesalers charge the pharmacy for a drug

certificate of medical necessity form to be completed and signed by the prescriber for insurance payment for diabetic supplies

co-insurance a percentage-based insurance plan whereby the patient must pay a certain percentage of the prescription price

computer an electronic device for inputting, storing, processing, and/or outputting information

coordination of benefits (COB) online billing of both a primary and a secondary insurer

co-payment (co-pay) the amount that the patient is to pay for each prescription

credit card a method of online payment that is a type of loan, either paid totally at the end of the month or partially with a finance charge added

database management system (DBMS) application that allows one to enter, retrieve, and query records

days supply the duration of time (number of days) a dispensed medication will last the patient and often required on drug claims submitted for insurance billing

debit card a method of online cash payment that instantly deducts the cost of the purchase from the customer's bank account

deductible an amount that must be paid by the insured before the insurance company considers paying its portion of a medical or drug cost

diet supplement a category of nonprescription drugs that include vitamins, minerals, and herbals that are not regulated by the FDA

discount a reduced price

doughnut hole insurance coverage gap in Medicare Part D programs by which the patient must pay 100% of the cost of the medication

dumb terminal a computer device that contains a keyboard and a monitor but does not contain its own storage and processing capabilities

durable medical equipment (DME) Medical equipment such as hospital beds, wheelchairs, canes, or crutches that may be covered under Medicare Part B insurance

Flex card a medical and prescription insurance credit card

gross profit the difference between the purchase price and the selling price; also called markup

health insurance coverage of incurred medical costs such as physician visits, laboratory costs, and hospitalization

inventory the entire stock of products on hand for sale at a given time

inventory value the total value of the entire stock of products on hand for sale on a given day

just-in-time (JIT) purchasing involves frequent purchasing in quantities that just meet supply needs until the next ordering time

markup the difference between the purchase price and the selling price; also called gross profit

Medicaid a state government health insurance program for low-income and disabled citizens

Medicare Part D a voluntary insurance program that provides partial coverage of prescriptions for patients who are eligible for Medicare

online adjudication real-time insurance claims processing via wireless telecommunications

over-the-counter (OTC) drug a medication that the FDA has approved for sale without a prescription

perpetual inventory record unit-by-unit accountability, often required for Schedule II controlled inventory records

posting the process of reconciling the invoice and updating inventory

prescription benefits manager (PBM) a company that administers drug benefits from many insurance companies

prime vendor purchasing an agreement made by a pharmacy for a specified percentage or dollar volume of purchases

prior authorization (PA) approval for coverage of a high-cost medication or a medication not on the insurer's approved formulary, obtained after a prescriber calls the insurer to justify the use of the drug; must be obtained before the drug is dispensed by the pharmacy in order to be covered by insurance

profit the amount of revenue received that exceeds the expense of the sold product

purchasing the ordering of products for use or sale by the pharmacy

receipt a printout that is a proof of purchase

receiving a series of procedures for accepting the delivery of products to the pharmacy

remote computer a minicomputer or a mainframe that stores and processes data sent from a dumb terminal

Schedule V drug a medication with a low potential for abuse and a limited potential for creating physical or psychological dependence; available in most states without a prescription

smart terminal a computer that contains its own storage and processing capabilities

tiered co-pay an escalating cost or co-pay for a generic drug, a preferred brand name drug, and a nonpreferred brand name drug

Tricare a federal government health insurance program for active and retired military and their dependents

workers' compensation insurance provided for a patient with a medical injury from a job-related accident; also called workers' comp

wholesaler purchasing the ordering of drugs and supplies from a local vendor who delivers the product to the pharmacy on a daily basis

Chapter Summary

- The pharmacy technician has an important role in helping with the business operations of the pharmacy.
- The technician has an important responsibility in assisting customers in locating needed OTC drugs, diet supplements, and medical supplies.
- Some OTC drugs, such as Schedule V cough syrups, decongestants containing pseudoephedrine, and Plan B contraceptives, require specific procedures prior to sales.
- The technician can assist the diabetic patient who needs syringes, needles, test strips, glucometers, and related medical supplies.
- The technician must be competent in all cash register management functions, including sales by cash, check, credit card, debit card, and Flex card.

- The technician's responsibilities in inventory management include the purchasing, receiving, and return of drugs; the technician must understand these responsibilities in order to run a profitable pharmacy.
- Purchasing, receiving, inventorying, and recordkeeping of controlled substances require specific legal and paper trail procedures.
- Calculating the markup on the products and computing any discounts is often the responsibility of the technician.
- Understanding the concept of average wholesale price is necessary for billing insurance companies.

- A basic knowledge of both computer and mathematical skills is necessary for the technician to manage pharmacy business functions successfully.

- The technician must have an understanding of various private and government insurance programs and the knowledge to process online claims for prescriptions successfully.

Chapter Review

Checking Your Understanding

 Additional Quiz Questions

Choose the best answer from those provided.

1. OTC drugs are regulated by
   a. the FDA.
   b. the DSHEA.
   c. the CDC.
   d. state laws.

2. Garlic capsules are regulated by
   a. the FDA.
   b. the DSHEA.
   c. the CDC.
   d. state laws.

3. A computer software application that can enter, retrieve, and query records is a(n)
   a. spreadsheet.
   b. word processing system.
   c. database management system (DBMS).
   d. Internet Web browser.

4. Online claims processing of prescriptions to insurance is done by
   a. wireless telecommunications.
   b. completing a universal claim form.
   c. telephoning the insurance company.
   d. using a patient's Flex card.

5. A PBM is best described as a(n)
   a. insurance company.
   b. company that contracts with several insurance companies.
   c. drug wholesaler.
   d. prime vendor.

6. If an insurance company has three different co-pays for each class of medications, then its payment structure is best described as
   a. average wholesale price.
   b. out-of-pocket.
   c. tiered co-pay.
   d. dual co-pay.

7. Who is eligible for Medicare Part D?
   a. patients with incomes below the poverty line
   b. disabled patients
   c. any patient eligible for Medicare
   d. retired military personnel and their families

8. How do most community pharmacies maintain their daily inventory of drugs?
   a. purchasing directly from the drug manufacturer
   b. purchasing using the Internet
   c. purchasing from a local wholesaler
   d. borrowing from the hospital pharmacy

9. A DEA 222 form must be used to order and receive which controlled substance?
   a. Schedule II
   b. Schedule III
   c. Schedule IV
   d. Schedule V

10. The average price that wholesalers charge a pharmacy for a medication is also called
    a. AWP.
    b. usual and customary.
    c. markup.
    d. discount.

Thinking Like a Pharmacy Tech

1. Create a diagram outlining the steps from receipt of a prescription through online adjudication. What key pieces of information are needed from the patient insurance card to process the claim?

2. Solve the following business math problems:

   a. Eye drops with antihistamine are purchased in cases of 36 drop-dispenser bottles. The pharmacy desires a markup of $1.75 per bottle. The purchase price is $111.60 per case. What is the selling price per bottle?

   b. Identify the markup and the selling price of an oral antibiotic suspension that costs the pharmacy $15.60 per bottle if the markup rate is 25%.

   c. A month's supply of an asthma tablet costs the pharmacy $24.80, and the selling price is $30.75. Calculate the markup rate.

   d. John's Drug Shop purchases five cases of dermatologic cream at $100 per case. The invoice specifies a 15% discount if the account is paid in full within 15 days. What is the discounted price?

   e. In question d, each case contains 24 tubes of cream. You are to markup each tube by 20% based on the discounted cost. What is the selling price per tube?

   f. A prescription is written for a tube of ointment. The AWP is $62.00. Smith's Pharmacy purchases the tube at AWP, and Jones's Pharmacy purchases the tube at AWP minus 10%. The insurer reimburses at AWP plus 2% plus a $1.50 dispensing fee. How much profit does each pharmacy make?

   g. Sinus tablets have an AWP of $37.50 per 50 tablets. The Corner Drug Store dispensed prescriptions for a total of 300 sinus tablets during May. They were purchased at AWP minus 15%. The insurer reimburses at AWP plus 1.5% plus a $2.00 dispensing fee. Fifteen prescriptions of 20 tablets each were filled that month. How much profit was made?

   h. Review the following inventory list and calculate the necessary purchases to reestablish maximum inventory. Write your answers in the *Purchased* column.

John's Drug Shop Inventory

Drug	Maximum Level	Dispensed Today	Minimum Level	Current Inventory	Purchased
Eucerin cream, jars	10	1	3	3	
Ampicillin, capsules	4500	500	4000	2400	
Eyedrops, bottles	24	4	4	4	
Nystatin oral solution	1000 mL	100 mL	200 mL	400 mL	
Sterile saline	600 mL	315 mL	100 mL	75 mL	

3. Calculate the days supply for insurance billing on each of the following prescriptions.

a.

R
    ProAir MDI #1 (200
    inhalations per MDI)

    Sig: 2 sprays q6 h prn
    wheezing

c.

R
    Gentamicin Ophthalmic
    Solution 7.5 mL

    Sig: 2 gtts in each eye qid
    for 7 days

b.

R
    Fluticasone Nasal Spray #1
    (120 sprays per canister)

    Sig: 2 sprays in each nostril
    daily for allergies

d.

R
    Keflex 250 mg/5 mL
    100 mL

    Sig: ¾ tsp po tid for 10 days

Communicating Clearly

1. A pharmacy technician working in a retail environment should be familiar with various terms related to health insurance. Patients often have a difficult time understanding how their insurance works, and the technician can often act as an intermediary and advocate for the patient with regards to prescription drug benefits. Research the following insurance terms and define them in words that would be easily understood by a customer of your pharmacy.
   a. major medical insurance
   b. Medicare, Parts A, B, and D
   c. Medicaid
   d. deductible
   e. co-pay
   f. co-insurance
   g. preferred vs. nonpreferred brand
   h. prescription benefits manager (PBM)
   i. usual and customary
   j. dual and tiered co-pays
   k. prior authorization

2. Visit a community pharmacy and identify two or three sugar-free cough or cold products that would be safe to recommend to a parent with a young child who is diabetic. What information is found on the OTC label?

3. Compare the cost and features of three glucometers stocked in a community pharmacy. Are rebates offered—if so, how much? Also compare the cost of test strips that go with each meter. How much would a month's supply of strips (box of 100) cost?

Researching on the Web

1. Visit the AmerisourceBergen Web site at www.amerisourcebergen.net and Cardinal Health at www.cardinal.com. Compare and contrast the type of services that these wholesalers provide to a community pharmacy.

2. Go to www.dea.gov. Check for contact phone numbers for your state and for local or regional news on drug enforcement.

Check the most recent federal drug seizures in your state for cocaine, heroin, methamphetamine, marijuana, ecstasy, and meth labs. What schedule was hydrocodone in 1971? How many prescriptions have been written for hydrocodone in the past five years?

3. Go to http://www.diabetes.org/risk-test.jsp and take the diabetes risk test.

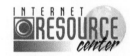

For further study of chapter-related topics, explore the Web links in the Web Center at www.emcp.net/pharmpractice4e.

Nonsterile Pharmaceutical Compounding

8

Learning Objectives

- Define the term *compounding*, describe common situations in which compounding is required, and identify examples of nonsterile compounding.

- Review and follow good compounding practices in the pharmacy.

- Distinguish terminology, such as manufactured product vs. compounded preparation.

- Identify quality standards for nonsterile compounding contained in USP Chapter 795, including product selection and beyond-use or expiration dating.

- Distinguish the components and purpose of a master control record from a compounding log.

- Understand and calculate common mathematical problems that occur in a compounding pharmacy.

- Identify and describe the equipment used for the weighing, measuring, and compounding of pharmaceuticals.

- Explain the proper techniques for weighing pharmaceutical ingredients, measuring liquid volumes, and compounding nonsterile preparations.

- Define the term *percentage of error* and understand how the concept relates to accuracy in the compounding pharmacy.

- Explain the common methods used for comminution and blending of pharmaceutical ingredients.

- Discuss the techniques by which solutions, suspensions, ointments, creams, powders, suppositories, and capsules are prepared.

- Identify the steps that are necessary in the compounding process.

- Identify references with a specialty focus on compounding.

Preview chapter terms and definitions.

Compounding remains an important part of pharmacy practice, and pharmacy technicians assist in this important task. This chapter deals with the compounding of nonsterile preparations (also known as extemporaneous compounding) that are not commercially available. The equipment, techniques, and terminology, as well as the laws, regulations, and standards, differ from those for other types of pharmacy practices. This chapter also outlines how a technician functions within a community pharmacy with a compounding practice. Compounding of sterile preparations, such as intravenous solutions, is covered in Unit 3, *Institutional Pharmacy*.

The Need for Compounding

Until the emergence of modern, large-scale pharmaceutical manufacturing in the mid-nineteenth century, pharmacists routinely prepared (i.e., compounded) a majority of all prescriptions from raw pharmaceutical ingredients extracted from plants. With advancements in large-scale manufacturing practices, the need for compounding lessened, but recent trends indicate that the practice may be increasing. Approximately 30 to 40 million prescriptions are compounded in the United States each year. Pharmacists and their technicians are increasingly being called on to prepare a recipe or compounded preparation in doses or strengths for human or veterinary use.

Compounding is defined as the process of preparing a prescribed medication for an individualized patient from bulk ingredients by a pharmacist in order to treat a specified medical condition. The compound is made according to a prescription by a licensed prescriber. Compounding is the production of a medication on demand, in an appropriate quantity and dosage form, from pharmaceutical products that are not commercially available. According to the FDA, compounding does not include reconstituting a pediatric antibiotic powder with distilled water per the directions of the manufacturer.

Compounding may be nonsterile or sterile. **Sterile compounding** is used in the production of medications that must be free of microorganisms such as those used for injection or instillation in the eye. **Nonsterile compounding** is used in the production of capsules, tablets, ointments, and creams.

In a compounding pharmacy, the pharmacist must develop a written policy and procedure manual (similar to that in hospital pharmacies) and follow all state and federal laws, regulations, and national standards for preparing nonsterile (and sometimes sterile) preparations. Only high-grade pharmaceutical ingredients can be used. Quality control programs must be included in the manual to enhance both patient care and safety. Documentation and recordkeeping are important components meeting professional standards.

A need truly exists for pharmaceutical compounding. Many high-volume chain pharmacies (and even most independent pharmacies) do not have the time, space, or expertise for compounding. As a result, a national trend exists: a growing number of independent community pharmacies are initiating or specializing in a compounding service. These pharmacies have the necessary equipment, space, and expertise to prepare compounded prescriptions safely. Both pharmacists and technicians require special training and certifications to work in a compounding pharmacy. The future trend for compounding pharmacies is for each compounding practice to pass national accreditation standards.

The technician often assists the pharmacist in the time-consuming and labor-intensive task of preparing products for pharmaceutical compounding, checking and ordering quality inventory ingredients, and maintaining a clean work environment. When working in the compounding pharmacy, the technician does not have as much direct contact with the customer as in the community pharmacy setting, but the position requires attention to detail; eye, hand, and motor coordination; and good math skills for precise

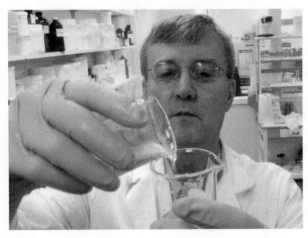

A pharmacy technician mixes a compound. Compounding, or the art of pharmacy, involves combining patient-specific medications.

calculations. Job opportunities for certified pharmacy technicians working in compounding pharmacies continue to increase as this industry grows. If you like making recipes in the kitchen, then you will enjoy learning the art of pharmaceutical compounding.

Sterile Compounding

Most sterile compounding is performed in the hospital pharmacy. Sterile compounding includes the preparation of any parenteral product to be injected, although most solutions are for intravenous use. Other routes of administration, such as intramuscular and subcutaneous injection, must also be prepared under controlled environmental conditions to minimize the risk of contamination. Sterile compounding also commonly occurs in specialized pharmacies, such as home healthcare and nuclear pharmacies.

More and more community pharmacies that dedicate their practice to compounding also prepare sterile products. The compounding of sterile preparations requires special equipment, space, and expertise. If a community pharmacy compounds both sterile and nonsterile preparations, then all necessary USP guidelines and regulations must be followed. The guidelines for nonsterile compounding (Chapter 795) are discussed later in this chapter, whereas the guidelines for sterile compounding (Chapter 797) are discussed in Chapter 10, *Infection Control*.

Nonsterile Compounding

Solutions, suspensions, ointments and creams, powders, suppositories, and capsules are examples of nonsterile compounding preparations in the community pharmacy. Some community pharmacies focus primarily on compounding prescriptions. Many physicians, especially dermatologists and gynecologists, prefer to individualize their prescriptions for their patients. Physicians from hospice care, or care for the terminally ill, and pain management clinics often use the services of a compounding pharmacy to meet specific patient needs. Pharmacists also compound prescriptions from dentists and from veterinarians for animals of all sizes and types.

Some examples of situations that require nonsterile compounding include the following:

Safety Note

Products compounded for veterinary use cannot be used in humans.

- The prescription calls for doses smaller than those that are commercially available, as is sometimes the case with pediatric medications. For example, a prescription might call for 10 mg per dose of a medication, but that medication is available only in unscored tablets containing 30 mg of the active ingredient. To match the 10 mg prescribed dose, the pharmacist might have to pulverize, or triturate, the tablets and then mix the resultant powder with an inactive powder to fill 10 mg capsules.
- A medication normally available in a solid dosage form might have to be prepared in another dosage form, such as a liquid, suspension, or suppository, for administration to a patient who cannot or will not swallow the solid form. For example, tablets may need to be triturated in a mortar and pestle, with a suitable suspending agent added.
- A noncommercially available medication may need to be prepared for a veterinary application, such as a thyroid medication for a cat.

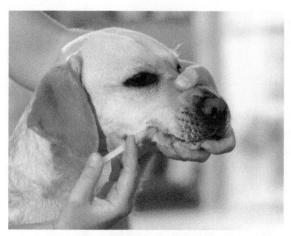

Compounding pharmacies often prepare a drug in a special formulation for a pet.

- An oral medication with an unpleasant taste might have to be prepared in a more palatable, flavor-masking syrup base to ensure compliance by a pediatric patient.
- An oral medication may have adverse effects on the stomach, such as causing an ulcer. If an ulcer-causing oral medication can be formulated into a topical gel formulation, then the patient can experience the therapeutic benefits of the drug without the risk of adverse effects. An example of a formula for a topical anti-inflammatory compounded preparation is shown in Figure 8.1.
- A medication may be available only in commercial forms containing preservatives, colorings, or other materials for patients with allergies. An alternative without the unwanted ingredients needs to be prepared.
- A dosage form other than those commercially available may be desired to customize the rate of delivery, rate of onset, site of action, or other pharmacokinetic properties of the drug. Postmenopausal women may have differing needs for hormone replacement therapy than commercially available fixed-dose tablets and may be concerned about side effects. A compounded mixture of hormones, in a cream or gel formulation, can be individualized to a patient to relieve symptoms without the risk of side effects.

Solutions As defined in Chapter 4, a solution is a liquid dosage form in which the active ingredients are dissolved in a liquid vehicle. The vehicle that makes up the greater part of a solution is known as a *solvent*. An ingredient (medication) dissolved in a solution is known as a *solute*. Solutions may be aqueous (or water), alcoholic, or hydroalcoholic. Hydroalcoholic solutions contain both water and alcohol, which may be needed to dissolve some solutes. Solutions are prepared by dissolving the solute in the liquid solvent or by combining or diluting existing solutions. Colorings or flavoring agents may be added to solutions if needed. A simple syrup, known as *Syrup NF*, can be made by combining 85 g of sucrose with 100 mL of purified water.

An example of a recipe or master control record for an otic solution to remove ear wax is contained in Figure 8.2. The master control record is discussed later in the chapter.

Suspensions In a suspension, as opposed to a solution, the active ingredient is not dissolved in the liquid vehicle but rather is dispersed throughout it. An obvious prob-

---

FIGURE 8.1
Master Control Record for Topical Compound

Safety Note

The abbreviation *qs* means to add "as much as necessary" to the specified amount. To minimize a medication error, use text words rather than abbreviations.

Compound Title
ketoprofen 10% and ibuprofen 2.5% in pluronic lecithin organogel

Compound Ingredients

ketoprofen ....10 g
ibuprofen ....2.5 g
lecithin:isopropyl palmitate 1:1 solution...............................22 mL
Pluronic F127 20% gel qs to total ....100 mL

Compounding Procedure

Mix the ketoprofen and ibuprofen powders with propylene glycol to form a smooth paste. Incorporate the lecithin:isopropyl palmitate solution and mix well. Add sufficient Pluronic F127 gel to volume and mix using high-shearing action until uniform. Package and label.

FIGURE 8.2
Master Control Record for Otic Solution Compound

Compound Title
urea and hydrogen peroxide otic solution

Compound Ingredients
carbamide peroxide ....6.6 g
glycerin, as much as necessary to total ....100 mL

Compounding Procedure
Dissolve the carbamide peroxide in sufficient glycerin to volume; then package and label. A beyond-use date of up to 6 months can be used for this preparation.

lem with suspensions is the tendency of the active ingredient to settle. To avoid settling of the insoluble drug, a suspending agent is added after vigorous trituration or grinding of the tablets into a powder. Such suspending agents include tragacanth, acacia, and carboxymethylcellulose (CMC).

Many pediatric suspensions that are commercially unavailable can be prepared in the pharmacy from adult tablets or capsules. A good example is compounding a suspension of captopril for a pediatric patient less than 6 years of age. The drug is only available in 12.5 mg, 25 mg, 50 mg, and 100 mg oral tablets. The pediatric dose is approximately 0.2 mg/kg. For a patient weighing 10 kg (22 lb), the dose is 2 mg. Tablets must be crushed, and a suitable suspending agent and flavoring agents must be identified for stability and palatability. The auxiliary medication container label "Shake Well" should always be added to a suspension.

The point (and rate) at which the suspending agent is added in the mixing procedure can be crucial. Therefore the technician must always remember to add the ingredients in the proper order, according to the formula or recipe. Flavoring agents may sometimes be incompatible with the active ingredient because of pH or acid/base ratio. Many vendors provide flavoring vehicles that have been proven to be safe and effective in children for both reconstituted solutions and nonsterile compound preparations.

Ointments and Creams Ointments, creams, and lotions are semisolid dosage forms that are meant for topical application. Gynecologists in particular are requesting more compounded formulations to individualize hormone treatments for their patients. An ointment is a water-in-oil (w/o) emulsion that is occlusive, greasy, and not water washable. A cream is an oil-in-water (o/w) emulsion that is nonocclusive, nongreasy, and water washable. A lotion is a liquid suspension or oil-in-water emulsion used topically in areas of the body such as the scalp, where a lubricating effect is desirable. A cream is best prepared with glass equipment, whereas an ointment is best prepared using water-repellent plastic equipment.

Water-soluble bases are commonly called *creams* even though they are officially defined as *ointments*. Water washability and absorption relate to cosmetic appearance such as vanishing creams. Polyethylene glycol is an example of a water-soluble base. The properties of "ointment" bases such as lanolin, petrolatum, and Aquaphor vary in their degree of occlusiveness, emolliency, water washability, and water absorption. An occlusive base has the ability to hold moisture in the skin and is best used when additional hydration is needed, such as for a patient with dry skin. An emollient base has the ability to soften skin, such as in bath oils. White petrolatum is an example of a lipophilic base with high occlusive and emollient properties. Most ointment bases are commercially available from a wholesaler or pharmacy compounding vendor.

Powders In the past the pharmacist commonly prepared prescription medicines in the form of powders. Often the pharmacist dispensed powders that were prepared, measured, mixed, divided into separate units, and placed on pieces of paper that were then folded and given to the patient. However, powders dispensed in bulk amounts had the disadvantage of leading to inaccuracy in the dose taken by the patient. With the exception of single-agent OTC Goody's Powders, the dispensing of medicines in the dosage form of divided powder is rare. Fresh herbs are commonly prepared in this manner in herb shops in this country and in China.

To a layperson, a powder is any finely ground substance. To a pharmacist, a powder is a finely divided combination, or admixture, of drugs and/or chemicals ranging in size from extremely fine to very coarse. Official definitions of powder size include very coarse (No. 8 powder), coarse (No. 20 powder), moderately coarse (No. 40 powder), fine (No. 60 powder), or very fine (No. 80 powder), according to the amount of the powder that can pass through mechanical sieves made of wire cloth of various dimensions (e.g., No. 8 sieves, No. 20 sieves).

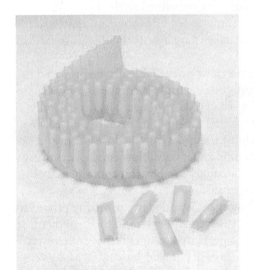
Disposable suppository molds are commonly used to dispense and shape suppositories.

Suppositories Suppositories are solid dosage forms that are inserted into bodily orifices, generally the rectum or the vagina or, less commonly, the urethra. They are composed of one or more active ingredients placed into one of a variety of bases, such as cocoa butter, hydrogenated vegetable oil, or glycerinated gelatin, which melts or dissolves when exposed to body heat and fluids. Suppositories are produced by molding and by compression. The preparation of suppositories involves melting the base material, adding the active ingredient(s), pouring the resultant liquid into a mold, and then chilling the mold immediately to solidify the suppository before the suspended ingredients have time to settle. Technicians must have experience to make a high-quality suppository preparation or defer to the pharmacist. Patients should be advised to refrigerate suppositories to minimize premature melting of the active ingredients.

Capsules A capsule is a solid dosage form consisting of a gelatin shell that encloses the medicinal preparation, which may be a powder, granules, or a liquid. Nonsterile compounding of ingredients for capsules is often done to provide unusual dosage forms, such as those containing less of an active ingredient than is readily available in commercial tablets or capsules.

Hard gelatin shells are made of gelatin, sugar, and water and consist of two parts: (1) the body, which is the longer and narrower part, and (2) the cap, which is shorter and fits over the body. In some cases capsules have a snap-fit design, with grooves on the cap and the body that fit into one another to ensure proper closure (Figure 8.3).

Hard gelatin shells commonly contain powders or granules and are used for extemporaneous (i.e., made-to-order) hand-filling operations. Hard-shell capsules come in standard sizes indicated by the numbers 000, 00, 0, 1, 2, 3, 4, and 5 (from largest to smallest). The largest capsule, size 000, can contain about 1040 mg of aspirin; the smallest, size 5, contains about 97 mg (Figure 8.4).

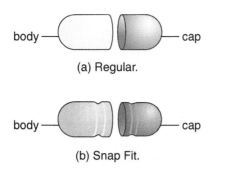

(a) Regular.

(b) Snap Fit.

FIGURE 8.3　Types of Hard-Shell Capsules

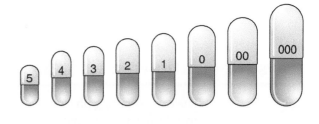

FIGURE 8.4　Hard-Shell Capsule Sizes

The sizes in which hard-shell capsules are available range from 5, the smallest, to 000, the largest.

Most hard-shell capsules are meant to be swallowed whole, but a few are meant only as conveyances for granules or powders to be sprinkled on food or in drink. Capsules should only be used in this manner when specifically intended for this purpose, because opening the capsule can adversely affect the capsule's controlled-release properties or may upset the stomach.

Bio-Identical Hormones　Many commercially available hormones are available in a fixed dose synthetic formulation. **Hormone replacement therapy (HRT)** consists of some combination of estrogen, progestin (female), and androgen (male) to relieve specific postmenopausal symptoms. **Estrogen replacement therapy (ERT)** consists of female hormones and is sometimes used in postmenopausal women and premenopausal women who have had complete hysterectomies. Many women may have concerns about the long-term safety of taking oral synthetic hormones.

A specialist may wish to individualize these hormones in a compound prescription. Such a prescription for bio-identical hormones attempts to match the individual requirements for each woman in a compounded cream or gel formulation. Table 8.1 lists the most common abbreviations for the various estrogen hormones contained in a compound prescription. The dose is often based on symptoms, clinical observations, and laboratory analyses of serum, saliva, or urine levels.

A woman maintains a symptom diary while on the hormone therapy, so the dose can be fine-tuned if necessary. A compounded cream or gel formulation may release the active ingredients more slowly and provide more long-lasting relief than a commercially available preparation. Because the various hormones in a topical formula-

TABLE 8.1　Abbreviations on Bio-Identical Hormone Compound Prescriptions

Bio-Identical Hormone	Abbreviation	Percentage
Estrone	E1	100%
Estradiol	E2	100%
Estriol	E3	100%
Biestrogen	E3/E2	80%/20%
Triestrogen	E3/E2/E1	80%/10%/10%

tion do not have to be eliminated through the liver like an oral tablet, it is much safer to use, although the long-term effects are unknown. Even with topical hormone compounds, the risk vs. benefit must be assessed by the physician on an annual basis.

Laws, Regulations, and Standards for Compounding

The compounding pharmacy must be licensed by both the state board of pharmacy and the federal government (if the pharmacy is dispensing controlled substances), as for a retail pharmacy. The Food and Drug Administration (FDA) Modernization Act of 1997 allows pharmacists to compound nonsterile or sterile medications for an individual patient if these medications meet established United States Pharmacopeia (USP) standards. Compounding a preparation that is commercially available is generally prohibited in most circumstances.

Federal and state laws and national standards also address quality issues by defining and requiring the adoption of good compounding practices within a compounding pharmacy. **Good compounding practices (GCP)** is composed of standards in many areas to ensure a high-quality compounded preparation (Table 8.2). Being able to compound by following GCP is a skill that is learned in the classroom, as well as through experience during on-the-job training. The pharmacist's duty is to ensure that all compounded products are prepared using GCP. For more information on good compounding practices, see the latest edition of the *Pharmacists' Pharmacopeia*.

In most cases, compounds are prepared for an individual patient and are not prepared until the prescription is received by the pharmacy. Pharmacies are allowed to

TABLE 8.2 USP Good Compounding Practices

Components of GCP	Standards
facility	designated area with adequate space; separate area for sterile compounding
personnel	all possess education, training, and proficiency in this specialized area; protective clothing must be worn
equipment	appropriate design, size, and space of balances and measuring equipment; must be cleaned and calibrated
ingredient selection	only high-grade chemicals, used and stored appropriately
compounding process	each step reviewed, with final check by the pharmacist
packaging and storage	for all ingredients, containers, and proper labeling
controls	quality control programs by the pharmacist must be in place
labeling of excess product	quantity and lot number
beyond-use dating	stability (and sterility in some cases) of preparation after compounding reflected in beyond-use dating
records and reports	including master control, compounding, equipment maintenance, and ingredients records
patient counseling	how to take and store the preparation safely

prepare excess product, called **anticipatory compounding**, as long as quantities are reasonable. These preparations must be labeled with lot number and beyond-use dating (discussed later in this chapter). Pharmacies are allowed to advertise their compounding services, but not the compounding of a specific preparation.

Federal laws also have an impact on those pharmacies specializing in making the prescription product in bulk in advance and selling to other pharmacies or healthcare professionals. If a community pharmacy is selling compounded drug products directly to health professionals (rather than to an individual patient), including to out-of-state pharmacies, then it must apply to the FDA for a manufacturing license. A manufacturing license requires many more regulations, additional procedures, and quality control checks. It is not feasible for most small compounding pharmacies to comply with these requirements.

USP Chapter 795

The United States Pharmacopeia (USP) has developed uniform standards to enhance patient safety and to protect pharmacists from litigation involved in both nonsterile (Chapter 795) and sterile compounding (Chapter 797, discussed in Chapter 10). Although it is not affiliated with any governmental agency, the FDA elects to use and enforce USP standards in the inspection of compounding pharmacies.

Definition of terms is important. Pharmaceutical manufacturers such as Eli Lilly and Merck produce **manufactured products**, whereas pharmacies produce **compounded preparations**. Chapter 795 states that a pharmacy must meet minimum standards (GCP) in terms of adequate space, as well as have the necessary equipment to compound medications. Equipment must be properly maintained, used, calibrated, and cleaned.

The USP guidelines focus on written policies and procedures for quality control, verification, and patient counseling. The quality of source ingredients must be verified. Quality control includes not only the ingredients for compounding but also training of personnel, maintaining stability and consistency of the finished preparation, preventing errors, and documenting expiration dates of compounded preparations. There must be evidence of the stability of the compound and documentation for beyond-use dating.

Product Inventory The quality of the ingredients is important to prepare a high-quality product that is both efficacious and safe. Chapter 795 specifies that only USP or National Formulary (NF) grade ingredients should be used. If such ingredients are not available, then pharmacists should secure a high-grade, purified product that is accompanied by a certificate of analysis (indicating that it is certified by the American Chemical Society).

The pharmacist often makes the decision about what source is used for ingredients—both active and inactive—in compounded medications. The decision is based on cost, quality, and purity of product. The reputation of the manufacturer and the support that the manufacturer provides also influence the choice of products selected for use in the compounding pharmacy. Many large-volume compounding pharmacies use their membership with the Pharmaceutical Compounding Centers of America (PCCA) as a primary source of product, because these centers have been certified after undergoing extensive research and scientific testing. PCCA also provides a reputable source for information and research on compatibility and stability of prepared or new compounds. Often the pharmacist must balance the higher cost of PCCA source ingredients with other lower-cost sources that also provide certified USP- or NF-grade ingredients.

Safety Note

A certificate of analysis provided by the American Chemical Society ensures that an ingredient is a high-grade, purified product.

TABLE 8.3 Bulk Product Contacts

Organization	Phone Number	Web Address
PCCA	800-331-2498	www.pccarx.com
Paddock Laboratories, Inc.	800-328-5113	www.paddocklabs.com
Hawkins Pharmaceutical	800-375-0009	www.hawkinsinc.com
Spectrum Chemical	800-342-6615	www.spectrumchemical.com
Medisca Inc.	800-932-1039	www.medisca.com
Letco Medical	800-239-5288	www.letcoinc.com

Pharmacists should have more than one source of quality ingredients, in case of a shortage, back order, or drug product recall. Table 8.3 contains a representative list of sources of bulk product and contact information for the pharmacy technician. On request, manufacturers of bulk ingredients will provide a certificate of analysis of their products.

Ingredients are commonly ordered by the technician two or three times per week, depending on volume and inventory of the compounding pharmacy. The ingredients are received the next day from one of several overnight mail services and stored by the technician. A **Material Safety Data Sheet (MSDS)** needs to be filed by the technician for all bulk chemicals or drug substances that are stored in the pharmacy. The MSDS contains important information on hazards and flammability of chemicals and procedures for treatment of accidental ingestion or exposure. The MSDS is discussed in more detail in Chapter 11, *Preparing and Handling Sterile Products and Hazardous Drugs*.

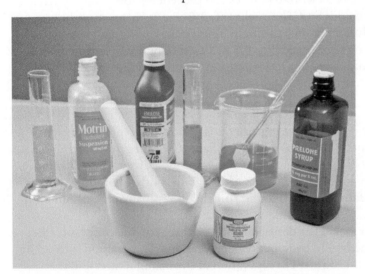

Common ingredients and equipment used in a compounding pharmacy.

Storage is generally in tight, light-resistant containers at room temperature. If the technician or pharmacist is unsure, then he or she should refer to the USP or NF compendia for temperature requirements. The technician should always check expiration dates prior to mixing any ingredients listed in the master control record. The technician should always list the source of ingredient and the NDC number on the compounding record, especially if the manufacturer has recently changed.

Beyond-Use Dating One of the key requirements of USP 795 (nonsterile preparations) and USP 797 (sterile preparations), as well as accreditation, is to have a written policy and procedure for beyond-use dating. Manufactured products have expiration dates; compounded preparations have **beyond-use dating**.

Beyond-use dating is initiated at the time of compounding, but not at the time of dispensing; this is another reason why preparations should be prepared as close to the time of patient dispensing as possible. For example, a compound prescription may have two or more active or inactive ingredients. Each one has a different manufacturer expiration date. What beyond-use dating should be used for the final compounded preparation?

In the case of nonsterile compounded products, there must be documentation of product stability. **Stability** is defined as the extent to which a product retains the same properties and characteristics that it possessed at the time of preparation. Some allowable variation (i.e., +/–2%) is to be expected. Stability includes physical properties (i.e., appearance, taste, uniformity, dissolution, and suspendibility) and chemical properties (potency). Stability also includes microbial sterility for any sterile preparation.

Chapter 795 provides estimates for beyond-use dating. For example, a refrigerated aqueous solution has a beyond-use date of 14 days. Solids (i.e., tablets and capsules) and nonaqueous solutions have a beyond-use date of 6 months or less, depending on the ingredients making up the compound. All other formulations are labeled with a 30 day beyond-use date or duration of therapy, whichever is earlier. If a manufactured or bulk drug is used, then the dating is 25% of the remaining expiration date or 6 months, whichever is earlier. If dates differ between ingredients, then the earliest date is always used. Examples 1 and 2 demonstrate the calculation of beyond-use dating for two nonsterile preparations.

Example 1

A pediatric suspension of a blood pressure medication is combined with a suspending agent on March 30, 2010, with the following source drug and expiration date:

Drug	Source of Drug	Expiration Date
Lisinopril	Manufacturer	July 2010
Suspending agent	Bulk chemical	October 2011

What should the beyond-use date be?

The labeled date should be April 30, 2010. This is 25% of the 4 months that elapse between the date that the compound was made (March 30, 2010) and the expiration date of the manufactured drug (considered to be July 31, 2010).

Example 2

A bio-identical cream is formulated with two different hormones on March 30, 2010, with the following source drugs and expiration dates:

Drug	Source of Drug	Expiration Date
Hormone A	Bulk chemical	July 2011
Hormone B	Bulk chemical	October 2011

What should the beyond-use date be?

In this case, both ingredients are bulk chemicals. The labeled date should be July 31, 2010, or 25% of the earlier expiration date of Hormone A. If Hormone A had an expiration date of October 2011, then the beyond-use date is September 30, 2010, or 6 months after the product was formulated.

The integrity of the final compounded preparation must be verified by scientific research if other beyond-use dating is used. If the compounding pharmacy has verifiable data from the PCCA or an outside analytical laboratory to extend the beyond-use dating, then the preparation can be used. The cost of testing each compounded preparation would be prohibitive for a small compounding pharmacy. Thus conservative guidelines in USP Chapter 795 are most often used. The technician should always check with the pharmacist to be sure that the labeled beyond-use dating is in accordance with the standards.

In the case of sterile compounded preparations, the requirements from Chapter 797 are, as expected, stricter. There must be documentation not only for product stability but also for sterility, or "being free from microorganisms." Most compounded sterile preparations do not contain a preservative. In a community pharmacy, the sterile preparation may only be allowed to have 24 hour or 72 hour beyond-use dating. Patients must be counseled on the labeling requirements, especially if they will be using the medication beyond the labeled dating. The patient information emphasizes the need for correct aseptic technique in a clean room environment using specialized equipment, which is further discussed in Chapter 10.

Accreditation of Compounding Pharmacies

Many compounding pharmacies today are seeking national accreditation to protect their patients and their businesses from legal challenges and to differentiate their practices from those of other pharmacies. The organization responsible for accreditation is the **Pharmacy Compounding Accrediting Board (PCAB)**. The primary role of PCAB is to provide quality standards for compounding through voluntary accreditation. The pharmacy must agree to follow specified principles as well as meet all specified standards, such as USP Chapters 795 and 797, in order to receive a "seal of accreditation." PCAB includes standards for both nonsterile and sterile compounded preparations. An accredited compounding pharmacy has a competitive advantage in the marketplace.

Continuous quality improvement (CQI) is a process of written procedures in the PCAB standards designed to identify problems and recommend solutions. As a part of CQI procedures of an accredited compounding pharmacy, there is a monthly or quarterly spot check of the technician's work. A random product is selected and sent to an outside analytical lab for analysis and exact measurement of the components. The product generally must be +/- 2% of the potency of the individual ingredients. If the steps in a procedure were not followed or if the technician needs additional training as a result of the analysis, then the corrective action must be documented and dated by the pharmacist.

Certification of Pharmacy Technicians

In addition to successfully passing a broad national certification examination (see Chapter 14, *Your Future in Pharmacy Practice*), the pharmacy technician who aspires to work in a compounding pharmacy must complete minicertifications and laboratory training in nonsterile and sterile (if preparing IV preparations) compounding . The knowledge and skills necessary to pass these specialty certifications are commonly developed as workshops and labs by Pharmacy Compounding Centers of America (PCCA). Certifications by all technicians may be necessary to attain or maintain PCAB accreditation of the pharmacy. Any compounding tasks undertaken by the technician must, in any case, be directly supervised (in the same room) and checked by the pharmacist.

Documentation of Nonsterile Compounding

Compounding is done in accordance with specific, documented instructions. Documentation of all active and inactive ingredients, as well as the proper sequence and procedure for mixing, is crucially important in preparing a high-quality preparation. All calculations for the amounts of individual ingredients must be made initially by the pharmacist, double-checked by the pharmacy technician, and verified by the pharmacist after the preparation has been compounded.

The Master Control Record

The compounding of a medication requires the addition and mixing of several necessary ingredients. The compound requires a formula (or recipe) before the technician can begin to prepare the product. After a prescription has been received by the pharmacist, the instructions for making the compound are retrieved or developed by the pharmacist. This recipe is a **master control record**, which is available either in the computer database or as a hard copy on recipelike cards. Figure 8.5 is an example of a computerized master control record.

The master control record is prepared (for a new compound) and reviewed by the pharmacist or provided by a subscriber compounding service such as the PCCA. The pharmacist uses his or her best professional judgment to assess the safety and suitability for the prescription to be compounded, as well as its intended use, especially on new orders for which a recipe must be created. Physicians are open to suggestions from the pharmacist to improve the quality or safety of their prescription.

The master control record lists the drug's name, strength, and dosage form; the ingredients and their quantities; and mixing instructions. Because of wastage, the master control record usually accounts for some overage in the weights of all of the ingredients needed. This record also includes recommended beyond-use dating and storage and labeling requirements.

Other examples of a master control record are shown in Figures 8.1 and 8.2.

FIGURE 8.5
Computerized Master Control Record

This master control record is created using PK software.

ingredients and quantities

mixing instructions

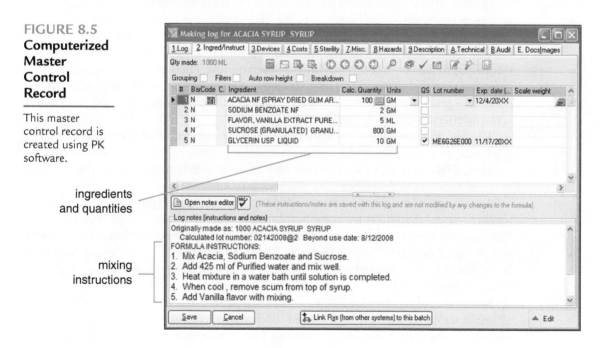

FIGURE 8.6
**Compounding
Log**

This record
is for Magic
Mouthwash, a
commonly made
formula.

Patient Name _____   Date Prepared _12/2/20XX_____

Rx # _____   Master Control Record # _____

Compounding Formula for Magic Mouthwash

Ingredient Name	Amount Needed	Manufacturer	NDC #	Lot #	Expiration Date	Prepared By	Checked By
Lidocaine 2% viscous	60 mL	HiTech	50838-0775-04		12/10/20XX		
Diphenhydramine 12.5 mg/mL	60 mL	Walgreens	00363-0379-34		07/12/20XX		
Mylanta, generic	60 mL	Qualitest	00603-0712-57		03/12/20XX		
Nystatin suspension	60 mL	Qualitest	00603-1481-58		09/11/20XX		
Total quantity	240 mL						

Prepared by _____

Approved by _____

Date _____

Directions _____

Auxiliary Labeling: SHAKE WELL

The Compounding Log

From the master control record, a printed **compounding log** is generated for each
compound to be prepared. The compounding log is unique for each prescription and
is thus intended for a specific patient. The pharmacist uses the compounding log to
complete the initial mathematical calculations and documents those calculations on
the printout. The pharmacist also identifies on the log any special equipment for the
technician to use when compounding the preparation. This compounding log is then
turned over to the pharmacy technician to direct the preparation of the product. A
computer-generated copy of the log, called the **prescription record**, is also stored and
is thus retrievable for future refills.

The compounding log lists all ingredients of the compounded preparation; quantity made; date of compounding; manufacturer; wholesaler source; and assigned lot
number, NDC number, and expiration date for each ingredient; as well as the initials
of the pharmacist and compounding technician.

An example of a manual compounding log is provided in Figure 8.6 listing the
ingredients and directions for compounding a preparation called *Magic Mouthwash*.
This formula has many variations in different regions of the country and is commonly
compounded in community pharmacies. This is an example of a basic compound that
is prepared by mixing together ingredients of existing commercially available liquids
or suspensions.

Before starting to prepare a compound for a patient, the technician should gather
all necessary ingredients and equipment. Each step of the process is checked and
initialed by the pharmacist and technician. The technician must double-check the

calculations by the pharmacist and those contained in the master control record. Any calculations completed by the technician should be written on the compounding record and checked by the pharmacist. A printout of the weight of each ingredient is usually attached to the compounding record or log sheet for pharmacist verification so that each weight in the preparation of the compound can be double-checked. It is also important to document the beyond-use date of a prepared compound.

If the compounding pharmacy receives prescriptions for hospice care or pain management patients, then it may be necessary to compound controlled substances. As expected, the procedures and recordkeeping for C-II compounds is much more detailed and extensive. Each and every milligram of the narcotic must be accounted for on the compounding record and additional log sheets. As with C-II prescriptions in the community pharmacy, the pharmacist is accountable and usually personally prepares such compounded preparations. The written manual of the pharmacy should outline the exact procedures to follow in order to meet state and federal requirements.

Calculations in the Compounding Pharmacy

The pharmacy technician practicing in a compounding pharmacy must have a knowledge of mathematical conversions and a good aptitude for performing calculations accurately. Although the pharmacist is legally responsible and checks all calculations made by the technician, a double-check of both the pharmacist's calculations and those contained in the master control record is recommended. The following examples illustrate how a technician uses calculations in a compounding practice.

Example 3

A prescription for a pediatric patient calls for 60 mL of a suspension of Coreg at a concentration of 5.5 mg/mL. Coreg is not available commercially as a suspension, but only as tablets in strengths of 3.125 mg, 6.25 mg, 12.5 mg, and 25 mg. How would you compound this prescription?

Step 1. Determine how many milligrams of Coreg are needed to compound this prescription using the ratio-proportion method.

$$\frac{x \text{ mg}}{60 \text{ mL}} = \frac{5.5 \text{ mg}}{1 \text{ mL}}$$

$$\frac{(60 \text{ mL}) \, x \text{ mg}}{60 \text{ mL}} = \frac{(60 \text{ mL}) \, 5.5 \text{ mg}}{1 \text{ mL}}$$

$$x \text{ mg} = 330 \text{ mg}$$

Step 2. Determine the tablet sizes and number of each that must be triturated (or ground) with the mortar and pestle to equal approximately 330 mg.

$$12 \text{ tablets} \times 25 \text{ mg/tablet} = 300 \text{ mg}$$

$$2 \text{ tablets} \times 12.5 \text{ mg/tablet} = 25 \text{ mg}$$

$$1 \text{ tablet} \times 6.25 \text{ mg/tablet} = 6.25 \text{ mg}$$

$$300 \text{ mg} + 25 \text{ mg} + 6.25 \text{ mg} = 331.25, \text{ which is close to the desired 330 mg}$$

Step 3. After trituration, 60 mL of suspending agent is slowly added to the pulverized tablets, a small amount (usually ½ to 1 dropperful) of flavoring agent is added, and then the product is labeled with beyond-use dating and the following instructions: "Shake Well" and "Refrigerate."

Example 4

A prescription is received to prepare a gel or cream formulation using 30 g of Ketoprofen 10%, 30 g of Gabapentin 10%, and 30 g of Lidocaine 3%. Calculate the amount of each bulk ingredient needed and then prepare the compound.

Step 1. Determine how many grams of each bulk ingredient are needed.

Ketoprofen
10% × 30 g = 3 g of Ketoprofen needed

Gabapentin
10% × 30 g = 3 g of Gabapentin needed

Lidocaine
3% × 30 g = 0.9 g, or 900 mg of Lidocaine needed

Step 2. Weigh out these amounts of each medication.

Step 3. Mix these powders, add a sufficient amount of propylene glycol to dissolve them, and then add the powdered glycol mixture to a gel or cream base formulation to make 90 g of final product.

Example 5

A prescription is received to prepare a compound for three ingredients in a ratio of 1:1:6 = 80 g. How much of each of the three ingredients is needed?

A = 10 g
B = 10 g
C = 60 g

1:1:6 = total of 80 g

10 g : 10 g : 60 g = 80 g

The total amount of the preparation equals 80 g, with ingredient C added at six times the amount of ingredients A and B.

Example 6

Using 10% oral viscous Lidocaine to make *Magic Mouthwash*, how many milligrams in 1mL of 10% viscous Lidocaine?

Because a 1% concentration = 10 mg/mL, a 10% concentration = 100 mg/mL.

Example 7

How much Nitrobid 2% ointment is required to make 100 g of a 0.2% ointment?

Nitrobid is commercially available as a 2% ointment, but the prescription calls for a 0.2% ointment. The desired concentration is one-tenth or 10% of the commercially available product. Mix 10 g of 2% Nitrobid (10% of 100 g) ointment with approximately 90 grams of ointment base to make a final preparation of 100 g of 0.2% ointment.

Safety Note

Remember that a 1% concentration equals 10 mg/mL. A 20% concentration equals 200 mg/mL. This conversion is often used to make sterile preparations in the hospital and in the home health-care environment.

In this example, you could also use the alligation method discussed in Chapter 5, with 2% Nitrobid combined with 0% active ingredients of the ointment base. Remember that 2% Nitrobid is equivalent to 20 g, and 0.2% Nitrobid is equivalent to 2 g.

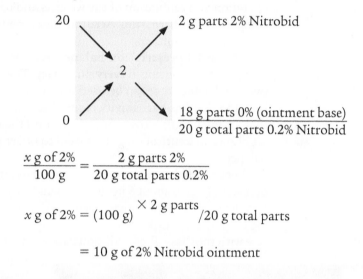

$$\frac{x \text{ g of } 2\%}{100 \text{ g}} = \frac{2 \text{ g parts } 2\%}{20 \text{ g total parts } 0.2\%}$$

$$x \text{ g of } 2\% = (100 \text{ g}) \times 2 \text{ g parts} / 20 \text{ g total parts}$$

$$= 10 \text{ g of } 2\% \text{ Nitrobid ointment}$$

Example 8

Nystatin powder has an activity of 100,000 units/g. How many milligrams of nystatin would you use in each capsule if the final preparation is supposed to be 1,500,000 units per capsule?

Step 1. Convert 100,000 units/g to units per milligram.

$$100,000 \text{ units/g} \times 1 \text{ g}/1,000 \text{ mg} = 100 \text{ units/mg}$$

Step 2. Determine the amount of milligrams needed in each capsule using the ratio-proportion method.

$$\frac{x \text{ mg}}{1,500,000 \text{ units}} = \frac{1 \text{ mg}}{100 \text{ units}}$$

$$\frac{(1,500,000 \text{ units}) \, x \text{ mg}}{1,500,000 \text{ units}} = \frac{(1,500,000 \text{ units}) \, 1 \text{ mg}}{100 \text{ units}}$$

$$x \text{ mg} = 15,000 \text{ mg}$$

Equipment for Weighing, Measuring, and Compounding

Proper compounding by the technician requires an intimate knowledge of various kinds of pharmaceutical equipment to weigh, measure, reduce, and combine ingredients. An appreciation for allowable percentage of error in weighing and measuring ingredients is also discussed in this section.

Weights and Balances

Many types of balances are used to weigh pharmaceutical ingredients accurately. The type of balance used often is based on the volume of pharmaceutical compounding and the cost of balances. The pharmacy technician must become familiar with the operation and calibration of the weights and balances used in the community and compounding pharmacies. Accurate measurements are required in order to produce a quality preparation.

A **Class III prescription balance**, formerly known as a *Class A prescription balance*, is required equipment in every pharmacy. The Class III prescription balance is a two-pan balance that can be used for weighing small amounts of material (120 mg or less) and that has a sensitivity requirement (SR) in the range of +/-6 mg. This means that a 6 mg weight moves the indicator on the balance by 1 degree. A standardized set of pharmaceutical weights is used to offset the ingredient weight with a Class III balance.

A **counterbalance** also contains two pans but is used for weighing larger amounts of material, up to about 5 kg. It has a sensitivity requirement in the range of +/-100 mg. Because of its lesser sensitivity, a counterbalance is not used in prescription compounding but rather for tasks such as measuring bulk products (e.g., Epsom salts). As is the case with the Class III prescription balance, a standardized set of pharmaceutical weights is used to offset the ingredient weights on a counterbalance.

Ingredients (and weights if using a Class III or counterbalance) should always be placed on a **weighing paper** or powder paper. Weighing paper is placed on the balance pan to avoid contact between pharmaceutical ingredients and the balance tray. Typically, glassine paper is used. Glassine paper is a thin paper that has been coated with a nonabsorbent paraffin wax. The paper on each balance pan should be of exactly the same size and weight. The edges of the paper on the pan may be folded upward to hold the ingredient to be weighed.

A **digital electronic analytical balance** uses a single pan and is easier to learn to use and more accurate than a Class III balance or a counterbalance. However, electronic balances tend to be much more costly ($2,500 or more) and are typically used in large-scale or dedicated pharmacy compounding labs and hospitals.

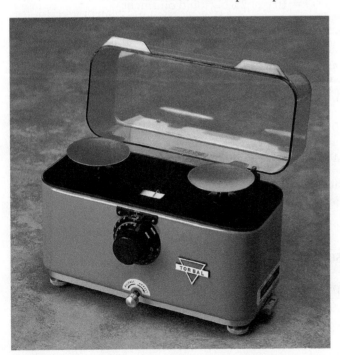

The Class III prescription balance is a two-pan balance for weighing small amounts of ingredients.

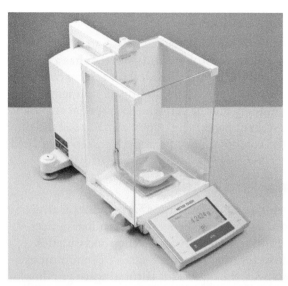

A digital electronic balance is very accurate, with a capacity of 100 g or more and a sensitivity as low as +/–1 mg.

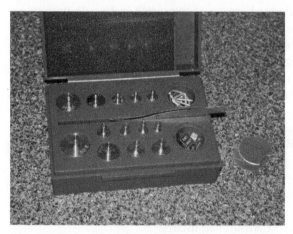

A set of pharmacy weights. Metric weights are in the front row and apothecary weights are in the back row.

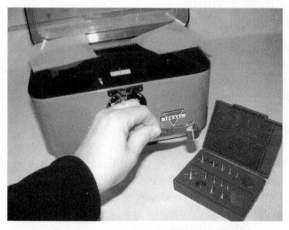

Weights should be transferred using forceps and should not be touched with bare skin. Moisture or oils affect their accuracy.

Pharmaceutical Weights

Pharmaceutical weights may be used with two-pan balances. Weights are generally made of polished brass and may be coated with a noncorrosive material such as nickel or chromium. Sets contain both metric and apothecary weights. (For information about the metric and apothecary measurement systems, see Chapter 5.) Typical metric sets contain gram weights of 1, 2, 5, 10, 20, 50, and 100 g, which are conically shaped, with a handle and flattened top. Fractional gram weights (e.g., 10, 20, 50, 100, 200, and 500 mg) are also available. These are made of aluminum and are usually flat, with one raised edge to facilitate being picked up using forceps.

Avoirdupois weights (see Chapter 5) of $\frac{1}{32}$, $\frac{1}{16}$, $\frac{1}{8}$, $\frac{1}{4}$, $\frac{1}{2}$, 1, 2, 4, and 8 oz may also be used. Weights come in a container in which they should be stored when not in use. Care should be taken not to touch or drop a weight or otherwise expose it to damage or contamination. Weights are used for both measurement and calibration of equipment. Electronic balances generally do not need to use the pharmacy weights.

Forceps and Spatulas

Weights should not be transferred using the hands and fingers. A **forceps** is an instrument used for grasping small objects, such as pharmaceutical weights. Forceps are used for picking up smaller weights and transferring them to and from measuring balances to avoid transferring moisture or oil to the weights. Over time moisture and oil can change the weight of the weights and become a potential source of error in preparing small doses, such as for pediatric patients. A cloth may be used to transfer larger weights.

A **spatula** is an instrument used for transferring solid pharmaceutical ingredients to weighing pans and for various compounding tasks, such as preparing ointments and creams or loosening material from the surfaces of a mortar and pestle and placing the final preparation in a container. A spatula may be made of stainless steel, plastic, or hard rubber. Hard rubber spatulas are used when corrosive materials, such as iodine and mercuric salts, are handled.

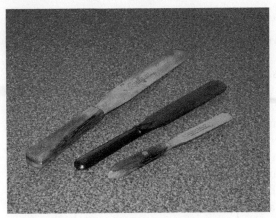

Spatulas are a common tool in a compounding pharmacy.

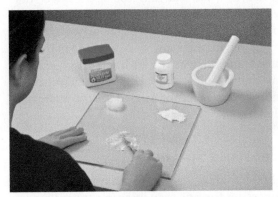

A compounding slab is used to prepare specialized prescriptions for creams and ointments.

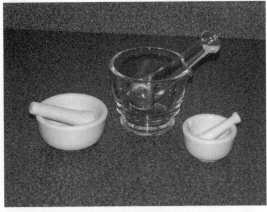

The mortar and pestle are used to mix or grind substances.

Compounding Slab

A **compounding slab**, also known as an ointment slab, is a plate made of ground glass that has a flat, hard, nonabsorbent surface ideal for mixing compounds. In lieu of a compounding or ointment slab, compounding may be performed on special disposable nonabsorbent parchment paper, which is discarded after the compounding operation has been completed.

Mortar and Pestle

A **mortar and pestle** are used for grinding and mixing pharmaceutical ingredients. These familiar devices come in glass, porcelain, and Wedgwood varieties. Paradoxically, the coarser the surface of the mortar and pestle is, the finer is the triturating, or grinding, that can be done. As a result, a coarse-grained porcelain or Wedgwood mortar and pestle set is used for triturating (or pulverizing) crystals, granules, and powders, whereas a glass mortar and pestle, with its smooth surface, is preferred for mixing of liquids and semisolid dosage forms such as creams, ointments, and gels. A glass mortar and pestle also has the advantage of being nonporous and nonstaining.

An electro mortar and pestle is often used in a high-volume compounding pharmacy to reduce particle size and to mix the pharmaceutical compound more thoroughly after the weighing and manual manipulation of ingredients with a spatula. This equipment can be calibrated to a specific product if necessary, but it generally produces a pharmaceutically elegant cream or ointment after 3 minutes of constant automated mixing.

Graduate Cylinders, Pipettes, and Beakers

A **graduate cylinder** is a glass or polypropylene flask used for measuring liquids. The flasks come in two varieties: (1) conical and (2) cylindrical. Conical graduates have wide tops and narrow bases and taper from the top to the bottom. These graduates are calibrated in both metric and apothecary units. Cylindrical graduates are more accurate and have the shape of a uniform column. Cylindrical graduates are generally calibrated in metric units (in other words, cubic centimeters). Both kinds of graduate cylinders are available in a wide variety of sizes, ranging from 5 mL to more than 1000 mL.

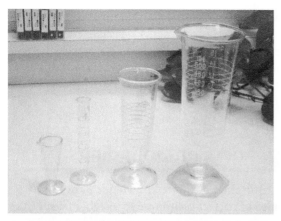

Graduates are available in a variety of sizes and shapes. Cylindrical graduates are more accurate than conical graduates. The second graduate from the left is cylindrical.

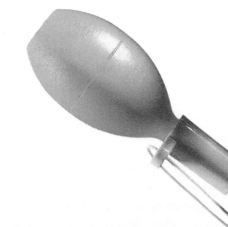

A suction device is used on a pipette to withdraw hazardous liquids.

Glass beakers such as those that you may have used in the chemistry lab are available in various sizes; they are used to measure larger volumes of liquids (usually 8 fluid ounces or more); beakers are not as accurate as graduate cylinders and are only used when an exact measurement of liquid is not required. Remember that milliliters (abbreviated as mL) and cubic centimeters (abbreviated as cc) are equivalent and interchangeable terms of liquid measurement.

A **pipette** is a long, thin, calibrated hollow tube used for measurement and transfer of volumes of liquid less than 1.5 mL. A pipette is like a glass straw. A pipette filler, which is like a suction device, is used instead of the mouth for drawing up a hazardous solution, such as an acid, into the pipette.

Other Equipment

A myriad of other equipment is used in the pharmacy compounding operation. Freezers and refrigerators are required to store some ingredients and final products. The technician needs to check and document equipment temperatures, as well as room temperature, on a daily basis.

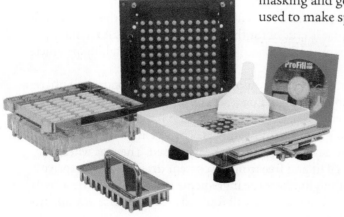

To prepare tablets a powder container hood with special masking and gowning is required. A convection oven may be used to make special tablet formulations, such as pellets and rapid-dissolve compounds. A single-punch tablet press is used to blend active and inactive ingredients (or excipients). The powders can be weighed and placed in a die; when the handle is lowered, an individual tablet is produced by compression. A pellet press is used to compound an implantable urethral pellet of medication. A capsule machine with multiple metal plates may be used to replace the one-at-a-time punch-and-fill method discussed later in this chapter; a capsule machine can make 100 capsules within a short period.

A small capsule-filling unit may be used in a compounding pharmacy.

If sterile preparations are compounded, then additional equipment and space are needed. An autoclave may be used to sterilize metal instruments. Specialized equipment and a clean room environment are essential if sterile products are prepared. An incubator may be used to culture products, surfaces, or air for microbial contamination; most growth, if present, occurs in the first 48 hours, but the product is checked again after 2 weeks of in-house sterility testing.

Technique for Weighing, Measuring, and Compounding

Proper compounding by the technician requires an intimate knowledge of not only various pharmaceutical equipment but also of correct technique to weigh, measure, reduce, and combine ingredients. An error in measuring ingredients could result in serious drug toxicity. Special attire requirements are indicated for the pharmacy technician working in a compounding pharmacy.

Attire and Preparation Requirements

Before measuring and preparing ingredients, the technician must meet minimum attire standards. Although the standards are not as rigid as requirements for making sterile preparations, the technician should follow the attire guidelines as specified in the policy and procedure manual of the community pharmacy. Clean protective clothing should be worn during any compounding operation to protect drug products from contamination. Generally, the minimum requirements for nonsterile compounding include a hairnet, long lab coat, and gloves. If hazardous chemicals are used, then eye goggles, mask, and double gowning may be necessary; an eyewash station must be available in case of an accidental exposure.

USP Chapter 795 also specifies that all personnel must wash hands, even for nonsterile compounding. Hands must be washed with a liquid antimicrobial soap with a brisk rubbing action for a minimum of 15 seconds; the hands should be rinsed well and dried off with paper towel that is appropriately disposed of after each procedure. Hands should be washed and disposable gloves should be discarded after each compounded preparation. No food items should be stored or consumed in the staging area.

Technique for Weighing Pharmaceutical Ingredients

Accurately weighing ingredients is one of the most essential parts of the compounding process and a technique that is crucial for the technician to learn. A technician must continually practice to feel confident and comfortable with weighing products on various prescription balances.

The electronic balance is the preferred equipment for most compounding pharmacies. An electronic balance should be placed on a secure, level, nonvibrating surface, at waist height. It must be perfectly level, both side to side and front to back. Leveling is often the most time-consuming process for beginners. The levelness should be checked often throughout the day if the balance is heavily used. The area where the balance is placed should be well lit and free from air current drafts, dust, corrosive vapors, or high humidity that might affect the ingredients or the weight measurements. These balances are usually enclosed on all four sides to minimize any air current impacts during the weighing process.

The procedure for measuring using an electronic balance are outlined in the steps shown in Table 8.4.

TABLE 8.4 Steps for Using an Electronic Balance

1. Locate the zero point, including the weight of the weighing or powder paper.
2. Place a small amount of chemical or drug to be measured (from the compounding record) onto the paper on the pan, using a spatula to transfer it.
3. Once a nearly precise amount of material has been transferred to the pan, a very small adjustment upward can be made by placing a small amount of material on the spatula, holding the spatula over the paper, and lightly tapping the spatula with the forefinger to knock a bit of the substance onto the pan; this is done with the balance unlocked and the balance beam free to move.
4. Read the digital weight measurement.
5. Lock the balance before removing the measured substance.

The electronic balance should be warmed up for 30 minutes after the AC adapter is plugged in, and then it should be calibrated each day prior to use. Many electronic balances produce a hard-copy printout of the weights of the individual ingredients that the technician has measured. This printout is then attached to the compounding record for the pharmacist to check the final compounded preparation. A pharmacist or an experienced certified technician may need to check the technician's weighing technique and results for a while after initial training, especially if no printout for the weights of ingredients is available.

The balance should be in the locked or "arrested" position when it is not in use and when it is being moved. Avoid spilling materials onto the balance. If any materials are spilled on the balance, then wipe them off immediately with the balance in the locked position. Do not place materials onto the balance while it is released (in other words, unlocked), because doing so may force the pan down suddenly and cause damage to the instrument. Balances must be cleaned after each use, with documented daily calibration.

A Class III prescription balance is sufficiently accurate for infrequent compounding in a community pharmacy. The correct technique is demonstrated in Figure 8.7. However, variations in technique could easily result in a small but serious error, resulting in a subtherapeutic or toxic dose of medication.

Weighing the exact amount prescribed is essential because the product cannot be easily checked for content once mixed. A pharmacist must visually check the weight measurements of all ingredients that the technician has weighed.

FIGURE 8.7 Weighing with a Class III Prescription Balance

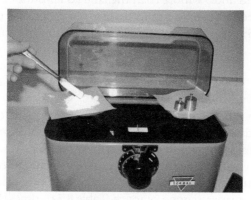

(a) Transferring a substance to the scale.

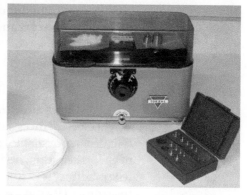

(b) The final measurement is taken with the lid closed.

Chapter 8 *Nonsterile Pharmaceutical Compounding*   253

Calculating Percentage of Error

Percentages are used in a variety of ways in the preparation of medication doses. As discussed in Chapter 7, percentages are used when doing the business of the pharmacy (i.e., calculating percentage of sales, discount, or markup). In the compounding pharmacy, percentages are used in determining the possible percentage of error and the least weighable quantity of a substance for safe preparation.

Error in measurement in nonsterile preparations is expected, and allowances are made for a certain **percentage of error** over or under the target measurement. The percentage of error within this range is not consequential for most compounded medications. Pharmacy scales are generally very accurate; however, knowing the margin of error or sensitivity of a balance is important. Most balances are marked with their degree of accuracy. When any substance is weighed, the scale will appear to have measured correctly. However, too small a sample may have an unacceptable margin of error.

Most nonsterile compounded preparations, such as tablets, capsules, ointments, creams, and gels, are prepared in larger quantities than the original prescription from the physician, especially if refills are written. For example, instead of preparing 30 capsules of a medication each month, the master control record may call for a minimum quantity of 100 capsules to be made. The reasons include both the costs in terms of personnel preparation time and the lowered percentage of error in the measuring and mixing of ingredients. The stock bottles for the excess product must be labeled with quantity, lot number, date made, and beyond-use dating, as well as the initials of the pharmacist and compounding technician. The technician must check the stock medication on the shelf monthly for expiration dates or as specified in the policy and procedure manual.

If a substance was weighed or measured incorrectly and an instrument is available to remeasure the amount in question more accurately, then we can determine the percentage of error. This can be found by using the following formula:

$$\frac{\text{amount of error}}{\text{quantity desired}} \times 100 = \text{percentage of error}$$

In this equation, the amount of error is the difference between the actual amount and the quantity desired, or

$$\text{actual amount} - \text{quantity desired} = \text{amount of error}$$

For example, a new brand of vitamins claims to have a range of 9% bioavailability of a national brand of 1000 mg vitamin C. The range of error is +/–90 mg or 910 mg to 1090 mg. This is 9% less and 9% more than the labeled amount of 1000 mg. Some more potent compounded drugs may require a narrower range of error, usually less than or no greater than 5%. Sterile compounded preparations may have an error range of less than 2%.

Technique for Measuring Liquid Volumes

Liquid volumes are often much easier to measure than solid ingredients that must be weighed on balances, and a wide variety of containers such as beakers and graduate cylinders are available to assist in volumetric measurement. A general rule of thumb is to always select the device that yields the most accurate volume. Selecting a container that is at least half full during measurement, or using the smallest device that holds the required volume, is considered good practice. Table 8.5 outlines the procedure for measuring liquid volumes.

TABLE 8.5 **Measuring Liquid Volumes**

1. Choose a graduate cylinder with a capacity that equals or very slightly exceeds the total volume of the liquid to be measured. Doing so reduces the percentage of error in the measurement. In no case should the volume to be measured be less than 20% of the total capacity of the graduate. For example, 10 mL of liquid should not be measured in a graduate cylinder exceeding 50 mL in capacity. The closer the total capacity of the graduate is to the volume to be measured, the more accurate the measurement will be.

2. Note that the narrower the column of liquid is in the graduate, the less substantial any reading error will be. Thus, for very small volume measurements, a pipette is preferable to a cylindrical graduate, and, for larger measurements, a cylindrical graduate is preferable to a conical graduate, and a conical graduate may be preferable to a glass beaker.

3. Pour the liquid to be measured slowly into the graduate, watching the level of the liquid in the graduate as you do so. If the liquid is viscous, or thick, then you should attempt to pour it toward the center of the graduate to avoid having some of the liquid cling to the sides.

4. Wait for liquid clinging to the sides of the graduate to settle before taking a measurement.

5. Read the level of the liquid *at eye level* and read the measure at the bottom of the meniscus (see Figure 8.8).

6. When pouring the liquid out of the graduate, allow ample time for all of the liquid to drain. Depending on the viscosity of the liquid, more or less clings to the sides of the graduate. For a particularly viscous liquid, some compensation or adjustment for this clinging may have to be made.

Safety Note

Always measure liquids on a solid, level surface at eye level.

FIGURE 8.8
Meniscus

Liquid in a narrow column usually forms a concave meniscus. Measurements should be taken at the bottom of the concavity when read at eye level.

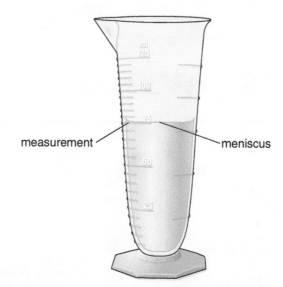

measurement — — meniscus

On the upper surface of the liquid is a **meniscus**, or moon-shaped body (in other words, slightly concave or bowed inward toward the center) (Figure 8.8). The level of the liquid is slightly higher at the edges; therefore, do not measure the level by looking down on the graduate. Instead measure at eye level. Read the level of the liquid at the *bottom* of the meniscus.

Techniques for Mixing Compounded Drugs

Before preparing a drug for compounding, the technician should gather the master control record, ingredients, equipment, glassware, packaging material, and mixing directions. Providing adequate and uninterrupted time to the person who is compounding the prescription is also very important to minimize measuring or calculation errors.

After the technician has accurately weighed or measured out the individual ingredients in a compounded prescription, he or she must learn the best technique to mix the active and inactive ingredients for a tablet, capsule, cream, ointment, gel, or other formulation. The mixing directions should include the need for diluting or sequencing the addition of ingredients. The best technique for mixing a given set of compounded medications should be included in the master control record or suggested by the experienced pharmacist.

Comminution and Blending **Comminution** is the act of reducing a substance to small, fine particles. **Blending** is the act of combining two substances. Techniques for comminution and blending include trituration, levigation, pulverization, spatulation, sifting, and tumbling. With repetition and experience, the technician can become more proficient in the preparation of a high-quality, pharmaceutically elegant, compounded preparation.

Trituration is the process of rubbing, grinding, or pulverizing a substance to create fine particles, generally by means of a mortar and pestle. A rapid motion with minimal pressure provides the best results. As discussed previously, various types of mortar and pestles are available for different ingredients.

When mixing solids and liquids, reducing the particle size of the solid by gently heating the liquid (if the liquid is stable or nonvolatile) on a hot plate generally makes the solid dissolve faster and more uniformly. In addition, there will be less precipitation or clinging together of the solute into particles of unacceptably large size.

Figure 8.9, *a,* shows an example of a compounding log for a prescription for a dog. To prepare this medication, the technician follows the steps in Table 8.4 for weighing

FIGURE 8.9

Preparing a Solution for Sparky the Dog

(a) Compounding log. (b) Weighing the potassium bromide. (c) Potassium bromide and beef flavoring. (d) Partially triturated. (e) Adding distilled water. (f) Prepared prescription waiting for pharmacist approval.

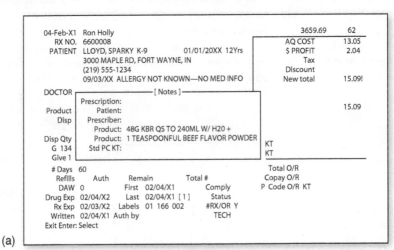

(a)

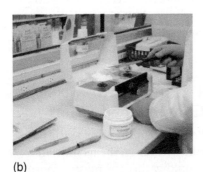

(b)

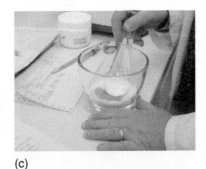

(c)

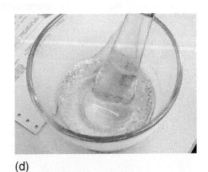

(d)

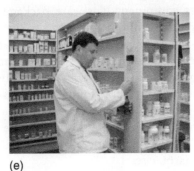

(e)

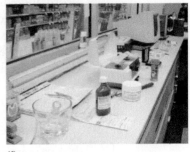

(f)

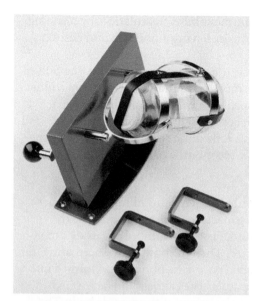

A manual powder mixer enhances the mixing of two powders needed for a compounded prescription.

the product (potassium bromide) (Figure 8.9, *b*). Then, the product is placed in a mortar to be triturated and combined with the flavoring (Figure 8.9, *c*). Figure 8.9, *d*, shows the mixed ingredients, but, at this stage, more trituration is needed to get the particles to a more even texture. The mixed and triturated ingredients are put into an amber bottle, using a glass funnel. In Figure 8.9, *e*, a wall-mounted source of distilled water (also used to reconstitute antibiotic powders) is added to mix the veterinary prescription. Then, the bottle is shaken well and labeled, and the preparation is laid out to be checked by the pharmacist (Figure 8.9, *f*).

Levigation is typically used when reducing the particle size of a solid during the preparation of an ointment. A paste is formed of a solid material and a tiny amount of a liquid levigating agent, such as castor oil or mineral oil, that is miscible, or mixable, with the solid. The amount of levigating agent added to the final preparation is included in the compounding record. The paste is then triturated with a glass mortar and pestle to reduce the particle size and added to an ointment base.

Pulverization by intervention is the process of reducing the size of particles in a solid with the aid of an additional material in which the substance is soluble—a volatile solvent such as camphor, alcohol, iodine, or ether. The solvent is added per mixing directions on the master control record, and then the mixture is triturated. The solvent is permitted to evaporate so it does not become part of the final product.

Spatulation is the process of combining and mixing substances by means of a spatula, generally on an ointment slab or tile. **Sifting** is a process not unlike the sifting of flour in baking. It can be used to blend or combine powders. Powders can also be combined by **tumbling**—placing the powders into a bag or container and shaking it.

Compounding Ointments and Creams Dermatologic therapies may call for combining existing ointments or creams. Most ointments and creams are prepared via mechanical incorporation of materials, levigation, or mixing in a mortar and pestle.

In other cases, the dry ingredients of an ointment or cream may have to be triturated, or reduced to a fine powder, in a mortar and pestle before being added to the ointment or cream base. This is to avoid a gritty, nonuniform appearance of the preparation. When placing a powder into an ointment, adding the powder in small amounts and constantly working the mixture in with the spatula or pestle to reduce particle size to obtain a smooth, nongritty product is important. An electro mortar and pestle or automated ointment mill can be used if available to maximize the mixing of ingredients and to improve the appearance of the final preparation.

If mixing three or more ingredients to the ointment or cream base, then adding them sequentially rather than mixing them together is important; this allows for more drug stability and a more pharmaceutically elegant end preparation. When an ointment slab and spatula are used, the edge of the spatula should press against the slab to provide a shearing force, which allows for a smoother preparation.

Compounding Powders Powders are combined and mixed by a variety of means, including spatulation, trituration, sifting, and tumbling in a container or blending machine. Powders may also be levigated (formed into a paste using a small amount of liquid) in preparation for being added to an ointment base. Spatulation, or blending with a spatula, is used for small amounts of powder having a uniform and desired particle size and density.

In order to create an oral solid pediatric dose, the pharmacist might have to pulverize, or triturate, commercially available tablets, mix the resultant powder with a diluent powder, and use that powder mixture to fill capsules. A **diluent powder** is an inactive ingredient(s) that is added to the active drug in compounding a tablet or capsule. Tumbling is used to combine powders that have little or no toxic potential. The powders to be combined are placed in a bag or in a wide-mouthed container and shaken well; alternatively, manual mixers may be used.

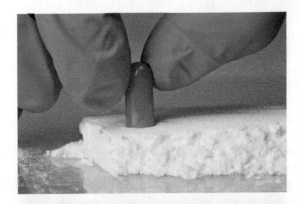

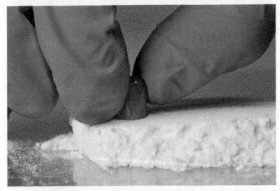

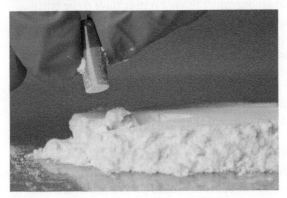

In the punch method for extemporaneous filling of capsules, the body of the capsule is filled by "punching" into a cake of the powder. The filled capsule is then weighed to verify the dose.

Filling Capsules When hand-filling a capsule with powder, a pharmacist or technician may use the **punch method**. First, the number of capsules to be filled is counted. Then the powder is placed on a clean surface of paper, porcelain, or glass and formed into a cake with a spatula. The cake should be approximately ¼ to ⅓ the height of the capsule body. The body of the capsule is then punched into the cake repeatedly until the capsule is full. The cap is then placed snugly over the body. Granules are generally poured into the capsule body from a piece of paper. Hand-operated capsule-filling machines are often used in higher volume compounding pharmacies.

Geometric Dilution Method Often a mortar and pestle is used to combine more than one drug using a **geometric dilution method**. Place the most potent ingredient, which is most likely the ingredient that occurs in the smallest amount, into the mortar first. Then add an equal amount of the next most potent ingredient and mix well. Continue in this manner, adding, each time, an amount equal to the amount in the mortar, until successively larger amounts of all the ingredients are added. Then add any excess amount of any ingredient and mix well.

This technique can be used when mixing toxic or potentially insoluble liquids. Trituration is used when a potent or hazardous drug is mixed with a diluent powder. At first, equal amounts of the potent drug and the diluent are triturated with a mortar and pestle. When these are thoroughly mixed, more of the diluent is added, equal to the amount already in the mortar. This process is continued until all of the diluent is incorporated into the compound.

The same concept can be used when mixing incompatible liquids. When mixing two liquids, a possible precipitation of solutes within the liquids can sometimes be avoided by making each portion as dilute as possible before mixing the liquids together.

The Compounding Process

Table 8.6 summarizes the 14 steps required by USP Chapter 795 to compound a nonsterile preparation. These steps, or something similar, should appear in the policy and procedure manual for the compounding pharmacy. If these steps are followed on each and every compound prescription, then the quality and efficacy of the preparation will be maximized and the risk of medication error minimized. Following these steps also minimizes legal liability and ensures continuing accreditation status.

The following sections discuss further the proper selection of medication containers, labeling, recordkeeping, and cleanup requirements, as well as the final check process by the pharmacist and the counseling of the patient. Issues related to insurance coverage for compounded products are discussed at the end of this section.

Safety Note

Compounding should never be rushed.

TABLE 8.6 Steps in the Compounding Process

1. The pharmacist judges the suitability of the prescription to be compounded in terms of safety and intended use.
2. The pharmacist retrieves and reviews the master control record in the computer.
3. The pharmacist prints out a compounding record or log sheet for the technician to make the nonsterile preparation.
4. The pharmacist performs all necessary mathematical calculations and identifies the necessary equipment for the technician; the technician double-checks all calculations.
5. A medication container label is typed or created by the computer software using information in the compounding log.
6. The pharmacy technician uses appropriate protective clothing and handwashing technique.
7. The technician gathers all necessary active and inactive ingredients, as well as prepares and calibrates any necessary equipment.
8. The technician weighs and adds all ingredients for the preparation, initials each step, and adds documentation (such as source and NDC number) to the compounding record.
9. The technician labels and stores the medication in a suitable container.
10. The pharmacist reviews the compounding record (with the printout of the weights of all ingredients) and medication container label and assesses appropriate physical characteristics of the preparation, such as any weight variations, adequacy of mixing, clarity, odor, color, consistency, and pH.
11. The technician prepares a medication container label, affixing it to the proper container. The label includes the following:
    a. Patient name
    b. Physician name
    c. Date of compounding
    d. Name of preparation
    e. Internal ID or lot number
    f. Beyond-use date
    g. Initials of compounding technician and pharmacist
    h. Directions for use, including any special storage conditions
    i. Any additional requirements of state or federal law
12. The pharmacist signs and dates the compounding record and/or prescription, files the records (computer entry and printed copy), and places the compounded preparation in a storage bin for patient pickup.
13. The technician cleans all equipment thoroughly and promptly, reshelves all active and inactive ingredients, and properly labels and stores any excess preparation.
14. The pharmacist counsels the patient at the time of pickup.

Selecting Medication Containers

With so much emphasis on chemical stability, it is important for the pharmacy technician to select the appropriate container to extend the beyond-use dating as much as possible. Standards for packaging the most common compounds are provided by USP in the *Pharmacists' Pharmacopeia* (see under Reference Sources for the Compounding

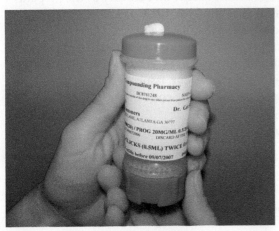

The TopiClick is a patented delivery system to dose hormone creams and gels accurately.

Pharmacy). For tablets and capsules, amber-colored prescription vials are used to protect the product from light. Ointments and creams may be placed in ointment jars in various sizes. Suppositories and pellets may be dispensed in cardboard boxes.

Bio-identical hormones in a cream or gel formulation are often dispensed in an oral syringe, with the dosage calibrated to milliliters on the syringe. An easier-to-use, unique weight-to-weight delivery system, called TopiClick, has recently been patented. This system resembles a deodorant dispenser: each turn or click delivers a given amount (250 mg) of medication. Using TopiClick, a patient can easily and accurately dispense the correct amount of medication and the method appears to be well accepted by physicians as an alternative to oral syringes.

Labeling and Cleanup

After the compounding operation, the preparation must be labeled with a prescription label (in other words, medication container label) containing all information required by the governing laws and regulations of the state and federal government. The ingredients of the compound and the amounts of these ingredients should be clearly stated on the medication container label. The label should also included beyond-use dating (often labeled "discard after"), the lot number, and the date of the compounding. If commercial products are used, then the generic names and the names of inactive ingredients, should be listed on the medication container label. No abbreviations of active drug ingredients should be used (in the rare event that the drug must be identified in an emergency).

The prescription balance, when not in use, should be placed in the locked position and covered, and weights must be placed back in their original container. Once the compounding operation is completed for each product, equipment and the work area should be thoroughly cleaned, and ingredients should be returned to their proper places in storage.

Many active pharmaceuticals and bulk ingredients used in compounding are considered hazardous chemicals. This designation may reflect chemical ignitibility, corrosivity, reactivity, or toxicity. These chemicals are prepared in very small doses in compounded preparations and thus are not generally considered to be hazardous. These compounds can be mailed without special precautions and labeling if proper storage conditions can be maintained. The technician must pay special attention to correct cleanup disinfectants and procedures to minimize cross-contamination and potential allergic reactions.

Any expired or discarded product including a hazardous chemical should be placed in a sealed container in a designated biohazard container (not the wastebasket) per written policy and procedure. After the contents have been verified and signed off by the pharmacist, an outside vendor takes receipt and discards the materials per state and federal regulations.

Final Check by the Pharmacist

The pharmacist is legally responsible for checking the final product, including ensuring that the correct master control record was used, that mathematical calculations were accurate on the compounding record, and that printouts on all weighed ingredients (if available) were verified. The medication container label must also be checked. A careful record of the compounding operation, including ingredients and amounts of ingredients used, the preparer of the compound, and the name of the supervising pharmacist, should be kept. Compounding logs provide a means of keeping such records in the computer and as printed copy.

Finally, the pharmacist checks the **pharmaceutical elegance** (or how the product looks) by performing a physical inspection of the preparation. The pharmacist uses his or her knowledge and experience to review the adequacy of mixing, odor, color, consistency, and pH (acid or base balance) if necessary. The pharmacist initials the compounding record and the label and places the product under proper storage conditions for pickup by the patient.

After the product is prepared by the technician and checked by the pharmacist, a printed copy of the compounding record is filed with the original prescription, for later retrieval or recall if necessary. Prescriptions are filed in accordance with state, federal, and other legal regulations. Easy retrievability is important if there is a drug recall of any ingredients or if an adverse effect occurs in the patient. In addition to printed copies of the formula and prescription, most records are stored on a CD or hard drive of the computer on-site or, preferably, through an off-site vendor.

Patient Counseling by the Pharmacist

The pharmacist should communicate to the patient that his or her prescription has been individually prepared and compounded. In addition, the compounded preparation information should be typed on the medication container label. The patient should be aware of the ingredients contained in the compound prescription and their expected therapeutic and potential adverse effects.

As with all prescriptions, the pharmacist must offer counseling to all patients regarding compounded preparations. The pharmacist must be sure that the patient understands how to take the medication, especially if an unusual delivery system is used. For example, how does the dosage compare to the milliliters or cubic centimeters on a syringe or to the clicks on a TopiClick? How is this delivery device primed or how often does it need to be primed? The pharmacist must also communicate the proper storage conditions for the compounded preparation, as well as the labeled beyond-use or expiration dating.

Reimbursement

Insurance generally does not cover the cost of a compounded preparation. This is a major reason for the growth of specialized compounding pharmacies as insurance has squeezed much of the profit from an independent community pharmacy. The patient cost for a compounded medication is based on the time and experience of the pharmacist and technician rather than on the costs, which are usually minimal, of the active and inactive ingredients. Most compounded prescriptions take a minimum of 30 to 60 minutes to prepare.

Some insurance companies allow the pharmacy to submit a universal claim form (UCF), complete with NDC numbers of each ingredient for reimbursement. Patients often pay out-of-pocket and then are reimbursed by their insurance at a later date.

A compounding pharmacy provides all necessary information for a patient on a Universal Claim Form for a Compound Medication to bill insurance. The success of reimbursement for a compounded medication may be greater if the patient, rather than the pharmacy, submits the claim billing a third-party insurer.

Reference Sources for the Compounding Pharmacy

Nonsterile compounding requires specialty training, certification, and experience. In addition to receiving advice from the supervising pharmacist, the pharmacy technician can refer to standard reference works on the subject, such as *Remington: The Science and Practice of Pharmacy* by Gennaro, and at the following:

- Professional Compounding Centers of America (PCCA)
- United States Pharmacopeia
- *Secundum Artem: Current and Practical Compounding Information for the Pharmacist*
- International Academy of Compounding Pharmacists

As discussed earlier in the chapter, PCCA is a source supplier of high-quality USP- and NF-grade ingredients. The PCCA also holds national and regional educational and certification seminars in sterile and nonsterile compounding for pharmacists and pharmacy technicians. Membership entitles access to the master formulas that have been developed and proven safe and effective over the years. PCCA is also a source of pharmacy software as well as marketing and business consultations.

As discussed in Chapter 2, the USP is a private, nongovernmental organization that is responsible for setting standards, such as Chapter 795, that are recognized by the government (FDA) and by private organizations (such as the Joint Commission discussed in Chapter 9, *Hospital Pharmacy Practice*). The USP has recently published a *Pharmacists' Pharmacopeia*, which is a reference for pharmacy personnel involved in sterile and nonsterile compounding. This text includes approved monographs for 120 compound preparations, as well as all necessary guidelines and standards for the safe preparation, packaging, and storing of compound prescriptions.

The interested and motivated student is encouraged to go to the Paddock Labs Web site (www.paddocklabs.com) and view its archives of helpful compounding information in the *Secundum Artem* series. Another helpful local source of information for the compounding community pharmacist is a hospital pharmacy, especially a pediatrics hospital pharmacy, where a pharmacist may have a needed recipe or formula and has experience compounding and flavoring formulations for neonates, infants, and pediatric patients.

The International Academy of Compounding Pharmacists is a political action group; membership is open to both pharmacists and pharmacy technicians. It keeps compounding pharmacies alert to legislative challenges that have an impact on their profession. For example, the FDA has suggested that all compounded preparations should be considered new drugs and thus subject to undergoing a new drug application process similar to the requirements for pharmaceutical manufacturers. If such legislation were passed, then compounding pharmacies would cease to exist—with the erosion of a basic right of the profession for more than 200 years.

Chapter Terms

anticipatory compounding preparing excess product (besides an individual compound prescription) in reasonable quantities; these preparations must be labeled with lot numbers

beyond-use dating the documentation of the date after which a compounded preparation expires and should no longer be used

blending the act of combining two substances

Class III prescription balance a two-pan balance used to weigh material (120 g or less) with a sensitivity rating of +/–6 mg; also known as a Class A balance

comminution the act of reducing a substance to small, fine particles, including trituration, levigation, pulverization, spatulation, sifting, and tumbling

compounded preparation a patient-specific medication prepared on-site by the technician, under the direct supervision of the pharmacist, from individual ingredients

compounding the process of preparing a prescribed medication for an individual patient from bulk ingredients created by a pharmacist in order to treat a specified medical condition according to a prescription by a licensed prescriber

compounding log a printout of the prescription for a specific patient, including the amounts or weights of all ingredients and instructions for compounding; used by the technician to prepare a compounded medication for a patient

compounding slab a flat, hard, nonabsorbent surface used for mixing compounds; also known as an ointment slab

continuous quality improvement (CQI) a process of written procedures designed to identify problems and recommend solutions

counterbalance a two-pan balance used for weighing material up to 5 kg with a sensitivity rating of +/–100 mg

digital electronic analytical balance a single-pan balance that is more accurate than Class III balances or counterbalances; it has a capacity of 100 g and sensitivity as low as +/–1 mg

diluent powder an inactive ingredient that is added to the active drug in compounding a tablet or capsule

estrogen replacement therapy (ERT) treatment consisting of some combination of female hormones

forceps an instrument used to pick up small objects, such as pharmacy weights

geometric dilution method the gradual combining of drugs using a mortar and pestle

good compounding practices (GCP) USP standards in many areas of practice to ensure high-quality compounded preparations

graduate cylinder a flask used for measuring liquids

hormone replacement therapy (HRT) therapy consisting of some combination of estrogen and progestin (female) and androgen (male) hormones

levigation a process usually used to reduce the particle size of a solid during the preparation of an ointment

manufactured products products prepared off-site by a manufacturer

master control record a recipe for a compound preparation that lists the name, strength, dosage form, ingredients and their quantities, mixing instructions, and beyond-use dating

Material Safety Data Sheet (MSDS) contains important information on hazards and flammability of chemicals used in compounding and procedure for treatment of accidental ingestion or exposure

meniscus the moon-shaped or concave appearance of a liquid in a graduate cylinder used in measurement

mortar and pestle equipment used for mixing and grinding pharmaceutical ingredients

nonsterile compounding the preparation of a medication, in an appropriate quantity and dosage form, from several pharmaceutical ingredients in response to a prescription written by a physician, such as tablets, capsules, ointments, or creams; sometimes referred to as extemporaneous compounding

percentage of error the acceptable range of variation above and below the target measurement; used in compounding and manufacturing

pharmaceutical elegance the physical appearance of the final compound preparation

pharmaceutical weights measures of various sizes made of polished brass, often used with a two-pan Class III prescription balance; available in both metric and apothecary weights

Pharmacy Compounding Accrediting Board (PCAB) an organization that provides quality standards for a compounding pharmacy through voluntary accreditation

pipette a long, thin, calibrated hollow tube used for measuring liquids less than 1.5 mL

prescription record a computer-generated version of the compounding log that documents the compounding recipe for a specific prescription and patient

pulverization the process of reducing particle size, especially by using a solvent

punch method a method for filling capsules in which the body of a capsule is repeatedly punched into a cake of medication until the capsule is full

sifting a process used to blend powders through the use of a sieve

spatula a stainless steel, plastic, or hard rubber instrument used for transferring or mixing solid pharmaceutical ingredients

spatulation a process used to blend ingredients, often used in the preparation of creams and ointments

stability the extent to which a compounded product retains the same physical and chemical properties and characteristics it possessed at the time of preparation

sterile compounding the preparation of a parenteral product in the hospital, home healthcare, nuclear, or community pharmacy setting; an example is an intravenous antibiotic

trituration the process of rubbing, grinding, or pulverizing a substance to create fine particles, generally by means of a mortar and pestle

tumbling a process used to combine powders by placing them in a bag or container and shaking it

weighing paper a special paper that is placed on a weighing balance pan to avoid contact between pharmaceutical ingredients and the balance tray; also called powder paper

Chapter Summary

- Nonsterile compounding is used today to prepare medications in strengths, combinations, or dosage forms that are not commercially available.
- Compounding is used to prepare solutions, suspensions, ointments, creams, powders, suppositories, and capsules according to a formula contained in the master control record.

- The standards for nonsterile compounding practices are found in USP Chapter 795.
- Beyond-use dating is the assignment of an expiration date on a compounded preparation that meets USP guidelines or is supported by independent scientific research.

- Product quality for bulk ingredients is important in compounding a high-quality product.
- The master control record and the compounding log document that the correct ingredients, equipment, and technique have been used to prepare a quality preparation.
- Calculations for individual ingredients and the final compounded preparation must be double-checked by the pharmacist.
- Instruments for extemporaneous compounding include the Class III prescription or electronic balances, pharmaceutical weights, forceps, spatulas, weighing papers, compounding or ointment slab, parchment paper, mortar and pestle, graduate cylinders, and pipettes.
- Mortars and pestles are available in glass, Wedgwood, and porcelain varieties. Graduates are available in various sizes in both conical and cylindrical shapes, the latter being the more accurate.
- Proper technique and use of the correct measuring devices are crucial when weighing pharmaceutical ingredients.
- The compounding process includes selecting the most appropriate medication container, affixing a label, keeping accurate prescription records, and cleaning up.
- The pharmacist is legally responsible for the final check of the compounded prescription and for counseling the patient.
- Pharmacy technicians often need additional training and certification to practice in a compounding pharmacy.
- Nonsterile compounding is an art to be learned under the tutelage of an experienced pharmacist.

Chapter Review

Checking Your Understanding

Choose the best answer from those provided.

 Additional Quiz Questions

1. Beyond-use dating is the expiration date of
   a. the manufactured product.
   b. the compound preparation.
   c. the individual ingredients.
   d. pharmacy technician certification.

2. The most accurate balance used in a compounding pharmacy is a(n)
   a. Class III prescription balance.
   b. Class A prescription balance.
   c. counterbalance.
   d. electronic balance.

3. An alternative to the ointment slab is
   a. weighing paper.
   b. parchment paper.
   c. a graduate cylinder.
   d. a pipette.

4. A Class III prescription balance is unlocked, temporarily, when the technician
   a. adds weighing papers to the trays.
   b. adds pharmaceutical ingredients to the trays.
   c. moves the balance from one place to another.
   d. checks a measurement.

5. When measuring the amount of liquid in a graduate, read the level of the liquid at eye level and read the level of the meniscus from the
   a. top.
   b. bottom.
   c. back.
   d. front.

6. When using the geometric dilution method, the most potent ingredient, usually the one that occurs in the smallest amount, is placed into the mortar
   a. half at the beginning and half at the end.
   b. in stages throughout the compounding process.
   c. last.
   d. first.

7. An ingredient such as a powder dissolved in a solution is known as a
   a. suspension.
   b. precipitate.
   c. solute.
   d. solvent.

8. A suppository mold is chilled immediately after filling to
   a. solidify the compound before its volatile components evaporate.
   b. reduce the possibility of spoilage.
   c. prevent contamination of the compound.
   d. solidify the compound before suspended ingredients have time to settle.

9. The punch method is used for filling
   a. hypodermics.
   b. capsules.
   c. suppositories.
   d. caplets.

10. An appropriate auxiliary label for all liquid suspensions is
    a. "Take with food."
    b. "For topical use only; do not swallow."
    c. "Shake well before using."
    d. "May cause drowsiness."

Thinking Like a Pharmacy Tech

1. Practice using a Class III prescription balance and a mortar and pestle to prepare the following amounts of ingredients. Combine the ingredients and use the punch method to fill capsules with this "pumpkin pie spice" compound. What size of capsule should be used? How many capsules will this fill?
   a. 2.75 g ground cinnamon
   b. 8.5 g sugar
   c. 7.5 g ground nutmeg
   d. 1.5 g allspice
   e. 2.5 g triturated anise seed or clove

2. Explain why using proper techniques and weighing ingredients with accuracy are important for compounding preparations in the pharmacy.

3. You are instructed to weigh 80 g of a cream base for a topical compound. Your error range is 3%. What is the least acceptable amount and the largest acceptable amount within this accepted error range?

4. Select the most appropriate size of graduate to measure the following volumes. You have the following available in the pharmacy: 1 fl oz (30 mL), 2 fl oz (60 mL), 4 fl oz (120 mL), 8 fl oz (240 mL), 500 mL, and 1000 mL.
   a. 45 mL
   b. 75 mL
   c. 125 mL
   d. 450 mL
   e. 550 mL
   f. 890 mL

5. You are to dispense 453 mg of a powder. The original measurement is 453 mg. When you double-check the amount using a more accurate scale, the actual amount is 438 mg. What is the percentage of error of the first measurement?

6. Calculate the beyond-use dating for the *Magic Mouthwash* compound in Figure 8.6.

Communicating Clearly

1. The art of compounding uses a unique language, and you have been asked to describe the following terms to a pharmacy student who is visiting your pharmacy. Use simple terms.
   a. levigate
   b. punch method
   c. triturate
   d. spatulation
   e. diluent
   f. tumbling
   g. solute
   h. solvent
   i. geometric dilution
   j. comminution

2. A patient has arrived at the pharmacy where you work. She has a prescription for a compound that your pharmacy often makes. You are very busy and will not be able to get to this compound for at least 1 hour. The patient, frustrated from waiting so long at the physician's office, is now frustrated that you cannot prepare her prescription immediately. What do you tell this patient? Explain why special compounded prescriptions take longer than other prescriptions. Write out your responses.

Researching on the Web

1. Visit the Web site for *Secundum Artem: Current and Practical Compounding Information for the Pharmacist* at www.paddocklabs.com and choose articles that discuss one of the following topics. Choose a topic that you or a member of your family may have a personal interest in. Use the information in the articles to write a summary of the issues involved in compounding the product you selected.

   acne
   ear or otic illnesses
   rectal disorders
   scalp disorders
   sports injuries
   stomach or GI disorders
   superficial fungal infections
   wound care

2. Visit the PCAB Web site at www.pcab.org and find four specific mission statements for this organization.

3. Visit the Web site for your state board of pharmacy and research rules for compounding by the pharmacy technician. Select a neighboring state and compare how laws and regulations may differ.

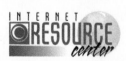

For further study of chapter-related topics, explore the Web links in the Web Center at www.emcp.net/pharmpractice4e.

Unit

3

Institutional Pharmacy

Hospital Pharmacy Practice

9

Learning Objectives

- Describe the classifications and functions of a hospital and the role of the director of pharmacy.
- Identify services that are unique to a hospital pharmacy in contrast to a community pharmacy.
- Contrast a medication order with a unit dose profile.
- Identify the advantages of a unit dose drug distribution system.
- Explain the proper procedure for repackaging of medications.
- Identify the process of medication dispensing and filling in a hospital pharmacy.
- Discuss the advantages of an automated floor stock system for medication, including narcotics.

- Describe specialty services, such as intravenous admixtures and total parenteral nutrition.
- Describe a medication administration record.
- Identify the roles of major hospital committees.
- Describe the role of the institutional review board (IRB) in approving investigational drug studies.
- Explain the major role and standards of the Joint Commission.
- Discuss the role of automation and inventory control in the hospital.

Preview chapter terms and definitions.

This chapter provides an overview of the organization of a hospital and the responsibilities of the director of pharmacy. Inpatient drug distribution systems are described, including unit dose, repackaging, floor stock, narcotic inventory, and intravenous admixtures. The chapter also explains the responsibilities of the pharmacy technician in the inpatient drug distribution system. The use of automation in the drug distribution system and on the patient care unit will play an increasingly important future role in minimizing medication errors. Chapter 10, *Infection Control*, discusses the use of aseptic technique, and Chapter 11, *Preparing and Handling Sterile Products and Hazardous Drugs*, discusses the techniques and procedures used in the preparation of parenterals and the proper handling and disposal of hazardous agents.

Hospital Organization

The hospital pharmacy exists as part of a much larger and more complex organization called the *hospital* that provides needed emergency, trauma, surgical, and medical services to a community. Hospitals are often described according to bed capacity. In addition, hospitals may be classified in several ways, including the following:

- type of service, such as general and specialized
- university (i.e., teaching) and private (i.e., nonteaching)
- lengths of stay into short-term care (i.e., less than 30 days) and long-term care (i.e., 30 days or more)
- governmental (i.e., Veterans Administration [VA]) and nongovernmental
- for-profit and nonprofit

Hospitals employ hundreds if not thousands of employees, including pharmacy technicians. In fact, pharmacy technicians have been heavily used in this setting since the 1960s. Some of the functions of a hospital are listed in Table 9.1. Regardless of type, function, and size of hospital, nearly all contain a hospital pharmacy.

An overview of the typical hospital structure is important to better understand the roles and responsibilities of the hospital pharmacy. Traditionally, a president, or chief executive officer (CEO), runs the hospital and reports to a board of directors. Reporting to the CEO are the vice presidents of various departments. The vice president for professional services usually oversees the departments responsible for anesthesiology, clinical services, laboratory testing, medical records, pharmacy, psychiatry, radiology, rehabilitation, respiratory care, and social services.

The Director of Pharmacy

The **director of pharmacy** is the pharmacist-in-charge, with overall responsibility for the hospital's pharmacy services. This includes managing the budget, hiring and firing personnel, developing a strategic vision, complying with all federal and state regulations and laws, and developing policy and procedures to comply with hospital policies and accreditation standards. The director of pharmacy generally reports to the vice president for professional services (or similar title).

The director of pharmacy works closely with the director of nursing and the chief of staff in medicine to provide high-quality patient care. Depending on the hospital size, additional assistant or associate directors with more specific responsibilities within the hospital pharmacy may work under the director. In a small rural hospital,

---

TABLE 9.1 Functions of a Hospital

- diagnosis and testing
- treatment and therapy, including surgical intervention
- patient processing (including admissions, recordkeeping, billing, and planning for postrelease patient care)
- public health education and promotion, provided through a variety of programs, including smoking cessation programs, weight loss programs, support group programs, and screenings of community members (including mammographies and testing of blood pressure and cholesterol)
- teaching (i.e., training health professionals)
- research (i.e., carrying out programs that add to the sum of medical knowledge)

only one or two pharmacists may make up the pharmacy staff, yet the overall responsibilities remain the same.

The director of pharmacy determines the level and scope of services offered by the hospital pharmacy. Examples include the following:

- type of medication distribution systems such as
  □ presence of IV admixture and total parenteral nutrition (TPN) or nutrition service
  □ satellite or small pharmacies located on a patient care unit within the hospital
- service availability 24 hours, 7 days a week, or less
- pharmacy participation in emergency codes
- provision of specialty services
  □ outpatient pharmacy services or outsourcing
  □ clinical pharmacists making rounds with physician and monitoring patients
  □ drug information center or service provided by staff

The pharmacy director is responsible for submitting a budget and complying with that budget. Drug budgets can be difficult to predict, especially 1 to 2 years in advance. Newer, more expensive drugs may come into the marketplace to replace lower-cost alternatives, or a new transplant service may be implemented in the hospital, requiring the use of expensive immune-suppressing drugs.

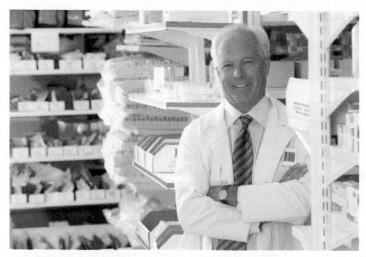

The director of pharmacy is responsible for overseeing the drug distribution and specialized services within the hospital.

Because of budget or staffing restrictions, some hospital pharmacies may elect to outsource some distribution or clinical services. Outsourcing may include contracting with a pharmacy outside the hospital to provide services. For example, an IV admixture or nutrition service may be located off-premises, with products delivered to the hospital, or a hospital may contract with a local community pharmacy to lease space and provide outpatient pharmacy services in the hospital. In any case, safety and quality of care must never be compromised.

The director is also responsible for developing adequate and consistent written policies and procedures for every aspect of the operation, including state and federal laws. Pharmacy technicians should study this manual; often a technician may need 2 months or longer to function in an adequately independent manner in a hospital pharmacy.

The hospital's human resources department generally advertises for personnel positions and screens candidates; however, the director of pharmacy makes the final decision when pharmacy staff is hired. Because of access to pharmaceuticals, the hospital commonly requests criminal background checks for all personnel before hiring. Many pharmacy technicians may be hired on a contingency basis (i.e., their performance is reevaluated after 3 or 6 months). Applicants with prior hospital experience or formalized training or certification are considered to be more qualified than other applicants without such experience or training. Interviewing strategies for a pharmacy technician are discussed in Chapter 14, *Your Future in Pharmacy Practice*.

TABLE 9.2 Hospital Pharmacy Services

- filling medication orders (as opposed to prescriptions)
- routinely preparing 24–72 hour supplies of patient medications in a form appropriate for a single administration to a patient (as opposed to a 30 or 90 day supply)
- prepackaging medications for patient use
- delivering stat orders or emergency medications to the patient care unit or patient room
- stocking patient care unit with floor stock medications and supplies
- preparing parenteral products using aseptic techniques
- following universal precautions in the IV room (see Chapter 10)
- ensuring that biological and hazardous agents are handled and disposed of properly
- auditing pharmacy services for evaluation of service accuracy and quality
- maintaining a drug information service and providing drug information to the other healthcare professionals in the institution
- preparing and maintaining a formulary—a select list of approved drugs
- conducting drug use evaluations, such as appropriate use of antibiotics
- providing in-service drug-related education to nurses and physicians
- taking and documenting medication histories on admission
- monitoring patient outcomes
- counseling patients at discharge from the hospital
- participating in clinical drug investigations and research
- providing expert consultations in such areas as pediatric pharmacotherapy, nutritional support, and pharmacokinetics

Hospital Pharmacy vs. Community Pharmacy

Many of the functions carried out in the community pharmacy discussed in Unit 2 are also carried out in hospital pharmacy settings. With the exception of insulin and some blood thinners, most prescriptions dispensed in the typical community pharmacy are oral medications or prepackaged specialty medications, such as inhaled drugs for the lungs, ophthalmics for the eye, otics for the ear, and topicals for the skin. The hospital pharmacy dispenses not only these types of medications but also parenteral drugs, biological agents, and potentially hazardous chemotherapy medications.

As you learned in Chapter 1, pharmacists and pharmacy technicians work in a wide variety of practice settings. Some similarities exist between the functions of a hospital pharmacy and those of a community pharmacy. Services unique to a hospital pharmacy are listed in Table 9.2. The hospital pharmacy technician plays a key role in preparing and delivering the right drug to the right patient at the right time.

Inpatient Drug Distribution Systems

Safety Note

All computer systems must protect patient privacy.

The inpatient drug distribution system in many hospital pharmacies consists of a unit dose, floor stock, IV admixture, and TPN service. Automation is having a major impact on improving the efficiency and quality of pharmacy services and minimizing medication errors in the hospital pharmacy. A computer system within a hospital pharmacy is most often networked with that of other departments, such as nursing, laboratory, and administration. A computer system provides the opportunity for transmitting and sharing information, including patient data, laboratory results, medication orders, pharmacy literature, and adverse reaction reports.

Examples of how automation improves efficiency and safety in each area of the inpatient drug distribution areas are discussed throughout this chapter.

Medication Orders

In the hospital pharmacy, a prescription is in the form of a **medication order**. Medication orders are processed differently in the hospital than in the community pharmacy. Medication orders may be listed in admission, new, or continuation orders. An **admitting order** is written by the physician upon patient admission to a hospital. A new medication order is like a new prescription. A **stat order** is an emergency order that must receive priority attention and be immediately input into the pharmacy database, filled, checked, and transported to the patient care unit for administration. A **continuation order** is the equivalent of approval to continue the originally prescribed medications, like a refill. Most hospitals have a policy that a physician must review and approve all medication orders at least weekly.

The hospital pharmacy receives copies of all hospital orders written for an individual patient by the physician. Computer-generated or handwritten hospital orders may include diagnosis, allergies, diet, activity level, x-ray, vital signs, and lab tests, as well as medications. Medication orders may consist of regularly scheduled oral, parenteral medications, IV fluids, as well as "prn," or "as needed," medications (see Figure 9.1).

FIGURE 9.1
Admitting Hospital Order

DATE	HOUR	PHYSICIAN'S ORDERS	DO NOT USE THIS SHEET UNLESS RED NUMBER SHOWS
9-1-20XX		Admit to: Dr. Smith	
		Diagnosis:	
		1. Lower abdominal pain with history of diverticulitis	
		2. Asthma	
		3. Chronic back pain	
		4. Anxiety	
		Condition: Fair	
		Vitals: per routine	
		Labs: Chem 12, Electrolytes, ABG	
		X-ray: Lungs	
		Allergies: Codeine, Floxin, Biaxin, PCN, Ceclor, Doxycycline	
		Diet: Clear liquids, Low salt, 1800 kcal/day	
		IVFs: NS @ 125 mL per hour	
		Meds: Phenergan 25 mg IV q6 h prn nausea/vomiting	
		Levaquin 500 mg IV daily	
		Levsin 0.125 mg po tid	
		Ambien 10 mg po q pm prn sleep	
		Soma 350 mg po tid prn muscle spasm	
		Advair 250/50 1 puff bid	
		Singulair 10 mg po daily	
		Lorcet 10 mg po bid	
		Pepcid 40 mg po bid	
		Albuterol 0.083% 1 unit via nebulizer q6 h prn	
		Nasonex 2 sprays in each nostril daily	
		Zoloft 100 mg 2 tabs po daily	

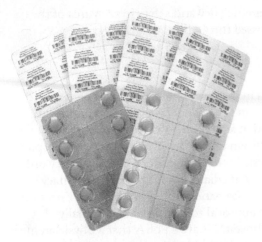

A unit dose is an individually prepared medication and dose for a specific patient. The lot number (on the labeling) from the manufacturer is needed in case of a drug recall. A bar code is often used for scanning in the pharmacy or patient care unit.

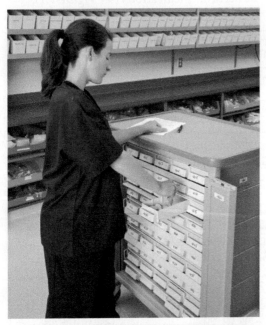

A unit dose cart has individually labeled drawers that contain medications for patients assigned to a designated patient care unit.

The pharmacist or experienced pharmacy technician must review all written hospital orders to determine which ones are for medications that must be input into the pharmacy computer database. The pharmacist verifies the accuracy of the transcription by the technician with the original physician order before any medication is sent to the patient care unit. Once the medication order is approved by the pharmacist, the technician can provide the necessary drugs to fill the order. After the pharmacist checks the filled order, the nurse is then responsible for administering the medication to the patient and documenting this in the patient's medical record.

Unit Dose

Beginning in the early 1960s, hospitals have made use of a unit dose drug distribution system for dispensing medications. A **unit dose** is an amount of a drug prepackaged for a single administration. In other words, it is an amount of medication in a dosage form that is ready for administration to a particular patient at a particular time. Unit dose is an important part of the **inpatient drug distribution system**, in which a supply, for 24 hours or more, of individual doses for many medications is prepackaged or specially prepared and sent to each patient care unit, where the medications are administered.

A unit dose drug distribution system increases efficiency by making the drug formulation as ready to administer as possible, rather than requiring nurses to prepare doses from multiple-dose containers. Most common oral medications, such as tablets and capsules, are commercially available in a unit dose formulation. Unit dose labels include the following minimum information:

- generic or brand name of the drug
- strength of the dose
- bar code of the product
- lot number from the manufacturer's packaging
- expiration date

The hospital pharmacy technician uses a computer-generated fill list to add unit doses for each individual patient. Each patient on each patient care unit has a designated removable drawer of medication that is delivered to the patient care unit in a moveable **unit dose cart** that typically has two sets of removable drawers—one for use on the patient care unit and a replacement for filling next-day medication orders by the technician in the hospital pharmacy.

Each drawer in the unit dose cart is labeled with a specific patient's name and room number. Typically, a patient's drawer is designated for that patient until the patient is discharged from the hospital or transferred to another patient care unit.

Each drawer of the cart contains medication container label(s) inside, created using information from the computer-generated list. Medications are usually provided for 24 hours, although smaller hospitals may exchange patient drawers less frequently.

The cost of one dose of medication is proportionately higher in a hospital than one dose from a retail pharmacy. A patient is typically charged for each dose administered; the cost may include pharmacy and nursing personnel costs in addition to the cost of the drug and unit dose packaging.

Safety Note

Only unopened unit doses can be returned to stock.

Despite its higher packaging costs, a unit dose system has been demonstrated to save time and money. It provides increased security for medications, reduces medication errors, reduces nursing time, and makes administration, charging, and crediting easier. Unit doses returned in their original unopened packages may be returned to drug stock for reuse, thus minimizing drug wastage.

In larger hospital pharmacies, an automated robotic system may be used to fill unit dose medication orders. All of the unit dose medications are packaged with an identifying bar code. Both solid and liquid oral medications, as well as prefilled syringes and vials, are packaged in the bar-coded plastic devices. A robotic arm uses suction and pneumatic air to pull the medication and transfer it to a collection area. Patients' individualized medication orders are then placed in an envelope or plastic tray for delivery.

Automation can minimize dispensing errors, more accurately track and manage drug inventory, dispense medication for multiple hospitals, and implement medication administration verification at patient bedside consistent with modern bar-code technology. The primary role for the technician working in a pharmacy using automation technology is to stock the robotic system. Automation allows the pharmacy staff to shift from time-intensive preparation of unit doses to repackaging, inventorying floor stock, and preparing IV admixtures.

With the advent of more sophisticated automated floor stock systems (discussed later in the chapter), there is less need for the traditional preparation and delivery of unit dose medications to the nursing unit. In many hospitals unit dose preparations are limited to infrequently used medications or those that are not commercially available.

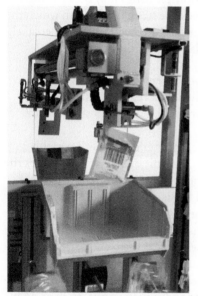

A robotic device fills prescriptions using the downloaded prescription orders and bar-coded unit dose medication packages.

Repackaging Medications into Unit Doses Because manufacturers do not prepare all drugs in a unit dose form and because individual medication orders may call for nonstandard doses, the hospital pharmacy staff often needs to repackage medications. A **medication special** is a single dose preparation made for a particular patient. Oral tablet, capsule, or liquid medication specials are examples of drug formulations that are typically prepared and packaged in a unit dose form. The process of creating patient-specific unit doses is labor intensive and is often the responsibility of a pharmacy technician.

Pharmacies may use a variety of time- and cost-saving devices to assist in the preparation of medications. Hospital pharmacies may purchase the product in bulk and use a packaging machine to prepare individual doses. Other repackaging equipment may involve the use of counting trays, automated packaging machines, and a liquid-filling apparatus. Typical unit dose packaging includes heat-sealed zip-lock bags, adhesive-sealed bottles, blister packs, and heat-sealed strip packages for oral solids, as well as plastic or glass cups, heat-sealable aluminum cups, and plastic syringes labeled "For Oral Use Only" for oral liquids. The packaging provides an airtight and light-resistant delivery system to ensure physical stability of the drug.

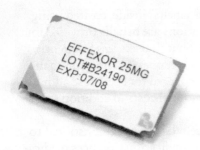

Labeling of customized unit doses that have been repackaged in the hospital pharmacy should include the drug name, strength, lot number, and expiration date.

Repackaged medications must be carefully labeled. In addition to labeling, it is also important, and legally required, to carefully record and document information about the medications that have been repackaged in the hospital pharmacy. The repackaging documentation is made using the **repackaging control log** (Figure 9.2), which contains the following information:

- date of repackaging
- internal lot number
- drug, strength, dosage form
- manufacturer's name
- manufacturer's lot number and expiration date
- quantity or number of units packaged
- initials of the repackager and the pharmacist who has checked the repackaging

Additional information may be required for repackaged drugs, depending on hospital policy, state guidelines, and accreditation standards. Multiple drugs may be repackaged and listed on the log sheet. The pharmacist should check the stock bottle from which the pharmacy technician obtained the medication, the unit dose medication container label, and the packaging of the final product before it is added to the unit dose cart.

Medication Filling Medication orders that have been received by the hospital pharmacy and entered into the pharmacy database are filled on a regular basis, every 24 hours or less, until the patient is released from the hospital. Figure 9.3 shows examples of medication orders for hospital patients.

After the medication orders are entered into the computer database, a patient-specific **unit dose profile** is created (see Figure 9.4). The unit dose profile includes the name and strength of the medication and the route and time of administration. A printout of all unit dose profiles results in a **cart fill list** (see Figure 9.5). This list identifies the unit dose or repackaged medications and the administration times needed by each patient in the hospital. The cart fill list is usually printed out each morning by the pharmacy technician to prepare doses to be sent to the patient care unit (assuming that the medication is not in automated floor stock—see next section).

The unit dose profile and cart fill list include a detailed dose administration schedule. Each hospital has a standard time for various dose administrations, such as q4 h, q6 h, q8 h, q12 h, bid, tid, and qid. As discussed in Chapter 5, hospitals commonly use

FIGURE 9.2
Repackaging Control Log

						Initials	
Date Repackaged	Pharmacy Lot Number	Drug Name Strength Dosage Form	Manufacturer and Lot Number	Expiration Date	Quantity of Units	Prep. By	Approved By

Repackaging Control Log
Department of Pharmaceutical Services

FIGURE 9.3
**Medication
Orders**

Patient Name	Order	Room #
Charlene Landers	labetalol 200 mg IV q8 h	825
	Phenergan 25 mg IV q6 h prn	
	D5 ½ NS 20 mEq KCl at 50 mL/h	
	npo after 12M	
John Henry	gentamicin 20 mg IV q8 h	432
	baby powder	
	ASA gr V po q6 h	
Oscar Wilder	Nitrostat SL prn	503
	Capoten 25 mg po STAT, then bid	
Tim Turner	10,000 units heparin IV stat	407
	gentamicin 60 mg IVPB tid	
	Bentyl 10 mg po tid prn	
Nancy Lynch	continue Rocephin 1 g IV q24 h	335
	continue Zithromax IV 500 mg q24 h	

military or international time for scheduled dose administration times. For instance, IV penicillin q6 h is usually administered at 0600 (6:00 a.m.), 1200 (noon), 1800 (6:00 p.m.), and 0000 (midnight).

If an order is received after the unit dose medications have already been delivered to the floor, then the pharmacist or pharmacy technician supplies sufficient medication until the next cart fill. For example, if Zantac 300 mg q8 h is ordered at 1:00 p.m. (1300), then two doses need to be delivered for the 2:00 p.m. (1400) and 10:00 p.m. (2200) dose administrations, and a third dose is placed in the patient's unit dose cart drawer for the next morning. A total of 3 doses are needed until the next cart change.

In a 300 bed hospital, more than 90,000 oral doses may be administered per day! Unit dose medications may not be administered to the patient for a variety of reasons. For example, a patient may be undergoing a procedure such as an X-ray at the time medication is scheduled, cannot take oral medications prior to surgery by the physician's order, or may have become nauseous, so an oral medication was changed to an injectable form. Although a dose may have been skipped intentionally, it

FIGURE 9.4
**Unit Dose
Profile**

℞ **Bill Hopkins   Room 535**
ciprofloxacin 500 mg PO
Q12 H   1700   0500

FIGURE 9.5
Cart Fill List

℞ **Bill Hopkins   Room 535**
ciprofloxacin 500 mg PO
Q12 H   1700   0500

Marla Waters   Room 532
Flexeril 10 mg PO
Q8 H   0800   1600   0000

Lowell Goodman   Room 638
Lyrica 150 mg PO
Q HS   2200

Lisa Reynolds   Room 714
amoxicillin-clavulanate 875 mg PO
TID   0800   1400   2200

The label "NPO" indicates that nothing be given by mouth. Patients with this designation cannot be given oral medications.

may also have been missed accidentally and not administered by the nurse. Some pharmacy departments use the medications remaining in the patient drawer in the unit dose cart as a quality assurance tool: remaining medications instigate an investigation into why the medication was missed. The pharmacy technician plays a crucial role in bringing missed doses of selected drugs to the attention of the pharmacist.

To comply with regulations and minimize illegal drug diversion, no Schedule II drugs are dispensed during a unit dose cart fill; in many hospitals Schedule III/IV drugs may not be dispensed in the unit dose drawer per policy. Instead, they are obtained from the narcotic cabinet or locked automated floor stock system by the nurse at the time of administration to the patient.

Floor Stock

Floor stock is an inventory of frequently prescribed drugs that is stored on the patient care unit. Historically, floor stock was usually limited to selected drugs used on a prn (*pro re nata*, or as needed) basis and included mostly OTC medications. Ointments, creams, ear drops, and eye drops are considered bulk items that are supplied as floor stock and placed at bedside on request by a physician's order.

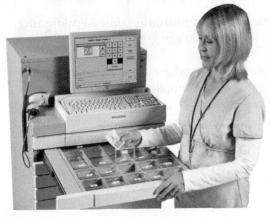

This automated delivery system dispenses stock drug items on the patient care unit.

With the advent of automated delivery systems, such as AcuDose-Rx (McKesson) and Pyxis (Cardinal), floor stock can consist of frequently used medications, including controlled substances and IV fluids that can be tailored to the individual needs of the patient care unit. The automated delivery systems are extensions of the unit dose delivery system. They allow secure, locked storage of the medications, free up nursing time, capture all charges for dispensed medications, and have the capability to track all medications by type of drug, patient, and caregiver. In addition, such systems often alert the nurse to potential drug allergies.

Incorporating automation in the hospital pharmacy increases the assurance that the right drug will get to the right patient, at the right time, in the right dose. Each dose in the floor stock system must be matched with a medication order. The initials of the nurse who retrieves the floor stock medication is recorded; any discrepancies must be resolved by the nurse or the pharmacist.

A perpetual inventory is maintained for most medications (all controlled and expensive drugs) in the computerized inventory database. The hospital pharmacy assumes responsibility for maintaining inventory through a floor stock replacement system. Patient care units send reports, sometimes called out-of-stock reports, to the hospital pharmacy throughout the day requesting inventory to be replaced. A pharmacy technician often maintains this floor stock inventory according to predetermined levels. In addition, the pharmacy technician inspects the floor stock to do the following:

No food items can be placed in a refrigerator that is dedicated to storing medications.

- check for expired drugs
- remove excess inventory
- confirm that all medications are stored properly, including items requiring refrigeration
- ensure that the refrigerator temperature is correct

FIGURE 9.6
Controlled Drug Administration Record

SCHEDULE II DRUG ADMINISTRATION FORM					
Drug Demerol	**Strength** 100 mg	**Quantity** 25	**Form** ☐ Tablet ☐ Capsule ☑ Injection ☐ Liquid		**Control Number** A 3735
Issued By R Anderson			**To Station** CCU		**Date Issued** 10/10/20XX
Received By (Nurse in Charge) Nancy Ter Haar					**Date Received** 10/10/20XX

Date	Time	Patient Name	Room No.	Medication	Dosage Given	Wasted	Physician	Administered By	BAL
10/11/20XX	0550	Ruth	CCU	Demerol	100 mg		Schnars	Lynn	24
10/12/20XX	1245	Henry	CCU	Demerol	100 mg		Fields	Roberts	23
10/14/20XX	1625	Wilder	CCU	Demerol	90 mg	10 mg	Vantle	Matthews	22
10/15/20XX	1130	Turner	CCU	Demerol	75 mg	25 mg	Archer	Ter Haar	21

RECORD OF WASTE AND SPOILAGE					
Dose No	**Date**	**Amount**	**Explain Wastage**	**Signature #1**	**Signature #1**
	10/15/20XX	25 mg	defective syringe	*Ter Haar*	*Roberts*

Narcotics in a Hospital Pharmacy

As in the community pharmacy, all Schedule II controlled substances in a hospital pharmacy must be secured in a locked cabinet or safe, whether stored in the pharmacy or at the patient care unit. Narcotics are commonly included in the floor stock inventory of each patient care unit in the hospital. A careful audit trail must exist to account for each medication. The date and time that the narcotic is administered to a specific patient must be verified with the written medication order, nursing notes in the patient chart, and a **Schedule II drug administration record**. An example of such a form is provided in Figure 9.6. This record is a balance of each remaining dose of narcotic and may be manual or automated.

In a manual system, the record must be reconciled at each nursing shift. The names of the prescribing physician and the nurse administering the medication must be recorded, as well as amount of the drug given; if any amount is wasted (or drug destroyed), then the record must be witnessed by another health professional. The nurse and pharmacist have to reconcile each dose of each narcotic drug administered in the hospital.

With the advent of automated systems, the primary function of the pharmacy department is to resupply the floor stock on each patient care unit. When delivery is made to the patient care unit, then the name of the pharmacy technician as well as that of the receiving nurse must be recorded for each dose of each narcotic drug.

Automation has also simplified the narcotic inventory and tracking records. Narc-Station by McKesson is an example of one kind of automated system. It provides a compatible software tracking system to maintain the recordkeeping, reporting, and transaction date for all controlled substances from the wholesaler to the patient care unit. Automated systems provide real-time reports and immediate access to information that identifies trends in narcotic usage in a patient care unit. The pharmacy technician is responsible for reporting to the pharmacist any unusual increases in delivery or use of controlled substances. Discrepancies involving controlled drugs must be resolved with a witness. A pharmacist may also be responsible for checking and reconciling the narcotic inventory records, especially if discrepancies cannot be resolved on the patient care unit; discrepancies must be immediately resolved.

Intravenous Admixture Service

Nearly all hospital pharmacies provide an intravenous (IV) admixture or an IV additive service for the preparation of many injectable medications, including antibiotics, thrombolytics (or clot busters), nutrition, and cancer chemotherapy.

An **IV admixture service** is defined as the preparation of such medications and IV solutions in a sterile, germ-free work environment in the pharmacy. Many medications ordered in the hospital are reconstituted or dissolved in sterile water or normal saline (salt solution) and then added to an IV solution. These medications are commonly administered to the patient by IV infusion over several hours. Many medications for infusion are prepared in a small volume of IV fluid and then piggybacked (IVPB), or connected to the existing tubing of a plastic bag with a large volume of IV fluid that the patient is receiving. More details are provided on preparing IVPBs in Chapter 11.

The IV admixture service is staffed by specially trained pharmacists and pharmacy technicians. In addition to maintaining sterility to reduce microbial contamination, these medications can be more accurately and safely prepared and labeled in a clean room environment in the pharmacy, resulting in fewer medication errors and less risk of contamination. Some potentially hazardous drugs—such as those used for cancer chemotherapy—must be prepared using specialized equipment in a special work environment.

Many hospital pharmacies have a **total parenteral nutrition (TPN)** service as part of the IV admixture service. A TPN service often consists of a specially trained or certified physician, nurse, nutritionist, and pharmacist. A TPN is a specially formulated IV parenteral solution that provides for the entire nutritional needs of a patient who cannot or will not eat. A TPN solution may contain more than twenty ingredients, including amino acids, carbohydrates, fats, sugars, vitamins, electrolytes, and minerals. Sterility is critically important because the TPN is administered directly into the patient's vein and because it may be hanging at room temperature for up of 24 hours. TPN solutions are used in patients of all ages, in both hospital and home healthcare environments. A pharmacy technician must be certified and may need to complete additional training for the preparation of TPN solutions.

In an IV admixture service, it is critically important for the pharmacy technician to understand the importance of conducting a physical inspection of the end product before any IV solution or TPN is sent to the patient care unit. The product is checked under special lighting, by both the technician and the pharmacist, for particulate matter or physical incompatibility of the drugs. For example, a physical incompatibility results if an acid salt is added to a basic salt. Particulate matter also includes "coring" of a part of the rubber stopper from a vial of medication. If a defective IV product is administered, then it could cause a severe adverse or allergic reaction in a patient.

Larger hospital pharmacies also use automation to make IV admixtures and TPNs. This technology allows the pharmacy to operate more efficiently, minimizing medication errors and significantly reducing inventory. In addition, the technician can spend more time preparing IV compounds. Both pharmacists and technicians are responsible for correctly operating the equipment and maintaining inventory supplies used in the automation process.

Safety Note

Although automation reduces errors, technical errors must still be monitored.

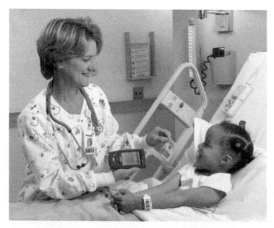

Automation and bar-code scanning technologies on the patient care unit reduce errors in medication administration. The right drug and the right dose must be delivered to the right patient.

Medication Administration Record

When a nurse administers any medication—oral, IV, or prn—it is recorded in the patient's medical record on a form called a **medication administration record (MAR)**. Each record is patient specific and includes prescription numbers or medication orders, names of all drugs, doses, routes of administration, administration times, start and stop dates, and special instructions for the hospital staff. The exact time that each dose of each drug is administered is recorded and initialed by the nurse on the MAR. A separate listing in the MAR is kept for prn, or as needed, drugs. An example of an MAR is included in Figure 9.7.

Technology has been developed to help nurses document the administration of drugs accurately and quickly. An **electronic medication administration record (eMAR)** documents the administration time of each drug to each patient, often using bar-code technology. In hospitals using an eMAR, medication orders are input in handheld computer devices by the physician at the patient's bedside. Patients wear wristbands with bar

FIGURE 9.7
Medication Administration Record (MAR)

Patient Name: John Henry **Physician:** Trondheim **Allergies:** Codeine sulfate
Hospital ID: 5522103   CCU **Diagnosis:** (1) Gastroenteritis, (2) Renal failure
Gender: M
Age: 46

Order No.	Medication		Start	Stop	Days 0700 to 1859	Nights 1900 to 0659
433800	PANTOPRAZOLE SOD IV IVP EVERY 24 HOURS	40 MG	09/10 0800 OCW	12/09 0800	0800	
448842	DEMEROL IM EVERY 4 HOURS	100 MG	09/12 1000 PLH	12/11 1000	0800 1200 1600	2000 0000 0400
448891	ENOXAPARIN INJ SC ONCE A DAY	40 MG/0.4 ML	09/12 1000 PLH	12/11 1000	1000	
449100	NEUTRA-PHOS PO TWICE A DAY MIX CONTENTS WITH 2.5 OZ OF WATER OR JUICE STIR WELL AND GIVE PROMPTLY	1 PACKET	09/12 1000 PLH	12/11 1000	1000	2200
458037	CHLORDIAZEPOXIDE HCL CAP PO EVERY 8 HOURS WARNING: DOSE IS 50 MG = 2 CAPS	25 MG	9/13 1400 RGC	09/20 1400	1400	2200 0600
435135	VANCOMYCIN-AV SODIUM CHLORIDE AV 0.9% 250 ML IVPB EVERY 24 HOURS, INFUSE OVER 60 MIN	1 GRAM	09/11 0800 OCW	09/18 0800	0800	

codes that identify them and link them to their corresponding eMAR. Once a physician inputs the order, it is electronically transmitted to the hospital pharmacy. After the order is checked by the pharmacist, filled by the technician, and sent to the patient care unit, the nurse scans the bar code on the patient wristband and compares it to the bar code on the medication to minimize the potential of administration errors. Medication errors are further reduced by more than 50% by using an eMAR system.

Hospital Committee Structure

An extensive committee structure is needed to support the functions of a hospital. The main committees relating to pharmacy include pharmacy and therapeutics (P&T), infection control, and institutional review board (IRB). The important role of the infection control committee is discussed in Chapter 10. A pharmacy technician often represents the pharmacy department on one or more hospital committees. The roles of these hospital committees are discussed in more detail in the following sections.

Pharmacy and Therapeutics Committee

In the hospital setting, the **pharmacy and therapeutics (P&T) committee** reviews, approves, and revises the hospital's formulary and maintains the drug use policies of the hospital. The P&T committee routinely meets on a monthly (or quarterly) basis and usually consists of multiple members from the medical staff, as well as representatives from the hospital and nursing administration. The director of pharmacy and, in a large hospital, the drug information pharmacist often represent the pharmacy department on the P&T committee. The director of pharmacy often acts as the secretary and is responsible for recording and disseminating the minutes of the meeting; the drug information pharmacist is responsible for researching and making unbiased recommendations to the committee.

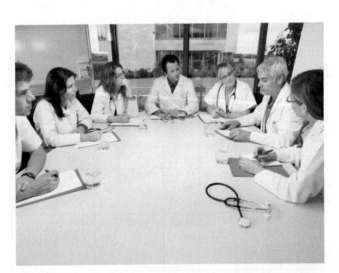

Members of the P&T committee meet primarily to discuss drug formulary changes as well as review medication error reports.

If a medical staff member wants the P&T committee to consider a new drug to be added to the hospital formulary, then he or she must complete and submit an extensive medication application form. The drug information pharmacist then reviews this initial information and completes a search of the medical literature. The cost, advantages, and disadvantages of the new drug are then compared with an existing formulary drug, and these findings are presented to the entire committee for their consideration.

At times, formulary approval may be restricted to a specific medical service. For example, a new, high-cost antibiotic with limited indications and high resistance patterns may be restricted to the *infectious disease service*. A physician not on this service is not allowed to write this prescription (and the pharmacy cannot fill the order) unless it is approved and signed by an infectious disease physician.

The formulary system is based on providing effective medications while limiting patient and hospital costs. If a physician writes a prescription for a *nonformulary* drug—

one not on the approved list—then he or she must justify to the chairperson of the P&T committee or an attending physician the necessity of such a drug for this patient.

The P&T committee is also responsible for reviewing the following:

- studies on the appropriate use of drugs within the hospital
- investigational study drugs for hospital use
- any medication error reports

The drug information center is often responsible for evaluating medication errors and adverse drug reactions and reporting them to the P&T committee. When the committee reviews a medication error report, their focus is not to fix blame, but to identify and correct the problem so that the error does not reoccur.

Institutional Review Board

The **institutional review board (IRB)** is the committee that ensures that appropriate protection is provided to a patient in terms of investigational drugs or procedures. Another name for the IRB is the *human use committee*. Any clinical research investigational study requires approval by the IRB before enrollment can begin. This committee consists of representatives from medicine, pharmacy, nursing, and hospital administration, as well as a consumer member. Most committees in a large hospital meet every month.

An **investigational drug** is defined as a drug that is being used in clinical trials and has not yet been approved by the Food and Drug Administration (FDA) for a specific indication in the general population. The investigator usually submits an application outlining the study, including number of subjects, age of subjects, and type of subjects (i.e., patients vs. healthy volunteers), as well as an informed consent form. An **informed consent** is a document written about the study in terms that are understandable to the lay public. The informed consent for the study must specify the risks vs. the benefits, reimbursement (if any), and follow-up responsibilities and procedures in case of an adverse event.

The IRB protects the patient by assuring both adequate knowledge of the risks of the study and confidentiality of medical information. Adverse events must be reported to the IRB, which reevaluates the approval of the study if necessary. Special procedures exist for neonates, pediatrics, underage women of childbearing age, and patients with mental health problems. The investigator and the IRB must also meet regulations at the state and federal level.

The IRB protects patient confidentiality for participation in investigational studies. In addition to the physician, who sees the medical data? The answer to this question must be specified in the application and protocol. Most commonly, patients are assigned a number (separate from their hospital number) to maintain anonymity. Investigational data may be collected, collated, and sent outside the hospital to a government agency or private company; however, the individual patient's identity and medical data must remain protected. Patient confidentiality is discussed in more detail in Chapter 13, *Human Relations and Communications*.

The Joint Commission

The **Joint Commission**, previously called the Joint Commission on Accreditation of Healthcare Organizations (JCAHO), is an independent, not-for-profit group that sets and measures the standards for quality and safety of health care through an accreditation process. **Accreditation** is like a Good Housekeeping stamp of approval; it means that the hospital has met specific standards of quality and safety. The desired result of the work of this commission is to save patient lives, to provide better health care and quality of life for patients, and to lower healthcare costs.

The Joint Commission evaluates a hospital's performance in specific areas, compares that performance against the defined standards, and then awards a hospital accreditation if the hospital meets those standards. These evidence-based standards of care used as part of the accreditation process are developed in consultation with healthcare experts, providers, and researchers. Medicare and other third-party insurance companies now require accreditation for coverage of services provided by hospitals.

All departments, including the pharmacy, need to have an up-to-date policy and procedure manual, as required by the Joint Commission. In addition, all pharmacy personnel, including pharmacy technicians, should be trained and updated on all policies and procedures outlined in the policy and procedure manual. Annual documentation of such training is required. The percentage of technicians who are certified may be used as a surrogate measure of competency.

The inspection of a hospital for pending Joint Commission accreditation, sometimes referred to as a survey, requires an extensive, multi-day, on-site visit. The inspection is completed at random and is unannounced. A pharmacy technician may be interviewed by a member of the survey team, and the process requires a thorough review of each department's policy and procedure manual, to be sure that it is in compliance with quality and safety standards.

The Joint Commission acts as a patient advocate, making sure that a hospital is following the appropriate standards and procedures. The process is not meant to be punitive, but to ensure patients that all standards are being met or improvements are being instituted for the hospital to be in compliance. For example, if a hospital pharmacy has received multiple budget cuts that may compromise the quality of care or the level of safety of its procedures, then the Joint Commission survey team has the authority to require prompt corrective action by hospital administration.

The objective of the on-site survey is not only to evaluate the hospital but also to provide education and guidance to improve the hospital's overall performance. The survey team includes healthcare professionals who are extensively trained and certified and who receive continuing education to keep them informed about advances in quality-related performance evaluation. The survey team generally provides a summary report to the hospital administrative staff and employees. The final accreditation report is available on the Joint Commission's Web site for review by any consumer or healthcare professional.

Quality of Care Standards

The Joint Commission has National Quality Improvement Goals, which provide standards for quality of patient care in select patient populations. The Joint Commission requires hospitals to report on the key indicators of quality of care in areas such as heart attack, heart failure, community-acquired pneumonia, and surgical infection rates.

The survey team requests a number of medical charts to randomly review for compliance with national quality standards of care. For example, in assessing the hospital performance for the care of the heart attack patient, the following medication-related factors are evaluated, measured, and compared with those at other hospitals that have been accredited by the Joint Commission:

- use of aspirin, prescribed on arrival and at discharge because it decreases the risk of recurrent blood clots and improves survival

- use of certain heart drugs, called *beta blockers,* within the first 24 hours and at discharge to minimize damage to the heart
- timely use of thrombolytic or clot buster therapy within 30 minutes of arrival to reduce heart muscle damage
- timely use of PCI or balloon angioplasty for heart blockage within 120 minutes of arrival
- use of certain heart drugs called angiotensin-converting enzyme inhibitors (ACEIs) or angiotensin receptor blockers (ARBs) at discharge if the patient has a diagnosis of heart failure
- documentation that the physician discussed smoking cessation programs with patients who smoke
- comparison of rates of inpatient mortality for heart attack patients

The performance is compared to that of other hospitals of similar size that are accredited by the Joint Commission. Comparative analysis is performed at a state level and nationwide and is made available to employers and patients. For example, inappropriate antibiotic use could lead to an increase in surgical site infections, resistance patterns within the hospital, and healthcare costs.

Safety-Related Standards

Almost 50% of the Joint Commission's standards are *directly* related to safety. Standards involving the hospital pharmacy include reconciling a patient's medication profile upon admission to the hospital with medication orders and improving safety of medication use and drug infusion pumps. These standards address a number of significant patient safety issues, including the implementation of patient safety programs, the response to adverse events when they occur, and the prevention of accidental harm. Medicare no longer reimburses hospitals for the additional cost of treating preventable medication errors, injuries, and infections, so a strong economic incentive exists.

The Joint Commission may recommend a safety program to improve communications with physicians and nurses in the ordering, preparation, and dispensing of medications to minimize medication errors. Other examples are implementation of policies prohibiting the use of nonapproved abbreviations or policies requiring computer checks and balances with sound-alike drugs to ensure that the right drug, in the right dose, is given to the right patient. The survey team is most interested in measuring changes in the implemented safety program. For example, the use of nonapproved abbreviations was reduced from 19% in 2006 to 7.5% in 2008.

The Joint Commission's safety-related standards are based on the assumption that, if a preventable medication error occurs, investigating the cause and making necessary corrections in policy or procedure are much more important than fixing blame on an individual. When the cause of the error is identified, a repeat medication error may be prevented in the future. The standards also require that the hospital outline its responsibility to advise a patient about adverse outcomes of the care received.

Inventory Management

As much as 70% of the budget of a hospital pharmacy department is spent on pharmaceuticals. Budgetary planning and an accurate inventory tracking system are extremely important responsibilities of the director of pharmacy. In addition to pharmaceuticals, the budget often includes IV solutions, sets, and pumps, as well as medical supplies. Storage space is often limited, so having sufficient inventory without shortages is important to provide good patient care. Similar to the community pharmacy, in a hospital pharmacy the pharmacists and technicians usually perform a physical inventory of their drugs annually.

Purchasing

Most hospital pharmacies purchase their pharmaceuticals from a primary wholesaler and their IV solutions and administration sets directly from the manufacturer. Pharmacists must ensure that their patients receive the highest quality pharmaceuticals at the lowest cost. In many large hospitals, an inventory control pharmacist or technician works closely with pharmacy administration to develop specific criteria based on projected use for budget planning. These criteria are used as the basis for a confidential, sealed bid process, which includes suppliers and manufacturers of drugs and IV solutions. These bids are very competitive, especially in large hospitals where hundreds of thousands of units of some products may be used each year.

Pharmacy technicians may be responsible for collecting information for the drug-bidding process. Many states require a separate bidding process and a separate physical inventory if the hospital operates an outpatient community pharmacy.

The bid process determines the source of approved drug products that are listed in the hospital formulary. Most accepted bids lock in the medication cost for 1 year. Changing brands of medication too often may cause confusion to the pharmacist, nurse, and physician, because the color, shape, or packaging may differ from that of previously stocked medication. The bid contract on IV solutions may be for a longer period because changing IV solutions and sets and educating all nurses every year on the changes are not feasible or cost-effective and may increase the risk for medication administration errors.

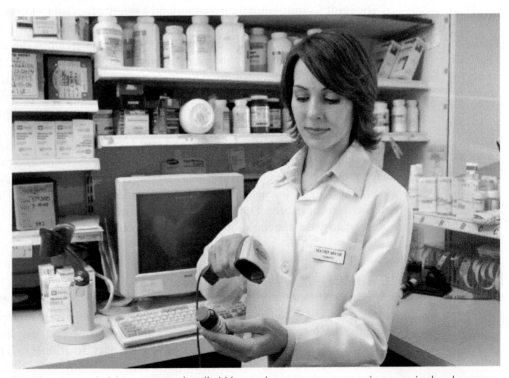

The pharmacy technician may use a handheld bar-code scanner to manage inventory in the pharmacy.

Ordering

An important part of the technician's position is the receipt, storage, and ordering of pharmaceuticals; discrepancies in the order from the wholesaler or pharmaceutical manufacturer should be resolved. Automation from the pharmacy wholesalers is making inventory management more accurate and less costly. Computerized hand-held systems help manage inventory in each area of the hospital by collecting data using bar-code scanning devices and sending this information to the hospital pharmacy. Inventory and labor costs are reduced with the efficiencies of this technology.

At times a hospital pharmacy may need to borrow a medication from another hospital or from a community pharmacy; the policy and procedure manual should outline the process, and the borrowed drug should be returned when more is received from the wholesaler. Because both the hospital pharmacy and retail pharmacy may borrow during the month, the net balance of the borrowing at the completion of the month is paid. Careful documentation with proper signatures is needed in the rare event that controlled substances are borrowed between institutions to provide a paper audit trail.

Receiving and Storage

Once the drugs from the wholesaler are received and the invoice verified, the drugs must be properly stored. The technician should not accept receipt for any potentially damaged goods, so inspection of the box or container may be indicated. Stock on the shelves should be rotated so that the most recent inventory is not used first. For some drugs, refrigeration or even freezing may be necessary. Plastic bags of IV solutions must be removed from boxes and wiped down before placement in the IV storage area in order to keep the room clean and free of dust. The technician should check all special orders (medications not routinely stocked in the pharmacy) and out-of-stocks in case a patient needs a newly acquired medication.

Two types of pharmaceuticals require special consideration in inventory control: (1) controlled substances and (2) investigational drugs. The Controlled Substances Act (CSA) defines ordering inventory, filing, and recordkeeping requirements for controlled substances. Purchase of Schedule II controlled substances must be authorized by a pharmacist and executed on the Drug Enforcement Administration (DEA) 222 form as discussed in Chapter 7. A physical inventory of Schedule II substances is required every 2 years. Any destruction of C-II drugs must be witnessed and documented in the department records.

As discussed earlier in the chapter, all investigational drug studies must be approved by the institutional review board, or the human use committee. Investigational drugs require special ordering, handling, and recordkeeping procedures by the pharmacy technician. Investigational drugs must be maintained in a secure area of the pharmacy until a valid written medication order is received. In most of these research studies the drug is not labeled with a name or strength, but it still requires identification with lot number and expiration date.

Another important area of responsibility for the technician is the storage and return of expired drugs for credit from the manufacturer. This also includes drugs subject to FDA or drug manufacturer recall. One of the primary responsibilities of the pharmacy technician is to identify expired drugs, remove them from storage in the pharmacy or patient care unit, and return them to the wholesaler for credit. If the manufacturer or the FDA recalls a drug, then the technician often compares the lot number of the drug in the recall letter or notice with inventory in pharmacy storage. Generally a form indicating drug, strength, amount, and lot number is completed, signed, and returned to the wholesaler with the drugs for credit. Returns of C-II drugs must be recorded on a special DEA 106 form.

Chapter Terms

accreditation the stamp of approval of the quality of services of a hospital by the Joint Commission

admitting order a medication order written by a physician on admission of a patient to the hospital; may or may not include a medication order

cart fill list a printout of all unit dose profiles for all patients

continuation order a medication order written by a physician to continue treatment; like a refill of medication

director of pharmacy the chief executive officer of the pharmacy department

electronic medication administration record (eMAR) documents the administration time of each drug to each patient often using bar-code technology

floor stock medications stocked in a secured area on each patient care unit

informed consent written permission by the patient to participate in an IRB-approved research study in terms understandable to the lay public

inpatient drug distribution system a pharmacy system to deliver all types of drugs to a patient in the hospital setting; commonly includes unit dose, repackaged medication, floor stock, and IV admixture and TPN services

institutional review board (IRB) a committee of the hospital that ensures that appropriate protection is provided to patients using investigational drugs; sometimes referred to as the human use committee

investigational drugs drugs used in clinical trials that have not yet been approved by the FDA for use in the general population or drugs used for nonapproved indications

IV admixture service a centralized pharmacy service that prepares IV and TPN solutions in a sterile, germ-free work environment

Joint Commission an independent, not-for-profit group that sets the standards by which safety and quality of health care are measured and accredits hospitals according to those standards; previously called the Joint Commission on Accreditation of Healthcare Organizations (JCAHO)

medication administration record (MAR) a form in the patient medical chart used by nurses to document the administration time of all drugs

medication order a prescription written in the hospital setting

medication special a single dose preparation not commercially available that is repackaged and made for a particular patient

pharmacy and therapeutics (P&T) committee a committee of the hospital that reviews, approves, and revises the hospital's formulary of drugs and maintains the drug use policies of the hospital

repackaging control log a form used in the pharmacy when drugs are repackaged from manufacturer stock bottles to unit doses; the log contains the name of the drug, dose, quantity, manufacturer lot number, expiration date, and the initials of the pharmacy technician and pharmacist

Schedule II drug administration record a manual or electronic form on the patient care unit to account for each dose of each narcotic administered to a patient

stat order a medication order that is to be filled and sent to the patient care unit immediately

total parenteral nutrition (TPN) a specially formulated parenteral solution that provides nutritional needs intravenously (IV) to a patient who cannot or will not eat

unit dose an amount of a drug that has been prepackaged or repackaged for a single administration to a particular patient at a particular time

unit dose cart a movable storage unit that contains individual patient drawers of medication for all patients on a given nursing unit

unit dose profile the documentation that provides the information necessary to prepare the unit doses, including patient name and location, medication and strength, frequency or schedule of administration, and quantity for each order

Chapter Summary

- The hospital is a complex organization.
- The director of pharmacy is the chief executive officer of the pharmacy department and is responsible for its safe and efficient operation.
- Hospital pharmacies carry out a number of unique activities, such as managing the unit dose drug distribution system; repackaging; maintaining floor stock, including narcotics; and providing IV admixture and TPN services.
- In the hospital setting, a prescription is called a medication order; it is written as an admitting, new, or continuation order.
- A unit dose drug distribution system saves money and reduces the chance of medication errors.
- A cart fill list is used by the technician to fill medication needs for a hospitalized patient.
- The pharmacy technician is often responsible for preparing repackaged units of medications that are not commercially available in unit dose packaging.
- Most hospitals today have an extensive floor stock system, consisting of frequently used unit dose drugs as well as narcotics and IV solutions.
- An intravenous (IV) admixture service may reduce the chance of medication dosage and calculation errors and the risk of contamination.

- Many hospital pharmacies have a centralized TPN service in which electrolytes and vitamins are added to a variety of IV nutrition solutions.
- A medication administration record or MAR is used by a nurse to document the administration time of each medication to each patient.
- The pharmacy and therapeutics (P&T) committee is primarily responsible for making the final decision on the medications included in the hospital's drug formulary.
- The institutional review board (IRB) is responsible for protecting the patient in investigational studies undertaken in the hospital.
- The primary mission of the Joint Commission is to assess hospital suitability for accreditation ensuring quality care and patient safety in the hospitals that are accredited.
- The pharmacy technician assists in the ordering, purchasing, and receiving of medications.
- Automation is widely used in the hospital pharmacy in filling inpatient and outpatient medication orders, preparing IV and TPN solutions, documenting floor stock and medication administration, and in inventory control.

Chapter Review

Checking Your Understanding

Choose the best answer from those provided.

 Additional Quiz Questions

1. A formulary is a
   a. list of approved drugs available through a hospital pharmacy.
   b. description of the contents and pharmacological characteristics of manufactured drugs.
   c. set of formulae for extemporaneous compounding.
   d. set of formulae for preparation of common parenteral admixtures.

2. Patient confidentiality for participation in investigational studies is a function of the
   a. P&T committee.
   b. Infection Control committee
   c. institutional review board (IRB)
   d. Joint Commission.

3. A unit dose is
   a. a supply of medication prepared for a hospital patient care unit.
   b. an amount and dosage form appropriate for a single administration to a single patient.
   c. the average recommended dose for an adult male.
   d. the dose recommended by the United States Pharmacopeia (USP).

4. A function unique to a hospital pharmacy, compared to a community pharmacy, would include
   a. maintaining drug treatment records.
   b. ordering and stocking medications and medical supplies.
   c. dispensing and repackaging medications.
   d. handling sterile parenteral hazardous drugs.

5. The Joint Commission is primarily interested in patient safety and
   a. quality of care.

---

   b. patient satisfaction.
   c. decreasing hospital costs.
   d. drug information services.

6. The primary function of the P&T committee is to
   a. maintain a formulary of approved drugs.
   b. approve investigational drug protocols.
   c. establish policies on proper use of antibiotics.
   d. set the drug budget for the pharmacy department.

7. In the hospital, a prescription is commonly referred to as a
   a. medication order.
   b. MAR.
   c. protocol.
   d. prn or floor stock medication.

8. When the pharmacy technician receives a *stat* order, the medication should be sent to the nurse
   a. immediately.
   b. within the next 1 to 2 hours.
   c. at the next shift change.
   d. the next morning.

9. Physical inventory of drugs in the hospital pharmacy is usually conducted every
   a. month.
   b. 6 months.
   c. year (annually).
   d. 2 years.

10. The provision of the entire nutritional needs of a patient by means of intravenous (IV) infusion is known as
    a. an eMAR.
    b. the IRB.
    c. the Joint Commission.
    d. a TPN.

Thinking Like a Pharmacy Tech

Write out a complete description, not using abbreviations, of the following medication orders.

Patient Name	Order	Room #
1. Tom Smith	ascorbic acid 500 mg po daily	230
	Basaljel po prn ac and hs	
	Toradol 10 mg po q4-6 h	
	Demerol 50 mg IM q4 h prn	
2. Natalie Wang	Lunesta 3 mg po q hs	311
	Zyrtec 1 tsp po q am	
	MOM 30 mL po prn	
	Humalog 70/25 30 u subcutaneously in AM ac and 20 units in PM ac	
3. Kathy Sooner	Lipitor 40 mg po q hs	402
	Ducolax 5 mg po q24 h	
	hydrocodone 5/500 1-2 tab q6 h prn pain	
	Amoxicillin 1 g IVPB q6 h	
	Gentamicin 80 mg IVPB q8 h	
	D5 ½ NS 1L @ 125 mL/h	
4. Wesley Elmore	atenolol 100 mg q am	321
	MOM 10 mL po q pc	
	Colace 150 mg po hs	
	Ativan 2 mg IM 2 h prior to surgery	
5. Jennie Conners	Minitran 0.2 mg/h apply q am	401
	Fleet prep kit ut dict 1 h prior to colonoscopy	
	ASA 650 mg po q4 h	
	Cipro 500 mg IVPB q12 h	
	NS 500 mL with KCl 20 mEq @ 100 mL/h	

Communicating Clearly

1. Communicating in the hospital setting often means working with a wide variety of other healthcare providers. Understanding what roles they play in the patients' health care is essential to effective communication. What duties does each of the following have?
   a. physician
   b. anesthesiologist
   c. registered nurse
   d. licensed practical nurse
   e. nurse's aide
   f. housekeeping aide
   g. social services aide or worker
   h. respiratory therapist
   i. phlebotomist
   j. medical lab technician

Researching on the Web

1. Visit the ASHP Web site.
   a. What types of training does ASHP offer?
   b. What are the benefits of technician membership?
   c. How do you become a member?

2. Go to www.ashp.org/bestpractices and identify nine advantages of a unit dose drug system over alternative distribution systems.

3. Pharmacy techs working in a hospital setting are often responsible for the repackaging of drugs into a unit dose package. Go to www.ashp.org/bestpractices and find "Single Unit and Unit Dose Packages of Drugs." Then identify and describe in detail the seven parts of a label for a repackaged drug.

4. The Joint Commission focuses on patient safety. In the hospital pharmacy that includes the prevention of medication errors. Go to www.jointcommission.org and find "Statistics in Sentinel Events." Look for year trends in Medication Errors.

5. Visit www.hcahealthcare.com and review the emphasis on patient safety. List two ways that this group of hospitals has reduced medication errors.

6. Go to the www.jointcommission.org Web site and identify the list of "do not use" symbols and abbreviations.

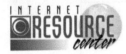

For further study of chapter-related topics, explore the Web links in the Web Center at www.emcp.net/pharmpractice4e.

Infection Control

10

Learning Objectives

- Explain the role of pathogenic organisms in causing disease.

- Distinguish among bacteria, viruses, fungi, and protozoa.

- Discuss the advantages and disadvantages of various forms of sterilization.

- Identify sources and prevention of common causes of contamination.

- Discuss the importance of the Centers for Disease Control and Prevention (CDC) guidelines on preventing the transmission of infectious disease within the hospital.

- Contrast hand washing and hand hygiene practices when in a sterile work environment.

- Discuss the importance of vaccinations for healthcare workers.

- Contrast a manufactured sterile product with expiration dating vs. a compounded sterile preparation (CSP) with beyond-use dating according to USP Chapter 797 guidelines.

- Identify procedures to minimize airborne contamination with CSPs.

- Apply contamination risk level designations and appropriate beyond-use dating for CSPs.

- Identify the role of the infection control committee.

- List common universal precautions to protect hospital employees.

Preview chapter terms and definitions.

ospitals and home healthcare pharmacies (and some compounding pharmacies) commonly compound or prepare sterile preparations. To understand what a sterile preparation is, one needs to know something of the study of microbiology and the germ theory of disease. A comprehension of the potential dangers of contaminants makes the processes of sterilization and aseptic technique more easily understood. The consequences of not following correct technique can increase the risk for the development of serious hospital-acquired infections, which can lead to patient mortality.

The roles of the Centers for Disease Control and Prevention (CDC) and United States Pharmacopeia (USP) are extensively discussed in this chapter. The USP has published guidelines for the preparation of compounded sterile preparations (CSPs) that have been adopted by accrediting organizations as national standards. The infection control committee is responsible for implementing these guidelines within the hospital setting. The pharmacy technician must be educated and trained in proper aseptic technique and follow these guidelines, which are contained in the department policy and procedure manual.

Identifying and Controlling the Source of Infection

Infection control is extremely critical in a hospital setting. Patients with severe disease may have a compromised immune system and may thus be more susceptible to serious and sometimes life-threatening infections. Also, microorganisms have a greater ability to adapt and become resistant to potent antibiotics in the hospital than in the community setting. It is important to understand how infection spreads and how hospitals can employ special techniques and procedures to limit the possibility of contamination.

The Development of the Germ Theory of Disease

Until relatively recently, the causes of illness—especially infectious diseases—were not fully understood. Disease was attributed to evil influences, and knowledge of the actual causes of infectious disease progressed slowly over the centuries. In the seventeenth century, the Dutch merchant Anton van Leeuwenhoek made the first crude microscope. In 1673 he observed through his microscope what are today called microorganisms. Although van Leeuwenhoek observed microbes, the Englishman Robert Hooke used a microscope to observe the walls of dead plant cells. Hooke called the pores between the walls "little cells." His discovery of cell structure marked the beginning of cell theory.

Until the second half of the nineteenth century, it was generally believed that some forms of life could arise spontaneously from matter. This process was known as spontaneous generation. People thought that toads, snakes, and mice could be born from moist soil, that flies could emerge from manure, and that maggots could arise from decaying flesh. In 1668 the Italian physician Francesco Redi demonstrated that maggots could not arise spontaneously from decaying meat by conducting a simple experiment in which jars containing meat were left open, sealed, or covered with a fine net. Redi showed that maggots appeared only when the jars were left open, allowing flies to enter to lay eggs.

As discussed in Chapter 3, in 1798 Edward Jenner discovered the principle of immunization against disease. He noticed that milkmaids who had caught cowpox from cows were then immune to contracting smallpox from humans. By infecting healthy persons with cowpox, Jenner successfully inoculated them against smallpox. However, because microorganisms had not yet been identified as disease-causing agents, the reasons behind the success of Jenner's immunizations were not fully understood.

The French research scientist Louis Pasteur was instrumental in proving the germ theory and furthering the advances of Jenner in vaccine research. Pasteur demonstrated that the fermentation process is caused by the growth of microorganisms in the nutrient broth, not by "spontaneous generation," which was the common belief at the time. In 1861 Pasteur demonstrated that microorganisms are present in the air and that they can contaminate seemingly sterile solutions, but that the air itself does not give rise, spontaneously, to microbial life.

To disprove the spontaneous generation theory, Pasteur filled several short-necked flasks with beef broth and boiled ham. Some flasks were left open and allowed to cool.

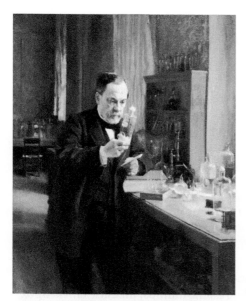

Pasteur demonstrated that microorganisms are present in the air and can infect animals and humans.

In a few days, these flasks were contaminated with microbes. The other flasks, sealed after boiling, remained free of microorganisms.

Pasteur also noted that microorganisms can contaminate fermenting beverages. In his time, the quality of winemaking was inconsistent. One year the wine was sweet, but the next year it was sour. No uniform method had been discovered to ensure the same quality year after year. While experimenting along the lines used in his broth experiment, Pasteur discovered that if grape juice was heated to a certain temperature, cooled, and treated with specific yeast, then the wine would be more consistent year after year. Based on this work Pasteur developed a process to kill most bacteria and mold in milk called **pasteurization**. To his credit, pasteurization is still used today.

Beverage contamination led Pasteur to conclude that microorganisms infected animals and humans as well. The idea that microorganisms cause diseases came to be known as the **germ theory of disease**. Pasteur, the originator of the theory, designed experiments to prove it. The germ theory also led Pasteur and other scientists to link the activity of microorganisms with physical and chemical changes in organic materials. Pasteur proposed preventing the entry of microorganisms into the human body.

Joseph Lister, an English surgeon, built on Pasteur's work and applied it to human medicine. Lister knew that carbolic acid (or phenol) kills bacteria, so he began soaking surgical dressings in a mild carbolic acid solution. Lister then developed antiseptic methods in surgery. These meticulous washing and gowning methods form the basis of sterile technique, which was widely and quickly adopted and is still in use in hospitals and pharmacies. His sterile surgical techniques significantly reduced postoperative infections and saved thousands of lives.

In 1876 Robert Koch defined a series of steps, known as Koch's postulates, that could be taken to prove that a certain disease was caused by a specific microorganism. Koch discovered rod-shaped bacteria in cattle that had died from anthrax. He cultured the bacteria in artificial media and used them to infect healthy animals. When these animals became sick and died, Koch isolated the bacteria in their blood, compared them with the bacteria originally isolated, and found them to be the same.

Microorganisms and Disease

Since the days of Pasteur, Lister, and Koch, thousands of pathogenic, or disease-causing, microorganisms have been identified. Not all microorganisms cause disease. Some, in fact, perform essential functions, such as creating by-products that are used as medicines, in fermenting wine, to fix nitrogen in the soil, and to help the body break down various food substances. For example, yogurt consists of good bacteria that can reestablish normal flora in the gastrointestinal (GI) tract and reduce diarrhea that may be caused as a side effect of antibiotics. However, some organisms may be pathogenic.

Bacteria A **bacterium** is a type of small, single-celled microorganism; bacteria can exist in three main forms when viewed under the microscope: spherical (i.e., cocci), rod shaped (i.e., bacilli), and spirochetes (Figure 10.1). In the microbiology lab, after Gram

FIGURE 10.1
**Characteristic
Bacterial Shapes**

(a) Round cocci.

(b) Rodlike bacilli.

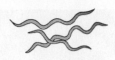
(c) Spiral-shaped
spirochetes.

staining, some bacteria are identified as either Gram positive (blue or purple) or Gram negative (red). Normal human skin is colonized by several bacteria. Bacteria cause a wide variety of illnesses, such as food poisoning, strep throat, ear infections, rheumatic fever, meningitis, pneumonia, tuberculosis, pinkeye, and acne.

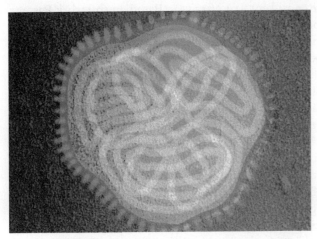

An electron micrograph of a virus. The virus is much smaller than a bacterium and can only be viewed with an electron microscope. It does not have all of the components of a cell and requires other living cells to replicate itself.

Viruses A **virus** is a very small microorganism that consists of little more than a bit of genetic material enclosed by a casing of protein. Viruses need a living host in which to reproduce and cause a wide variety of diseases, including colds, mumps, measles, chickenpox, influenza, hepatitis, and human immunodeficiency virus (HIV).

Fungi A **fungus** is a parasite on living organisms (by feeding on dead organic material) that reproduces slowly by means of spores. Spores and some fungi are microscopic plants that can occur as molds, mildews, or mushrooms and that travel through the air. Some molds are the source of antibiotics such as penicillin. Others are implicated in mild conditions such as athlete's foot, ringworm, or vaginal yeast infection or in more serious systemic fungal infections in the hospital, which can be potentially life threatening.

Protozoa A **protozoa** is a microscopic organism made up of a single cell or a group of more or less identical cells. Protozoa live in water or as parasites inside other creatures. Examples of protozoa include paramecia and amoebae. Amoebic dysentery, malaria, and sleeping sickness are examples of illnesses caused by protozoa.

Asepsis and Sterilization

The scientific control of harmful microorganisms began only about one hundred years ago. Before that time, epidemics or pandemics caused by microorganisms (that is to say, smallpox or cholera) killed millions of people. Three different bubonic plagues killed 137 million people in Europe (caused by fleas spreading the bacteria from diseased black rats). In addition, European diseases such as smallpox and syphilis decimated the native population of the Americas. Before the modern era, as many as 25% of delivering mothers died of infections carried by the hands and instruments of attending nurses and physicians. During the American Civil War, surgeons sometimes cleaned their scalpels on their boot soles between incisions. The flu epidemic of 1918 killed over 25 million people worldwide, including 650,000 in the United States. The source of this epidemic was a bird virus that was transmitted to humans. There are concerns today that a reactivation of this avian flu could cause a pandemic and

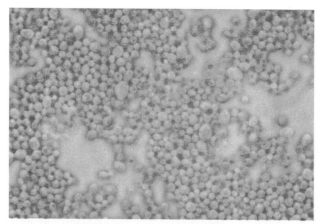

A photomicrograph of a fungus. Fungi are multicellular organisms, unlike bacteria or viruses.

high mortality. Developing an efficacious vaccine is a global major health priority.

Asepsis is the absence of disease-causing microorganisms. The condition of asepsis is brought about by **sterilization**—any process that destroys the microorganisms. When an object such as a medical instrument is sterilized, no need exists to identify the species of microbes on it, because sterilization kills even the most resistant microbial life forms present. Many types of sterilization exist: heat, dry heat, mechanical, gas, and chemical. Many of these methods may be used in a large hospital setting. A brief overview of commonly used sterilization techniques is provided for the pharmacy technician.

Heat Sterilization One traditional method for killing microbes is heat sterilization or boiling. Heat is available, effective, economical, and easily controlled. Boiling kills vegetative forms, many viruses, and fungi in about 10 minutes, but more time is required to kill other organisms, such as fungus spores and the hepatitis viruses. If water supply in the home is compromised, then the recommendation is to boil water before drinking. Automatic dishwashers loosely borrow from the concept of heat sterilization during their drying cycle.

Heat sterilization uses an **autoclave**, a device that generates heat and pressure, to sterilize. When moist heat of 121 °C (or 270 °F) under pressure of 15 psi (pounds per square inch) is applied to instruments, solutions, or powders, most known organisms—including spores and viruses—are killed in about 15 minutes. At home, pressure cookers use the concept of heat and pressure to sterilize vegetables. Heat sterilization is being used less frequently in the hospital setting, partly because of space requirements, equipment expense, and personnel training issues.

Dry Heat Sterilization Dry heat, such as direct flaming, also destroys all microorganisms. Dry heat is impractical for many substances but is used for the disposal of contaminated objects, which are often incinerated. For proper sterilization using hot, dry air, a temperature of 170 °C must be maintained for nearly 2 hours. Note that a higher temperature is necessary for dry heat, because a heated liquid more readily transfers heat to a cool object.

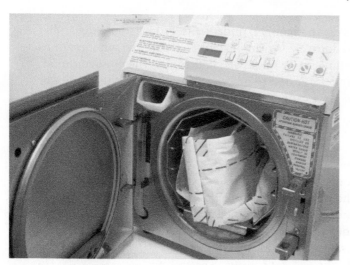

An autoclave generates heat and pressure to sterilize; it kills most known organisms in about 15 minutes.

Mechanical Sterilization Mechanical sterilization is achieved by means of filtration, which is the passage of a liquid or gas through a screenlike material with pores small enough to block microorganisms. This method of sterilization is used for heat-sensitive materials such as culture media (used for growing colonies of bacteria or other microorganisms), enzymes, vaccines, and antibiotic solutions. Filter pore sizes are 0.22 micron for bacteria and 0.01 micron for viruses and some large proteins. Filters may be used in pharmaceutical manufacturing plants as well as hospital pharmacies. Filters are discussed more in Chapter 11, *Preparing and Handling Sterile Products and Hazardous Drugs*.

Gas Sterilization Gas sterilization, which makes use of ethylene oxide, is used for objects that are labile, or subject, to destruction by heat. Gas sterilization requires special equipment and aeration of materials after application of the gas. This gas is highly flammable and is used only in large institutions and manufacturing facilities that have adequate equipment to handle the gas. Many prepackaged IV fluids and bandages are manufactured and sterilized using this type of sterilization. Ethylene oxide leaves a slight, nonharmful residue that can be detected as an odor.

Chemical Sterilization Chemical sterilization is the destruction of microorganisms on inanimate objects by chemical means. Few chemicals produce complete sterility, but many reduce microbial numbers to safe levels. A chemical applied to an object or topically to the body for sterilization purposes is known as a **disinfectant**. Iodine, isopropyl alcohol (IPA), and chlorinated bleach are often used as topical disinfectants.

Contamination

Harmful microorganisms, especially bacteria, are everywhere in large numbers. Bacteria or other contaminants can be introduced extremely easily onto a sterile object or device or into a sterile solution.

For the pharmacy technician working in the preparation of sterile IV products, the prevention of contamination is crucial. The introduction of contaminated IV solution into a patient at surgery or with a compromised immune system can cause serious infection or even death. In a hospital pharmacy, contamination can occur by three primary means: (1) touch, (2) air, and (3) water. Understanding these modes of contamination helps explain the reasons for the procedures followed in the hospital pharmacy to reduce or eliminate contamination.

Touch

Millions of bacteria live on skin and hair and under nails. Proper scrubbing and following strict aseptic procedures are very important to reduce the numbers of bacteria on the hands before handling sterile materials. Touching is the most common method of contamination and the easiest to prevent. In addition to the practice of frequent washing, the use of gloves and caps or hairnets can minimize touch contamination.

Air

Microorganisms are commonly found in the air, in dust particles, and in moisture droplets. Sterile materials should be prepared in a designated area in which the numbers of possible contaminants are maintained at a low level. Special equipment, called a laminar flow hood or workbench, can control airflow and minimize contamination; this equipment is discussed later in this chapter.

Water

Even tap water is not free of microorganisms. Moisture droplets in the air, especially after a sneeze or cough, often contain harmful microbes. Sterile materials should not be contaminated by exposure to droplets of tap water or other sources of contaminated moisture. A pharmacy technician with a common cold should notify the pharmacist supervisor; often a change in work functions for that day is recommended. Protective plastic shields on equipment and use of masks minimize moisture contamination.

The Centers for Disease Control and Prevention

The **Centers for Disease Control and Prevention (CDC)** is a governmental agency that provides guidelines and recommendations on infection control. The CDC publishes reports on the sensitivity and resistance of various bacteria to antibiotics in different regions of the country, providing guidelines on the drug of choice, the dosage, and the duration of treatment for many common infectious illnesses.

A major focus of the CDC is the prevention of transmission of infectious agents in the hospital to protect both patients and healthcare workers. Failure to follow proper procedures or inadequate personnel training could produce a high incidence of healthcare-associated infections (HAIs), with tragic consequences. With the emergence of new, dangerous, or pathogenic strains of bacteria that are resistant to multiple drug therapies, all healthcare personnel must follow policies and procedures strictly. The Joint Commission carefully reviews infection control procedures in its accreditation process. HAIs, or nosocomial infections, are discussed later in the chapter under the Infection Control Committee.

The CDC updates and publishes guidelines to protect the patient and the healthcare worker from infectious disease. The following sections highlight the guidelines concerning hand hygiene, protective clothing, and the importance of vaccinations for the healthcare worker.

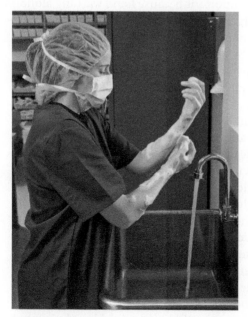

Hand washing minimizes touch contamination and reduces the transmission of disease.

Hand Hygiene

According to the CDC, simple hand washing and hand hygiene are the single most important practices to minimizing touch contamination and reducing the transmission of infectious agents. **Hand washing** is defined as using plain or antiseptic soap and water. To be effective, plain detergent soaps with minimal antimicrobial activity must be used for at least 30 seconds, the time needed to rub off the transient skin microorganisms effectively. **Hand hygiene** is defined as using special alcohol-based rinses, gels, or foams that do not require water. Unless the hands are visibly dirty, the alcohol-based products are preferred because of their superior antimicrobial activity, quick drying effect, and convenience. Studies have demonstrated that proper hand hygiene can minimize the transmission of infections within the hospital.

The effectiveness of hand hygiene in infection control may be affected by technique (see Table 10.1), as well as the presence of artificial fingernails and jewelry, which can harbor microorganisms. Hand hygiene is required even if gloves

TABLE 10.1　Hand Washing and Hand Hygiene Guidelines

- When washing hands with soap and water, wet hands first with water, apply an amount of product recommended by the manufacturer to hands, and rub hands together vigorously for at least 15 (preferably 30) seconds, covering all surfaces of the hands and fingers. Rinse hands with water and dry thoroughly with a disposable towel. Use towel to turn off the faucet. Avoid using hot water; repeated exposure to hot water may increase the risk of skin irritation.

- Liquid, bar, or powdered forms of plain soap are acceptable when washing hands with a nonantimicrobial soap and water. When bar soap is used, small bars of soap and soap racks facilitating drainage should be used.

- Dry hands with single-use towels, or air dry. Multiple-use cloth towels of the hanging or roll type are not recommended for use in healthcare settings, because they can transfer infectious agents.

- When decontaminating hands with an alcohol-based hand rub, apply product to palm of one hand and rub hands together, covering all surfaces of hands and fingers, until hands are dry. Follow the manufacturer's recommendations regarding the volume of product to use.

Source: The Centers for Disease Control and Prevention (CDC), www.cdc.gov.

are used or changed. The adherence to proper technique in the hospital has averaged only 40% in several clinical studies. Alcohol-based hand hygiene products are usually readily available throughout the hospital, including the cafeteria and patient waiting rooms, for use by both healthcare professionals and visitors.

Gloves

The CDC recommends that healthcare workers, such as pharmacy technicians working in the IV area, use gloves, primarily to prevent the transmission of normal or pathogenic skin flora to patients. Gloves are important because hand washing alone may not prevent the transmission of microorganisms if the hands are heavily contaminated. Personnel who use gloves may be less likely to use correct hand hygiene practice. Obviously, hand washing and glove use by physicians, nurses, and phlebotomists involved in direct patient contact is even more important.

Gloves are generally made of latex or vinyl; either material appears to offer comparable protection. However, because many healthcare workers and patients may be sensitive to latex, alternative latex-free gloves should be available. Some latex-free gloves are powdered; after their removal, the residual powder may interact with the alcohol-based antiseptic to cause an uncomfortable gritty feel. Using petroleum-based ointments or creams may decrease the integrity of the gloves. Gloves should never be washed or reused. Used gloves should be discarded in a designated area per hospital procedure.

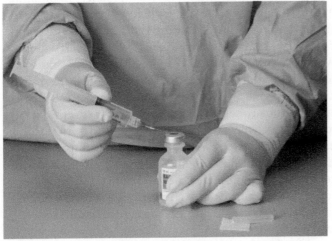

Gloving by the pharmacy tech in the preparation of sterile products provides an additional safeguard to touch contamination.

Vaccination

You may not think that getting a flu shot is important to your health, especially if you are young and healthy. However, if you are working in a hospital setting, then the CDC recommends that you receive an annual flu shot (usually free of charge) to keep you, your family members, and hospitalized patients healthy. Vaccination keeps you productive by reducing the number of sick days needed. The flu shot also reduces the amount of inappropriate or unnecessary use of antibiotics. Inappropriate antibiotic use can produce drug-resistant organisms.

Studies have demonstrated that many healthcare workers have evidence of exposure to the influenza virus even if they are asymptomatic themselves. This exposure may be passed on to family members or patients in the hospital who have compromised or weakened immune systems. Influenza exposure to a frail older patient or an infant can be fatal. However, studies have shown that only 40% of healthcare workers take advantage of the opportunity of getting an annual flu shot.

Flu vaccines are normally 70% to 90% effective; they are not 100% effective because the virus mutates or changes every year. Thus, this year's flu vaccine is often based on the antigenic strains from last year's flu virus. This is why you must get a shot every year. The best time to get the vaccination is October or November each year, because the immune system can take a few weeks to respond fully. Use of oral or intranasal antiviral drugs is not as effective as the injectable vaccine.

Vaccination is even indicated for healthcare workers who are pregnant. Only personnel who have an acute febrile illness or are hypersensitive to eggs should not receive the vaccine; however, once the fever has subsided, the vaccine should be administered. Minor illnesses, such as a cold, are not valid reasons for not getting the vaccine. Contrary to popular myth, you cannot get the flu from the vaccine, because the virus is an inactivated or killed virus. Severe adverse effects are rare.

Occasionally a virulent pathogenic influenza virus can appear and cause a regional pandemic or even worldwide epidemic. The avian bird flu is an example of a virus that may, in the future, mutate or directly infect humans. In the case of any such outbreak, all healthcare workers should be fully vaccinated in order to protect themselves and to allow them to provide care for the sick.

USP Chapter 797 Standards

In 2004, the United States Pharmacopeia (USP) developed the first official and enforceable requirements for sterile preparation compounding to improve the quality standards in the pharmacy. The Joint Commission has adopted these guidelines and evaluates their compliance in hospital pharmacies on future accreditation visits. The original guidelines were modified and updated in 2007 and approved in 2008. Some variance with compliance to the recommendations contained in Chapter 797 results from space limitations and hospital size, staffing, and budget; however, most hospital pharmacies are striving for full compliance.

The standard, known as **USP Chapter 797**, focuses on the sterility and stability of a compounded sterile preparation. A **compounded sterile preparation (CSP)** is defined as a sterile product that is prepared outside of the pharmaceutical manufacturer's facility. Sterility refers to the CSP being free from microorganisms, whereas stability refers to chemical and physical characteristics of the CSP, such as pH, degradation, formation of precipitates (or salts), or unexpected color changes. Both sterility and stability are important considerations.

As expected, requirements for sterile compounding are more stringent than for nonsterile compounding (discussed in Chapter 8). Differences include the following.

- working in a defined clean-room environment
- additional requirements for personnel garbing
- personnel testing and training in principles and practices of aseptic technique
- environmental quality specifications
- disinfection of gloves and surfaces

The 797 standards pertain to all personnel—pharmacy technicians and pharmacists—involved in the preparation, storage, and transportation of CSPs prior to administration to the patient. In addition to drugs, CSPs include biologicals, diagnostics, nutrients, and radioactive pharmaceuticals. The impact of these standards on the preparation, storage, and handling of TPN and hazardous drugs is discussed further in Chapter 11. The Chapter 797 standards also apply to all practice settings, including a compounding, nuclear, home health, or long-term healthcare pharmacy, as well as clinics and physicians' offices. If a hospital pharmacy outsources, or sends out, its orders for the preparation of IV additives and/or TPNs, then all 797 requirements must be met by the off-site pharmacy.

Environmental Quality and Standards

Compounding facilities are physically designed and environmentally controlled to minimize airborne contamination. The 797 standards use the **International Organization for Standardization (ISO)** classification system for defining the amount of particulate matter (i.e., potential airborne contamination) allowed in room air where CSPs are prepared. The lower the ISO number is, the less particulate matter is present in the air. Hospital pharmacy labs must conform to the air quality requirements, and workflow patterns must be limited in order to protect the sterility of the area where the sterile compounding work is done.

As shown in Figure 10.2, the sterile compounding area or IV room is divided into three main areas: the ante area, the buffer area, and the direct compounding area. In small hospital pharmacies that prepare low-risk CSPs, the ante and buffer area may be one room. The **ante area** is where personnel hand washing and garbing procedures, staging of components, order entry, CSP labeling, and other high-particulate-generating activities are performed. The air quality of the ante area should be maintained at ISO Class 7 or 8. The **buffer area** is where the supplies for CSPs (such as IV bags and administration sets) are stored for later use. The buffer area should have an air quality of no more than ISO Class 7. The air quality level in the staging area, outside the laminar airflow workbenches (LAFW), must be maintained at ISO Class 5; the staging area is used to assemble necessary supplies for making a CSP for an individual patient. The most sterile area is the **direct compounding area (DCA)**, where the compounding is performed under a LAFW.

The air quality of the entire compounding lab, including the DCA, is controlled with a high-efficiency particulate air (HEPA) filter system. The pharmacy technician working in this setting is responsible for maintaining the air filtration system and the overall cleanliness of the IV area. Carts, counters, cabinets, and shelves used in all areas of the compounding area should be designed to minimize contamination. The floor, ceiling, and walls should be sealed to provide for easy cleaning and to prevent the harboring of microorganisms. Only furniture, equipment, and supplies necessary for the preparation of CSPs should be allowed in the defined areas of the compounding area.

FIGURE 10.2
Sterile Compounding IV Room Layout

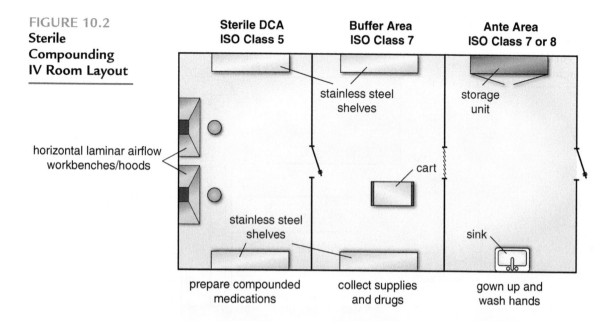

Sterile DCA ISO Class 5	Buffer Area ISO Class 7	Ante Area ISO Class 7 or 8

horizontal laminar airflow workbenches/hoods

stainless steel shelves

storage unit

cart

stainless steel shelves

sink

prepare compounded medications

collect supplies and drugs

gown up and wash hands

Together, the direct compounding area and the buffer area make up the **clean room**. The clean room is physically segregated from the rest of the pharmacy to minimize airflow. In addition, access to a clean room is restricted to those personnel trained to prepare CSPs. Personnel with certain medical conditions or wearing sheddable cosmetics are not allowed to work in the direct compounding area because of increased risk of shedding of skin and microorganisms. No food or drink can be taken into any of the areas of the compounding lab, and no chewing gum should be used by personnel entering or working in these areas.

No long-term storage (i.e., use of IV boxes) is permissible in the clean room. Packaged supplies such as IV bags, administration sets, or syringes should be taken out of their original cartons and cleaned and disinfected in the ante area before passage into the buffer area. Similarly, only specific items used for the sterile compounding can be taken into the DCA. Expiration dates and packaging defects are inspected first in the buffer area before the items are brought into the DCA.

Special Equipment

An important tool for maintaining the ISO Class 5 air quality in the IV clean room are the laminar airflow workbenches (LAFW). The LAFW is considered the aseptic work area within the DCA where CSPs are prepared. A **horizontal laminar airflow workbench (LAFW)** is used to prepare nonhazardous CSPs, whereas a vertical LAFW is used to prepare hazardous CSPs. A horizontal positive-pressure LAFW cannot be located in the same clean room as a vertical negative-pressure LAFW: the airflow patterns would increase the risk of employee exposure to dangerous contaminants. The institution must ensure proper positioning of the workbenches away from high-traffic areas, doorways, air vents, or other locations that could produce air currents contaminating the working area.

Horizontal LAFW As shown in Figure 10.3, in a horizontal LAFW, air from the room is pulled into the back of the hood. Air flows from the back of the hood, across the work surface, and out into the room. As the air passes through the hood, it is prefiltered with

FIGURE 10.3
**Horizontal
Laminar Airflow
Workbench**

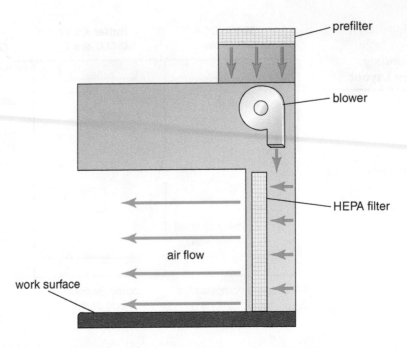

an air-conditioner–like **high-efficiency particulate air (HEPA) filter** to remove large particles. The HEPA filter removes 99.97% of all particles 0.3 micron or larger.

The horizontal LAFW is enclosed on all but one side (the front), and personnel must work at least 6 inches into the hood to avoid working within the mix of filtered air and room air at the front of the hood. Before personnel start to do IV preparations, all items needed (ampules, vials, syringes, IV bags, and so on) should be placed within the aseptic work area, which is at least 6 inches from the front or 3 inches from either side. No objects should be placed so as to impede airflow while work is being done in the LAFW. Blockage from objects placed between the HEPA filter and sterile objects creates an air disturbance that is three times the diameter of the blocking object; placed next to the back of that hood, the air disturbance is as much as six times the diameter.

Note that the clean area created within the LAFW provides a very clean environment but does not prevent all means of contamination, especially those caused by human error and touch. The LAFW work surface must be cleared of all nonsterile extraneous items (pens, labels, scissors, and so on). Items stored in nonsterile cardboard containers should be wiped with isopropyl alcohol (IPA) before personnel enter the LAFW. Outer packaging should be removed at the edge of the aseptic work area.

Vertical LAFW The **vertical laminar airflow workbench (LAFW)** is used for the preparation of hazardous CSPs, such as cancer chemotherapy drugs. In a vertical laminar airflow workbench (Figure 10.4), the air flows from the top of the hood down, through a prefilter and a HEPA filter, and onto the work area. The air is then recirculated through another HEPA filter and vented 100% to outside air to minimize human exposure. The front of the hood is partially blocked by a glass shield. The pharmacy technician is often responsible for checking and documenting the status of the operation, hourly air exchanges (minimum 12 hourly), and HEPA filters for the vertical LAFW.

The technician should wear eye protection, a mask, and proper apparel—gown, gloves, and hair covering—even when cleaning the vertical laminar airflow hood. The procedures for working with hazardous drugs are designed to protect the hospital pharmacy technician as well as the patient. The preparation, storage, and handling of hazardous drugs are further discussed in Chapter 11.

Safety Note

Coughing and talking should be directed away from the hood and workbench.

FIGURE 10.4
**Vertical Laminar
Airflow
Workbench**

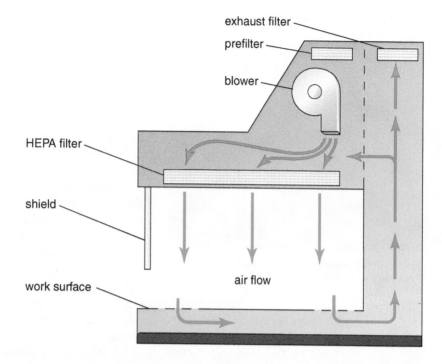

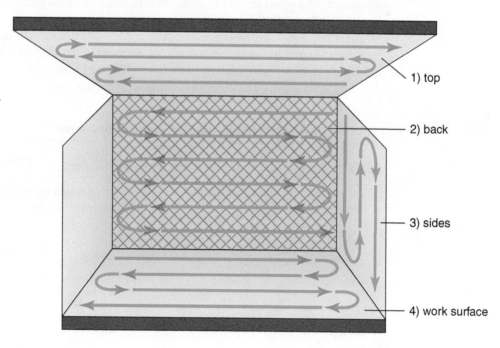

Maintenance The routine cleaning of both the horizontal and vertical LAFWs is an important responsibility of the IV technician. During cleaning, the blower in the laminar flow hood should remain on, and the technician should be in full protective garb. The entire LAFW should be cleaned with 70% IPA daily. The cleaning motion depends on the part being cleaned. The top, back, and work surface should be cleaned from side to side and back to front. The sides should be cleaned from top to bottom and back to front. The parts of the hood should be cleaned in the order shown in Figure 10.5—top, back, sides, and work surface—and recorded on a log sheet. The clear Plexiglas protective sides should be cleaned with sterile water and then with 70% IPA.

FIGURE 10.5
**Laminar Airflow
Workbench and
Hood Cleaning
Order**

1) top
2) back
3) sides
4) work surface

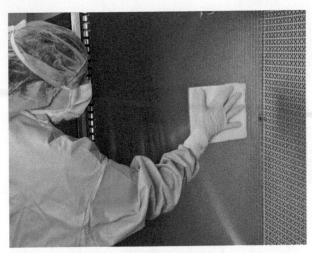
An IV technician in full protective clothing must clean the entire LAFW before each shift.

The work surface of the LAFWs must be cleaned prior to each shift; the IPA should remain in contact with the surface for 30 seconds and be fully dry before preparation of a CSP begins. Avoid excessive use of alcohol to disinfect the work surface to avoid buildup of alcohol vapors in the cabinet. A lint-free, plastic-lined pad is used to absorb small particles or spills. Cleaning the work surface with IPA should be repeated after all spills within the LAFW.

Laminar airflow workbench hoods are normally kept running all the time. If the hood is turned off for installation, repair, maintenance, or relocation, then it should be operated for at least 30 minutes before being used to prepare CSPs. The hospital pharmacy technician working in the IV sterile area is often responsible for checking and documenting the status of the HEPA filters for the laminar airflow hoods. These air filters should be changed to comply with requirements from the manufacturer.

Table 10.2 summarizes the frequency of cleaning of various sites within the IV compounding area. The pharmacy technician should confirm and document that the ante and buffer areas are cleaned at least monthly.

Personnel Cleansing and Garb

Personnel must remove all outerwear, such as coats, sweaters, hats, and so on, prior to entry into the ante area of the compounding area. A designated order progresses from the dirtiest to the cleanest activity. The process starts with hand washing and donning protective garb (booties, head covering, gown, and facial mask in this order) in the anteroom. The gown should be a disposable, clean, nonshedding one, with the arms fitting snugly around the wrists.

After donning the protective garb, the process continues with appropriate hand hygiene, initiated in the buffer room area. Antiseptic washing with alcohol or chlorhexidine gluconate is indicated; allow the antiseptic to dry before donning sterile, nonpowdered gloves. The gloves are the last protective garb to be donned (in the

TABLE 10.2 Cleaning in the IV Compounding Area	
Site	**Frequency**
LAFWs and other equipment in the direct compounding area	at the beginning of each shift or immediately after each spill
counters and easily cleanable work surfaces	daily
floors	daily
walls	monthly
ceilings	monthly
storage shelving	monthly

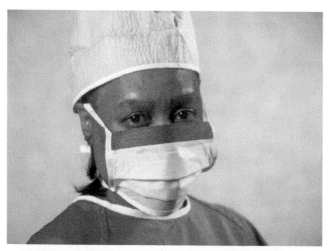

To work in the IV area, a pharmacy technician must wear full protective clothing to prevent contamination of the CSP.

buffer area), because they must be the cleanest, to avoid microbial touch contamination. Every time that a glove touches a nonsterile surface, it must be disinfected again with 70% IPA. Additional protection is necessary for preparing hazardous drugs in a vertical LAFW; eye mask protection and double gloving are recommended to protect the technician.

The technician should immediately replace any gloves having tears or punctures. If he or she leaves the room (i.e., to use the restroom, to go to lunch, or so on), then the entire process must be repeated; the exception is that, if the gown is clean, then it may be left in the ante area (for that shift only) and donned again before entering the clean room. If the technician is working with hazardous drugs, then a new gown should be worn each time that the clean room area is entered. The technician should discard all garb in a designated area at the end of the shift.

Contamination Risk Levels

Risk levels are assigned to each CSP based on the probability of microbial, chemical, or physical contamination. As defined in Chapter 8, beyond-use dating is the expiration date of a compounded sterile preparation. How does a CSP differ from a manufactured sterile product? For example, an IV bag of dextrose and water is a sterile product approved by the FDA, with a manufacturer's **expiration date**, or shelf life. An IV bag of dextrose and water with an antibiotic such as IV penicillin is a CSP compounded in a licensed pharmacy with beyond-use dating.

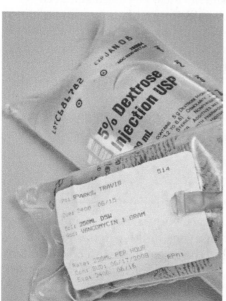

Expiration dating refers to a manufactured product whereas beyond-use dating refers to a CSP.

For CSPs, beyond-use dating is a conservative estimate based on contamination risk or specific sterility testing provided by the hospital or manufacturer. Risk levels for CSPs are defined as low, medium, and high. Documentation of sterility testing and assignment of beyond-use dating becomes more comprehensive and restrictive with high-risk CSPs (see Table 10.3) compared to low-risk CSPs.

- Low-risk CSPs include sterile products that have been manipulated using aseptic technique for a single-volume transfer, such as the transfer of a sterile solution withdrawn from an ampule, a vial or bottle, or a bag with a sterile syringe and needle. This level also includes the transfer, measuring, and mixing of a CSP containing three or fewer ingredients.
- Medium-risk CSPs include multiple sterile products combined using automated devices or transferred from multiple sterile containers into a final sterile container such as an IV bag. Unlike low-risk CSPs, those at this level involve multiple-volume transfers and more complex aseptic technique. An example is a TPN solution containing more than three electrolytes or vitamins.

TABLE 10.3 Default Beyond-Use Dating vs. Risk Level*

Risk Level	Room Temperature	Refrigerator	Freezer
low	48 hours	14 days	45 days
medium	30 hours	9 days	45 days
high	24 hours	3 days	45 days

*If reliable scientific testing data are available, then the beyond-use dating can be adjusted.

- High-risk CSPs include products that have been compounded from nonsterile ingredients and sterile products without preservatives or those exposed to inferior air quality. All high-risk CSPs must be sterilized by using a 0.22 micron filter to remove particulate matter, by autoclaving, or by dry heat. The method of sterilization chosen is dependent on the chemical stability of the product. Examples include dissolving nonsterile ingredients into a CSP and filtering prior to patient use.

Table 10.3 lists the suggested beyond-use dating of various CSPs by risk level and storage temperature. Some small hospital pharmacies may only be involved in the preparation of low- and medium-risk CSPs. Immediate-use CSPs, such as mixing drugs during a resuscitation code, are exempt from compliance with standards.

Training Required to Work with CSPs

A pharmacy technician working in the hospital pharmacy IV area clearly holds an important and responsible position and has a lot to learn. This chapter provides a brief overview of USP guidelines, but the skills and experience necessary to practice in a clean-room environment are extensive. Background reading, interactive learning modules, orientation, and supervised training must be completed before a technician can prepare CSPs. Written tests and skills assessments must be passed and documented, usually on an annual basis, to meet USP guidelines and Joint Commission accreditation standards. The technician may be required or encouraged to acquire additional certifications for sterile compounding. With such certifications and experience, the technician may be rewarded in salary for CSP-related responsibilities.

In a home healthcare setting, the patient or a caregiver may be responsible for the administration of a CSP. The USP Chapter 797 standards require that a formalized training program be in place to ensure proper understanding and compliance with this complex procedure.

Infection Control Committee

Infection control is the responsibility of all healthcare workers. Patients and employees are only safe from infectious processes when everyone working in the hospital follows good infection control techniques. Within the hospital, the **infection control committee (ICC)** provides leadership and acts as a clearinghouse of information for the hospital. This committee also plays a major role in ensuring that the hospital is in compliance with the Joint Commission accreditation standards as well as with the guidelines from the CDC and USP Chapter 797.

The ICC is generally made up of physicians, nursing staff, infection control practitioners, quality assurance personnel, and risk management personnel, as well as representatives from microbiology, surgery, central sterilization, and environmental services. A pharmacist with an interest and expertise in antibiotics is also a member of the team. The goal of this interdisciplinary team is to bring together individuals with expertise in different areas of health care.

The primary role of the ICC is to prevent, identify, and control nosocomial infections, as well as infections from the community brought into the hospital. A **nosocomial infection**, also called a healthcare-associated infection (HAI), occurs when bacteria found in the hospital from any source cause a patient to develop an infectious disease. Some nosocomial infections are resistant to antibiotic treatment and can be life-threatening. According to the CDC, 1.7 million patients develop new infections in the hospital each year, resulting in 99,000 deaths! Adherence to recommended infection control guidelines can significantly decrease the transmission of infectious agents. The hospital pharmacy technician, especially when preparing CSPs, must rigidly follow guidelines designed to protect the technician as well as the patients.

This committee sets infection control policy and is involved in planning, monitoring, evaluating, updating, and educating. This is accomplished by the following.

- surveillance of nosocomial infections
- antibiotic and other product evaluations
- investigation of infection outbreaks and infection clusters
- development of infection control procedures for all departments and staff
- patient education concerning medical waste management

The committee may be involved in evaluating which disinfectant should be used in the surgical operating room or which kind of sterilization is best for medical instruments. If resistance of microorganisms to an antibiotic is increasing, then the committee may review whether the antibiotic is being used inappropriately or in a dosage that is too small. If an outbreak should occur, then the committee undertakes an investigation to determine the cause of the problem and recommends the necessary education or changes in protocols.

Annual educational programs are conducted for all hospital employees on general infection control guidelines, and mechanisms to update and disseminate new information to staff are designed. Another policy of importance to the pharmacy technician may include the handling and disposal of medical waste, as well as the proper discarding of sharps (a **sharp** is a used needle) into a special and appropriately labeled container.

In addition to preventing hospital workers from spreading infectious disease to patients, the hospital is also responsible for preventing workers from contracting infectious diseases from patients. The ICC is responsible for educating all hospital employees about the importance of following necessary procedures to minimize employee exposure.

Bacteria or viruses may be carried in the blood and other bodily fluids such as saliva, semen, gastrointestinal (GI) fluid, lymphatic fluid, sebum, mucus, and excrement. Examples of diseases that can be spread by means of bodily fluids include tuberculosis (TB), human immunodeficiency virus (HIV), and hepatitis B. Procedures followed in all healthcare settings to prevent such infection as a result of exposure to blood or other bodily fluids are known as **universal precautions**. Table 10.4 provides a list of the general guidelines that make up the universal precautions. All hospital workers should be fully up-to-date on their immunizations.

TABLE 10.4   Universal Precaution Guidelines

- Universal precautions apply to all persons within the hospital.
- Universal precautions apply to all contact or potential contact with blood, other bodily fluids, or body substances.
- Disposable gloves must be worn when contact with blood or other bodily fluids is anticipated or possible.
- Hands must be washed thoroughly after removing the latex gloves.
- Blood-soaked or contaminated materials, such as gloves, towels, or bandages, must be disposed of in a wastebasket lined with a plastic bag.
- Properly trained custodial personnel must be called if cleanup or removal of contaminated waste is necessary.
- Contaminated materials, such as needles, syringes, swabs, and catheters, must be placed in red plastic containers labeled for disposal of biohazardous materials. Proper institutional procedures generally involve incineration.
- A first-aid kit must be kept on hand in any area in which contact with blood or other bodily fluids is possible. The kit should contain, at minimum, the following items.
  - adhesive bandages for covering small wounds
  - alcohol
  - antiseptic or disinfectant
  - bottle of bleach, which is diluted at the time of use to create a solution containing 1 part bleach to 10 parts water, for use in cleaning up blood spills
  - box of disposable latex gloves
  - disposable towels
  - medical tape
  - plastic bag or container for contaminated waste disposal
  - sterile gauze for covering large wounds

Universal precautions are applied more by those healthcare workers with direct patient contact or by those who handle patient body fluids and tissues—such as physicians, nurses, laboratory staff, and respiratory care technicians. Pharmacy personnel generally do not have direct patient contact but should be cautious and cover an open wound or cut. Following the procedures outlined in this chapter protects personnel and hospitalized patients from unnecessary risk of infection.

Chapter Terms

ante area the area of the IV room used for hand washing and donning protective garments, among other high-particulate-generating activities

asepsis the absence of disease-causing microorganisms

autoclave a device that generates heat and pressure to sterilize

bacterium a small, single-celled microorganism that can exist in three main forms, depending on type: spherical (i.e., cocci), rod-shaped (i.e., bacilli), and spiral (i.e., spirochetes)

buffer area the area of the IV room used for the storage of components and supplies (such as IV bags and administration sets) that are used for compounding CSPs; also area for hand hygiene and donning protective gloves

Centers for Disease Control and Prevention (CDC) a governmental agency that provides guidelines and recommendations on health care, including infection control

clean room an area that includes the buffer and staging areas and the sterile, direct compounding area (DCA) of the IV compounding lab

compounded sterile preparation (CSP) a sterile product that is prepared outside the pharmaceutical manufacturer's facility, typically in a hospital or compounding pharmacy

direct compounding area (DCA) the sterile, compounding area of the IV room, in which the concentration of airborne particles is controlled with a HEPA filter providing ISO Class 5 air quality

disinfectant a chemical applied to an object or topically to the body for sterilization purposes, such as rubbing alcohol

expiration date the date after which a manufacturer's product should not be used

fungus a single-celled organism similar to human cells; marked by the absence of chlorophyll, a rigid cell wall, and reproduction by spores; feed on living organisms (or on dead organic material)

germ theory of disease the idea that microorganisms cause diseases

hand hygiene the use of special dry, alcohol-based rinses, gels, or foams that do not require water

hand washing the use of plain or antiseptic soap and water with appropriate time and technique

high-efficiency particulate air (HEPA) filter a device used with laminar flow hoods to filter out most particulate matter to prepare parenteral products safely and aseptically

horizontal laminar airflow workbench (LAFW) a special biological safety cabinet used to prepare IV drug admixtures, nutrition solutions, and other parenteral products aseptically

infection control committee (ICC) a committee of the hospital that provides leadership in relation to infection control policies

International Organization for Standardization (ISO) a classification system to measure the amount of particulate matter in room air; the lower the ISO number, the less particulate matter is present in the air

nosocomial infection an infection caused by bacteria found in the hospital from any source that causes a patient to develop an infectious disease; also called healthcare-associated infection (HAI)

pasteurization a sterilization process designed to kill most bacteria and mold in milk and other liquids

protozoa a single-celled organism that inhabits water and soil

sharp a used needle, which can be a source of infection

sterilization a process that destroys the microorganisms in a substance, resulting in asepsis

universal precautions procedures followed in healthcare settings to prevent infection as a result of exposure to blood or other bodily fluids

USP Chapter 797 guidelines on the sterility and stability of CSPs developed by the United States Pharmacopeia (USP) that have become standards for hospital accreditation

vertical laminar airflow workbench (LAFW) a special biological safety cabinet used to prepare hazardous drugs, such as cancer chemotherapy drugs, aseptically

virus a minute infectious agent that does not have all of the components of a cell and thus can replicate only within a living host cell

Chapter Summary

- The identification of microorganisms as a cause of infectious disease is a surprisingly recent development.
- Bacteria, viruses, fungi, and protozoa are examples of microorganisms that can be harmful.
- Various types of sterilization are available to kill microorganisms from medical instruments, devices, and surfaces.
- The CDC publishes guidelines to minimize the transmission of infectious disease within the hospital environment.
- Proper hand washing and hand hygiene practices are the most important ways to minimize touch contamination.
- Respiratory illness may limit the ability of the pharmacy technician to work in a sterile clean room environment.
- Every healthcare worker should have up-to-date immunizations.
- The USP 797 Guidelines provide official and enforceable requirements for improving the quality of compounded sterile preparations (CSPs).

- The proper use of a LAFW can minimize airborne contamination.
- A vertical laminar airflow workbench is required for the preparation of hazardous IV drugs.
- A compounded sterile preparation requires special aseptic techniques to minimize contamination.
- A CSP has more restrictive beyond-use dating than a manufactured sterile product or a nonsterile preparation.
- The assignment of beyond-use dating for CSPs depends on contamination risk level and type of sterile container.
- The major role of the infection control committee (ICC) is the prevention of hospital-associated infections.
- Universal precautions are used to prevent infection when a hospital worker comes into contact with blood or other bodily fluids.

Chapter Review

Checking Your Understanding

Choose the best answer from those provided.

 Additional Quiz Questions

1. A pathogen can cause
   a. a heart attack.
   b. an embolism.
   c. a thrombosis.
   d. an infectious disease.

2. The principle of immunization against disease was discovered by
   a. Robert Hooke.
   b. Edward Jenner.
   c. Anton van Leeuwenhoek.
   d. Louis Pasteur.

3. Small microorganisms that consist of little more than some genetic material surrounded by a protein case are known as
   a. bacteria.
   b. protozoa.
   c. viruses.
   d. fungi.

4. The absence of disease-causing microorganisms is known as
   a. sterilization.
   b. asepsis.
   c. hand hygiene.
   d. mechanical sterilization.

5. Which type of sterilization do intravenous bags and administration sets require?
   a. dry heat
   b. mechanical
   c. chemical
   d. gas

6. The most common cause of contamination is by
   a. touch.
   b. air.
   c. water.
   d. dust.

7. The best way to minimize touch contamination with a CSP is by
   a. not wearing jewelry in the clean room.
   b. hand washing and hand hygiene.
   c. wearing latex gloves.
   d. working in a laminar airflow hood.

8. USP Chapter 797 deals primarily with
   a. infection control policies within the hospital.
   b. sensitivity testing for antibiotics to prevent nosocomial infections.
   c. documentation of controlled drugs.
   d. prevention of contamination of compounded sterile preparations.

9. The primary role of the infection control committee (ICC) is to
   a. approve antibiotics for the hospital formulary.
   b. purchase antibiotics.
   c. verify correct dosages on all medication orders for antibiotics.
   d. prevent nosocomial infections.

10. Universal precautions deal with infections by disease-causing microorganisms found in
   a. tap water and other liquid sources.
   b. blood and other bodily fluids.
   c. emergency rooms.
   d. pharmacies.

Thinking Like a Pharmacy Tech

1. If your instructor can access petri plates, then experiment with the common sources of contamination, such as touch, air, and water. Incubate the petri plates overnight at a controlled temperature and check for bacterial growth over the next few days.

2. If you have access to a lab, demonstrate for your instructor correct hand washing and hand hygiene technique. Which disinfectant should be used on the surface of the LAFW, and how long must it be in contact before the technician makes a CSP?

Communicating Clearly

1. What is the possible role for each of these members of the infection control committee?
   a. physician
   b. pharmacist
   c. nurse
   d. hospital administrator
   e. representative of the housekeeping staff

2. The Joint Commission is scheduled for a visit, and the director of pharmacy would like you to review and recommend a policy on pharmacy personnel who come to work with a cold. What written procedures would you implement to reduce the transmission of viral disease?

Researching on the Web

1. Check the following Web site for information: www.ashp.org/bestpractices. Review the guideline for aseptic technique and product preparation and training and education.

2. Go to www.ashp.org/bestpractices. In Medication Therapy and Patient Care, find the ASHP Statement on the Role of the Pharmacist in Infection Control. List 10 ways that the pharmacy department can reduce the risk of transmission of infections.

3. Go to www.cdc.gov and see what immunizations are recommended for healthcare workers who elect to work in a hospital.

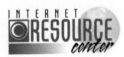 For further study of chapter-related topics, explore the Web links in the Web Center at www.emcp.net/pharmpractice4e.

Preparing and Handling Sterile Products and Hazardous Drugs

11

Learning Objectives

- Identify two common methods of delivering IV preparations.
- Describe common characteristics of intravenous solutions, including solubility, osmolality, and pH.
- Identify common vehicles for intravenous solutions.
- Identify the difference between large-volume and small-volume parenteral solutions.
- Discuss the preparation of TPN, frozen products, and closed system transfer devices (CSTDs).
- Differentiate expiration dating and beyond-use dating.
- Summarize the steps necessary for aseptic technique in a hospital pharmacy.

- Describe the correct procedure used in preparing compounded sterile preparations (CSPs) from vials and ampules.
- Identify the role and function of equipment used in IV preparation and administration, including catheters, controllers, syringes, needles, IV sets, and filters.
- Identify the components of an intravenous administration set.
- Calculate intravenous flow rates.
- Discuss the importance of and techniques for preparing, handling, and disposing of hazardous agents.

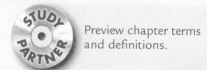

Preview chapter terms and definitions.

Compared with a community pharmacy, a hospital pharmacy carries out unique activities, such as the routine preparation of sterile preparations and the preparing, handling, and disposing of hazardous drugs. A major responsibility of the pharmacy technician is the preparation of these compounded sterile preparations (CSPs) that may contain electrolytes, vitamins, minerals, medications, or nutrition for patients with serious illnesses.

This chapter describes the technique and equipment used in the preparation of various IV products from vials and ampules. Special IV solutions—such as TPNs, frozen antibiotics, and medications available in innovative, closed system transfer devices—are covered. All techniques in preparation of IV products must be in compliance with the revised USP Chapter 797 guidelines. This chapter contains examples for calculating IV flow rates in IV and nutrition solutions.

Preparing Intravenous Products

IV fluids and medications may be administered by immediate bolus or slow infusion over minutes or hours. In a bolus injection or **IV push (IVP)**, the medication is rapidly administered with a syringe into an IV line or catheter, usually in the patient's arm. On the other hand, the slow IV infusion delivers large amounts of liquid into the bloodstream over prolonged periods (usually more than 1 hour). This route of administration is used to deliver blood; water; other fluids; nutrients, such as lipids and sugars; electrolytes; and drugs. Medications are prepared and administered in large- or small-volume parenteral IV solutions, as discussed later in the chapter. Some cancer medications cannot be given by bolus injection because of their toxicity. These cancer agents can often be administered through IV infusion into the bloodstream because the infusion dilutes the drug sufficiently to avoid causing adverse effects.

The intravenous (IV) route of administration is used for a variety of reasons, including the following.

- to facilitate reaching therapeutic drug serum levels
- to guarantee that the drug is administered
- to administer drugs requiring high tissue levels
- to administer drugs with unreliable gastrointestinal (GI) absorption
- for the patient who needs nutrition and can have nothing by mouth (NPO)
- for the patient who is unconscious or uncooperative
- for rapid correction of fluids or electrolytes

Pharmacists and technicians compound sterile IV preparations, consisting of drugs and IV solutions, in a form that is ready to be administered to a patient. To be in compliance with USP Chapter 797 guidelines, CSPs must be prepared in a laminar airflow hood using correct aseptic technique. When personnel are working in the laminar flow hood, they should be free from interruptions in order to maintain a sterile environment. They need to stay mentally focused on IV preparation tasks to minimize contamination and medication errors.

Products used during the preparation must always be sterile and handled in such a manner as to prevent contamination. Most parenteral products are introduced directly into the bloodstream and must be sterile and free of air or particulate matter; otherwise, complications can occur. IV preparations have many physical characteristics, including solubility, osmolality, pH, and stability.

Characteristics of IV Products

Intravenous (IV) preparations are solutions in which ingredients are dissolved or, much less commonly, emulsions, which are mixtures of two immiscible, or unblendable, solutions. The body is primarily an aqueous, or water-containing, vehicle, and thus most IV preparations introduced into the body are made up of ingredients placed into a sterile water medium.

Some preparations, however, may be oleaginous, or oily. For example, an emulsion containing fat may be administered in some cases to supply extra calories to patients who cannot or will not feed themselves and who need more calories than can be supplied by dextrose in water and/or amino acids in total parenteral nutrition (TPN) solutions. Examples of commercially available parenteral emulsions used for nutritional support are Intralipid, Liposyn II/III, and propofol. Fat emulsions have the advantage over typical TPN solutions in that they do not require the insertion by the physician of special central-line catheters.

IV preparations must also have chemical properties that do not damage vessels or blood cells or alter the chemical properties of the blood. Generally speaking, an IV must be iso-osmotic (i.e., the same number of particles in solution per unit volume) and isotonic (i.e., the same osmotic pressure) as blood. **Osmotic pressure** is the pressure required to maintain equilibrium, with no net movement of solution.

Osmolarity is a measure of the milliosmoles of solute per liter of solution (mOsm/L). Tonicity is the effective osmotic pressure equivalent. Osmolarity and tonicity are similar and interchangeable terms, even though the membrane of blood cells is more or less permeable to various chemical substances. The osmolarity or tonicity of blood is approximately 285 mOsm/L. An example of an **isotonic solution** (i.e., a solution with the same number of particles as blood) is 0.9% normal saline (NS). An isotonic solution is in the range of 280–310 mOsm/L.

Pharmacists sometimes have to adjust the tonicity of parenteral preparations to ensure that they are near isotonic. A parenteral solution of greater than normal tonicity (greater than 285 mOsm/L) is said to be hypertonic. A **hypertonic solution** (or hyperosmolar solution) has a greater number of particles than the blood cells themselves. An example of a hypertonic solution is 50% dextrose or 3% sodium chloride. On occasion, it is necessary to administer hypertonic solutions, but this must is done very slowly and cautiously by the nurse or physician. A TPN nutrition solution with an osmolarity of greater than 900 mOsm/L is another good example of a hypertonic solution; it cannot be given in a peripheral vein but must be administered through a central catheter into a large subclavian vein so that it can be sufficiently diluted by the blood. A solution of less than normal tonicity (less than 285 mOsm/L) is said to be hypotonic. A **hypotonic solution** (or hypoosmolar solution) has fewer numbers of particles than blood cells. An example of a hypotonic solution is 0.45% NS.

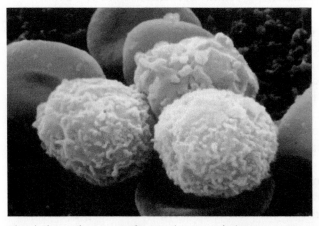

Blood plasma has a pH of 7.4 and an osmolarity near 285 mOsm/L. Most IV solutions have a neutral pH and are isotonic (280–310 mOsm/L) or near isotonic, so as not to damage red blood cells.

The degree of acidity or alkalinity of a solution is known as its **pH value**. If a solution has a pH of less than 7, then it is acidic. If it has a pH value of more than 7, then it is alkaline. Blood plasma has a pH of 7.4; therefore it is slightly alkaline. The blood pH must stay very close to this pH for the patient to stay healthy. IV solutions should have a pH that is neutral (or near 7.0); otherwise, they may adversely affect the pH of the blood.

Occasionally, more than one drug must be added to an IV solution. Once those medications are reconstituted with sterile water, the proper dose is withdrawn and added to the IV solution. If one medication is an acidic salt and the other an alkaline salt, then once the two medications are combined, a solid precipitate may be formed. For example, if sodium bicarbonate is added to a solution with potassium chloride, then the resulting solution contains potassium bicarbonate and sodium chloride or salt. A solid precipitate is not desirable, and all final solutions are visually inspected by the pharmacist and technician to confirm that precipitates are not present. The introduction of particles from an incompatible IV solution can cause an embolism, or blood clot, in a vessel. A useful reference for physical drug incompatibility is the latest edition of *Trissel's Stability of Compounded Formulations*, which is found in most hospital pharmacies. Most medications today are administered in separate IV minibags, so physical incompatibilities are rare.

A final physical characteristic of an IV solution is its stability under various storage conditions. Many IV medications must be refrigerated (or even frozen) after being compounded to maintain their activity; the preparation and beyond-use dating of these drugs are discussed later in the chapter. Other IV solutions must be covered with an amber-colored bag to protect the drug from exposure to light. An example of a light-sensitive agent is an IV infusion of the antifungal drug amphotercin B.

IV Solutions

There are multiple IV solutions that are available in plastic bags and various volumes of fluid. The vehicles most commonly used for IV infusions are dextrose in water, normal saline, or a dextrose in saline solution. The pharmacy technician who compounds sterile preparations in the hospital, home healthcare, or compounding pharmacy setting must become familiar with abbreviations for terms used in medication orders for IV solutions and in preparing parenteral solutions (Table 11.1).

The two main types of IV solutions are small-volume parenterals and large-volume parenterals (LVPs). A **small-volume parenteral (SVP)** usually contains less than 250 mL and is typically used for delivering medications at a controlled infusion rate. In some cases, an infusion is prepared specifically to deliver a medication. In other cases, a medication is "piggybacked," or added onto a running IV. An **IV piggyback (IVPB)** involves the preparation of a small amount of solution, usually 50 to 100 mL, in a minibag. The volume of solution needed is dependent on the dose and solubility of the medication. The piggybacked solution is then infused into the tubing of the running IV, usually over a short time (from 30 minutes to 1 hour). Some medications that are given intermittently may also be mixed in a larger amount of fluid (150 mL, 250 mL, or 500 mL) in order to obtain a more dilute concentration to avoid vein irritation and patient discomfort.

A **large-volume parenteral (LVP)** is used to replenish fluids and to provide drugs, electrolytes, and nutrients such as vitamins, minerals, and glucose. LVPs are commonly available in 250 mL, 500 mL, and 1000 mL sizes. An LVP usually contains one or more electrolytes that are added (hence the term "IV Additive Service") to the IV solution. Potassium chloride is the most common additive, but other salts of potassium, as well as magnesium or calcium can be added based on the requirements of the individual patient. An IV solution that contains a specific mixture of electrolytes called "lactated Ringer's solution" may be used alone or in combination with a dextrose or NS solution. Examples of such drugs requiring an LVP include vancomycin and many cancer drugs. An example of a special LVP that contains glucose, amino acids, vitamins, minerals, and trace elements is called a total parenteral nutrition (TPN). TPNs are usually contained in 1000 mL or 2000 mL volumes to provide nutritional support for 12 to 24 hours. More information on TPNs is contained in the following discussion. Figure 11.1 shows some typical physician orders for IV infusions of medications and electrolytes.

IV infusions may use any of a variety of IV pumps to regulate amount, rate, and timing of flow. Special IV solutions that are commonly prepared by the pharmacy technician include TPNs, frozen IV solutions, and closed system transfer devices, which are described in the following discussion.

Total Parenteral Nutrition (TPN) Solutions A special type of IV admixture is total parenteral nutrition (TPN). A TPN provides calories of the nutrition needs for a patient of any age who is unconscious or who cannot receive food or water or medication by mouth (NPO). An NPO designation can be as a result of surgery, infection, or inflamma-

TABLE 11.1 Commonly Used IV Products and Abbreviations

Component		Abbreviation
Fluids	2.5% dextrose in water	$D_{2.5}W$
	5% dextrose in water	D_5W
	5% dextrose and lactated Ringer's solution	D_5RL or D_5LR
	10% dextrose in water	$D_{10}W$
	5% dextrose and normal saline	D_5NS
	2.5% dextrose and 0.45% normal saline	$D_{2.5}\frac{1}{2}NS$
	5% dextrose and 0.45% normal saline	$D_5\frac{1}{2}NS$
	normal saline	NS
	0.45% normal saline	0.45% NS or ½NS
	lactated Ringer's solution	RL or LR
	sterile water for injection	SW for injection or SWFI
	bacteriostatic water for injection	BW for injection or BWFI
	sterile water for irrigation	SW for irrigation
	normal saline for irrigation	NS for irrigation
Electrolytes	potassium chloride	KCl
	potassium phosphate	K phos or KPO_4
	potassium acetate	K acet
	sodium phosphate	Na phos or $NaPO_4$
	sodium chloride	NaCl
Additives	multivitamin for injection	MVI
	trace elements (combinations of essential trace elements such as chromium, manganese, and copper)	TE
	zinc (a trace element)	Zn
	selenium (a trace element)	Se

tion in the gastrointestinal tract. TPNs are commonly prepared in the hospital but may also be prepared in a home healthcare pharmacy or outsourced to an off-site pharmacy.

A TPN commonly contains more than 50 components, such as protein, amino acids, and carbohydrates, as well as electrolytes, vitamins, minerals, trace elements, and medication (such as insulin). Although there are guidelines for typical adult daily requirements, the components of a patient's TPN are individualized to the patient, based on laboratory findings and clinical response, and are often changed daily. Specialized order sheets are available with a list of all common ingredients. Figure 11.2 is an example of a TPN request form for an adult patient.

To improve efficiency and reduce intensive labor costs, many large hospitals use an **automated compounding device (ACD)** to prepare multiple TPN solutions. With so many additives and calculations and multiple entries into a sterile IV solution, the

FIGURE 11.1
Physician's
Orders for IV
Infusions

℞ Mefoxin 1 g IV q6 h

℞ nafcillin 1 g IV q4 h

℞ penicillin 2 million units IV q4 h

℞ add 100 units Humulin R regular insulin to
500 mL NS @ 20 mL/hour (label ℞
concentration 0.2 units/mL)

℞ begin magnesium sulfate 5 g in 500 mL NS to
run over 5 hours × 1 dose only

℞ fluids to 0.45 NS with 20 mEq KCl @
125 mL/hour

need for a reliable, programmable, automated device to reduce medication errors and contamination is readily apparent.

The USP Chapter 797 guidelines specify that the hospital pharmacy must ensure both the accuracy and the precision of ACDs. The accuracy of the volume and the weight is tested by comparing with sterile water for injection. A validated chemical analysis of all ingredients of a TPN is usually outsourced to a laboratory with the proper equipment. The precision of the ACD is important, especially when adding electrolytes such as potassium chloride, which can be toxic. Daily records on calibration must be kept by the technician and reviewed by the pharmacist at least weekly. The testing, monitoring, and surveillance of ACDs are outlined in the written policy and procedure manual of the pharmacy department.

The administration of a TPN requires the insertion of a **central venous catheter (CVC)**, also called a central-line catheter, into the subclavian vein in the neck—as opposed to most IVs, which are administered by vein in the arm. A large vein is required for its administration because of the hyperosmolar or hypertonic concentration of the ingredients and the large amount of fluid (usually 2000 mL per day) that must be diluted in the bloodstream. The TPN solution is commonly administered via an infusion pump.

The IV tubing includes a special 0.22 micron in-line filter to filter contaminants and maintain sterility. Aseptic technique—in both TPN prepa-

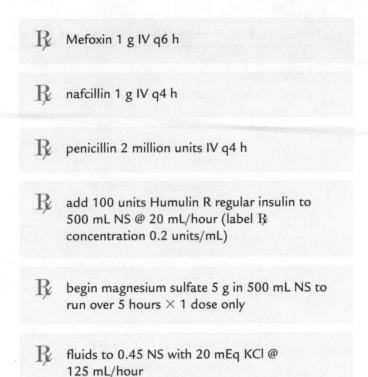

This automated compounding device (ACD) adds micronutrients to TPN solutions. This procedure is done within a laminar airflow workbench.

FIGURE 11.2
TPN Request Form

Adult Parenteral Nutrition Order Form
Mt. Hope Hospital
My Town, SC

Patient: _____
Room: _____

Date: _____ Time: _____

☐ Consult Nutritional Support Service (Beeper 0349)

☐ Conduct Indirect Calorimetry Test

Central Formula (per liter)		Peripheral Formula (per liter)	
Amino Acids	40 g	Amino Acids	25 g
Dextrose	17.5% (600 kcals)	Dextrose	6% (200 kcals)
Fat 20%	125 mL (250 kcals)	Fat 20%	200 mL (400 kcals)
Standard Electrolytes*		Standard Electrolytes*	
Trace Elements—4: 1 mL/day		Trace Elements—4: 1 mL/day	
Multivitamins—12: 10 mL/day		Multivitamins—12: 10 mL/day	
		Osmolarity: 740 mOsm/L	
Total Volume _____ mL/day		Total Volume _____ mL/day	

*Standard Electrolytes (per liter) Na: 50 mEq, Ca: 7.5 mEq, Cl: 45 mEq, Acetate: 45 mEq, Phos: 9 mM

Special Formulation (Indicate Total Daily Requirements) **Guidelines** **General Rule**

1. Amino Acids _____ g/day   0.5–2.5 g/kg/day   1 g/kg/day
   Type _____

2. Total Nonprotein
   Calories _____ kcals/day*   10–40 kcals/kg/day   25 kcals/kg/day

   Dextrose _____%   0–100%   65%
   Fat _____%   0–65%   35%
   100%   100%

3. Total Volume _____ mL/day   Minimum Volume: 1 kcals/1.0 mL
*Substrate must equal 100%.

Special Formulation—Electrolytes (check one)

☐ Standard Electrolytes/Liter   ☐ Standard Electrolytes plus
                                        Additional Electrolytes

☐ Standard Electrolytes/Liter—No Potassium   ☐ Custom Electrolytes

Sodium Acetate	_____ mEq/day	Potassium Acetate	_____ mEq/day
Sodium Chloride	_____ mEq/day	Potassium Chloride	_____ mEq/day
Sodium Phosphate	_____ mEq/day	Potassium Phosphate	_____ mEq/day
Magnesium Sulfate	_____ mEq/day	Calcium Gluconate	_____ mEq/day

Multivitamins—12: (10 mL) per _____   Other _____
Trace Elements—4: (1 mL) per _____   Other _____

HUMAN REGULAR INSULIN _____ units/day

Phytonadione (Vit. K) 10 mg IM per _____

OTHER _____

Special Instructions _____

M.D.   **Pharmacy Must Receive TPN Orders by 12 Noon**
76016153

ration by the pharmacy staff and proper catheter care by the nursing staff—is critical to avoid introducing bacteria directly into the bloodstream. The tubing is replaced with each new TPN bag (or bottle) to minimize bacterial contamination and infection. Many hospitals have special TPN teams of physicians, nurses, dieticians, and pharmacists who specialize in the care of such patients.

Frozen IV Solutions To minimize labor-intensive preparation and maximize expiration dating, many antibiotic sterile products are commercially available in IV minibags in a premixed frozen state. If these products are not available, then the technician may be preparing a CSP for later patient use. These products are kept in the freezer in the hospital pharmacy until a medication order is received. At that time, the product is thawed, a patient-specific label with expiration date is prepared and affixed to the bag, and the medication is sent to the nursing unit for administration. Thawing may consist of a sufficient time at room temperature or the use of a microwave thawing device. If the products are commercially available, then manufacturer recommendations for thawing, which vary with each product, must be followed by the IV technician.

Once thawed, the expiration dating varies with the drug and storage conditions. For example, an Ancef antibiotic solution has an expiration date of 48 hours at room temperature, or 10 days if stored under refrigerated conditions. The Zosyn antibiotic solution has an expiration date of 24 hours at room temperature, or 14 days if stored in the refrigerator. Once thawed, the preparation cannot be refrozen. If the antibiotic solution is a CSP that is unused and returned from the nursing unit, then the pharmacist must determine whether or not the product can be relabeled and used with new expiration dating. The decision to relabel or not is influenced by the storage conditions on the nursing unit. The nursing unit's storage conditions must be in compliance with USP 797 for the medication to be returned to pharmacy stock or relabeled. Most hospital pharmacies purchase commercially available frozen products (mostly antibiotics), because scientific studies indicate less wastage and longer expiration dating as results.

IV Medications in Closed System Transfer Devices (CSTDs) A **closed system transfer device (CSTD)** is a relatively recent innovation in packaging design and drug delivery systems used to minimize labor intensive preparation, contamination, and drug wastage. CSTD systems provide both a vial of medication and a specified IV solution that can be attached and prepared aseptically at patient bedside without the need to use a syringe and needle to reconstitute a dose of medication.

CSTDs are available under many trade names, such as ADD-Vantage, Mini Bag Plus, Add-A-Vial, Add-Ease, Vial Mate, Duplex, and so on. Only selected products—mostly antibiotics—are available in a CSTD system. CSTDs are not considered compounded sterile preparations (or CSPs) and thus do not come under the auspices of Chapter 797 guidelines for beyond-use dating. The technician is directed to follow manufacturer recommendations for diluent, storage, and expiration dating.

Each CSTD delivery system differs somewhat in design, but the concept is similar. The drug—which has not been reconstituted—is coupled (with or without an adaptor) with an appropriate volume of IV solution. Depending on the CSTD, many commonly used drugs in the hospital are available in 50 mL, 100 mL, and 250 mL minibags with many diluent options (D_5W, D_5NS, NS, lactated Ringer's, and so on).

The pharmacy technician is responsible for attaching or assembling the correct drug and dosage to the correct IV solution and volume, with proper patient labeling and expiration dating. The product is then activated aseptically by the nurse on the patient care unit just prior to patient administration and then transferred via a sterile, aseptic, closed system to the appropriate IV solution attached to the vial.

CSTDs are more efficient because doses are premeasured for rapid reconstitution and easy assembly by the nurse on the patient care unit. There is no need for freezing, thawing, or refrigeration in the pharmacy or nursing unit, because the product is immediately administered to the patient.

A CSTD also helps reduce waste. Doses that have not been activated may be returned to the pharmacy for reuse and relabeling. Depending on the CSTD, once the product has been removed from the sterile packaging, a 14 to 30 day shelf life is left in which to reuse the product. The manufacturer's product package insert should be consulted for expiration dating; the stability varies with the concentration of the drug, the diluent, and the storage conditions. Activated doses, however, cannot be refrigerated or refrozen and are often discarded.

Other advantages of CSTDs are improved safety and efficiency. In terms of safety, admixing errors are minimized, doses are standardized, and enhanced labeling and bar coding of both product and IV solution are provided. In other words, the nurse knows exactly what is in the IV solution. The closed system sterile packaging minimizes contamination, and CSTDs do not use needles, thus preventing the possibility of inadvertent needle sticks by the pharmacist, technician, or nurse. Personnel costs are saved because no admixing is necessary and no additional supply costs, such as for syringes, needles, alcohol wipes, gauze, and so on, are incurred. These advantages may well outweigh the additional cost per unit.

Often, a hospital pharmacy has to purchase more than one CSTD delivery system to cover a wider variety of drugs. Problems with drug availability from the manufacturer are not uncommon. Thus, the technician who can reconstitute a vial and add it to an IV solution remains the reliable backup delivery system. The CSTD systems differ slightly in their activation and the pharmacist or technician may need to provide an in-service to assist the nurses in the varying manipulation techniques of the commercially available CSTDs.

Aseptic Technique

As discussed in Chapter 10, asepsis is the absence of disease-causing organisms. **Aseptic technique** is defined as the manipulation of sterile preparations and devices in such a way as to avoid introducing disease-causing microorganisms. Sterile preparations include medications stored in single- and multiple-dose vials, ampules, and other containers that must be transferred to an IV solution for patient use. Sterile devices used to transfer medications include syringes, needles, and IV administration sets.

Pharmacy technicians prepare CSPs on the laminar airflow workbench (LAFW) following aseptic technique in the hospital pharmacy. Following proper procedure for handling sterile preparations and devices helps ensure an accurate microbial-free product. Proper aseptic technique in using vials and ampules is an essential skill for the pharmacy technician. Pharmacy technicians working for home healthcare, long-term care environments, and compounding pharmacies may also need to develop these skills for occasional IV product preparation. Table 11.2 summarizes the steps for preparing sterile preparations using aseptic technique.

The pharmacy technician often uses single-dose or multiple-dose vials or ampules in the preparation of CSPs in the IV area. Identification of beyond-use dating and expiration dating for the diluents, medications, and CSPs is an important responsibility for the IV area pharmacy technician.

Preparing CSPs Using Medication from Vials Not all parenteral drugs are available in a commercially available, ready-to-use syringe, frozen solution, or CSTD. This may be due to instability in a ready-to-use sterile solution because of instability and short expiration dating. Many times, a CSP must be prepared by the pharmacy technician under the LAFW, using correct aseptic technique. Before it is added to an IV bag, the drug must be taken up (or withdrawn) into the syringe from a single- or multiple-dose vial (MDV) or from a glass ampule.

Because the rubber stopper on a vial (or ampule neck) can harbor microorganisms, the technician must wipe these with 70% isopropyl alcohol (IPA) and let them dry. Entering or opening a multiple-dose vial begins when the rubber stopper is first punctured with a sterile needle. The technician must not touch the tip of the needle in the

When working in the pharmacy clean room, it is important to wear appropriate sterile gear, including shoe covers, face mask, full head covering, scrubs or gown with back closure, and gloves. Eye protection should be used if preparing hazardous drugs.

TABLE 11.2   Summary of Procedures to Maintain Aseptic Technique

1. Remove all jewelry (e.g., watches, rings, bracelets, necklaces).
2. Put on, in sequence, nonshedding coats, gowns, or coveralls (hospital scrubs); head and facial hair covers; face masks; and shoe covers. Note that it is important to follow the order of items indicated in this step.
3. Scrub hands and arms to the elbows thoroughly with soap and water.
4. Clean the laminar flow hood with isopropyl alcohol. The alcohol must remain in contact with the surface for 30 seconds prior to compounding any sterile product.
5. Place only essential materials in the airflow workbench—no paper, pens, or labels. Remove the selected syringe(s) from its packaging, attach a needle, and then discard the waste.
6. Scrub again with an antiseptic cleanser and put on gloves in a clean-room environment.
7. Swab or spray needle-penetration closures on vials, injection ports, and other materials with isopropyl alcohol.
8. Prepare the CSP by withdrawing the medication from vials or ampules and introducing it into the IV container.
9. Complete a quality check of the product for container integrity and leaks, solution cloudiness, particulates, color of solution, and proper preparation of product.
10. Present the CSP, the containers and devices used, and the label to a pharmacist for verification of the product before sending them to the patient care unit.

Safety Note

Inject an equal amount of air into the vial with the syringe and needle before withdrawing the medication.

sterile transfer of a diluent to prepare a CSP; if an inadvertent touch occurs, then the needle should be wiped with IPA or replaced. The needle bevel tip should penetrate the rubber closure at an angle, which is then straightened to 90 degrees so that as additional pressure is applied to the syringe, the bevel heel enters the closure at the same point as the tip. This technique prevents **coring**, or the inadvertent introduction of a small piece of the rubber stopper into the solution.

This process of adding diluent and/or withdrawing fluid via a syringe and needle produces a positive pressure inside the vial. Vials are closed systems; therefore the amount of air introduced should be equal to the volume of fluid removed, for most drugs. Table 11.3 details the procedures generally followed for using a syringe to withdraw liquid from a vial.

The pharmacy technician must pay close attention to beyond-use dating for vials used in the preparation of CSPs. A single-dose vial of diluent without a preservative must be used within an hour (under aseptic conditions) or discarded in order to remain in compliance with Chapter 797 guidelines. If the technician is working in a clean-room environment, then the beyond-use dating defaults to 28 days for an MDV. The drug may be chemically stable for more than 28 days, but the manufac-

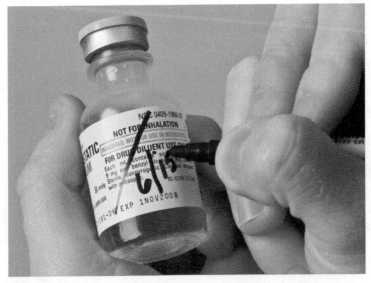

Even though a multiple-dose vial of diluent contains a preservative, it must be discarded after 28 days, because sterility cannot be ensured beyond this time.

TABLE 11.3   Using a Syringe to Draw Liquid from a Vial

1. Choose the smallest-gauge needle appropriate for the task. The smaller the needle, the less the chance of coring the rubber top of the vial and thus introducing particulate into the liquid within it.

2. Attach the needle to the syringe.

3. Draw into the syringe an amount of air equal to the amount of drug to be drawn from the vial.

4. Swab or spray the top of the vial with alcohol beforehand; allow the alcohol to dry. Puncture the rubber top of the vial with the needle bevel up. Then bring the syringe and needle straight up, penetrate the stopper, and depress the plunger of the syringe, emptying the air into the vial (Figure 11.3, *a*). Check for coring.

5. Invert the vial with the syringe still inserted.

6. Draw up from the vial the amount of liquid required (Figure 11.3, *b*).

7. Withdraw the needle from the vial. In the case of a multiple-dose vial, the rubber cap closes, sealing the contents of the vial.

8. The majority of liquids drawn up from a vial are added to an IV solution. In these cases, capping of the empty syringe is discouraged to avoid needlesticks. In the rarer cases in which an actual syringe is dispensed, remove and properly dispose of the needle, and then cap the syringe with a sterile syringe cap. If a capped syringe is sent to the patient care unit, then a new needle is attached at the time of injection into a patient.

FIGURE 11.3
Withdrawing Medication from a Vial

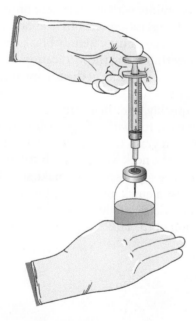

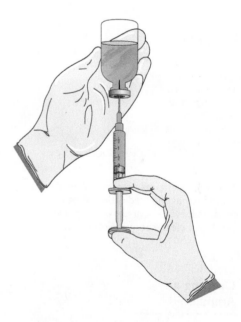

(a) Inject an amount of air into the vial equal to the volume of liquid needed.

(b) Withdraw the desired amount of medication into the syringe from the inverted vial.

turer cannot assure that the preservative will maintain sterility for more than 28 days. The technician should mark the beyond-use dating on the multiple-dose vial for future use by other pharmacy personnel and to ensure that the vials are stored under appropriate conditions.

The technician must remember that a manufactured sterile product (as opposed to a CSP), such as an antibiotic, does not follow 797 guidelines. The expiration dating is

Safety Note

Check the medication package insert to verify which diluent and what volume should be added to the medication vial to make a correct concentration of sterile solution.

based on scientific studies by the manufacturer and varies with the product, diluent, and storage conditions. The expiration dating can be found in the product package insert.

In some cases, as with lyophilized (or freeze-dried) powder, the solid drug in the vial may be reconstituted with a preservative-free diluent such as sterile water for injection (SWFI) or normal saline (NS). Many IV antibiotics are prepared in this manner. A **diluent** is the sterile fluid to be added to the medication powder to reconstitute or dissolve it. Some drugs may be reconstituted with a diluent in an MDV with a preservative. Once the drug is in solution, it can be withdrawn into a syringe and added to an IV fluid. Be sure to double-check the dosage, expiration date, and the amount of diluent to be drawn up into the syringe.

For example, Ancef is a commercially available antibiotic product. Various dosages are available in vials that contain inactivated powder. Once the powder is reconstituted, or activated with diluent, in the pharmacy, the vial of the product has an expiration date of 24 hours at room temperature; if the vial is refrigerated at 2 to 8 °C, then the expiration date is extended to 96 hours. However, if the reconstituted solution is immediately frozen (–20 °C), then the drug has an expiration date of 12 weeks. If the antibiotic is added to a minibag containing an IV fluid, then it becomes a CSP and is subject to USP 797 guidelines for beyond-use dating.

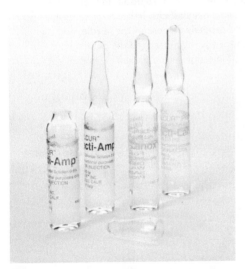

An ampule contains no preservative. Any unused remaining medication must be discarded, even if you are working under a LAFW in a clean-room environment.

Preparing CSPs Using Medication from Ampules Some drugs are available in solution in an ampule. An **ampule** is a drug container with a single dose only; it contains no preservative. The glass ampule offers another challenge because the technician must carefully break the top off the ampule before withdrawing the medication. Prior to breaking the ampule, the contents in the top must be moved into the body by swirling the ampule in an upright position, inverting it quickly, and then turning it back upright, or by tapping the top with a finger. Clean the neck with an alcohol swab; then grasp the ampule between the thumb and index finger at the neck with the swab still in place. The glass around the top is scored to make such breaking easy and clean. Use a quick motion to snap off the top (Figure 11.4). The ampule generally snaps at the neck. Do not break in the direction of the HEPA filter when in the LAFW.

FIGURE 11.4

Opening an Ampule

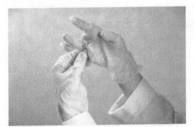

(a) Gently tap the top of the ampule to bring the medication to the lower portion of the ampule.

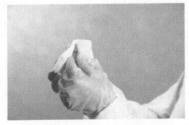

(b) Wrap a swab around the neck and top of the ampule.

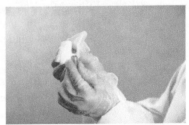

(c) Forcefully snap the neck away from you.

To withdraw medication from an opened ampule, tilt the ampule, place the needle bevel of a filter needle or the tip of a filter straw in the corner near the opening, and withdraw the medication. Use a needle equipped with a filter to screen out any tiny glass particles, fibers, or paint chips that may have fallen into the ampule. Before injecting the contents of a syringe into an IV, the needle must be changed to avoid introducing glass or particles into the admixture. If a standard needle is used to withdraw the drug from the ampule, then the needle must be replaced with a filter device before the drug is pushed out of the syringe. Filter needles are for one-directional use only.

Preparing a Label for an IV Admixture

When making an IV admixture, you must also prepare a medication container label (Figure 11.5). The label should contain the following information:

- patient's name and identification number
- room number
- fluid and amount
- drug name and strength (if appropriate)
- infusion period (e.g., infuse over 30 minutes)
- flow rate (e.g., 100 mL/hour)
- beyond-use date (or expiration date) and time
- additional information as required by the institution or by state or federal guidelines, including auxiliary labeling, storage requirements, and device-specific or drug-specific information, such as filters

In addition to the requirements previously discussed, a TPN label contains the dosages and volume of all ingredients, as well as the IV flow rate, beyond-use dating, pharmacist initials, and osmolarity of the final product (see Figure 11.6). In addition, the label includes specific nutrition information, including total calories as well as calories derived from protein, dextrose, or lipid (fat).

FIGURE 11.5
Large-Volume Parenteral (LVP) Label and Minibag Label

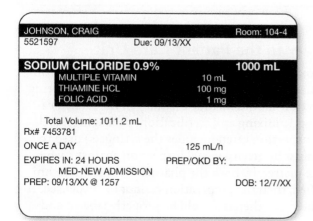

FIGURE 11.6
TPN Label

CAPS Rx: 0-327-0-2

Name: Michaels, James
Room: 129
Physician: Hurney
Order Volume: 2000 mL   Compound Volume: 2100 mL

CAPS Rx: 0-327-0-2
For: Michaels, James
Made: 09/13/20XX
Cont: BBRAUN TPN Bag 2.0 L
Volume   Code

CENTRAL MODIFIED TPN

AMINO ACIDS	90 g	945 mL	AMIN10 SF
DEXTROSE 70%	420 g	630 mL	D70W2L
--Additives--		QS 460.92 mL	H2O
SODIUM PHOSPHATE	2 mmol	0.70 mL	SODPHOS
POTASSIUM CHLORIDE	40 mEq	21 mL	POTCL2
POTASSIUM PHOSPHATE	5 mmol	1.75 mL	POTPHOS
POTASSIUM ACETATE	15 mEq	7.88 mL	POTACE2
CALCIUM GLUCONATE	8 mEq	18.06 mL	CALGLUO.46
MAGNESIUM SULFATE	2 mEq	0.52 mL	MAGSO450
MVI W/ VITAMIN K	10 mL	10.50 mL	MVI-INFUVI
M.T.E.-4	3 mL	3.15 mL	MTE4
INSULIN, REGULAR	50 units	0.53 mL	INSULH100

-- Approximate. Electrolyte Totals/Ordered

Na+	2.67 mEq	Cl-	40 mEq	
K+	62.33 mEq	PO4--	7 mmole	
Ca++	8 mEq	Ace-	15 mEq	
Mg++	2 mEq			

Nitrogen Content:	14.13 g	Protein Calories:	369 Kcal
Non-Protein Calories:	1428 Kcal	Dextrose Calories:	1428 Kcal
Total Calories:	1797 Kcal	Lipid Calories:	0 Kcal

RPh: PLH   Date: 9/13/XX   Time: 1252
Expires on 9/15/XX 0053
2000 mL at 83.33 mL/h will run for 24 hours
TPN Bag #   3
Approx. Osmolarity 1569.3 mOsm/L   Overfill Amount: 100 mL

Final Inspection and Delivery to the Patient Care Unit

The medication order, label, compounding procedure, preparation records, and all materials used to make the CSP must be inspected by the pharmacist prior to being sent to the nursing unit. The inspection should include accuracy in the identification and amount of ingredients, aseptic mixing and sterilization, packaging, labeling, and physical appearance. The inspection often includes the syringe(s) used to draw up the medication. All CSPs must be given a visual inspection against a white or black background for particulate matter, by both the pharmacist and the technician; if particulate matter is identified, then the preparation cannot be dispensed. If the CSP is to be administered for later use, then it should be properly labeled and stored in the refrigerator.

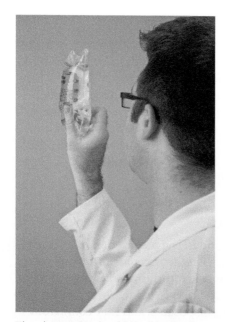

The pharmacist should double-check the technician's calculation and procedure and inspect the prepared IV bag to confirm that there are no visible impurities.

The CSP must be delivered to the hospital or nursing unit by such means that its packaging prevents damage, leakage, contamination, or degradation. If the CSP is sent off-site (to another hospital), then it should be sufficiently insulated and should be stored at the appropriate temperature. In the hospital, most CSPs are manually delivered to the nursing unit for immediate use or storage in the refrigerator on the nursing unit until use. The nurse must document the IV administration times in the medication administration record (MAR), which is similar to the documentation required of other administered oral and prn medications.

CSP Returns

What if a CSP is returned from the nursing unit? The patient may have been discharged, transferred to another hospital, or died, or the physician may have changed the medication order. CSPs can only be redispensed when the pharmacist or pharmacy technician is assured that it remained sterile and chemically stable during its storage on the nursing unit. Was the CSP stored under refrigeration and, if necessary, protected from light? Is there evidence of compromises in package integrity? The beyond-use dating (24 hours, 48 hours, and so on) remains the same. Extensions in beyond-use dating can only be approved if they are supported by scientific data. The pharmacist or technician must determine whether the beyond-use dating would occur before the next scheduled dose is administered. If the CSP will be used for another patient, then a new label must be generated.

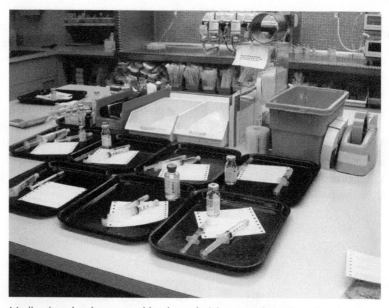

Medication that is prepared by the technician must be reviewed and approved by the pharmacist.

Equipment Used in IV Drug Preparation

A wide variety of sterile devices are used in the preparation and administration of intravenous (IV) medications by injection or infusion. Pharmacies use disposable plastic products to save time and money and to provide patients with inexpensive sterile products. Often the entire IV system sent out to the patient floors is composed of plastic. A thin, flexible, plastic **catheter** delivers the medication into the vein. In many cases, the only durable, nondisposable product used to deliver IV medication is an IV pump or controller that adjusts the rate of drug or fluid administration.

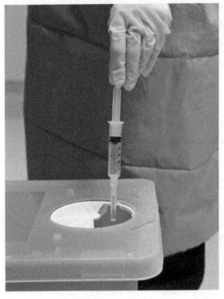

Used needles should be carefully discarded in a sharps container to minimize accidental needle sticks and risk of infection.

Syringes and Needles

Syringes, used for IV push and in the preparation of infusions, are made of glass or plastic. Glass syringes are more expensive, and their use is limited to medications that are absorbed by plastic. Plastic syringes, in addition to being less expensive, also have the advantage of being disposable, and they come from the manufacturer in a sterile packaging. Plastic syringes are used for preparing a majority of IV bolus or infusion preparations. Figure 11.7 shows the parts of a syringe.

The plunger and tip of the syringe are sterile and must not be touched. For greatest accuracy, use the smallest syringe able to hold the desired amount of solution. In any case, the syringe should be capable of holding more than twice the volume to be measured. A syringe is considered accurate to half the smallest measurement mark on its barrel. To get an accurate dose, observe closely the calibrations on the syringe barrel. Count the number of marks between labeled measurement units. If 10 marks are seen, then each mark measures off 1/10 of the unit. If 5 marks are seen, then each mark measures 1/5 of the unit. The volume of solution drawn into a syringe is measured at the point of contact between the rubber piston and the side of the syringe barrel. The measurement is not read at the tip of the piston.

A needle consists of two parts: (1) the cannula, or shaft, and (2) the hub, the part that attaches to the syringe (Figure 11.8). Needles are made of stainless steel or aluminum. Needle lengths range from 3/8 inch to 6 inches. Needles also come in gauges ranging from 31 (highest) to 13 (lowest). The higher the gauge is, the smaller the lumen, or bore, of the needle is. In the hospital pharmacy, 1 inch and 2 inch needles are commonly used, with a needle gauges ranging from 18 to 22. Remember that these needles are used by the technician only to prepare the medication—not to administer it to the patient.

Safety Note

Remember that the plunger and tip of the syringe are sterile and must not be touched.

Safety Note

After use, needles must be discarded in a designated sharps container.

FIGURE 11.7

Components of a Syringe

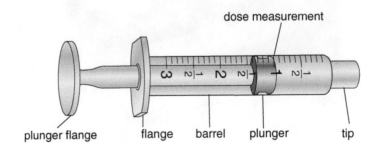

dose measurement

plunger flange   flange   barrel   plunger   tip

IV Sets

An **IV administration set** is a sterile, microorganism-free disposable device used to deliver IV fluids and medications to patients. The IV container is commonly a flexible, vented plastic bag. The set comes in sterile packaging and a sealed plastic wrap. Sets do not carry expiration dates, but they carry the following legend: "Federal law restricts this device to sale by or on the order of a physician."

Nurses generally have the responsibility for attaching IV tubing to the fluid container, establishing and maintaining flow rate, and managing overall regulation of the system during administration. Changes in regulations have forced pharmacy personnel to assess aspects of IV systems, including infusion sets. Pharmacy personnel need a complete understanding of IV sets and their operation for the following reasons.

- Pharmacists may be required to select sets that are optimal for prevention of incompatibilities in certain drug-drug or drug-fluid combinations.
- Pharmacists and other pharmacy personnel serving on cardiopulmonary resuscitation (CPR) or code teams may need to calculate dosages and drip rates for medications and prepare IV infusions, attach sets, and prepare the tubing.
- Pharmacy personnel may become involved in administration of IV medications to patients, including checking and changing lines, according to established guidelines at the hospital.
- Pharmacy personnel may have to provide in-service training for nurses to familiarize them with the proper use of new IV sets.
- Pharmacy technicians often use IV sets when transferring fluids from container to container under a laminar airflow hood.
- Pharmacy personnel use IV sets when making cancer chemotherapy to prime tubing for medication administration.

IV sets are sterile and **nonpyrogenic**, or free from microorganisms; however, in an operating room, the entire IV unit should be sterile. Such a unit is supplied in packaging that ensures sterility, generally in packages with peel-off cardboard on top and sealed plastic wrap. Some IV set packaging has a clear wrap for viewing the contents, whereas other packaging has an opaque package with a diagram of the enclosed set printed on the outside. A damaged package cannot ensure sterility. Discard sets that are in opened or damaged packages.

Most of the length of the IV tubing (and IV bags) is molded from a pliable polyvinyl chloride (PVC) and other plasticizers. Some drugs may be absorbed to some extent in the plastic bag or tubing, thus reducing the amount delivered intravenously to the patient. PVC sets should not be used for nitroglycerin, which is absorbed by the tubing. Special types of plastic sets are required for such infusions. Baxter Healthcare Corporation has developed AVIVA containers that are made of non-PVC film and contain no latex or DEHP [di(2-ethylhexyl)phthalate]. This system allows a fluid path-

Safety Note

Do not use PVC IV sets for nitroglycerin or fat emulsions.

FIGURE 11.8

Components of a Needle

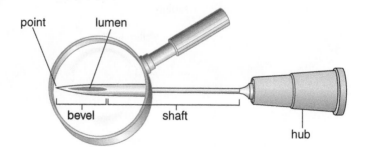

way in adults, pediatric patients, and neonates for those drugs that may be absorbed in plastic bags or tubing, such as the cardiac drug amiodarone.

The length of sets varies from extensions of 6 inches up to 110 to 120 inches. The longer sets are used in surgery. The priming of tubing depends on the length of the set—from 3 mL for the short extension up to 15 mL for longer sets. **Priming** is the action of flushing out the small particles in the tubing's interior lumen prior to medication administration and letting fluid run through the tubing so that all of the air is flushed out. Widespread use of in-line final filtration has reduced the need for flushing the line with the IV fluid before attaching the set to the patient. Standard sets have a lumen diameter of 0.28 cm. Varying the size of the lumen diameter achieves different flow rates. Regulation of flow rates is especially critical in neonates and infants but may also be useful in administering critical care drugs and limiting flow to a fluid-restricted patient.

Regardless of manufacturer, sets have certain basic components (Figure 11.9), which include a spike to pierce the rubber stopper or port on the IV container, a drip chamber for trapping air and viewing the drops per minute, a control clamp for adjusting the flow rate or shutting down the flow, flexible tubing to deliver the fluid, and an adapter for attaching a needle or a catheter. A catheter, or tube, may be implanted into the patient and fixed with tape to avoid having to repuncture the patient each time that an infusion is given.

FIGURE 11.9
Basic Components of an IV Set

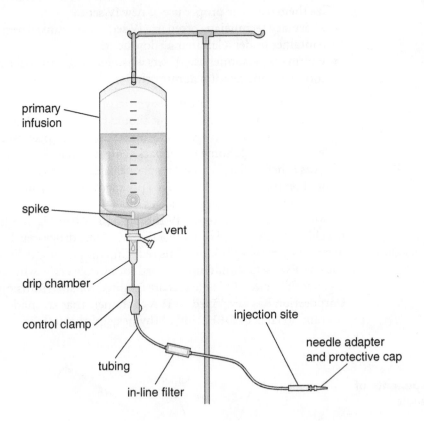

primary infusion

spike

vent

drip chamber

control clamp

tubing

in-line filter

injection site

needle adapter and protective cap

In addition to these parts, most IV sets contain at least one flange or a Y-site. A **Y-site** is one or more injection ports made of a rigid piece of plastic, with one arm terminating in a resealable port that is used for adding medication to the IV. Some IV sets also contain resealable in-line filters that offer protection for the patient against particulates, including bacteria and emboli. The port, once disinfected with alcohol, is ready for the insertion of a needle and the injection of medication. IV sets are commonly changed every 96 hours to minimize risk of infection.

The **spike** is a rigid, sharpened plastic piece used to pierce the IV container. The spike is covered with a protective unit to maintain sterility and is removed only when ready for insertion into the IV container. The spike generally has a rigid area to grip while it is inserted into the IV container. If an air vent is present on a set, then it is located below the spike. The air vent points downward and has a bacterial filter covering. The vent allows air to enter the bottle as fluid flows out of it.

A transparent, hollow chamber (the drip chamber) is located below the set's spike. Drops of fluid fall into the chamber from an opening at the uppermost end, closest to the spike. The number of drops it takes to make 1 mL identifies an IV set. This calibration is referred to as a **drop set**. The most common IV drop sets are 10, 15, 20, and 60, indicating 10 gtt/mL, 15 gtt/mL, 20 gtt/mL, and 60 gtt/mL, respectively (Figure 11.10). An opening that provides 10, 15, or 20 gtt/mL is commonly used for adults. An opening that provides 60 gtt/mL is used for pediatric patients and is called a minidrip set. The drip chamber prevents air bubbles from entering the tubing. Air bubbles generally rise to the top of the fluid if they form, rather than entering the patient. The chamber allows the attending nurse or pharmacist to set the medication flow or infusion rate by counting the drops.

The nurse administering the fluid starts the flow by filling the chamber with fluid from an attached inverted IV container. The chamber sides are squeezed and released.

FIGURE 11.10
Drop Sets

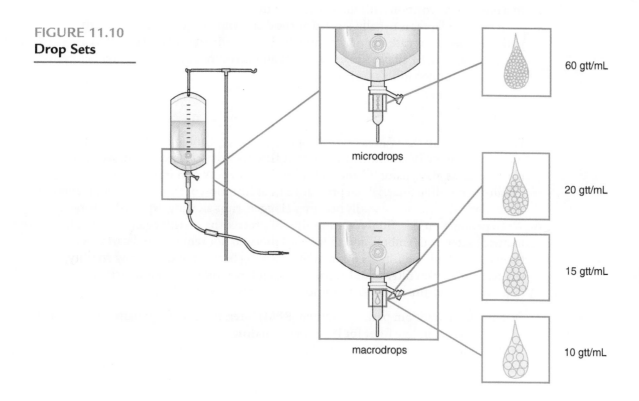

microdrops

60 gtt/mL

20 gtt/mL

15 gtt/mL

macrodrops

10 gtt/mL

Then fluid flows into the chamber. The procedure is repeated until an indicated level is reached or approximately half the chamber is filled. The entering drops are then counted for 15 seconds. Adjustments are made until the approximate number of drops desired is obtained. The rate should be checked five times, at intervals of 30 seconds, and again for a last count of 1 minute.

Clamps allow for adjusting the rate of the flow and for shutting down the flow. Clamps may be located at any position along the flexible tubing. Usually a clamp moves freely, allowing its location to be changed to one that is convenient for the health professional administering the medication.

Three types of clamps are commonly used for IV solutions: (1) slide clamps, (2) screw clamps, and (3) roller clamps.

- A slide clamp has an increasingly narrow channel that constricts IV tubing as it is pressed farther into the narrowed area. Slide clamps do not allow for accurate adjustment of flow rate but may be used to shut off flow while a more accurate clamp is regulated.
- A screw clamp consists of a thumbscrew that is tightened or loosened to speed or slow the flow.
- A roller clamp is a small roller that is pushed along an incline. The roller, when moved down the incline, constricts the tubing and reduces the fluid flow. Moving the roller up the incline, in contrast, increases the flow.

Creep and/or cold flow can affect clamp accuracy. **Creep** is the tendency of PVC tubing to return to its previous position. Tubing clamps are open during packaging and shipping. As a result, the tube tends to expand when the clamp constricts it. If, on the other hand, the tubing clamp has previously constricted the tubing, then as it is adjusted open, it tends to constrict with the reduced fluid flow, moving in the direction of its original position. **Cold flow** is a tendency of some clamps to return slowly to a more open position with increased fluid flow.

A needle adapter is usually located at the distal end of the IV set, close to the patient. A needle or catheter may be attached to the adapter. The adapter has a standard taper to fit all needles or catheters and is covered by a sterile cover before removal for connection.

Filters

Filters are used in the IV area of the hospital pharmacy for high-risk CSPs and are also included in many IV administration sets. A **filter** is a device used to remove contaminants, such as glass, paint, fibers, and rubber cores. An IV administration set may have a built-in or in-line filter, which provides a final filtration of the fluid before it enters the patient. A filter occasionally becomes clogged, thus slowing expected flow rates.

Depending on size, final filtration should protect the patient against particulate matter, bacteria, air emboli, and phlebitis. Filters do not remove virus particles or toxins. A 0.22 micron filter is optimal for blocking bacteria and ensuring sterility, whereas a 5 micron filter removes particles that block pulmonary microcirculation (but does not ensure sterility). Common filter sizes are as follows:

- 5.0 micron: random path membrane (RPM) filter, removes large particulate matter
- 0.45 micron: in-line filter for IV suspension drug
- 0.22 micron: removes bacteria and produces a sterile solution

Calculations in the Hospital Pharmacy

Safety Note

Always carefully check and double-check all calculations.

The pharmacy technician who prepares sterile IV preparations in the hospital or home healthcare setting should understand some math skills that are somewhat unique to these environments. In particular, the technician should double-check and triple-check calculations and flow rates for IV admixtures or TPN solutions, especially for neonatal or pediatric patients. This section focuses on the basic math skills needed to perform calculations in the areas of IV infusion flow rates and electrolyte replacement therapy.

IV Administration Flow Rates

IV flow rates are usually described as milliliters per hour or as drops per minute (expressed as gtt/minute). The pharmacy usually uses the milliliters per hour method, whereas nurses generally prefer drops per minute.

The formula used to determine the rate in drops per minute is as follows:

$$x \text{ gtt/minute} = \frac{(\text{volume of fluid} \div \text{delivery time in hours}) \times (\text{drop rate of administration set})}{60 \text{ minutes/hour}}$$

The following examples demonstrate the use of this equation.

Example 1

A physician orders 4000 mL of a 5% dextrose and normal saline (D_5NS) IV over a period of 36 hours. If the IV set delivers 15 gtts/mL, then how many drops must be administered per minute?

Begin by identifying the amounts to insert into the equation.

$$\text{volume of fluid} = 4000 \text{ mL}$$

$$\text{fluid delivery time} = 36 \text{ hours}$$

$$\text{drop rate of the administration set} = 15 \text{ gtts/mL}$$

$$x \text{ gtt/minute} = \frac{(\text{volume of fluid} \div \text{delivery time in hours}) \times (\text{drop rate of administration set})}{60 \text{ minutes/hour}}$$

$$= \frac{(4000 \text{ mL} \div 36 \text{ hours})}{60 \text{ minutes/hour}} \times (15 \text{ gtt/mL})$$

$$= \frac{(111 \text{ mL/hour}) \times (15 \text{ gtt/mL})}{60 \text{ minutes/hour}}$$

$$= 27.75 \text{ gtt/minute, rounded down to 27 gtt/minute}$$

Example 2 ─────── **If 500 mg of a drug is to be administered from a 50 mL minibag over 30 minutes using a 15 drop set, then how many drops per minute is that?**

Begin by identifying the amounts to insert into the equation.

$$\text{volume of fluid} = 50 \text{ mL}$$

$$\text{fluid delivery time} = 30 \text{ minutes or } 0.5 \text{ hour}$$

$$\text{drop rate of the administration set} = 15 \text{ gtt/mL}$$

$$x \text{ gtt/minute} = \frac{(\text{volume of fluid} \div \text{delivery time in hours}) \times (\text{drop rate of administration set})}{60 \text{ minutes/hour}}$$

$$= \frac{(50 \text{ mL} \div 0.5 \text{ hour}) \times (15 \text{ gtt/mL})}{60 \text{ minutes/hour}}$$

$$= \frac{(100 \text{ mL/hour}) \times (15 \text{ gtt/mL})}{60 \text{ minutes/hour}} = 25 \text{ gtt/minute}$$

Example 3 ─────── **You are to prepare 750 mg of medication in 75 mL for infusion over 30 minutes, using a 10 drop set. How many drops per minute is that?**

Begin by identifying the amounts to insert into the equation.

$$\text{volume of fluid} = 75 \text{ mL}$$

$$\text{fluid delivery time} = 30 \text{ minutes or } 0.5 \text{ hour}$$

$$\text{drop rate of the administration set} = 10 \text{ gtt/mL}$$

$$x \text{ gtt/minute} = \frac{(\text{volume of fluid} \div \text{delivery time in hours}) \times (\text{drop rate of administration set})}{60 \text{ minutes/hour}}$$

$$= \frac{(75 \text{ mL} \div 0.5 \text{ hour}) \times (10 \text{ gtt/mL})}{60 \text{ minutes/hour}}$$

$$= \frac{(150 \text{ mL/hour}) \times (10 \text{ gtt/mL})}{60 \text{ minutes/hour}} = 25 \text{ gtt/minute}$$

The number of hours that the IV lasts can be determined by dividing the volume of the IV bag (expressed in milliliters) by the flow rate (expressed in milliliters per hour). The following example demonstrates this calculation.

Example 4 ─────── **A 1 L IV is running at 125 mL/hour. How often does a new bag have to be administered?**

Begin by converting 1 L to 1000 mL, and then divide the volume by the volume per hour rate.

$$\text{hours the IV lasts} = \frac{1000 \text{ mL}}{125 \text{ mL/hour}} = 8 \text{ hours}$$

Electrolytes

Many IV fluids used in hospital pharmacy practice contain dissolved mineral salts; such a fluid is known as an **electrolyte**. These fluids are so named because they conduct an electrical charge through the solution when connected to electrodes. For example, the compound potassium chloride (abbreviated KCl) breaks down to K+ and Cl- ions in solution. Electrolyte solutions, in addition to being measured in the usual metric units such as milligrams, are also measured in milliequivalents (mEq). Milliequivalents (mEq) are related to molecular weight. Molecular weights are based on the atomic weights of common elements. A detailed discussion of these chemistry terms is beyond the scope of this text but is available on this text's Internet Resource Center at www.emcp.net/pharmpractice4e.

Example 5

You are requested to add 44 mEq of sodium chloride (NaCl) to an IV bag. Sodium chloride is available as a 4 mEq/mL solution. How many milliliters should you add to the bag?

Set up a proportion—comparing the solution that you need to create to the available solution—and solve for the unknown. Review examples in Chapter 5 if you are not sure how to solve a problem using the ratio-proportion method.

$$\frac{x \text{ mL}}{44 \text{ mEq}} = \frac{1 \text{ mL}}{4 \text{ mEq}}$$

$$\frac{(44 \text{ mEq}) \, x \text{ mL}}{44 \text{ mEq}} = \frac{(44 \text{ mEq}) \, 1 \text{ mL}}{4 \text{ mEq}}$$

$$x \text{ mL} = \frac{44 \text{ mL}}{4}$$

$$x \text{ mL} = 11 \text{ mL}$$

Hazardous Agents

Pharmacists and pharmacy technicians working in a hospital setting often come in contact with hazardous agents, such as cytotoxic drugs, requiring special handling and preparation. A **cytotoxic drug** can be a drug used in cancer chemotherapy, an antiviral drug for a patient with HIV, a biological hormone, a bioengineered drug, or a radioactive pharmaceutical. Although the benefit to the patient is greater than the risk of exposure and adverse effects, a healthcare worker may be adversely exposed to such an agent in the preparation process. Table 11.4 lists some commonly used cytotoxic and hazardous drugs.

TABLE 11.4 Commonly Used Cytotoxic and Hazardous Drugs

aldesleukin	doxorubicin	mercaptopurine
anastrozole	estramustine	methotrexate
asparaginase	etoposide	mitomycin
bleomycin	exemestane	mitotane
busulfan	floxuridine	mitoxantrone
carboplatin	fluorouracil	oxaliplatin
carmustine	ganciclovir	plicamycin
chlorambucil	hydroxyurea	procarbazine
cisplatin	idarubicin	streptozocin
cyclophosphamide	ifosfamide	temozolomide
cytarabine	irinotecan	thioguanine
dacarbazine	letrozole	thiotepa
dactinomycin	lomustine	topotecan
daunorubicin	mechlorethamine	vinblastine
denileukin diftitox	melphalan	vincristine

Risks of Exposures to Hazardous Agents

Four routes of exposure of personnel to hazardous agents include (1) trauma, (2) inhalation, (3) direct skin contact, and (4) ingestion, illustrated by the following examples.

- Trauma or injury. A technician using a syringe to add a drug to an IV bag might accidentally prick himself or herself with the needle or receive a cut from a broken container of the substance.
- Inhalation, or breathing in, of the hazardous substance. A technician might drop and break a bottle containing a volatile substance or use poor manipulation technique with a multiple-dose vial, releasing a fine mist of the medication from the container.
- Ingestion. A technician might ingest dust when crushing an oral tablet or cleaning a counting tray.
- Direct skin contact. A technician might accidentally spill a medication when pouring it from a large container into a smaller container or flask. Direct contact with some cancer drugs can cause immediate reactions.
  - Asparaginase may cause skin irritation.
  - Doxorubicin can cause tissue death and sloughing if introduced into a skin abrasion.
  - Nitrogen mustards can cause irritation of the eyes, mucous membranes, and skin.
  - Streptozocin is a potential carcinogen when it is exposed to skin. Accidental exposures in the pharmacy may occur through trauma, direct skin contact, and inhalation.

With exposure to hazardous agents, healthcare workers may suffer acute, chronic, and long-term risks to their health. Acute risks may be from contact resulting in skin rashes, allergic reactions, or perhaps even hair loss. In women of reproductive age, chronic exposure could result in infertility, spontaneous abortions, low-birth-weight infants, or even congenital malformations. Long-term risks with years of chronic exposure may include a higher risk for certain cancers, including leukemia.

Any woman of reproductive age who routinely works with hazardous agents should have confirmation in writing attesting to an understanding of the risks and the importance of taking additional precautions to prevent pregnancy. Pharmacy workers who are breast-feeding or trying to conceive should notify their supervisor so that extra precautions can be taken to minimize contact with any hazardous substances or to schedule a change in work responsibilities.

Inappropriate aseptic technique with nonhazardous CSPs may result in contamination and potential infection of the patient; sloppy technique with hazardous ones may be harmful to the employee's own health. The policy and procedures of the department, as well as guidelines and standards from USP Chapter 797, are designed to help protect the healthcare worker from unnecessary exposure and risks.

Receipt and Storage of Hazardous Agents

The pharmacy technician must wear gloves when receiving, stocking, inventorying, disposing, and preparing hazardous agents. Hazardous drugs should be delivered directly to the storage area and inventoried. Damaged packages should be inspected in an insulated area, such as a vertical airflow hood. The receipt of broken vials of drugs that have not been reconstituted should be treated as hazardous agent spills, discussed later in the chapter.

The inventory of these drugs should be separated from other medications to prevent contamination and exposure, as well as to reduce the potential error of pulling a look-alike container from an adjacent shelf or bin. Storage areas, such as drug cartons, shelves, bins, counters, and trays, should carry appropriate brightly colored warning labels and should be designed in such a way as to maximize product recognition and minimize the possibility of falling and breakage. For example, storage shelves should have a barrier at the front, carts should have rims, and hazardous drugs should be stored at eye level or lower. Ideal storage is in a room with frequent air exchanges and negative air pressure to dilute or remove potential airborne contaminants.

Hazardous drugs requiring refrigeration should be stored separately from other drugs, in bins that prevent breakage and contain leakage, should it occur. Access to storage areas and work areas for hazardous materials should be limited to specified trained personnel. A list of cytotoxic and otherwise hazardous drugs should be compiled and posted in appropriate locations in the workplace.

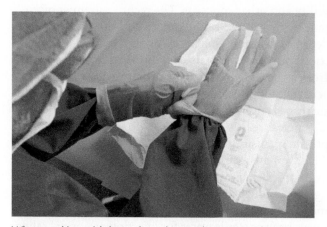

When working with hazardous drugs, pharmacy technicians must use double gloving and eye shields to protect themselves.

Protective Clothing

Protective clothing required for technicians working with cytotoxic drugs is similar to that discussed in Chapter 10 for preparing CSPs, but with additional requirements. A disposable, lint-free, nonabsorbent, closed-front gown with cuffed sleeves should be worn. Hair covers and shoe covers must be worn to reduce the potential for particulate contamination. Other protective clothing includes eye protection, mask, and use of latex gloves when disposing of damaged packages. Eye protection and double gloving are important additions when preparing hazardous agents.

Double gloving should be done after a thorough washing of the hands. Factors that influence glove permeability are glove thickness and exposure duration. All glove sizes should be available so that each worker has a good fit. The first pair of gloves should be tucked under the sleeve cuff of the gown, whereas the second pair should be placed over the top of the cuff. Gloved hands should then be washed to remove any powder that may be present, to prevent unnecessary particles in the hood. Gloves should be changed every 20 to 30 minutes with continuous use or immediately after a contamination or puncture occurs. Gloves should be turned inside out as they are removed and should be discarded in designated hazardous waste containers. As an alternative to double gloving, gloves are available, such as the ChemoBloc nitrile gloves, that are thicker than normal pairs, are latex-free, and can easily indicate any punctures in order to provide maximum protection for the technician.

Handling and Preparation of Hazardous Agents

CSPs of hazardous agents should always be prepared under conditions that protect the healthcare worker. Such agents should be prepared, per Chapter 797 guidelines, under a vertical laminar flow hood in an ISO Class 5 environment with the appropriate protective garb and meticulous aseptic technique. Wherever possible, unnecessary manipulation of hazardous agents should be avoided, even when the technician is working in a protective environment in the clean room.

In a small hospital, when the technician is preparing a small volume of hazardous CSPs (defined as fewer than 5 CSPs per week), certain allowances are made, but protection of the worker remains of paramount importance. If commercially available, a medication in a closed system transfer device (CSTD) is the preferred delivery system to minimize worker exposure; it should be assembled in a nonnegative pressure room (without a vertical LAFW), using appropriate protective garb and aseptic technique. The hospital pharmacy technician may also need to repackage an oral hazardous agent into unit dose bubble packaging.

Radioactive pharmaceuticals are often prepared in a nuclear pharmacy by a specially trained and certified nuclear pharmacy technician. The details of handling, preparation, and disposal of such agents are beyond the scope of this text but can be found in USP Chapter 823.

Handling Hazardous Agents in Vials Hazardous agents are not always available in a CSTD because of chemical stability and other concerns. The technician must often reconstitute powders of such agents with a suitable diluent and add the agent to an IV minibag. Reconstituting a powder of a hazardous substance by introducing a diluent (similar to sterile water for injection) produces a positive pressure inside the vial. The withdrawal of a cytotoxic drug from a vial differs from the procedure discussed with nonhazardous CSPs. The technician should introduce a volume of air that is less than the solution volume, thus producing a vacuum and preventing an aspirate when the needle is withdrawn from the rubber closure.

Drugs in vials may build up pressure, causing the drug to spray out around the needle thus increasing the risk of inadvertent aspiration of the hazardous drug. It is important that a slight negative pressure be maintained. To prevent excessive negative pressure, inject into the vial enough air to equal about 75% of the volume of drug to be withdrawn. Do not inject a volume of air equal to or greater than the amount of drug to be withdrawn. When adding a diluent such as sterile water for injection or normal saline to a vial, do so slowly, allowing pressure in the vial and syringe to equalize. Excessive negative pressure may cause leakage from the needle or cause the drug to splash back when the needle is withdrawn, creating a safety concern for the pharmacy technician.

For example, if you are to withdraw 4 mL of a cytotoxic drug from a multiple-dose vial, then you should inject no more than 3 mL of air (75%) before withdrawing the drug in the syringe. The use of a **chemo venting pin** also equalizes air pressure in the vial. Vials should not be vented unless a filter device is used. The rest of the technique for withdrawing medication is similar to that illustrated in Figure 11.3.

All syringes and IV containers should be labeled according to institutional guidelines. Syringes should be large enough so that the plunger does not separate easily from the barrel. If the medication is to be dispensed from the syringe, then the solution should be cleared from the needle and hub and the needle should be replaced with a locking cap. The syringe should be cleaned with a moistened wipe and then labeled. If the medication is to be added to an IV bag, then care should be used to prevent a puncture of the bag. The injection port and the bag should be wiped with a moistened alcohol wipe. The bag should be placed in a sealable container to contain leakage during transport.

The priming of IV administration sets with cytotoxic agents should always be performed in the vertical laminar airflow workbench in the hospital pharmacy. The bag should be primed with the base solution. The cytotoxic agent and tubing are then delivered to the nursing unit in a plastic bag. Common hospital procedure to minimize drug administration errors is for two nurses to double-check medication dose and labeling before administration to the patient. An incorrect dose, especially in a pediatric patient, could prove deadly. At the time of administration to the patient, the nurse must also wear a mask, gloves, and a special paperlike gown. Protective garb must be worn at the patient's bedside, even in the case of preparing and administering a chemotherapy drug in a CSTD system. Once the administration has been completed, the garb then must be discarded in a specially designated hazardous waste container.

Handling Hazardous Agents in Ampules When opening an ampule, tap the drug from the top of the ampule, wrap a pad around the ampule, and hold the ampule away from the face before breaking off the top. A 5 micron filter needle should be placed on the syringe to withdraw the solution from the ampule. The fluid should be drawn through the syringe hub. A standard needle is placed on the syringe. Excess drug and any air are ejected into the sterile vial until the correct volume is left.

Handling Hazardous Oral Drugs Hazardous oral drugs may be handled in both community and hospital pharmacy settings. During routine handling of hazardous oral drugs, workers should wear one pair of gloves of good quality and thickness, as well as a gown and respirator. The counting and pouring of these drugs (e.g., methotrexate) should be done carefully, and contaminated equipment such as counting trays should be immediately cleaned with detergent and rinsed. Tablet and capsule forms of hazardous materials should not be placed in automated counting or packaging machines. When the technician is crushing a hazardous drug in a unit-of-use package, the package should be placed in a small, sealable plastic bag and crushed with a spoon or pestle; the technician should use caution not to break the plastic bag. Compounding involving these drugs should be done in a protected area removed from air drafts and traffic.

Hazardous Agent Spills

The technician must be aware of the proper procedures in case of a hazardous agent spill and for disposal of a contaminated drug and clothing. The goal of the containment of a cytotoxic or hazardous material spill is ensuring that the healthcare setting, staff, patients, visitors, and environment (both inside and outside the medical facility) are not contaminated.

All spills—small or large—must be dealt with immediately. Cleanup and decontamination should be done with a spill kit. Spill kits contain materials to control and clean up spills of up to 1000 mL. A commercially available spill kit may be used, or one may be assembled with the following contents.

- nonabsorbent, lint-free gown
- gloves, two pairs
- respirator mask
- goggles, one pair
- absorbent towels
- chemo hazard labels
- spill control pillows or towels folded to work as pillows
- scoop and brush (for collecting glass fragments)
- plastic disposal bags labeled "Chemo Waste"
- "CAUTION: Chemo Spill" sign

A spill outside the clean room with a vertical LAFW should be posted with a warning sign. Proper attire must be worn, including gown, double gloves, goggles, and a mask or respirator for cleaning spills. Broken glass should be placed in the appropriate container—but never using bare hands. When cleaning up the spill, start from the edge of the spill and work inward, using absorbent sheets, spill pads, or pillows for the liquids and damp cloths or towels for solids. Use spill pads and water to rinse the area. Detergent should be used to remove residue.

Spills in the vertical LAFW require additional steps. The drain trough should be thoroughly cleaned and the cabinet decontaminated per manufacturer specification. All contaminated materials from a spill should be sealed in hazardous waste containers and placed in leak-resistant containers. The spill and cleanup and any personnel exposure must be documented.

Procedures in Case of Exposure

Every hazardous substance has a Material Safety Data Sheet (MSDS) outlining specific recommendations on how to handle an exposure (Figure 11.11). If the skin is exposed, then the affected area should be flooded with water immediately and thoroughly cleansed with soap and water. If the substance comes in contact with the eyes, then flush the affected eyes with large amounts of water or use an eye flush kit. Each hospital pharmacy should have a sink and/or eye wash area and eye flush kit accessible close to the clean room in the event of an accidental exposure to a hazardous drug.

Remove contaminated garments and/or gloves, and wash hands after removing the gloves. Dispose of contaminated garments appropriately in specially designated biohazard materials containers. No protective clothing should be taken outside the area where the exposure occurred. The exposed person should then be sent or escorted to the employee health or emergency room. Caution should be taken, including warning others, so as not to contaminate other persons or objects. Report any exposure incident to a supervisor, and complete an incident report.

FIGURE 11.11
MSDS Form

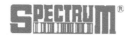

Material Safety Data Sheet

NFPA	HMIS	Personal Protective Equipment
2 1 0	Health Hazard — 2 Fire Hazard — 1 Reactivity — 0	 See Section 15.

Section 1. Chemical Product and Company Identification

Page Number: 1

Common Name/ Trade Name	**Methotrexate**	Catalog Number(s).	ME131, M1435
		CAS#	59-05-2
Manufacturer	SPECTRUM LABORATORY PRODUCTS INC. 14422 S. SAN PEDRO STREET GARDENA, CA 90248	RTECS	MA1225000
		TSCA	TSCA 8(b) inventory: Methotrexate
Commercial Name(s)	Amethopterin, Amethopterine, Antifolin, Methotrexat, Methylaminopterin, Methylaminopterium, Ledertrexate	CI#	Not available.
Synonym	4-Amino-4-deoxy-N(sup10)-methylpteroylglutamate; 4-Amino-4-deoxy-N(sup10)-methylpteroylglutamic acid; 4-Amino-N(sup10)-methylpteroylglutamic acid	IN CASE OF EMERGENCY CHEMTREC (24hr) 800-424-9300	
Chemical Name	N-[4-[[(2,4-Diamino-6-pteridinyl)methyl]methylamino]benzoyl]-L-glutamic acid		
Chemical Family	Not available.	CALL (310) 516-8000	
Chemical Formula	C20-H22-N8-O5		
Supplier	SPECTRUM LABORATORY PRODUCTS INC. 14422 S. SAN PEDRO STREET GARDENA, CA 90248		

Section 2. Composition and Information on Ingredients

Name	CAS #	Exposure Limits			% by Weight
		TWA (mg/m³)	STEL (mg/m³)	CEIL (mg/m³)	
1) Methotrexate	59-05-2				100

Toxicological Data on Ingredients	**Methotrexate:** ORAL (LD50): Acute: 135 mg/kg [Rat]. 146 mg/kg [Mouse].

Section 3. Hazards Identification

Potential Acute Health Effects	Hazardous in case of ingestion. Slightly hazardous in case of skin contact (irritant), of eye contact (irritant), of inhalation. Severe over-exposure can result in death.
Potential Chronic Health Effects	**CARCINOGENIC EFFECTS:** 3 (Not classifiable for human.) by IARC. **MUTAGENIC EFFECTS:** Mutagenic for mammalian somatic cells. Mutagenic for bacteria and/or yeast. **TERATOGENIC EFFECTS:** Not available. **DEVELOPMENTAL TOXICITY:** Not available. The substance may be toxic to blood, kidneys, lungs, liver, gastrointestinal tract, immune system, bone marrow. Repeated or prolonged exposure to the substance can produce target organs damage. Repeated exposure to a highly toxic material may produce general deterioration of health by an accumulation in one or many human organs.

Continued on Next Page

Courtesy of Spectrum Laboratory Products Inc., 2008.

Quality Assurance

How does the pharmacist or pharmacy technician know whether or not the sterile IV product that he or she prepared, labeled, checked, and sent to the nurse for the patient was accurate or free from microorganisms? If an ACD is used for TPN preparation, then is it accurate? Each hospital pharmacy must have a **quality assurance (QA) program** in its policy and procedure manual with which to check for medication errors or contamination.

A quality assurance program to detect and correct errors is important to ensure quality of care and employee safety and is required for accreditation. A QA program identifies the problem and tries to correct the problem so that it does not recur. The emphasis on QA programs in the hospital is not to affix blame, but to fix systems.

Recommendations for disinfecting the clean room and LAFWs are provided in Table 10.2. A quality control procedure for environmental monitoring of the clean room, LAFW, buffer area, and anteroom must be in place, as must training of all hospital personnel in proper aseptic technique and in the handling of hazardous drugs. As required by USP guidelines and the Joint Commission, sampling of the air, work surfaces, and glove tips should be routinely completed daily to monthly, depending on the contamination risk level of the CSP. Oversight for investigating hospital-acquired infections is provided by the infection control committee (ICC).

If breakdowns in accuracy or sterility are identified, then existing procedures must be reviewed and all pharmacy personnel may need refresher training. A breakdown in sterility in the pharmacy could lead to a serious breakout of nosocomial or healthcare-associated infections (HAIs) in the hospital.

Documentation of personnel training for aseptic technique and proper handling of hazardous agents is required by USP 797 guidelines and Joint Commission standards. All personnel in the hospital, including custodial workers, must have proper training in procedures involving identification, containment, collection, segregation, and disposal of cytotoxic and other hazardous drugs. This training must be completed and documented prior to working with these agents. Training for pharmacy personnel must cover the following areas:

- safe aseptic manipulation technique
- negative pressure techniques in a vertical laminar flow workbench hood
- correct use of CSTDs
- containment, cleanup, and disposal of breakage or spills
- treatment of personnel for contact and exposure

Training must be repeated and documented every year. For every new hazardous agent (new drug, new investigational drug), a Material Safety Data Sheet (MSDS) must be initiated, reviewed with the appropriate staff, and filed for reference. Any organization involved with cytotoxic or other hazardous drugs must have written procedures for proper handling and disposal of such drugs and should provide access to medical care and methods for documentation in the case of incidents of exposure. Environmental and air sampling for hazardous agents must be included in the department's quality assurance (QA) program. Government regulation is through the National Institute of Occupational Safety and Health (NIOSH), under the auspices of the CDC.

Working in the IV area requires training, experience, and certification. Following appropriate aseptic technique to minimize microbial contamination to a patient is very important. In the case of working with hazardous agents, use of proper technique may protect the technician's own health and well-being.

Chapter Terms

ampule a single-dose-only drug container; it contains no preservative

aseptic technique the manipulation of sterile products and devices in such a way as to avoid disease-causing organisms

automated compounding device (ACD) a programmable, automated device to make complex IV preparations such as TPNs

catheter a device inserted into a vein for direct access to the blood vascular system

central venous catheter (CVC) a catheter placed into a large vein deep into the body; also called a central line

chemo venting pin a device used to equalize pressure in the preparation of hazardous drugs

closed system transfer device (CSTD) a needleless delivery system by which medications are aseptically activated and added to an IV minibag at patient bedside

cold flow the tendency of a clamp on an IV administration set to return slowly to a more open position, with an increase in fluid flow

coring the act of introducing a small chunk of the rubber closure into the solution while removing medication from a vial

creep the tendency of a clamp on an IV administration set to return to its previous position

cytotoxic drug a hazardous drug that must be handled and prepared with extra precautions; such a drug may be used in cancer chemotherapy, an antiviral drug for a patient with HIV, a biological hormone, a bioengineered drug, or a radioactive pharmaceutical

diluent a sterile fluid added to a powder to reconstitute, dilute, or dissolve a medication

drop set the calibration in drops per milliliter on IV sets

electrolyte a dissolved mineral salt, commonly found in IV fluids

filter a device used to remove contaminants such as glass, paint, fibers, rubber cores, and bacteria from IV fluids

hypertonic solution a parenteral solution with a greater number of particles than the number of particles found in blood (greater than 285 mOsm/L); also called hyperosmolar, as in a TPN solution

hypotonic solution a parenteral solution with a fewer number of particles than the number of particles found in blood (less than 285 mOsm/L); also called hypoosmolar

isotonic solution a parenteral solution with an equal number of particles as blood cells (285 mOsm/L); 0.9% normal saline is isotonic

IV administration set a sterile, pyrogen-free disposable device used to deliver IV fluids to patients

IV piggyback (IVPB) a small-volume IV infusion (50 mL, 100 mL, 250 mL) containing medications

IV push (IVP) the rapid injection of a medication in a syringe into an IV line or catheter in the patient's arm; also called bolus injection

large-volume parenteral (LVP) an IV fluid of more than 250 mL that may contain drugs, nutrients, or electrolytes

nonpyrogenic the state of being free from microorganisms; a description of a packaged IV set

osmolarity a measure of the milliosmoles of solute per liter of solution (mOsm/L); for example, the osmolarity of blood is 285 mOsm/L; often referred to as tonicity for IV solutions

osmotic pressure the pressure required to maintain an equilibrium, with no net movement of solvent

pH value the degree of acidity or alkalinity of a solution; less than 7 is acidic and more than 7 is alkaline; the pH of blood is 7.4

priming the act of flushing out the small particles in the tubing's interior lumen prior to medication administration and letting fluid run through the tubing so that all of the air is flushed out

quality assurance (QA) program a feedback system to improve care by identifying and correcting the cause of a medication error or improper technique

small-volume parenteral (SVP) an IV fluid of 250 mL or less commonly used for infusion of drugs; with medication, also called an IV piggyback

spike the sharp plastic end of IV tubing that is attached to an IV bag of fluid

Y-site a rigid piece of plastic with one arm terminating in a resealable port that is used for adding medication to the IV

Chapter Summary

- Parenteral IV drugs can be administered by bolus injection or by infusion.
- IV infusions are used to deliver blood, water, other fluids, nutrients such as lipids and sugars, electrolytes, and drugs.
- IV preparations have many characteristics, including solubility, osmolality, and acid/base ratio or pH, that must be appreciated by the pharmacy technician.
- Many vehicles exist for IV solutions that are individualized to the need of the patient and the drug, such as dextrose in water, normal saline (NS), and dextrose in NS.
- Special IV solutions prepared or labeled in the pharmacy include TPNs, frozen IV solutions, and closed system transfer devices, or CSTDs.
- Medications for IV use must be prepared in a laminar airflow hood using proper aseptic technique and under the supervision of a licensed pharmacist.
- A pharmacy technician must become familiar with the components of each IV administration set, including controller clamps, drip chamber, and Y-sites.

- An in-line filter in the IV administration set protects the patient against particulate matter, bacteria, air emboli, and phlebitis.
- A technician must be able to compute drip and infusion rates for IV solutions.
- Hazardous drugs require special techniques, equipment, and procedures to protect the health of the employee, especially in women of childbearing age.
- Accidental exposures require immediate treatment, cleanup, reporting to the supervisor, and completion of an incident report.
- The pharmacy technician must undergo specific specialized training before working in a sterile environment with IV medications and hazardous drugs.
- A quality assurance program to detect and correct errors is important to ensure quality of care and employee safety and is required for accreditation.

Chapter Review

Checking Your Understanding

Choose the best answer from those provided.

 Additional Quiz Questions

1. An example of an isotonic solution is
   a. 0.9% normal saline (NS).
   b. dextrose 50%.
   c. sodium chloride (NaCl) 3%.
   d. 0.45% normal saline (NS).

2. The pH of blood is considered to be slightly
   a. acidic.
   b. alkaline.
   c. neutral.
   d. hypotonic.

3. A medication attached to a closed system transfer device is activated
   a. at time of manufacture.
   b. at time of receipt of medication in the hospital pharmacy from the wholesaler.
   c. by the nurse at the patient's bedside.
   d. by the technician inside a vertical LAFW.

4. For a pediatric patient, the flow rate of an IV administration set is commonly
   a. 10 gtt/minute.
   b. 15 gtt/minute.
   c. 20 gtt/minute.
   d. 60 gtt/minute.

5. What size of filter is needed to eliminate bacteria in the IV solution?
   a. 0.22 micron
   b. 0.45 micron
   c. 5 microns
   d. no filter is small enough to eliminate bacteria

6. The tonicity of a special IV solution, such as a TPN, is considered to be
   a. isotonic.
   b. hypertonic.
   c. hypotonic.
   d. hypoosmolar.

7. An IV order is received for $D_5\frac{1}{2}NS$ to be infused at a rate of 125 mL/hour. How many 1 L bottles must be prepared for use over the next 24 hours?
   a. one
   b. two
   c. three
   d. five

8. The expiration date for a medication in a CSTD delivery system once activated under refrigerated storage conditions is
   a. 24 hours.
   b. 48 hours.
   c. 14 days.
   d. per recommendation in product package insert.

9. To prevent excessive negative pressure, how many milliliters of air should be injected by syringe into a multiple-dose vial before drawing up a hazardous drug? Assume that you need to withdraw 2 mL of a cancer drug.
   a. 3 mL
   b. 2 mL
   c. 1.5 mL
   d. 0.75 mL

10. Cytotoxic drugs for IV administration must be prepared
    a. in a vertical laminar flow hood.
    b. in a horizontal laminar flow hood.
    c. at the nursing station just before administration to the patient.
    d. in the nonsterile extemporaneous compounding area.

Thinking Like a Pharmacy Tech

Using the following orders and the reconstitution chart in Table 11.5, answer the medication questions.

1. R̥ acyclovir 1 g q12 h
   a. In what fluid is the drug mixed?
   b. What is the expiration time at room temperature?
   c. Can it be refrigerated?

2. R̥ vancomycin 1.5 g q8 h
   a. What size of bag is used?
   b. What is the infusion time?
   c. What is the room temperature expiration?

3. R̥ Primaxin 500 mg q6 h × 3 days
   a. In what fluid is the drug mixed?
   b. What size bag is needed?
   c. How many bags are needed?

4. R̥ oxacillin 1 g × 5 days
   a. What size bag is needed?
   b. What fluid?
   c. If all bags are prepared today, then will the last one expire before the end of therapy?
   d. What is the infusion rate?

5. Solve the following IV rate and administration problems.
   a. A physician orders 3000 mL of a 10% dextrose and normal saline ($D_{10}NS$) IV over a 48 hour period. If the IV set delivers 15 gtt/mL, then how many drops must be administered per minute?
   b. A ½ L IV is running at a rate of 100 mL/hour. How long will the bag last?

6. Check a drug reference for guidelines on the reconstitution and stability of the following.
   a. 1 g cefazolin sodium for IV infusion in a minibag
   b. amphotericin B 50 mg vial added to a large-volume parenteral (LVP)
   c. cyclophosphamide 100 mg added to an LVP

TABLE 11.5 Minibag Administration Protocol

Agent	Volume	Infusion	EXP
Rate	EXP		
acyclovir (Zovirax)*	≤ 1 g; 50 mL	60 min	24 h RT
imipenem-cilastin (Pri-maxin)**	≤ 500 mg; 100 mL NS	60 min	10 h RT
	> 500 mg; 250 mL NS	60 min	48 h REF
oxacillin**	≤ 2 g; 50 mL NS	60 min	96 h RT
	> 2 g; 100 mL NS	60 min	7 day REF
vancomycin (Vancocin)	≤ 250 mg; 50 mL	60 min	96 h RT
	> 250 mg; 100 mL	60 min	
	> 1 g; 250 mL	60 min	

* Do not refrigerate.

** Denotes saline use only.

Note: Prepare each agent in D5W unless advised otherwise. RT indicates room temperature. REF indicates refrigeration.

Communicating Clearly

1. Communicating in the hospital setting often means working with a wide variety of other healthcare providers. Understanding what role they play in patient health care is essential to effective communication. What duties do each of the following have in IV and TPN therapy?
   a. physician
   b. nurse
   c. pharmacist
   d. pharmacy technician

2. Interview an IV hospital pharmacist or IV pharmacy technician about the applications of milliequivalents into IV admixtures and TPN solutions. Report to the class.

Researching on the Web

1. Visit www.ashp.org/bestpractices/draft_guidance/Gdl_Handling_HD-D1.pdf at the American Society of Health-System Pharmacists (ASHP) Web site and review the draft statement on cancer risks with improper handling of hazardous drugs.

2. Visit www.cdc.gov/niosh/docs/2004-165/ and review various exposure routes for cytotoxic drugs.

3. Check the infusion rates in adults and pediatrics for Intralipid or Liposyn II/III in the PDR or other reference.

4. Go to http://www.rxkinetics.com/iv_osmolarity.html and calculate the osmolarity in mOsm/L of the following IV fluid: 1 L of lactated Ringer's solution with 20 mEq of potassium chloride, 10 mEq of calcium chloride, 5 mEq of magnesium sulfate, and 5 mEq of sodium bicarbonate. Is this CSP isotonic, hypertonic, or hypotonic?

5. Go to http://www.spectrumchemical.com/MSDS/G5001.pdf and locate an MSDS for methotrexate USP. List first-aid measures for various exposures to this hazardous drug.

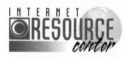

For further study of chapter-related topics, explore the Web links in the Web Center at www.emcp.net/pharmpractice4e.

Unit

4

Professionalism in the Pharmacy

353

Medication Safety

12

Kimberly Vernachio
PharmD, RPh

Learning Objectives

- Understand the extent of medical and medication errors and their effects on patient health and safety.

- Identify specific categories of medication errors.

- List examples of medication errors commonly seen in pharmacy practice settings.

- Apply a systematic evaluation to search for medication error potential to a pharmacy practice model.

- Define strategies, including use of automation, for preventing medication errors.

- Identify the common systems available for reporting medication errors.

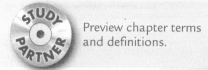

Preview chapter terms and definitions.

The pharmacy technician can play a crucial role in the prevention of medication errors in every pharmacy setting. Through categorizing the types of medication errors and their common causes, pharmacy personnel work to establish practices to promote safety throughout the prescription-filling process. Hospitals, accrediting agencies, and several state boards of pharmacy provide reporting systems to help document medication errors, to study their causes, and to prevent future errors. The Food and Drug Administration (FDA), the United States Pharmacopeia (USP), and the Institute for Safe Medication Practices have developed other medication error reporting systems.

Medical Errors

A **medical error** is any circumstance, action, inaction, or decision related to health care that contributes to an unintended health result. A medical error can be as simple as a lab test drawn at the wrong time, returning an inaccurate result, or as serious as a major surgical error that ends in death. A majority of what is known about medical errors comes from information collected in the hospital setting; however, hospital data make up only a part of a much larger picture. Generally, medical errors are difficult to define, because the circumstances that cause them are infinite.

Most health care is administered in the outpatient, office-based, or clinic setting. Although medical errors are more difficult to measure in these settings, the number of medical-related lawsuits readily provides a sense of the real scope of medical errors in the United States.

Several studies have attempted to measure the number and common causes of medical errors. These studies provide estimates on how many people die from medical errors. Examining only medical errors during hospitalization, one large government study suggested that as many as 98,000 people in the United States may die each year as a result of medical errors. This risk is greater than the risk of death from accident, diabetes, homicide, or human immunodeficiency virus (HIV) and acquired immunodeficiency syndrome (AIDS). Of note, Medicare no longer reimburses hospitals for the additional treatment costs for preventable medical errors; hospitals cannot bill the patient for these additional expenses either. Private insurers are expected to follow suit. Through accreditation and reimbursement, strong incentives exist for a hospital to place a high priority on the prevention of medical errors.

On the continuum of healthcare delivery, multiple sources for potential medical errors exist. Pharmacy technicians are an important part of the healthcare team; therefore, they should be constantly on the lookout for possible sources of medical errors and adopt safety-oriented work practices involving patients. When pharmacy technicians take steps to protect the safety of patients, they become an important barrier against an adverse patient outcome.

Medication Errors

The National Coordinating Council for Medication Error Reporting and Prevention defines a **medication error** as "any preventable event that may cause or lead to inappropriate medication use or patient harm while the medication is in the control of the healthcare professional, patient, or consumer. Such events may be related to professional practice, healthcare products, procedures, and systems, including prescribing; order communication; product labeling, packaging, and nomenclature; compounding; dispensing; distribution; administration; education; monitoring; and use."

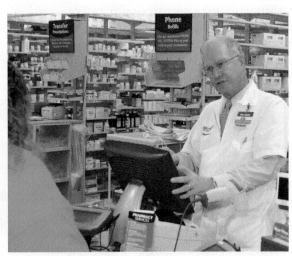

The profession of pharmacy exists to protect the safety of patients from medication errors and adverse effects of drugs. Automation assists the pharmacist and the technician in fulfilling this responsibility.

Medication errors are among the more common types of medical errors. The information on the effect of medication errors comes mostly from studies done in the hospital setting. From these studies, deaths from medication-related errors are estimated at about 7000 yearly.

In a report issued by the Institute of Medicine (IOM) in 2006, drug errors cause an estimated 400,000 preventable injuries in the hospital, with twice as many occurring in nursing homes. The IOM estimates that there are more than 500,000 preventable injuries among patients who are eligible for Medicare and are treated in outpatient clinics.

Far fewer studies of medication errors in community practice exist; however, a few studies give a sense of how large an issue medication errors can be in community practice. An estimated 1.7% of all prescriptions dispensed in a community practice setting contain a medication error: in other words,

4 out of 250 prescriptions contain a medication error of some type. Although not all medication errors result in harm to a patient, the same study estimated that 65% of the medication errors detected had an adverse effect on the patient's health.[1]

The results of medication errors cannot be easily measured. Lives are lost daily, patients are disabled or lose valuable time from work or school, and the direct and indirect cost to the healthcare system is conservatively estimated to be $3.5 billion annually. These costs are caused by additional hospitalizations, admissions to long-term care, physician visits, emergency room visits, and continuation of disease.

Patient Response

Most patients benefit from a medication's intended therapeutic response; however, an individual's unique physical and social circumstances make it impossible to predict which medication errors may cause harm.

Physiological Causes of Medication Errors Remembering that each patient has a unique response to medication can best highlight the importance of medication safety. Each person is genetically unique, and the speed at which a person can remove medications from the body varies tremendously. For instance, a patient may lack an enzyme that helps remove medications from the body, thus leading to serious harm or even death from a medication error. Even if this particular problem is caught and corrected before harm occurs, the result is still considered a medication error.

Another example of a physiological cause is an age-related decrease in kidney function. Kidney function also may be decreased in patients with chronic renal failure, high blood pressure, or diabetes. In the hospital setting, the kidney function may not be fully developed in neonates or prematurely born babies. Many medications rely on the kidney for their elimination from the body. If the dose is not lowered, then the drug could accumulate to toxic levels, causing an adverse reaction and medication error. This is one of many factors that the pharmacist must consider before approving and verifying a prescription.

Social Causes of Medication Errors Patients in the outpatient setting can also contribute to medication errors through incorrect self-administration. As a result, the medication does not work well, does not work at all, or may cause harm. Social causes of medication errors include failure to follow medication therapy instructions because of cost or noncompliance, failure to take therapy as the physician instructs, or misunderstanding instructions (perhaps because of language barriers). Patients can contribute to medication errors by doing the following:

- forgetting to take a dose or doses
- taking too many doses
- dosing at the wrong time
- not getting a prescription filled or refilled in a timely manner
- not following directions on dose administration
- terminating the drug regimen too soon

Such social causes may result in an adverse drug reaction or a subtherapeutic—or even toxic—dose. For example, over 50% of patients on necessary long-term medication are no longer taking their medication after one year. Not taking prescribed medication could result in progression of a chronic disease. Any of these circumstances

---

[1] Flynn, E. A., et al., "National Observational Study of Prescription Dispensing Accuracy and Safety in 50 Pharmacies." *Journal of American Pharmaceutical Association* 43 (2003): 191–200.

could result in lasting harm or in death, depending on the drug or the disease being treated. The technician should take note of the refill history when entering an order. If the patient appears to be noncompliant with the prescribed medication, then the noncompliance should be brought to the attention of the pharmacist for a potential counseling intervention. In any event, the results of all of these social circumstances are considered medication errors.

Categories of Medication Errors

An exact listing of medication errors is difficult to create, because the possible causes of a medication error can often be too numerous to count. However, categorizing errors into types or groups often aids in the identification and prevention of possible causes. Classic examples of medication errors are grouped into the following five major categories.

- An **omission error** occurs when a prescribed dose is not given. An omission occurs when the next dose is due, but the previous dose was not administered.
- A **wrong dose error** occurs when a dose is either above or below the correct dose by more than 5%.
- An **extra dose error** occurs when a patient receives more doses than were prescribed by the physician.
- A **wrong dosage form error** occurs when the dose formulation given to the patient is not the accepted interpretation of the physician order. Examples include a drug given by mouth for a drug ordered as an intramuscular (IM) injection, a capsule formulation dispensed instead of a tablet, or an immediate-release drug dispensed instead of a controlled or extended-release drug.
- A **wrong time error** occurs when any drug is given 30 minutes or more before or after it was prescribed, up to the time of the next dose. This is a common error in the hospital and nursing home; it does not include prn (i.e., as needed) orders.

Another way of categorizing medication errors is to define them according to what caused the failure of the desired result. The purpose of defining errors in this way is to identify clearly what the error was, where the error took place, and, through closer examination, what specifically caused it (i.e., the *why*). Medication errors can be categorized within three basic definitions of failure.

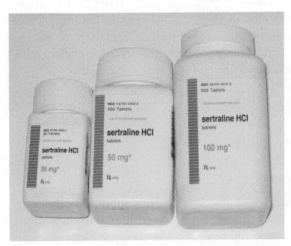

Because of similar packaging and labeling, a bottle for sertraline 100 mg may be inadvertently selected from the shelf instead of sertraline 50 mg, resulting in a serious dosage error.

- A **human failure** occurs at an individual level. An example of this type of error includes pulling a medication bottle from the shelf based on memory, without cross-referencing the bottle label with the shelf label and the medication order/prescription or National Drug Code (NDC) number. Human errors also include those made by the patient, such as noncompliance to prescribed drug therapy.
- A **technical failure** results from location or equipment. An example of this type of failure includes the incorrect reconstitution of a medication because of a malfunction of a sterile-water dispenser or failure to operate automated equipment properly, such as in the mass production of TPN solutions in the hospital pharmacy.

- An **organizational failure** occurs because of organizational rules, policies, or procedures. An example of this type of failure includes a policy or rule requiring the preparing or admixing of parenteral drugs, such as cancer chemotherapy, in an inappropriate setting without proper environmental controls.

Root-Cause Analysis of Medication Errors

Root-cause analysis is a logical and systematic process used to help identify what, how, and why something happened in order to prevent recurrence. Using some of the basic principles of root-cause analysis, a person can examine his or her own workflow to determine the potential for error and the type of failure that the potential error may involve. Using this analysis, it is possible to create a list of specific potential causes. Identifying the potential causes allows a person to take actions to prevent the error and to improve patient safety. The actions taken improve the quality of work being done, and thereby patient outcomes.

A medication error by handlers and preparers of medications has many causes. Three of the most common causes follow.

- An **assumption error** occurs when an essential piece of information cannot be verified; therefore an assumption is made. An example of an assumption error that a pharmacy technician might make is misreading a poorly written abbreviation on a prescription.
- A **selection error** occurs when two or more options exist, and the wrong option is chosen. An example of a selection error that a pharmacy technician might make is mistakenly using a look-alike or sound-alike drug instead of the prescribed drug or choosing an immediate-release formulation instead of an extended-release drug.
- A **capture error** occurs when focus on a task is diverted elsewhere and therefore the distraction captures attention, preventing the person from detecting the error or causing an error to be made. An example of a capture error might be taking a phone call in the middle of filling a prescription order and, as a result, dispensing the wrong number of tablets (i.e., the correct number was forgotten and not double-checked at the conclusion of the phone call).

In relation to capture errors, the work habits of the pharmacy technician can determine when and where in the prescription-filling process it is safe to allow focus on a task to be diverted. In other words, when the technician is completing a medication-related task, is there a point in the process at which stopping and answering the telephone is not appropriate? When is it appropriate to allow for such an interruption? Knowing when to allow interruptions and when not to do so is vitally important in maintaining individual safety practices.

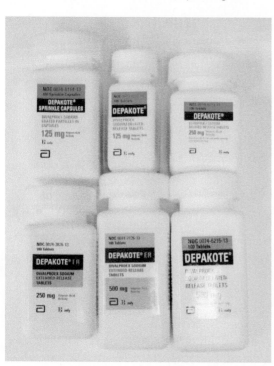

Because of identical names and similar look-alike packaging, the wrong dosage or formulation of the seizure drug valproic acid may be selected, resulting in a selection error. The technician should carefully check the original prescription and compare NDC numbers to prevent a medication error.

Prescription-Filling Process in Community and Hospital Pharmacy Practice

A thorough review of potential causes of medication error in work practices begins with outlining work tasks in a step-by-step manner. Figure 12.1 is an example of a step-by-step prescription-filling process for community and hospital pharmacy practice settings. For the most part, the filling process in both settings is identical; however, in the hospital setting, medications pass through an extra set of hands—the nurse's—before reaching the patient. This extra set of hands provides both an extra opportunity to prevent medication errors and an additional source of potential medication errors. In the community pharmacy, the technician is often the last check in the healthcare system before delivery of the medication(s) to the patient.

Once work practices are broken into individual steps, each step should be reviewed to determine what information is necessary to complete the step and what resources can be used to verify the information. In addition, consideration should be given to the possible errors that might result if information is missed or verification is not performed. Therefore, thinking of each step in terms of the following three parts is helpful.

- information that needs to be obtained or checked
- resources that can be used to verify information
- potential medication errors that would result from a failure to obtain or check the necessary information using the appropriate resources

FIGURE 12.1

Prescription-Filling Process

Although each step in this process can be a source of medication error, it is also an opportunity for pharmacy personnel to correct any such medication error.

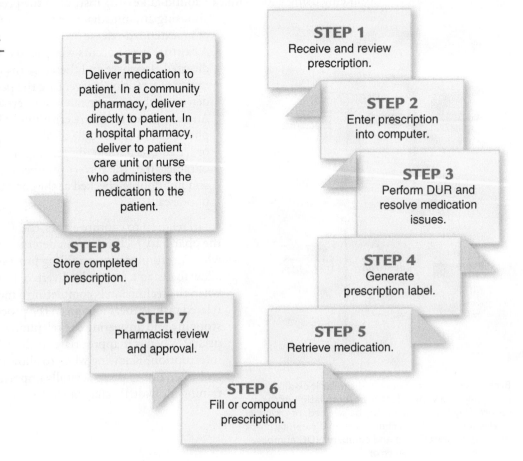

STEP 1
Receive and review prescription.

STEP 2
Enter prescription into computer.

STEP 3
Perform DUR and resolve medication issues.

STEP 4
Generate prescription label.

STEP 5
Retrieve medication.

STEP 6
Fill or compound prescription.

STEP 7
Pharmacist review and approval.

STEP 8
Store completed prescription.

STEP 9
Deliver medication to patient. In a community pharmacy, deliver directly to patient. In a hospital pharmacy, deliver to patient care unit or nurse who administers the medication to the patient.

Step 1: Receive and Review Prescription

Table 12.1 lists the information needed and the resources used to avoid potential errors in the first step of the prescription-filling process.

Before a new prescription enters the prescription-filling process, an initial check of all key pieces of information is vital. A thorough review substantially reduces the chances that an unidentified error will continue throughout the filling process.

The first and most basic part of prescription review begins by deciding whether or not all information involved is clear and legible. Can you read and understand it? Any unclear information should be clarified before any further action is taken. Another common cause of error is in the receipt of messages for verbal prescriptions of sound-alike drugs; if the caller did not spell out the name of the drug and the pharmacist (or technician, in some states) is unclear about the correct name, then the order should be clarified prior to computer entry and filling. If the nurse calls in the prescription, then the caller is encouraged to read back the phone order to minimize errors.

TABLE 12.1   Step 1: Receive and Review Information

Information to Check	Resources to Verify Information	Potential Errors Resulting from Failure to Check/Verify Information
Legibility: Can the prescription be read clearly?	physician, patient, independent reviewer, such as pharmacist or nurse	prescription misread
Prescriber information: Is the prescription valid? Did the prescriber sign the prescription? For narcotic prescriptions, is the prescriber's Drug Enforcement Administration (DEA) number listed? Are the prescriber's name, address, and phone number printed on the prescription?	physician, pharmacist, nurse	out-of-date (i.e., invalid) prescription filled; fraudulent prescription filled; patient receives medication intended for another patient
Patient information: Is all necessary information included? Is this prescription for this patient? Are the patient's name, date of birth, address, phone number, and allergies provided? Does the information match the profile?	physician, patient, immediate family member, patient profile, pharmacist, nurse	incorrect patient selected; contraindicated drug dispensed
Medication information: Is all necessary information included? Are drug name, dose, dosage form, route of administration, refills, directions for use, and dosing schedule included? Is the prescription dated?	patient, physician, family member, patient profile	wrong medication dispensed; wrong form/formulation dispensed; wrong dose dispensed; patient administers incorrectly; out-of-date (i.e., invalid) prescription filled

Safety Note

Careful review of the prescription or order is very important.

Before considering the details of the information contained in a prescription, determining whether the prescription is, in fact, a valid and legal prescription is important. The requirements for a valid prescription may vary from state to state, and every technician should be familiar with the requirements of the state in which he or she practices. Does the prescription contain all of the information necessary to be valid? For example, a prescription is valid for up to one year (less, in some cases) from the date of its writing. Validity cannot be determined if the prescription is not dated. If it is not determined to be valid, then the prescription should not be filled.

A prescription contains three basic types of information: (1) physician information, (2) patient information, and (3) medication information. Physician information should be sufficient to determine whether a licensed and qualified prescriber wrote the prescription. Generally, the physician's contact information should be included. No prescription or medication order is valid without the signature of the prescriber. In the community setting, prescriptions lacking a prescriber signature are not fillable (verbal prescriptions are an exception to this rule). Any verbal prescription order should include all of the information necessary to verify that the caller is, in fact, a valid prescriber or his or her designated agent. In hospital settings, a physician signature is still required to validate a prescription; however, orders given verbally are generally honored, provided that a signature is received within 24 hours.

Safety Note

A prescriber's signature is required for a written prescription to be considered valid.

Patient information should include enough detail to ensure that unique individuals can be pinpointed. Full names, addresses, dates of birth, and phone numbers give multiple points to cross-reference and separate patients who might otherwise have very similar information (e.g., patients with the same first and last names). Date of birth and allergies should always be included, because this information helps confirm the appropriateness of the medication. Comparing phone numbers may not be as helpful in identifying the patient as date of birth, because many people have both home and cellular phones.

Safety Note

A leading zero should precede values less than 1, but a zero should not follow a decimal if the value is a whole number.

Medication information should include the drug name, strength, dose, dosage form, route of administration, refills or length of therapy, directions for use, and dosing schedule. The absence of one of these pieces of information opens the way for medication errors, such as dispensing of the wrong medication, wrong formulation, wrong dosage or strength, or filling an invalid prescription. Prescribing errors include poor handwriting, using nonstandard abbreviations, confusing look-alike and sound-alike drug names (see Appendix B), and using "as directed" instructions. An "as directed" sig does not allow a pharmacist to verify normal recommended dose scheduling or to reinforce correct dosing regimen to patients. A leading zero should always precede a decimal point (e.g., 0.3). A zero should never follow a decimal (e.g., 3.0), because a tenfold error can occur if the decimal point is not detected.

Step 2: Enter Prescription into Computer

Table 12.2 lists the information needed and the resources used to avoid potential errors in the second step of the prescription-filling process.

Data entry is the act of moving important pieces of information from the hard copy of the prescription or medication order to the computer. The ability to perform this function accurately can make the difference between a patient receiving a correct and appropriate medication and a prescription that causes the patient serious harm or death. With so much at stake, concentration and focus on how information is entered is very important. As each piece of information is entered, the prescription should be compared with choices from the computer menu. Check the brand and

TABLE 12.2 Step 2: Enter Prescription into Computer

Information to Check	Resources to Verify Information	Potential Errors Resulting from Failure to Check/Verify Information
Are data choices from the computer menu and those on the prescription the same?	cross-check brand/generic names for identical spelling	look-alike or sound-alike drug selection error made
Does the spelling on the prescription match the drug selection options?		
Do the increments of measure on the drug selection options match those on the prescription (e.g., gram vs. milligram vs. microgram)?	cross-check measure prescribed with drug choices listed	patient given incorrect dose
For the dose selected, do available strengths or concentrations match?	cross-check dose written with available strengths or concentrations on selection menu; cross-check dose or concentrations that use decimals or leading or trailing zeros	patient given incorrect dose
Does the dose or concentration have leading or trailing zeros?		
Does it require a decimal?		
Do available forms match route selected?	match route to formulation choices (e.g., via injection to intravenous [IV] or intramuscular [IM] drugs; via oral route to capsule/tablet/liquid/lozenge)	inappropriate form or formulation selected

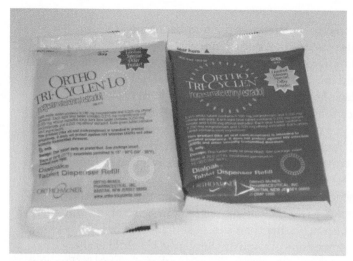

If the technician is not careful or has been distracted, then he or she may select Ortho Tri-Cyclen instead of Ortho Tri-Cyclen Lo at the time of computer entry, resulting in a potential medication error.

generic names and their spelling to determine whether the prescription and computer agree. Special attention should be paid to dosages, formulations, concentration, and the increments of measure. Prescriptions that contain unapproved, error-causing abbreviations must be confirmed with the prescriber.

A common example in the community setting is a prescription received for a brand name cough and cold remedy that the pharmacy does not carry or that the insurance does not cover. Most software lists a generic equivalent that the technician can substitute. However, because many of these agents contain multiple ingredients, it is often difficult to match up an exact generic equivalent. The phar-

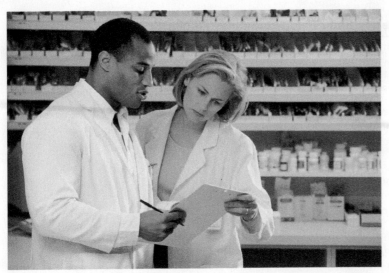

In the hospital pharmacy, it is important to confirm both the drug and the correct route of administration. An IM drug administered as an IV drug can cause a serious medication error.

macist may need to contact the prescriber or select a therapeutically equivalent product.

Does the form or formulation match the route of administration? Be aware that certain concentrations or formulations of a given medication may be associated with a particular route of administration. A common example of the potential for mismatching of form or formulation to route of administration is Depo-Medrol and Solu-Medrol. Both are injectables and have similar dosages, depending on the clinical situation. However, Depo-Medrol is for intramuscular (IM) administration only and is a cloudy suspension when reconstituted. Solu-Medrol is for intravenous (IV) administration and is a clear solution. A serious and potentially fatal medication error could occur if a suspension was inadvertently administered by the IV route. Other examples include ointments vs. creams in topical products or solutions vs. suspensions in ophthalmic medications.

Once computer entry of information has taken place, each data element of the completed entry should be compared with the same data elements on the original prescription before the entry process is finalized. This information should be checked by both the technician and the pharmacist. In the community pharmacy setting, after entry of prescription information into the computer, the medication is then billed to insurance.

Step 3: Perform Drug Utilization Review and Resolve Medication Issues

The potential for medication errors increase as the number of medications that a patient takes increases. This is a common occurrence with many older patients. For every prescription, a computerized drug utilization review (DUR) of the profile by the pharmacy technician should include a check for existing allergies and multiple drug therapy. A medication review should be performed by the pharmacist to check for drug interactions or duplication of therapy (see Table 12.3). For pediatric patients, especially those under two years of age, the dosage on the prescription (and entered into the computer) should be checked carefully. Conversely, patients who are older may require a lower dose because of age-related declines in liver and kidney function and other body changes.

For example, if the patient is allergic to codeine, then can the patient tolerate hydrocodone, a similar narcotic? Did the patient tell the physician about this allergy? Is the patient's allergy a "GI upset" rather than a rash, shortness of breath, or so on? Has the patient received hydrocodone previously? Similarly, if a child is allergic to penicillin, then there is a chance of cross-sensitivity with other antibiotics. The computer software generally flags allergies, but the technician should bring the potential problem to the attention of the pharmacist.

TABLE 12.3 Step 3: Perform DUR and Resolve Medication Issues

Information to Check	Resources to Verify Information	Potential Errors Resulting from Failure to Check/Verify Information
Drug screening: Does the prescribed medication interact with other conditions or medications listed on the profile?	patient, physician, family member, patient profile, interaction screening program, insurance provider electronic messages, drug information resources (e.g., books, call centers, package inserts, patient information handouts)	contraindicated drug dispensed; drug–drug or drug–disease interaction occurs
Pediatric dosing: Are the prescribed dose and frequency of dosing in a pediatric patient consistent with manufacturer recommendations and pharmacy references?	original prescription, physician, package inserts, electronic database, reference texts, pharmacist experience	serious overdose (or underdose) leading to side effects, adverse reactions, or treatment failure
Geriatric dosing: Are the prescribed dose and frequency of dosing in a geriatric patient consistent with manufacturer recommendations and pharmacy references?	original prescription, physician, package inserts, electronic database, reference texts, pharmacist experience	serious overdose leading to side effects or adverse reactions

If a patient receives an antibiotic prescription for Biaxin, then it may interfere and increase the risk of toxicity with other drugs, such as blood thinners and seizure medications. The pharmacist must decide whether to counsel the patient or contact the prescribing physician before approving the filling of this prescription. The computer software also flags duplicate therapy that may lead to serious adverse reactions. For example, is a patient taking both ibuprofen and etodolac? These are similar anti-inflammatory and pain medications that, if taken together for a long period, can then lead to a gastric bleed or ulcer.

Step 4: Generate Prescription Label

Table 12.4 lists the information needed and the resources used to avoid potential errors in the fourth step of the prescription-filling process.

Cross-check the label output from the computer with the original prescription to make sure that a typing error or inherent program malfunction did not alter the information. Is the correct patient name on the label? Are the drug, dose, concentration, and route information identical to those indicated in the original prescription?

Step 5: Retrieve Medication

Table 12.5 lists the information needed and the resources used to avoid potential errors in the fifth step of the prescription-filling process.

Products can contribute to errors by look-alike labels, similarities in brand or generic names, and similar pill shapes or colors. Use NDC numbers, drug names, and

TABLE 12.4   Step 4: Generate Prescription Label

Information to Check	Resources to Verify Information	Potential Errors Resulting from Failure to Check/Verify Information
Has the patient information been cross-checked?	compare label generated with original prescription	wrong patient, medication, or dose selected
Are the label and original prescription identical?	compare label generated with original prescription	wrong patient, medication, or dose selected
Are the leading or trailing zeros and unapproved abbreviations correct?	check with pharmacist or prescriber	incorrect dose selected
Do all the data elements match those of the original prescription (e.g., patient information, medication information, physician information)?	use additional information generated on label reference for verification (e.g., brand/generic names, National Drug Code [NDC], manufacturer name, addresses, phone numbers, age, date of birth)	inappropriate form or formulation selected

TABLE 12.5   Step 5: Retrieve Medication

Information to Check	Resources to Verify Information	Potential Errors Resulting from Failure to Check/Verify Information
Has the available information on the manufacturer's label been used to verify the medication selection?	original prescription, shelf- or bin-labeling systems, manufacturer names, NDC numbers, brand/generic name; pictographic medication verification references or computer programs	medication selection error made
Do the brand and generic name on the label match the product container?		
Do the dose strength and form on the label match those indicated on the product container?	original prescription, shelf- or bin-labeling systems, manufacturer names, NDC numbers, brand/generic name; pictographic medication verification references or computer programs	incorrect dose, form, or formulation selected
Do the National Drug Code (NDC) and manufacturer names match those listed on the label?	bin-labeling systems, NDC numbers; pictographic medication verification references or computer programs	incorrect dose, form, or formulation selected

other information available on manufacturers' labels or patient information handouts to verify selection of the correct product. Use both the original prescription and the generated label when selecting a manufacturer's drug product from the storage shelf. For example, Adderall and Inderal are similar brand names of medication, but a cross-reference of generic names reveals two very different names—amphetamine salts and propranolol.

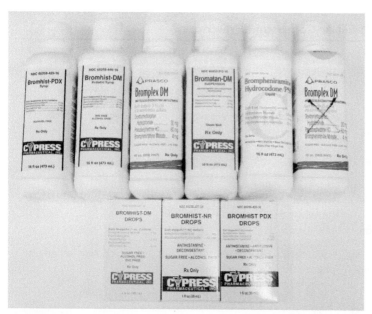

Many formulations and combinations of cough and cold medicine contain brompheniramine in both a syrup formulation for older children and drops for infants; always check the NDC number and original prescription to be sure that the right drug is selected. If you are not sure, then ask the pharmacist.

Wherever possible, use NDC numbers as a cross-check option, because each NDC number is specific to a particular form, packaging, and strength for each medication (discussed in Chapter 3). Therefore the NDC numbers of two forms of a medication, even at the same strength, do not match (nor do two different strengths of the same form of the same medication).

Accidental substitution of one drug or pharmaceutical ingredient for another is one of the most serious events that can occur in pharmacy practice. Because differences in potency or toxicity and failure to receive the drug prescribed for treatment or prevention all present to the patient significant risk of harm or possible death, extreme care must be taken not to substitute drugs that have similar names. Appendix B includes a list compiled by the Institute for Safe Medication Practices (ISMP) containing drug names that are near homonyms (i.e., words that sound alike) or homographs (i.e., words that are similar in spelling). The appendix also includes tips designed by ISMP to prevent dispensing errors.

In one infamous case, *Troppi vs. Scarf, 1971*, a pharmacist accidentally dispensed Nardil, an antidepressant, instead of Norinyl, a contraceptive. The woman who received the incorrect drug gave birth to a child, and the Michigan Court of Appeals held the pharmacist liable not only for the medical expenses incurred in the woman's pregnancy but also for the costs of raising the child.

Some pharmacy practices possess a computer-based pill identification program and use a shelf-labeling system to organize inventory. Such identification programs allow the pharmacist or technician to visually verify the medication dispensed, with a picture of the medication. These sources of information can be used to verify selection of the correct medication.

Step 6: Fill or Compound Prescription

Table 12.6 lists the information needed and the resources used to avoid potential errors in the sixth step of the prescription-filling process.

Calculation and substitution errors are frequent sources of pharmacy-related medication errors. A technician should write out the calculation and have a second person check the answer. Great care should be taken when reading labels and preparing compounded products. Using more than one container of product, preparing more than one product at a time, and paying attention to distractions or interruptions can all contribute to medication errors. Do not allow interruptions or distractions during filling or compounding. If you must stop before filling is complete, then be sure to start over from the beginning.

Safety Note

When compounding, do not allow interruptions. Prepare products one at a time.

TABLE 12.6   Step 6: Fill or Compound Prescription

Information to Check	Resources to Verify Information	Potential Errors Resulting from Failure to Check/ Verify Information
Have the amount to be dispensed and the increment of measure (e.g., gram, milligram, microgram) been reviewed?	amount dispensed (count twice), original prescription	incorrect quantity or incorrect dose dispensed
Does the prescription require a calculation or measurement conversion?	write out calculation and conversions; ask another person to review calculation	incorrect dose dispensed
If you are using equipment, then has the equipment been calibrated recently?	equipment (check calibration), pharmacist, patient information handout, package insert	incorrect dose dispensed
Does the medication dispensed require warning or caution labels?	pharmacist, patient information handout, package insert	administration error made by patient

In addition, all equipment should be maintained, cleaned, and calibrated on a regular basis. Use of technology presents its own unique potentialities for error. In most circumstances, errors caused by technology depend on the user; however, inherent technology malfunctions and program glitches happen. Therefore good safety practices should include a check for the accuracy of technology (e.g., computers, scales, pumps, dispensers) used in the prescription-filling process.

This principle is not limited to sophisticated equipment. The act of cleaning counting trays and spatulas on a regular basis is an important part of medication safety. Consider the potential for serious harm to a patient if the residue or dust from an allergy-causing medication contaminated the patient's prescription. For example, penicillins or sulfa-containing medications should be counted on dedicated counting trays because of the high prevalence of penicillin and sulfa allergy in the general population. If you are dispensing oral hazardous substances, such as methotrexate, then the counting tray must be cleaned to prevent contamination. Cleaning the counting tray with isopropyl alcohol after each of these drugs is dispensed is also recommended.

Caution and warning labels applied to a prescription container are intended to serve as reminders to patients about the most critical aspects of drug handling or administration. In most pharmacy settings with computerized systems, the caution and warning labels are generated with the label and coordinated with more detailed patient information handouts. These labels serve as an ever-present reminder of the most crucial aspects of proper medication administration and should always be included with prescription labeling. Before affixing the auxiliary labels to the prescription vial, ask the pharmacist which ones are priority. Often, as many as six labels are printed or needed but only three may fit on the vial. Be sure to ask about the policy at your practice site.

TABLE 12.7 Step 7: Pharmacist Review and Approval

Information to Check	Resources to Verify Information	Potential Errors Resulting from Failure to Check/ Verify Information
Did the pharmacist review the prepared medication?	original prescription, stock medication bottle or vial, calculations	invalid or out-of-date prescription filled
Can the pharmacist verify the validity of the prescription using the finished product and the information you provide?	original prescription	
Can the pharmacist verify the patient information using the finished product and the information you provide?	original prescription, patient profile, patient, physician or nurse	wrong patient given medication
Can the pharmacist verify the correctness of the prepared prescription based on the medication information provided?	physical appearance of prepared medication; calculations and conversions (provide them), original manufacturer's container, pictographic medication verification, programs, package insert	medication selection error made; incorrect dose, form, or formulation selected; incorrect medication administered

Step 7: Review and Approve Prescription

Table 12.7 lists the information needed and the resources used to avoid potential errors in the seventh step of the prescription-filling process. (Note: The pharmacist must be the one to review and approve the prescription in this step.)

The pharmacist is legally responsible for verifying the accuracy and appropriateness of any prescription that is filled, but it is not practical for pharmacists to verify each step in the filling process. Rather, a pharmacist verifies the quality and integrity of the end product. Thus, providing all available resources that are useful to ensure accurate verification is vital to patient safety. The easiest way to determine what information and resources are important to the verifying pharmacist is to ask whether the information provided with the medication filled allows the pharmacist to retrace the technician's steps in filling the prescription.

Can the pharmacist determine whether the prescription is valid, the patient information accurate, and the medication correctly prepared from the information provided with the finished product? For example, the stock bottle of medication should accompany the labeled medication container and original prescription. The information on the label should be compared to the information on the hard copy of the prescription written by the physician.

One useful exercise to help the technician become aware of what is needed by a pharmacist is to practice checking another's work. Trade finished products with another technician, if possible. Check each other's work. Can you retrace the steps taken to fill the prescription? Can you validate all of the key pieces of information? Undertaking this exercise on a regular basis helps highlight bad habits or short cuts that may open the way for medication errors.

TABLE 12.8 Step 8: Store Completed Prescription

Information to Check	Resources to Verify Information	Potential Errors Resulting from Failure to Check/ Verify Information
Are storage conditions appropriate for the medication (e.g., humidity, temperature, light exposure)?	package insert	medication becomes degraded
Are each patient's medications adequately separated?	physical review of medications placed in bags, boxes, or bins	patient receives medication not intended for him or her; patient fails to receive medication (i.e., omission)
Are storage areas kept neat and orderly?	use of organization systems (e.g., bins, boxes, bags, alphabetizing, numbering, consolidation)	patient receives medication not intended for him or her; patient fails to receive medication (i.e., omission)

Step 8: Store Completed Prescription

Table 12.8 lists the information needed and the resources used to avoid potential errors in the eighth step of the prescription-filling process.

Ensuring the integrity of medication is an important part of medication safety. Many medications are sensitive to light, humidity, or temperature. Failure to store medications properly may result in loss of drug potency or effect. In some cases, improper storage of a drug may result in a degraded product that causes serious harm. The following examples illustrate this type of problem.

- Freezing of certain insulins results in changes in the formulation and absorption by the body. Once the drug has been thawed and administered, the result is a drug that may demonstrate a different effect.
- Nitroglycerin is a product used for angina (i.e., chest pain). Nitroglycerin molecules adhere to plastics; therefore sublingual tablets must be stored in original glass containers under airtight conditions. Failure to maintain proper storage results in loss of drug effect.
- Overheating of fentanyl patches alters how the drug is released from the patch, resulting in a possible overdose.

Simple measures—such as well-organized and clearly labeled storage systems—can help keep a patient's medications together and separate them from those of other patients. Orderly storage decreases the chances that a patient will receive a prescription intended for someone else or not receive his or her own medication because it was given to another patient. Both scenarios are medication errors, and, depending on the drugs in question, each presents the potential to cause serious harm or death if the error goes undetected.

Step 9: Deliver Medication to Patient

Table 12.9 lists the information needed and the resources used to avoid potential errors in the ninth step of the prescription-filling process. In a community pharmacy setting,

TABLE 12.9 Step 9: Deliver Medication to Patient

Information to Check	Resources to Verify Information	Potential Errors Resulting from Failure to Check/Verify Information
Will the appearance of the pill be new to the patient or caregiver?	prescription label, patient, patient education handouts, patient profile	administration error made; patient noncompliant with medication instructions
Is the patient receiving medications intended for him or her?	patient, caregiver, original prescription, patient profile, bar-coding identification system	patient receives medication not intended for him or her; patient fails to receive medication (i.e., omission)
Does the patient or caregiver understand the instructions for use?	pharmacist, patient education handouts, drug information resources	administration error made; patient noncompliant with medication instructions; drug interactions, adverse reactions, degradation of medication occurs because of improper handling or storage
Does the patient or caregiver know what to expect?	pharmacist, patient education handouts, drug information resources	side effects and adverse reactions occur, clinical effect not achieved
Are all of the medications prescribed for the patient included?	consolidation of medications into one bag, bin, or box; use of organization systems (e.g., bins, boxes, bags, alphabetizing, consolidation)	patient fails to receive medication (i.e., omission); therapy not completed

the medication is ultimately received directly by the patient (or a designated representative), whereas, in the hospital, the medication is received by the nurse. In either case, the opportunity exists to verify the prescription information against the knowledge and expectations of the patient or the caregiver. In situations in which the patient directly receives the medication, it is often advised to confirm the patient's date of birth or address rather than name. For example, medications for both Richard C. Smith and Richard V. Smith may be in the storage bins; using a date of birth or an address ensures that the correct medication is dispensed to the correct patient.

Once patient identity is established, the technician should communicate the number of medications that he or she expects to receive and the patient's knowledge of their proper use. If the patient has questions on the medication, then the pharmacist should be consulted. Comparing the completed prescription against the information provided by the patient allows the pharmacist a final opportunity to capture potential errors that were unrecognized in the filling process, as well as potential errors resulting from

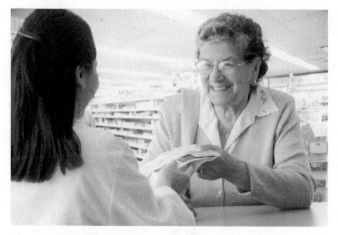

The technician should verify a date of birth or an address to be sure that the correct patient is receiving the correct drug.

gaps or misunderstandings in the patient's knowledge. In this way, errors—such as receipt of medications into the wrong hands or missing medications (i.e., omission of therapy), as well as drug, dosage form, and administration errors—are captured. Ask basic questions of the patient, such as "Do you know what your medicine is for and how to use it?" Call to the patient's attention the auxiliary warning and caution labels on the medication bottle. These inquiries may uncover unexpected drug interactions or side effects or indicate a patient in need of counseling to enhance his or her understanding of correct administration.

In some community pharmacies, a "show-and-tell" technique is employed to prevent medication errors and provide patient education. When the patient comes to the pharmacy to pick up the prescription, the pharmacy technician or pharmacist opens the vial and shows the drug product to the patient. This added step not only helps the patient identify the drug that he or she will be taking but also provides an extra opportunity for the technician or pharmacist to check that the correct drug product was put into the vial. If the patient notices that a refilled drug looks different from a previously filled drug, then the patient has a chance to point this out and have this discrepancy verified. Often the medication is refilled with a different manufacturer's brand of generic medication, which may look different. When the pharmacist relays this information to the patient, the patient will know that the incorrect medication was not dispensed in error. Medication errors can be caught before they ultimately reach the patient in this final check system.

In hospital settings, the medication passes through an extra set of hands (usually a nurse). Adding the caregiver to the medication delivery process provides an additional person to confirm the accuracy and appropriateness of the medication; however, the addition of a new step in the

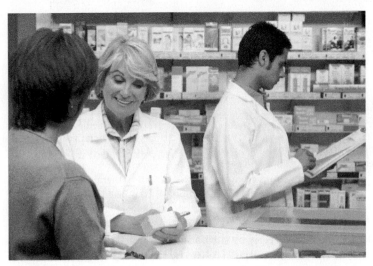

The technician is encouraged to use a "show and tell" technique to minimize medication errors. Showing the medication and reviewing the instructions can ensure that the correct drug was dispensed and that the patient understands the labeled directions.

process creates a new potential for a medication error. The task of medication delivery to the nursing station is mainly filled by technicians; therefore the technician is in the best position to search for potential errors. Take the time to notify the nurse that a newly prescribed medication has been delivered to the floor. This opens the door of communication to ask whether the nurse knows about the medication. Ask whether the medications delivered were all that were expected. If unit dose medication carts are returned to the pharmacy with unused regularly scheduled medication, then the pharmacist or pharmacy technician should follow up with the nurse to determine whether an error of omission occurred. Any discrepancies in the automated drug dispensing machines on the nursing unit should be resolved by the nurse with the technician or pharmacist.

In the treatment of certain diseases, such as cancer, multiple drug therapy combinations, including investigational medications, are prescribed together because they work in concert to treat the disease. If a particular drug is missing from the drug therapy combination, then treatment is incomplete. Like any omission, incomplete therapy is also a medication error. In addition, many of these drugs are extremely toxic. Any dose error could be fatal; therefore communication with the nurse or physician when these medications are delivered to the treatment area is also an opportunity to verify that doses prepared are, in fact, correct. All prescriptions and medication orders (and calculations) for chemotherapy and hazardous substances must be checked extra carefully by both the technician and the pharmacist because of their extreme toxicity.

Without the cooperative efforts of the pharmacy technician, pharmacist, and nurse to ensure safe medication use, a patient's well-being is not safeguarded, and the best health outcome cannot be achieved.

Medication Error Prevention

Learning to prevent medication errors means carefully examining potential points of failure and using available resources to verify information that is given or decisions that are made. Keeping in mind that the most common error in dispensing and administration is drug identification, a pharmacy technician becomes a very valuable asset in ensuring drug safety, for the pharmacy technician "owns" a substantial portion of the prescription-filling process. A pharmacy technician is often the person who first examines a prescription when it is entered into the computer and submitted for filling, and he or she is just as likely to be the last person to handle a medication before it reaches the patient. Consequently, the pharmacy technician often has the most opportunities to prevent a medication error. In addition, pharmacy technicians are also in a position to identify potential sources of error beyond prescription dispensing, because they are the ones who may interact with a patient or nurse when a prescription comes in or goes out of the pharmacy.

Many medication errors also occur during prescribing and administration. Prescriptions often pass through the hands of a pharmacy technician first once they are received from a physician or patient. Prescribers are responsible for ensuring the "five Rs," or five rights (Figure 12.2). In other words, they must ensure that the drug prescribed is the right drug for the right patient at the right strength, given by the

Safety Note

Incorrect drug identification is the most common error in dispensing or administration.

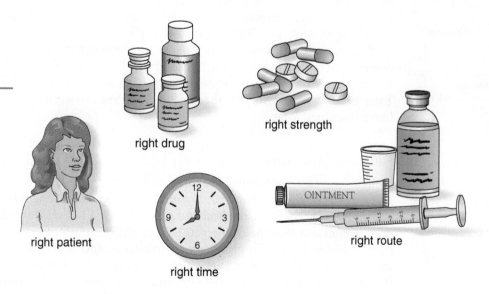

FIGURE 12.2
Five Rs for Patient Drug Administration

right drug

right strength

right patient

right time

right route

right route and administered at the right time. Pharmacy practice overlays physician responsibilities and thereby facilitates patient safety and error prevention by processes that verify the following.

- The correct patient is being given the medications, and other associated medications are correct.
- The correct drug is dispensed (e.g., Effexor vs. Effexor XL).
- The correct dose is prepared, whether for a child or adult, to maintain a correct body concentration or blood level.
- The correct route of administration is indicated (i.e., oral vs. sublingual).
- The appropriate dosage form is prepared (e.g., oral disintegrating tablets are dispensed for a child instead of oral tablets, and antibiotic suspensions are dispensed for administration to an infant). For a child or infant, a measuring device should accompany the medication to ensure that a correct dose is given. However, parents should be reminded to remove the oral syringe cap prior to administration of the medication.
- The correct administration times and the correct conditions for administration (e.g., medications that must be taken with or without food) are indicated.

The Responsibility of the Healthcare Professionals

Working in health care means making a commitment to "first do no harm." This means that healthcare workers must put safety first. As discussed in Chapter 1, the profession of pharmacy exists primarily to safeguard the health of the public. Because the effect of a potential medication error on the patient cannot be predicted, all professionals working in the healthcare system must focus on treating the patient, ensuring the best possible outcome by the safest possible means. As a result, no acceptable level of medication error exists, and each step in the task of filling medication orders should be reviewed with a 100% error-free goal in mind.

Additionally, proper packaging and instruction on medication use are essential to facilitate correct administration by a patient. Through careful listening and observation during a patient or medical staff interaction, a pharmacy technician can identify these potential sources of medication error on the patient's part and actively prevent the error by notifying the pharmacist. By constant surveillance for potential sources of medication error, pharmacy technicians become vital assistants to pharmacists and make a significant contribution to patient safety beyond the borders of the pharmacy.

Pharmacists are ultimately responsible for the accuracy of the medication-filling process, but technicians working in hospital and community pharmacy settings can assist in ensuring safety. By following some basic safe-practice guidelines listed in Table 12.10, pharmacists and pharmacy technicians can work together to create a larger margin of safety.

Patient Education

Patients and caregivers must have the basic knowledge needed to administer, handle, and support safe medication use. Pharmacy technicians can encourage patients to ask questions, relay complete medical and allergy history, and check medications (both prescription and over-the-counter [OTC]) carefully for information instructing when they should be taken. The pharmacy technician should be actively involved in monitoring for potential errors. Although pharmacy technicians cannot counsel patients, they can encourage patients to become informed about their conditions and to ask

TABLE 12.10 General Tips for Reducing Medication Errors

General Tips	■ Always keep the prescription and the label together during the fill process.
	■ Know the common look-alike and sound-alike drugs, and keep them stored in different areas (see Appendix B).
	■ Keep dangerous or high-alert medications in a separate storage area of the pharmacy.
	■ Always question illegible handwriting.
	■ Prescriptions/orders should be correctly spelled, with drug name, strength, appropriate dosing, quantity or duration of therapy, dosage form, and route. Missing information should be obtained from the prescriber.
	■ Use the metric system. A leading zero should always be present in decimal values less than 1.
	■ Question prescriptions/orders that use uncommon abbreviations. Avoid using abbreviations that have more than one meaning, and verify with the prescriber those of which you are unsure.
	■ Be aware of insulin mistakes. Insulin brands should be clearly separated from one another. Educate patients to verify their insulin purchase always.
	■ Keep the work area clean and uncluttered. Keep in the work area only those drugs that are needed for immediate use.
	■ Always verify information at each step of the prescription-filling process.
	■ The label should always be compared with the original prescription by at least two people.
Tips for Pharmacists	■ Check the original Rx, the NDC number, and the drug stock bottle.
	■ Initial all checked prescriptions.
	■ Visually check the product in the bottle.
	■ Cross-reference prescription information with other validating sources.
	■ Encourage documentation of all medication use, including over-the-counter (OTC) medications and diet supplements.
	■ Document all clarifications on orders.
	■ Maintain open lines of communication with patients, healthcare providers, and caregivers.
Tips for Technicians	■ Check the original prescription, the NDC number, and the drug stock bottle.
	■ Regularly review work habits, and actively look for actions to take that improve safe and accurate prescription filling.
	■ Verify information with the patient or caregiver when the prescription is received into the pharmacy and when the filled prescription is sent out of the pharmacy.
	■ Observe, listen to, and report pertinent information that may affect the safety or effectiveness of drug therapy to the pharmacist.
	■ Keep your work area free of clutter.

the pharmacist basic questions about the prescribed medications. Patients should understand the ten key pieces of information about every medication taken, as listed in Table 12.11.

By encouraging patients to ask questions and helping them connect with the pharmacist or appropriate healthcare provider, the technician assists patients in becoming more informed and empowers them to be advocates for their own safety and health.

TABLE 12.11 **Information Patients Must Know About Their Medications**

1. what the brand and generic names are
2. what the medication looks like
3. why they are taking the medication, and how long they will have to take it
4. how much to take and how often, and the best time or circumstances to take a medication
5. what to do if they miss a dose
6. what medications or foods interact with what they are taking
7. whether the medication prescribed is in addition to or replaces medication currently taken
8. what common side effects can be expected and what to do when they are encountered
9. what special precautions should be taken for each particular drug therapy
10. where and how to store the medication

TABLE 12.12 **Work Environment Practices to Promote Safety**

- Automate and bar-code all fill procedures.
- Maintain a clean, organized, orderly, and well-lit work area.
- Provide adequate storage areas with clear drug labels on the shelves.
- Encourage prescribers to use common terminology and only safe abbreviations.
- Provide adequate computer applications and hardware.

Innovations to Promote Safety

The physical work setting can make a major contribution to the overall safety of any pharmacy work environment. Adequate space and clean, well-lit conditions are just some of the basics, in addition to adequate staffing. Work shifts of 12 and 16 hours correlate directly with medication errors. Table 12.12 outlines work environment practices that a pharmacy can create to promote safety and to reduce errors.

Many efforts have been made to minimize the possibility of medication errors. An example in community pharmacy practice is the effort of Target pharmacies to visually redesign the packaging of dispensed medications to help patients take their medication more safely. The ClearRx design uses colored rings to help patients identify medications intended for them, as opposed to those intended for other family members. In addition, the medication container label is larger and more prominently displayed on the container. A consumer survey indicated a stronger preference (85%) for the ClearRx design over conventional labels and medication containers. Consumers felt that the new design improved safety and provided an easier-to-read label featuring better-organized warnings in larger type.

An example of using automation to minimize medication errors in the community pharmacy is the widespread use of bar-coding technology. Walgreens uses bar-coding technology throughout the medication filling process. The prescription information is

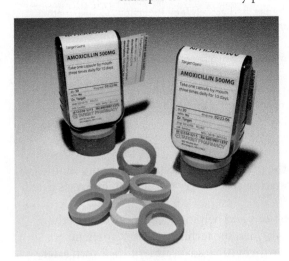

The Target ClearRx packaging is designed to help patients manage their medications by providing information in a clear, easy-to-read format.

entered into the computerized system and the pharmacy personnel scans the selected stock bottle's NDC number when the drug is selected from stock. The computer automatically compares the scanned number against the entered prescription information. If the prescription does not match the selected medication, the system indicates that an incorrect selection has been made. This minimizes the chance of selecting the incorrect drug or dose when filling a prescription. Walgreens also uses bar-coding technology in the final verification by the pharmacist. The computerized database includes images of the physical shape, color, and markings of the medication. The pharmacist can then compare the image on the computer screen against the bar code of the prepared medication to confirm that the appropriate medication was used. Many human errors are prevented by using such automation.

Moving from a paper-based system to an integrated computerized filling system is an easy and common example of how hospitals can also improve efficiency and allow resources to be redirected to increase patient safety and improve quality of patient care. When a pharmacist is actively involved in medication decisions, safety and outcomes for patients are clearly substantially improved.

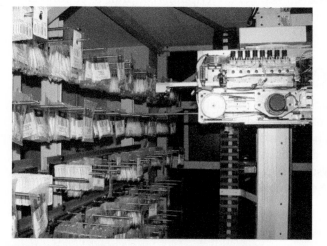

Robot-based medication dispensing increases efficiency and speed of medication delivery without compromising safety. The robot uses bar codes to validate drug selection, significantly reducing the chances of drug selection errors.

An example of this type of change and safety improvement occurred at Medcenter One Health Systems in Bismarck, ND.[3] Originally, the hospital operated a paper-based medication administration system. With this system, the hospital reported about 305 medication administration errors and estimated that an additional 50% went unreported. Pharmacists spent 90% of their time on order entry and distribution.

The Bismarck hospital converted its paper-based system to an electronic medication administration system (Admin-Rx), which used a computer-based bar code validation program that worked together with automated dispensing cabinets (AcuDose-Rx) and robotic filling systems (ROBOT-Rx). These technologic advances empowered the pharmacy technician staff to become more productive; as a result, pharmacists were freed to become more involved in patient care. Ultimately, medication-dispensing errors dropped from 11% to almost 0%.

An electronic medication administration record, or eMAR, is another example of how automation can minimize medication errors. Studies have estimated that 1.5 million medications errors occur each year, 50% of which are in nursing homes. At least 25% of these errors are preventable. As discussed earlier in the chapter, preventable medication errors can lead to the unnecessary deaths of 7000 patients per year.

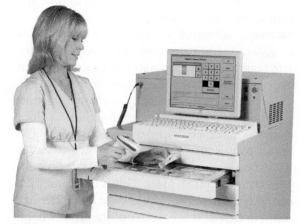

Automated dispensing cabinets such as this one are maintained primarily by technician staff. Use of bar-coding and scanning technology allows nurses to select the right medication.

[3] Personal communication, Dr. Marc Perlman, McKesson Provider Technologies.

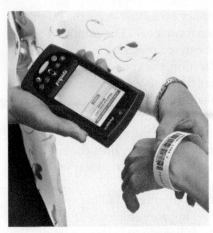

Bar-coding and scanning technologies ensure that the correct patient is receiving the correct medication.

With an **eMAR**, the administration of a medication is documented electronically rather than on paper. The physician directly inputs the medication order from a handheld personal computer or PDA. The order is sent electronically to the pharmacy where it is double-checked for accuracy by the pharmacist. The order is filled by the technician, checked by the pharmacist, and sent to the nursing unit. The medication is then administered to the patient by the nurse often matching the bar code of the medication with the bar code on the patient wristband. The nurse electronically documents that the medication was given.

Studies demonstrate that eMARs can reduce dispensing and administration errors by 75%. The Institute of Medicine encourages the adoption of eMAR technologies for all medication orders in all hospitals by 2011. Similar technologies using the electronic transmission of prescriptions continue to be adopted and encouraged in the community pharmacy.

Medication Error Reporting Systems

If "what is not known cannot be fixed," then the first step in the prevention of medication errors is collection of information and identification of problems. Fear of punishment is always a concern when an error arises; as a result, people may decide not to report an error at all, leaving the door open for the same error to occur again. For this reason, anonymous or *no-fault* systems of reporting have been established. The focus of no-fault reporting is on fixing the problem rather than on assigning blame.

State Boards of Pharmacy

Many efforts have been made to create a safe and comfortable atmosphere for individuals to report medication errors. Many states have mandatory error-reporting systems, but most officials admit that medical errors are still underreported, mostly because of fear of punishment and liability. States such as Florida, Texas, and California have worked to reduce the fear of reporting by passing new regulations that allow pharmacists to document errors and error-prone systems without worry of punishment so long as steps are taken to eliminate weaknesses that might allow such errors to continue. Most state boards of pharmacy do not punish pharmacists for errors, so long as a good faith effort was made to fill correctly. In addition, legislatures have proposed new laws that protect error reports from subpoena. These error reports must be separate from medical records, because all medical records can be subpoenaed, including prescription records.

The task of error reporting is best performed by the authority in charge; however, pharmacy technicians are an integral part of the process of error identification, documentation, and prevention. An understanding of the *what, when, where,* and *why* of error reporting is important for pharmacy technicians, as well as for pharmacists. The final and most important piece of medication error reporting is the delicate task of informing the patient that a medication error has taken place. This is commonly the task of the pharmacist. The circumstances leading to the error should be explained completely and honestly. Patients should understand the nature of the error, what (if any) effects the error may have, and how he or she can become actively involved in preventing errors in the future. Generally speaking, people are more likely to forgive an honest error, but rarely accept hiding of the truth.

The Joint Commission

Organizations also contribute to error-reporting efforts by creating a centralized point through which all members may channel information safely. A well-established example is the Sentinel Event Policy created by the Joint Commission in 1996. A **sentinel event** is an unexpected occurrence involving death, serious physical or psychological injury, or the potential for such occurrences to happen. When a sentinel event is reported, the organization (i.e., hospital, pharmacy, or managed-care company) is expected to analyze the cause of the error (i.e., perform a root-cause analysis), take action to correct the cause, monitor the changes made, and determine whether the cause of the error has been eliminated. Accreditation of hospitals is dependent on demonstrating an effective medical and medication error–reporting system. The Joint Commission supports the recommendations of the Institute of Safe Medication Practices (ISMP): (1) the elimination of certain abbreviations and (2) the education of healthcare professionals regarding frequently confused drug names in order to minimize errors (see Table 12.13).

TABLE 12.13 Problematic Prescription Abbreviations

Unapproved Abbreviation	Correct Form to Use	Potential Error
>	write out greater than	mistaken for number 7
<	write out less than	mistaken for letter L
cc	milliliter or mL	mistaken for units
μg	microgram or mcg	mistaken for mg
hs	half-strength or bed time	mistaken for other meaning
IU	International Unit	mistaken for IV
qd	every day; daily	mistaken for qid
qhr	every hour	nightly or at bedtime
qod	every other day	mistaken for qd
U	units	mistaken for 0 (zero) or V
$MgSO_4$	magnesium sulfate	mistaken for morphine sulfate
MSO_4	morphine sulfate	mistaken for magnesium sulfate
no leading zero (e.g., .2)	leading zero (e.g., 0.2)	mistaken for 2 (e.g.), creating a tenfold error
trailing zero* (e.g., 2.0)	no trailing zero (e.g., 2)	mistaken for 20 (e.g.), creating a tenfold error

*The trailing zero is allowed when required to indicate precision or significant figures, such as in laboratory reports or measurements. However, it should not be used in medication orders.

United States Pharmacopeia

Many professional organizations support patient safety efforts by gathering medical error information and using the data to create tools to support professionals in specific settings or situations. The United States Pharmacopeia (USP) supports two types of reporting systems for the collection of adverse events and medication errors, called MEDMARX and MERP.

The Internet-based program, used by hospitals and health systems, is known as MEDMARX. **MEDMARX** allows institutions and healthcare professionals to anonymously document, analyze, track, and trend adverse events specific to an institution. Since 1998, MEDMARX has received over 1.2 million reports of medication errors.

In 2008 USP published its eighth MEDMARX report, which tracked medication errors from 2003 through 2006. A total of 26,604 medication errors were reported, 1.4% of which caused patient harm; seven cases of death were caused or contributed to by a medication error. More than 60% of medication errors occurred during the dispensing process, with pharmacy technicians involved in 38.5% of the occurrences. Major contributing factors to the errors included distraction in the workplace, excessive workload, and inexperience.

The USP publishes a list of common look-alike and sound-alike drugs that often contribute to medication errors—for example, Prozac vs. Prilosec, Reminyl vs. Amaryl, and diazepam vs. diltiazem. If these medications are not spelled out during a telephone prescription, then an error could occur. The USP stresses awareness of such drugs and promotes adding a medical indication for each drug, as well as encouraging e-prescribing: for example, Reminyl is used for Alzheimer's disease, whereas Amaryl is used to lower blood sugar.

Institute for Safe Medication Practices

The **Institute for Safe Medication Practices (ISMP)** is a nonprofit healthcare agency whose membership is primarily comprised of physicians, pharmacists, and nurses. The mission statement of this organization is "to understand the causes of medication errors and to provide time-critical error reduction strategies to the healthcare community, policy makers and the public."

In concert with the USP, ISMP provides a national voluntary and confidential program called the **Medication Error Reporting Program (MERP)**. This program is designed to allow healthcare professionals to report medication errors directly. According to the program, medication errors include (1) incorrect drug, strength, or dose; (2) confusion over look-alike and sound-alike drugs, such as Adderall vs. Inderal (see Appendix B; (3) incorrect route of drug administration; (4) calculation or preparation errors; (5) misuse of medical equipment; and (6) errors in prescribing, transcribing, dispensing, or monitoring medications. Reports can be completed online. See Table 12.14 for the type of information collected.

ISMP makes the following recommendations to minimize dispensing errors.

- If possible, the order entry person should differ from the one who fills the order, thus adding an independent validation to the order entry process.
- Do not prepare prescriptions from the computer-generated label in case an error occurred at order entry; use the original prescription.
- Keep the original prescription, stock bottle, computer label, and medication container together in the filling process.
- The pharmacist should verify dispensing accuracy by comparing the original prescription with the labeled product with the NDC code of the manufacturer product.

TABLE 12.14 Information Needed for MERP

1. Describe the error or preventable adverse drug reaction. What went wrong?
2. Was this an actual medication error (it reached the patient), or are you expressing concern about a potential error that was discovered before it reached the patient?
3. Patient outcome (if an actual medication error).
4. Type of practice site (hospital, private office, retail pharmacy, drug company, long-term care facility, and so on).
5. The generic names of all products involved.
6. The brand names of all products involved.
7. The dosage form, concentration, or strength, and so forth.
8. How was the error discovered/intercepted?
9. Please state your recommendations for error prevention.

In most pharmacy programs, pharmacists and technicians are taught to check each prescription against the original prescription at least four times.

- check once when the medication is taken from the shelf
- check once during the computer entry and printing of the label
- check once during the filling of the prescription
- check the NDC number of stock bottle

See Table 12.15 for a list of high-alert medications, which have a high incidence of error, in the hospital and community pharmacy.

ISMP has sponsored national forums on medication errors, recommended the addition of labeling or special hazard warnings on potentially toxic drugs, and encouraged revisions of potentially dangerous prescription writing practices. For example, it first promoted the now common practice of using the leading zero. The Joint Commission has adopted many ISMP recommendations, including avoiding the use of common abbreviations, such as "U" or "IU" (spell out), and avoiding the use of the trailing zero when possible (i.e., Lisinopril 5 mg, not 5.0 mg).

ISMP is active in disseminating information to healthcare professionals and consumers, such as e-mail newsletters, journal articles, and videotape training exercises. The pharmacy technician should review the appendices to increase awareness of sources of medication errors. ISMP shares information with the FDA **MedWatch** program, a voluntary program run by the FDA for reporting serious adverse events, as well as the manufacturer. ISMP has both FDA safety and hazard alerts posted on its Web site.

TABLE 12.15 High Alert Medications

amiodarone	narcotic analgesics
chemotherapeutic agents	oral hypoglycemics
colchicine injection	Synthroid
Digoxin	TPN solutions
epidural or intrathecal medications	warfarin
hypertonic dextrose	Zantac liquid
morphine sulfate liquid	

Personal Prevention Strategies

Take care of yourself, and take care of your patients. Refusing to work a 12 or 16 hour shift is not always a realistic option, but there are ways recommended by HPSO (Healthcare Provider Service Organization) that you can take care of yourself to combat fatigue and help prevent errors.

- Get enough sleep. Experts say that 8 hours of sleep a night is best, so go to bed early enough. Avoid staying up until you cannot keep your eyes open any longer; as soon as you feel sleepy, turn out the lights and turn in.
- Exercise regularly. You may feel more tired at first, but regular exercise should eventually help boost your energy level. Plan to do your workout several hours before bedtime so that you are not keyed up when it is time to sleep.
- Take breaks at work. Even when things are busy, take breaks to relax and revitalize yourself, even if it means going outside to clear your head for a couple of minutes. You will not be much help if you cannot think clearly.
- Be wise about food. Eat a well-balanced diet for optimal energy. During your scheduled time, avoid sugar-laden snacks and choose complex carbohydrates for stamina.
- Avoid alcohol. A nightcap at home may relax you at first, but as the alcohol wears off, it disrupts your normal sleep patterns.
- Cut the caffeine. Coffee, tea, and other drinks that contain caffeine do not prevent fatigue; they just hide it. Limit your caffeine intake, especially near bedtime.

If you feel tired on the job, then do not be afraid to ask for help, such as having a colleague double-check your dosage calculations.

Chapter Terms

assumption error an error that occurs when an essential piece of information cannot be verified and is guessed or presumed

capture error an error that occurs when focus on a task is diverted elsewhere and therefore the error goes undetected

eMAR an electronic medication administration record, used to minimize medication errors

extra dose error an error in which more doses are received by a patient than were prescribed by the physician

human failure an error generated by failure that occurs at an individual level

Institute for Safe Medication Practices (ISMP) a nonprofit healthcare agency whose primary mission is to understand the causes of medication errors and to provide time-critical error reduction strategies to the healthcare community, policymakers, and the public

medical error any circumstance, action, inaction, or decision related to health care that contributes to an unintended health result

medication error any preventable event that may cause or lead to inappropriate medication use or patient harm while the medication is in the control of the healthcare professional, patient, or consumer

Medication Error Reporting Program (MERP) a USP program designed to allow healthcare professionals to report medication errors directly to the Institute for Safe Medication Practices (ISMP)

MEDMARX an Internet-based program of the USP for use by hospitals and healthcare systems for documenting, tracking, and identifying trends for adverse events and medication errors

MedWatch a voluntary program run by the FDA for reporting serious adverse events for medications and medical devices; serves as a clearinghouse for information on safety alerts and drug recalls

omission error an error in which a prescribed dose is not given

organizational failure an error generated by failure of organizational rules, policies, or procedures

root-cause analysis a logical and systematic process used to help identify what, how, and why something happened, in order to prevent recurrence

selection error an error that occurs when two or more options exist and the incorrect option is chosen

sentinel event an unexpected occurrence involving death or serious physical or psychological injury or the potential for occurrences to happen

technical failure an error generated by failure because of location or equipment

wrong dosage form error an error in which the dosage form or formulation is not the accepted interpretation of the physician order

wrong dose error an error in which the dose is either above or below the correct dose by more than 5%

wrong time error a medication error in which a drug is given 30 minutes or more before or after it was prescribed, up to the time of the next dose, not including as needed orders

Chapter Summary

- Pharmacy technicians play a crucial role in the prevention of medication errors.
- Knowing the potential causes and categories of medication errors is the first step toward preventing them from occurring.
- Medication errors caused by patients have physical and social causes.
- Once errors are identified, corrective measures should be put in place and permanent elimination of the source of error should be the goal.
- Each step of the medication-filling process has the potential to produce a medication error.
- Specific practices, careful work habits, and a clean work environment promote patient safety and decreases illness and injury caused by medication errors.
- Although pharmacy technicians cannot counsel patients concerning their medications, they can encourage them to ask questions of the pharmacist.
- Helping patients to become more informed also empowers them to be advocates for their own safety and health.
- Automation and technological advances can minimize medication errors.
- Several medication error reporting systems exist. Pharmacy personnel should be familiar with these sources and use them to confidentially report errors so that they do not occur again.

Chapter Review

Checking Your Understanding

Choose the best answer from those provided.

Additional Quiz Questions

1. For every 250 prescriptions dispensed in a community pharmacy, how many contain a medication error of some type?
   a. None
   b. 1
   c. 4
   d. 25

2. Which of the following scenarios is *not* a patient-caused medication error?
   a. The patient took an antibiotic with a meal when instructions said to take it on an empty stomach.
   b. The patient forgot an antibiotic dose yesterday, so he or she took an extra dose today.
   c. The patient did not receive a sufficient quantity of antibiotic suspension from the pharmacy.
   d. The patient took antibiotics left over from the last time that he or she was sick.

3. A wrong dose error occurs when a dose is either above or below the correct dose by more than
   a. 1%.
   b. 3%.
   c. 5%.
   d. 8%.

4. A patient applied a heating pad to an area where he or she also applied a potent narcotic skin patch, causing the patch to release all the medication at once, resulting in an overdose. This is an example of
   a. technical failure from improper application.
   b. human error.
   c. product defect error.
   d. physician prescribing error.

5. Filling a prescription with generic metoprolol when the drug requested was Toprol XL is an example of which type of error?
   a. assumption error
   b. selection error
   c. capture error
   d. None of the above

6. When receiving a new prescription, which of the following should a pharmacist or technician avoid doing?
   a. When handwriting is difficult to read, verify all drug information with the pharmacist, appropriate drug references, and/or the prescriber.
   b. Use a trailing zero when the dose written is for a whole number (i.e., 10.0 mg).
   c. Cross-check patient information on the written prescription with the patient.
   d. Verify that the patient has not experienced any new drug allergies and that all profile information is current and correct.

7. Which of the following sources of information is useful to verify that the correct medication has been selected from the shelf to fill the prescription order?
   a. generic and/or brand names on unit stock drug container
   b. NDC number
   c. drug name on original prescription
   d. All of the above

8. The most important factor in medication error reporting is to
   a. provide the medication at no cost to the patient.
   b. cover up the error from the pharmacist supervisor.
   c. immediately notify the USP.
   d. notify the patient.

9. At a minimum, patients and caregivers should understand ten key pieces of information about their prescription. Which of the following pieces of information is *not* included in those ten key pieces of information?
   a. the name of the medication
   b. best times to pick up the prescription
   c. where to store the medicine
   d. pill shape and color

10. A sentinel event is defined by the Joint Commission as
    a. an unexpected occurrence involving death or serious physical or psychological injury, or the potential for the occurrence to happen.
    b. an unexpected outcome as the result of a drug reaction or side effect.
    c. a computer program that looks out for medication errors in a hospital pharmacy.
    d. an adverse reaction with a vaccine.

Thinking Like a Pharmacy Tech

1. At a minimum, patients and caregivers should understand ten key pieces of information about their prescriptions. Name five of those key pieces of information.

2. Table 12.10 outlines activities that a pharmacist can do to reduce errors. Choose one and briefly describe how a pharmacy technician can support a pharmacist engaged in these activities to improve patient safety.

3. Using Appendix B, locate at least two pairs of drug names that are spelled similarly. Write a brief commentary on the differences between the drugs in each pair and what might happen if they were accidentally switched in the pharmacy and given to the patient. Would this mix-up be life-threatening?

Communicating Clearly

1. Many times, a patient has a question but may hesitate to ask the nurse, pharmacist, or physician because he or she is "so busy." Any time that a patient hesitates to ask a question or to understand his or her own condition better, a chance to improve the patient's health or to avoid an adverse event is lost. What could you do or say as a pharmacy technician to help the customer make the connection to the needed information?

2. Using Appendix B, locate at least two pairs of drug names that are sound-alike names when spoken out loud. Say them to a classmate across the room to see how easily they can be mistaken for each other. Repeat the exercise with other drug names and other students.

Researching on the Web

1. Choose a state, and visit that state's board of pharmacy Web site. Review the state regulations, and identify the information that must be present on a prescription to be valid in that state.

2. Visit the Target ClearRx Web site at www.target.com/pharmacy and click on "See What's New." Watch the video. What changes were made to improve Target medication vials? Discuss how these changes might improve patient safety.

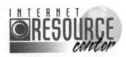 For further study of chapter-related topics, explore the Web links in the Web Center at www.emcp.net/pharmpractice4e.

Human Relations and Communications

13

Learning Objectives

- Explain the role of the pharmacy technician as a member of the customer care team in a pharmacy.
- State the primary rule of retail merchandising.
- Identify and discuss desirable personal characteristics of a pharmacy technician.
- Identify the importance of verbal and nonverbal communication skills.
- Provide guidelines for proper use of the telephone in a pharmacy.
- Identify and resolve linguistic and cultural differences in working with a customer.
- Identify and resolve problems related to mental and physical disabilities in working with a customer.
- Define discrimination and harassment, and explain the proper procedures for dealing with these issues.

- Identify examples of professionalism in the pharmacy.
- Explain the importance of managing change and being a team player in the pharmacy.
- Explain the appropriate responses to rude behavior on the part of others in a workplace situation.
- Define the role of pharmacy personnel in emergency situations in the community.
- Identify and discuss the important areas of the regulations of the Health Insurance Portability and Accountability Act (HIPAA).
- Discuss the importance of protecting patient privacy in the pharmacy.

 Preview chapter terms and definitions.

In addition to being an important part of the healthcare system, the community pharmacy is also a place of business, and the technician must be sensitive to customer service responsibilities similar to those appropriate in any retail setting. A customer service approach is important in the hospital setting as well, especially when providing support and information to other healthcare providers. Examples of providing first-rate customer service are provided for both retail and hospital pharmacy settings. In all pharmacy practice settings, maintaining patient confidentiality and following federal laws protecting patient privacy are crucially important.

Personal Service in the Contemporary Pharmacy

Since the Millis Study Commission Report in 1975 and the Hepler-Strand Report of 1990, the pharmacy profession has continued to undergo an extensive self-analysis and reevaluation of its duties and goals (see Chapter 1). The upshot of this reexamination of the profession has been an increased emphasis on patient-oriented pharmacy, with the provision of more information and counseling regarding medications. The pharmacist is now universally recognized as far more than a dispenser of drugs. The pharmacist has the following equally important duties.

- Identify known allergies, drug interactions, or other contraindications for a given prescription.
- Make certain that a given medication will not be harmful to a patient, given that patient's age and his or her medical and prescription history.
- Ensure that a patient understands what medication he or she is taking, why he or she is taking it, how it should be taken, and when it should be taken.
- Triage patient assessment of self-limited illnesses and recommend appropriate over-the-counter (OTC) or diet supplements to the patient.

Just as the pharmacist increasingly plays a more clinical role, so the pharmacy technician is increasingly expected to be much more than a cash register operator, a stock person, or an all-around pharmacy "gofer." Today the technician is viewed as an important part of the customer service team within the pharmacy.

In the 1960s and 1970s, at the height of the era of mass merchandising, customers became accustomed to large, impersonal supermarkets, department stores, and pharmacy superstores, with their numbered rows of merchandise and automated, barcoded checkout stations. In the 1980s, retail merchandisers began to realize that the mass-merchandising model adopted in the 1960s was terribly flawed. Customers missed the days of personal service (i.e., attending to the individual customer's needs) associated with the small, independent neighborhood pharmacy of the past, where everyone affectionately called the pharmacist "Doc."

For this reason, many of the large department store chains reorganized their operations to create separate small operational entities, known as *boutiques,* within their larger stores. They also began extensive training programs to improve the quality of customer service. In pharmacy, a new and welcome emphasis on personal service has also returned.

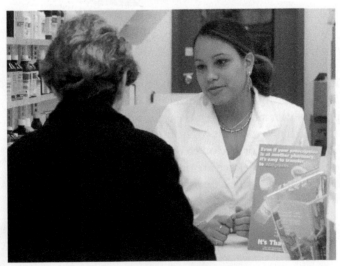

Courteous and attentive assistance makes a good impression on customers and influences their return to your pharmacy.

One mass-marketing research firm conducted an experiment involving bank tellers. In the experiment, one group of tellers was instructed to lightly touch customers on the hand or wrist at some point during each teller transaction. A second control group was instructed to carry out transactions as usual, without this "personal touch." Exit surveys of customer satisfaction were then conducted, with dramatic results. Although largely unaware that they had been touched during their teller transactions, those customers who had been touched reported a 40% higher satisfaction rate with the overall quality of service of their banks. The lesson to be learned from this research is not that one should make a habit of touching customers; indeed, touching should probably be avoided in most cases. However, a little personal attention goes a long way. A courteous tone of voice, a smile, eye contact, a listening ear, and a bit of assistance finding merchandise or holding a door can go a long way toward making customers think of the pharmacy in which you work as a pleasant place to visit and do business.

Even if the immediate task is not customer-oriented, the technician should then remember the primary rule of retail merchandising:

> At all times you are representing your company to the patient or customer. Remember that in a pharmacy you are, in a legal sense, an agent of your employer and entering into a contract to provide care to the patient. Your employer must "answer" for all of your actions.

Characteristics of the Pharmacy Technician

A successful pharmacy technician must possess a wide range of skills, knowledge, and aptitudes. He or she must have a broad knowledge of pharmacy practice and a dedication to providing a critical healthcare service to customers and patients. In addition, the pharmacy technician must have high ethical standards, eagerness to learn, a sense of responsibility toward patients and toward the healthcare professionals with whom he or she interacts, a willingness to follow instructions, an eye for detail, manual dexterity, facility in basic mathematics, good research skills, and the ability to perform accurately and calmly in hectic or stressful situations. The ability to accurately multitask (work on several projects at the same time) is a useful skill in every pharmacy environment. In addition to these skills, displaying a professional attitude with good communication and problem-solving skills is a very important characteristic for the pharmacy technician.

Attitude

Attitude is the overall emotional stance or disposition that a worker adopts toward his or her job duties, customers, employer, and coworkers. Attitude is extremely important in customer relations. In the hospital pharmacy, technicians often conduct their jobs behind the scenes, ordering and stocking items in the pharmacy area, retrieving stock for compounding operations, maintaining records, filling prescription or unit dose carts, making IVs, and cleaning. However, in a community pharmacy, the technician is on the front line of customer service. The technician should maintain a positive attitude, even on those days that are busier than usual and even when the technician's health may not be up to par.

Attitude also means taking pride in your workplace. The technician should provide feedback or offer suggestions to the supervising pharmacist or store manager on ways to improve the operation and serve customers better. Examples may include stocking OTC products, customer drop-off or pickup queue lines, insurance issues, ordering from wholesalers, work schedules, and so on. The technician should not criticize management but instead offer well-thought-out, constructive solutions. Being an invaluable asset to the overall pharmacy operation can often assist you in advancement and in negotiating a pay raise in the future.

Appear Professional **Appearance** is the overall look that an employee has on the job, including dress and grooming. Customers hope for a high degree of cleanliness and professionalism from their pharmacy. After all, they are entrusting their health or the health of their loved ones to the operation for which you work. Proper attire, grooming, and personal hygiene are important to convey a positive professional atmosphere to a customer. A pharmacy employee with unkempt hair or a uniform smock thrown over a pair of jeans makes a bad impression. The customer may not directly register these facts, and yet he or she goes away with a vague impression that the pharmacy is not a professional operation. The technician should wear a clean lab coat and name tag at all times. This sets the desired professional atmosphere and immediately identifies the technician as an employee of the pharmacy. However, the technician must follow the dress code of the pharmacy. The dress code may be crisp and professional or more relaxed and casual.

Respond to Customers Modern chain pharmacies are often large, complex places. When customers enter, often the first thing they do is stand in the middle of the floor, looking around for the part of the store where the product they seek is to be found. A good employee thus continually scans the area around him or her, looking for customers who are lost or confused or need help. In the hospital setting, your customer may be someone who is visiting a patient or a physician, a nurse, or another hospital worker who needs your help.

A pharmacy technician must be observant of customer needs. Often a customer is reluctant to ask for help, to avoid imposing on the technician or pharmacist's time. **Triage** customer needs in everyday practice by sorting requests or needs and ranking them by priority. In the community pharmacy, many things may be happening at once: you are cashiering a sale, the phone is ringing, a customer is waiting for help in the OTC aisle, and five patients are waiting to pick up their prescriptions. Acknowledge the customers by a simple statement such as, "I will be right with you." Then, when attending to their needs, you might say something like, "Thank you for waiting." Keeping your eye on the customer and meeting his or her needs applies to any retail operation. However, in other situations, such as a stat order in the hospital pharmacy, the order of requests needs to be ignored in response to a more urgent medical situation.

A major emphasis in modern pharmacy is to demonstrate professional caring or empathy toward the patient. Perhaps the patient who comes into your pharmacy has recently lost a loved one, or a loved one has become seriously ill, or the patient may have been recently diagnosed with a serious illness. Perhaps he or she has just been discharged from the hospital or spent the better part of a day or night at the emergency room. A recently widowed woman may approach the pharmacy with an inquiry about insurance plans; she may be confused about her Medicare Part D plan because her husband previously made all of the health insurance decisions.

Patients (and often pharmacy staff) are often confused with a myriad of insurance issues. Here are some common insurance questions that a technician may deal with in the community pharmacy.

- Why isn't this drug covered by my insurance?
- What do you mean my insurance is expired?
- Why isn't my new infant son covered on my insurance?
- What do you mean my insurance plan has changed?
- Why is my co-pay $60 on my antibiotic prescription?
- What is a prior authorization, and why do you need it?
- Why do you have to call the physician to clarify my prescription? I am in a hurry!

- What do you mean you cannot fill my [narcotic] prescription today?
- Why did you give me a 30 day supply when my physician wrote a 90 day supply of my medication?
- What do you mean you do not have my medication in stock?
- Why have you only filled my prescription with a 5 day supply?
- I am out of my heart medication and the physician's office is closed. What can I do?

The pharmacy technician is often the messenger of bad news when interacting with the patient. Take the necessary time to explain why the prescription could not be filled or was only partially filled. A pharmacy technician should always alert the patient to a change in manufacturer of a generic (different color or shape) or an out-of-stock or partial fill of their medication, and he or she should let the patient know when the medication will be in stock and available for pickup. At times, it may be necessary to fill the prescription with two different brands of the same medication; if so, then the patient must be alerted to this change at the time of pickup.

Know Your Pharmacy Few things are as frustrating to a customer as asking for help and getting an insufficient or inaccurate response. Often a customer is uncertain about what he or she is looking for or whom to ask for help. Once you spot that uncertain look, ask courteously, "May I help you?" Then, after the customer's response, you may have to ask some clarifying questions. If, for example, the customer is looking for aspirin, then he or she may need to know not only where OTC analgesic products are stocked in the store but also where to locate a specific analgesic (e.g., baby aspirin, aspirin for a migraine, liquid form for children, an enteric-coated form for those whose stomach cannot tolerate conventional analgesic dosage forms). If possible, escort the customer to the place where the merchandise is located and then help him or her find it.

In other cases, the customer may want to know whether to take aspirin or another OTC analgesic such as ibuprofen; or he or she may ask whether it is acceptable to take ibuprofen with blood pressure medication. The pharmacy technician can triage or sort out various requests by the customer: those involving product location, availability, or price can be handled by the technician. If there is a question requiring professional judgment, you may say to the customer, "That is a good question; let me have you speak with the pharmacist."

A pharmacy technician often helps customers find products in the retail pharmacy.

If a customer requests a product outside of the immediate pharmacy department area, then assist him or her by providing the aisle number and store location, or page a store manager if you are busy. If a customer requests a specific product that is not in stock, then check with the manager or consult the wholesaler notebook to see whether a special order can be made; if so, then let the customer know when the product should be received (usually the next day, unless on the weekend) and get his or her name and phone number for a courtesy call. If a product is out of stock, then be sure to apologize to the customer and offer a "rain check." Making an extra effort to provide customer service pays off in long-term dividends and return business for any retail operation.

Smile and Make Eye Contact The goodwill that you communicate always comes back to you in one way or another. Making a personal connection with the customer is important. Learning and greeting patients by name is especially important in a community pharmacy. Patients are far more likely to return to a pharmacy where they have received personal attention than to one where they have not. Some pharmacists have learned sign language so that they can communicate with patients who are hearing impaired.

Eye contact is especially important to older patients and patients who may be deaf or hard of hearing. A person who is hard of hearing learns to read lips informally to supplement the voice that he or she hears. If you speak with your head turned away, then the person may hear you but may not be able to interpret fully what you have said. This is especially important if your pharmacy has a drive-through window—it is often difficult to communicate over engine and ambient noise. Often you may need to repeat the customer request—whether it is verifying patient name, birth date, address, or other information. Remembering to make eye contact ensures that you are looking directly at the person. In addition, older generations of Americans often associate eye contact with honesty, sincerity, and respect.

Verbal and Nonverbal Communication

Communicating effectively takes practice. Once you have the knowledge and vocabulary needed to function effectively in the pharmacy, you can acquire the necessary verbal communication skills with time. Model yourself after someone whom you admire, but keep in mind that some of your coworkers have a different role and thus different communication needs and styles. Verbal communication skills take practice, and pronouncing medical terms and drug names is one hurdle that you can overcome with study. Listening and asking a coworker to pronounce words for you are the best ways to learn. Repeat difficult words to yourself several times. You may also find it helpful to keep a pocket-sized reference on drug names handy and make notes in it regarding pronunciation and usage.

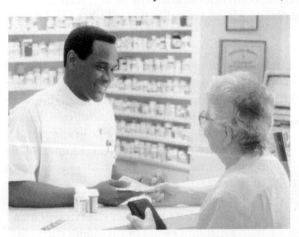
A pharmacy technician should maintain good eye contact and a pleasant attitude while talking with patients.

A pharmacy technician needs good verbal communication skills in the receipt of prescriptions and also when assisting the patient for an OTC medication. The technician performs a valuable service by gathering information and relaying this information to the pharmacist. One way to gather information from a patient is to ask well phrased questions, which is appropriate to the type of information needed. A **closed-ended question** is asked in a yes-or-no format, such as "Do you have a headache?" or "Have you tried aspirin?" An **open-ended question** allows the patient to share more information about his or her illness and is more helpful to the pharmacist in recommending the best treatment. Asking open-ended questions to the patient such as "Please describe your headache pain for me" is always preferable.

Nonverbal communication is easy to understand, and you need only pay attention to the other party to interpret what is being conveyed. As small children, people learn how to interpret nonverbal communication. Facial expression, eye contact, body position, and tone of voice are all methods of communicating without using words. Mannerisms and gestures often indicate agreement or disagreement. The mood of the other party can often be determined through nonverbal communication. Although each individual is unique and may exhibit unusual habits with certain moods, many generalizations can be made regarding nonverbal communication. Simple observation and listening can be effective ways to supplement the verbal portion of what you are hearing.

The following examples demonstrate nonverbal communication in the pharmacy.

Poor: Talk to a patient while filling a prescription or answering the phone.

Better: Ask the patient to wait a moment, complete filling the prescription or place the telephone caller on hold (or have another staff member take the call), and go down to the front counter or private counseling area and talk to the patient. Determine whether you can help the patient or direct the patient to speak with the pharmacist if necessary.

Poor: Show surprise through open-mouthed facial expressions when a patient shares a diagnosis with you (e.g., HIV, gonorrhea, syphilis, or depression).

Better: Be nonjudgmental, with minimal facial expressions, and assist the patient with the information or products that he or she needs. Be empathetic and show genuine concern. Remember that all patient medical information is confidential and protected by law.

Poor: Talk to a patient about an OTC recommendation with your arms crossed, at some distance from the patient.

Better: Move closer to the patient, ask open-ended questions, listen carefully, and be aware of both your body movements and those of the patient. Crossed arms often convey some barrier to communication, such as that you are too busy to help the patient.

The flip side of verbal communication is, of course, listening. Listening to the words and the voice that you are hearing is important. Maintain eye contact with the person speaking and send the speaker nonverbal signals indicating that you are genuinely interested in what he or she is saying. Learn to tolerate your own silence. Ask questions to clarify issues and repeat portions of the conversation to confirm that you have correctly heard what was said. Always use a nonjudgmental expression and tone of voice. Never let the patient feel that he or she is imposing or that your time is more valuable than the patient's.

Use Common Courtesies In every interaction with a customer, use courteous words and phrases. Begin and end interactions, even the briefest ones, with ceremonial courtesies such as "Good afternoon" and "Have a nice day." "Please" and "Thank you" should become a part of your regular vocabulary. Practice courteous speech, as demonstrated in these examples.

Poor: What do you need?

Better: May I help you?

Poor: It's over there.

Better: That's in aisle three. Follow me, and I'll show you.

Poor: It's $8.39.

Better: That will be $8.39, please.

Poor: Next?

Better: May I help whoever is next? *or* Hello, Mr. Stajich. Are you here to pick up or drop off a prescription?

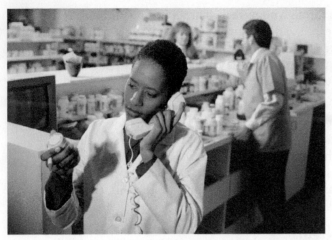

Pharmacy technicians need to be able to communicate effectively over the phone to both customers and healthcare professionals.

If a mistake was made in filling the prescription, then apologize immediately and bring it to the attention of the pharmacist according to the policy of the pharmacy. Make eye contact and admit an honest mistake instead of attempting to cover it up. The pharmacist will then explain to the patient how the mistake occurred and how it will be corrected. If no mistake was made, then the technician should be understanding and address patient concerns. If there is a delay in filling the prescription, then apologize to the customer for the inconvenience.

Telephone Courtesies Customers and healthcare professionals often contact pharmacies by telephone. The following are some guidelines for using the telephone properly.

- When you answer the phone, identify yourself and the pharmacy as follows: "Good morning, Oakhurst Pharmacy. My name is Ali. How may I help you?"
- Always begin and end the conversation with a conventional courtesy such as "Good morning" and "Thank you for calling." Stay alert to what the caller is saying and use a natural, conversational voice. You should be friendly but not too familiar with the caller. When speaking to patients who are hard of hearing, speak clearly, pronounce each word distinctly, and be prepared to repeat yourself.
- If the caller is calling in a new prescription, then you may need to turn over the phone to a pharmacist. In most states, technicians are not allowed by law to take prescriptions over the telephone. However, you should learn the regulations for the state in which you are employed.
- If the caller has questions about the administration or effects of a medication or about a medical condition, adverse reaction, or drug interaction, then place the customer on hold and refer the call to a licensed pharmacist.
- Make sure that any information you provide is accurate. Giving incorrect directions to a customer in need of a prescription can be a life-threatening mistake.
- If the caller is requesting a refill, then politely ask for his or her name or prescription number. After verifying that the prescription can be refilled and dispensed, give the patient an approximate time when it will be ready for pickup, and thank him or her for calling ahead.
- Depending on the regulations in your state and the procedures of your pharmacy, you may be authorized to handle prescription transfers or to provide information related to prescription refills. Follow the procedures outlined by your supervising pharmacist.
- If a customer is calling about a medical emergency or a prescription error, then refer the call to your supervising pharmacist.

Be Sensitive to Cultural and Language Differences and Disabilities Often pharmacies are located in areas catering to a diverse customer base. Differences in age, gender, ethnicity, language, culture, economic status, educational background, and disability will be part of your everyday practice in the pharmacy. Some male customers may feel more comfortable discussing questions on condom use or erectile dysfunction drugs with a male technician or pharmacist. Similarly, female issues may arise in the case of a female customer. What is most important is that the patient feels comfortable and receives the correct information.

If you cannot understand a customer because of a language difference, then do not speak louder or in a deliberate, slow, and punctuated manner. Simply enunciate your words and avoid using slang terms or abbreviations, because the person may not be familiar with them. Apologize courteously for your language deficiency if necessary, and find another store employee who can communicate in the customer's native tongue. If a translator is not available, then the pharmacist may have counseling sheets that use drawings, diagrams, and clocks made especially for this purpose. Some computer software programs print patient information in different languages. If you have special skills, such as other languages, then be sure to add that information to your résumé. See Appendix C for common Spanish phrases that may be used in pharmacy.

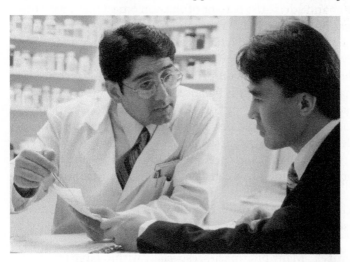

Pharmacy staff need to be able to assist customers from other cultural groups.

Ethnicity and cultural differences should also be taken into account. If the pharmacy where you are employed has a large group of patients from a particular ethnicity or culture, then you should make an effort to become familiar with that culture's diet, health habits and beliefs, and courtesies. For example, Hispanic patients may rely more on self-care, OTC medications, and diet supplements and less on physician visits. Patients from the Far East have a stronger belief in herbs than prescription medicines because herbal medicine is a major part of their culture. If you practice in rural America, then you may see and hear more about home remedies. Knowing more about the culture helps you provide higher-quality service and shows customers that you care about them. The pharmacy technician should be sensitive to these issues and try to overcome barriers.

Some patients may have varying degrees of mental or physical disabilities. If you are interacting with a mentally challenged patient, then you may need to be understanding in obtaining necessary demographic, insurance, and health information. Medication counseling by the pharmacist should be directed at the appropriate level—do not use medical jargon that may confuse the patient. If you see a patient on crutches in obvious pain in the waiting room, or a parent with a sick child, then alert the pharmacist so that the patient's prescriptions can be filled as expeditiously as possible.

A patient may be blind or partially blind, deaf or hard of hearing. These disabilities challenge the creativity of any technician. Older patients may have difficulty hearing, reading labels or printed information, or opening prescription vials. Careful listening, large print, and non-childproof lids may resolve some of these problems. If you have a particular skill, such as knowing sign language or Braille, then you could be a tremendous asset to your community.

Many patients may not have prescription drug insurance for various reasons, such as being unemployed, employed part-time without benefits, or unable to pay the high cost of self-insurance. If you can offer some lower-cost alternatives, such as store brand generics or calling the physician's office to find an alternative lower-cost prescription, then the patient often appreciates your help. If you have a free clinic or community health center in your area, then you might suggest these to the patient.

Observe whether or not the patient comprehends the information. What is most important is that patients without insurance coverage should not be treated differently from anyone else.

Problem Solving

Being a good problem solver for patient or workplace issues is a valuable asset for the pharmacy technician. One of the more important skills to develop is handling the difficult patient. Calming a patient who does not want to wait the estimated time or, more often, who does not understand a prescription insurance plan may be difficult. For example, if there is an insurance problem (such as those discussed previously), then offer to call the patient's insurance plan and resolve the problem; if you are busy, then offer to call the plan later and advise the patient of the outcome. Or if a patient needs an out-of-stock medication today, then it is common practice (and generates goodwill) for the pharmacy staff to call around to a neighboring pharmacy and send the patient to that pharmacy to have the prescription filled.

Problem solving might have an impact on your personal life. For many technicians, working in the pharmacy must be carefully balanced with home life (spouse and children), as well as going back to school. Staying focused and organized is critically important. Problems at home or school should not interfere with your performance at work; a lack of focus could lead to a serious medication error. If you need to work less often, or need to take some time off to deal with personal issues, then be sure to talk to your pharmacy supervisor so that allowances can be made without disrupting patient care.

Problem solving may include following written or unwritten policies and procedures in the pharmacy or resolving potential conflicts with management.

Follow Policies and Procedures Many pharmacies, especially within large retail chains and hospital pharmacies, have polices and procedures covering a wide range of activities, including technician responsibilities in customer care. A written manual is often necessary in a pharmacy with multiple pharmacists and pharmacy technicians so that all employees are on the same page with regard to procedures and customer service. A **policy and procedure manual** outlines all activities in the pharmacy; the larger the pharmacy and the more complex the organization, the more important it is for each employee to follow departmental guidelines.

Make sure that you are thoroughly familiar with these guidelines and abide by them in your routine interactions. For example, if you have a prescription to be filled for yourself or a family member, then it may be store policy that you do not fill or process that prescription yourself; violations could result in job termination. Deviations from other written procedures could also have adverse consequences in a legal case in which a medication error occurred. Individual pharmacists also have preferences about how prescriptions are prepared and dispensed under their guidance; although not always written, these guidelines should be learned and followed as you are trained in a particular pharmacy.

Conflict Resolution Disputes involving duties, hours, pay, and other matters are common occurrences in occupations of all kinds. Try to resolve work-related disputes through rational, calm, private discussion with the parties involved. If you are seeking a raise in pay, then prepare for the meeting by outlining your accomplishments; most pharmacies invest a significant amount of time in training a pharmacy technician and do not want to lose such a valuable employee.

A pay raise may be possible with added certifications or if you offer to take on additional responsibilities as a senior technician or to plan work scheduling or training new staff. If a pay raise is not possible, then you may be able to negotiate for additional fringe benefits, such as health insurance, vacation, or scheduled time off on weekends. Your interactions with your supervisor should always be professional and nonthreatening.

Discrimination and Harassment As with any job, bear in mind that **discrimination** (i.e., preferential treatment or mistreatment) and **harassment** (i.e., mistreatment, sexual, or otherwise) are not only unethical but also against the law. Discrimination—whether based on age, gender, ethnicity, or religion—is not tolerated in the workplace. If preferential hiring or promotion fails to follow proper written procedures and guidelines, then the pharmacy or hospital may be subject to a lawsuit.

The law requires all businesses, pharmacies included, to post information related to workplace discrimination and harassment. In the past, sexual harassment was defined as unwanted physical contact or as the act of making sexual conduct a condition for advancement, preferential treatment, or other work-related outcomes. However, the Supreme Court has redefined sexual harassment more generally as the creation of an unpleasant or uncomfortable work environment through sexual action, innuendo, or related means. Thus, you do not have to put up with off-color or crude jokes if you do not wish to hear them; be aware that you must not contribute in any way to creating an environment that is uncomfortable for your coworkers. One person's innocent remark, made in the spirit of fun, can be the basis for another person's grounds for a legal action.

Generally speaking, romantic or sexual involvements with coworkers, and especially with coworkers in supervisory or subordinate positions, are inadvisable. If you find yourself the object of discrimination or harassment, then first try to resolve the issue with the person or persons involved. Do your best to maintain your composure and to express your discomfort calmly and rationally. If discrimination or harassment persists, then you may need to discuss the matter with a supervisor. If the problem is not resolved, then follow up first with store management and then, if necessary, with upper-level management. Most chain pharmacies have a written policy and procedure in such matters; follow the established protocol. If you are unsuccessful, then, as a last resort, make inquiries regarding the discrimination and harassment laws and procedures in your state.

Other Aspects of Professionalism

Other aspects of professionalism include appropriate behavior in the workplace, teamwork, interacting with other health professionals, refusal to dispense medical advice, and emergency preparedness. Ethical behavior is also an important aspect of professionalism and is discussed in more detail in Chapter 14, *Your Future in Pharmacy Practice*.

Professional Behavior

Healthcare professionals at all levels are expected to abide by both written laws and ethical guidelines. **Decorum** means proper or polite behavior or that which is in good taste in the pharmacy workplace. Arguing with your supervisor in public is an example of inappropriate decorum. Another set of unwritten rules to be followed is often referred to as etiquette. **Etiquette,** defined as unwritten rules of behavior, is difficult to describe and is often recognized most easily when it is not being followed. For example, being disrespectful to a physician is an obvious violation of etiquette.

Respect should be shown to all who work in any healthcare facility, because each person has an important job to do that contributes to the overall health care provided to the patient. However, additional respect should be shown to those with a high level of medical training and those responsible for managing the facility where you are employed. Intimate personal relationships with coworkers or pharmacists are also discouraged in most practice settings.

Personal telephone calls and visits should be made only during breaks. Telling ethnic or off-color jokes and making disparaging comments about others is not acceptable or tolerated. When in doubt as to the expected behavior in a situation, be quiet, watch, and learn from someone else in the pharmacy who is a suitable model, and perform your assigned task. If you are not sure, then ask questions of the senior pharmacy technician or supervising pharmacist.

Teamwork

Pharmacy technicians and pharmacists must work together for 8 hours or more each day as a cohesive healthcare team to provide quality care and to process prescriptions for patients efficiently and safely. In a large chain pharmacy, you work with personnel of all ages and different gender, ethnic, and religious backgrounds. Personalities differ and sometimes clash. Is someone too talkative or loud? or too quiet and passive? Are some personnel too obsessive and compulsive? Do some seek patient contact and communication whereas others would rather fill prescriptions and minimize patient contact? These differences cannot be allowed to interfere in the workplace. There must be respect for other personnel, both individually and with respect to their roles in the pharmacy. Unresolved issues should be brought to the attention of the supervising pharmacist privately.

Any criticism of an individual's quality of work should be constructive and a learning experience. The problem may be simply a typo on a computer entry of the prescription or a more serious error, such as selecting the wrong patient or wrong drug or typing incorrect directions. Pharmacists often consult with their technicians on insurance problems because the technicians are often better versed in the nuances of the various plans. Common courtesies—such as "Could you please call the insurance plan and verify coverage?" or "Thanks for staying over to help us" when you are very busy and/or understaffed—can make a difference. In nonbusy times, share interest in coworkers' personal lives: "Where did you go on vacation?" "Did you have a fun weekend?" Simply put, all personnel must pitch in and share the workload to work together for the good of the patient. Studies also indicate that support from your employer, supervisor, and coworkers improves your job satisfaction.

A more experienced pharmacy technician may act as a mentor for a new technician.

Teamwork may also mean managing change. By definition, health care is dynamic—always changing. The pharmacy work environment also reflects dynamic change. The change may be in management or a last-minute change in work or vacation schedules, a change in policies and procedures, or a change in insurance plan coverage, not to mention the never-ending changes in drugs—new generics, new formulations, new dosages, and so on. Are you willing to come in on your day off and cover for a colleague who unexpectedly called in sick? Are you willing to work over your scheduled time even if you do not receive overtime pay? Managing change and being a team player are positive attributes in a pharmacy technician.

Interprofessionalism

In the course of their duties, pharmacy technicians encounter, personally or on the telephone, many other professionals and paraprofessionals, including pharmacists, physicians, nurses, medical assistants, administrators, store managers, sales representatives, insurance personnel, and other technicians. Health care is a demanding industry, often requiring long hours and involving stressful, emergency situations. As a result, practitioners in the industry often suffer from fatigue and stress. Sometimes this stress shows itself in unintentionally rude behavior. Rarely, it may present as abuse of alcohol or prescription drugs.

Unfortunately, busy healthcare professionals sometimes speak to subordinates in an inappropriate and nonprofessional manner. The degree to which you maintain your courtesy and respect, even in the face of rudeness, is a measure of your professionalism. If you return rudeness with kindness, then you often find that, immediately or over time, the quality of your interactions improves. If you answer the telephone and someone barks a command at you, then demonstrate your professionalism by attending to the content of the message and not to its tone.

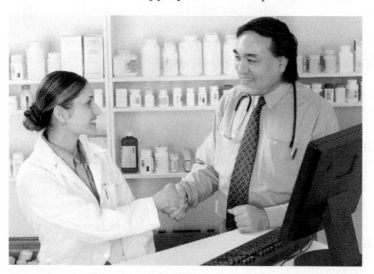

Pharmacy technicians should always interact with other professionals with respect.

Always refer to physicians, chiropractors, osteopathic professionals, and dentists using the title "Doctor." In the presence of patients, refer to the pharmacist as "Doctor" if he or she has achieved a Doctor of Pharmacy degree. Some states have designated all pharmacists as "Doctors" in recognition of their professional experience. When the technician refers to the pharmacist as "Doctor," this raises the level of customer respect not only for the pharmacist but also for the technician, who is "Doctor's Assistant." Refer to other supervisors using appropriate courtesy titles, such as "Mr., Mrs., or Miss," plus the last name, or "Sir," "Madam," or "Ma'am." A degree of formality is always in order until you are requested to use more informal modes of address in day-to-day operations.

New customers also arrive at the pharmacy and speak or inquire about physicians, specialists, and other healthcare professionals. General information may be given, but opinions on the competence of a particular physician or healthcare provider should not be given out by anyone in the pharmacy. At all times, avoid making disparaging comments about other healthcare providers. If such comments are made and the person's professional reputation is questioned, then that person may sue you for slander.

Do Not Dispense Medical or Pharmaceutical Advice

Safety Note

Do not provide medical advice. Direct such questions to the pharmacist.

A pharmacy technician is not trained or licensed to advise customers with regard to medications (including OTC drugs and diet supplements) and their use. Use common sense to determine whether a given query from a customer exceeds the bounds of common knowledge. As a rule of thumb, refer to a pharmacist any questions involving patient assessment, the proper administration, dosage, uses, or effects of a medication, whether prescription, OTC, or diet supplement, as well as any questions that require a professional opinion or judgment.

Of course, a technician should use common sense with regard to providing customers with information. In the case of OTC medications, sometimes customers need basic information that is readily available on the OTC packaging. For example, a customer might ask what an analgesic is, when an enteric-coated analgesic is appropriate, which alternative brands are available, or other routine questions that can be safely answered without referring the customer to the pharmacist.

Do not be afraid of admitting your lack of expertise. Customers appreciate that you are concerned enough to make sure that they receive accurate information. When a question deals with the effects or administration of a medication, ask the customer to wait for a moment while you get someone who can provide a professional answer to the question. In some instances, technicians may provide medication-related information when providing refills and when directed to do so by a pharmacist.

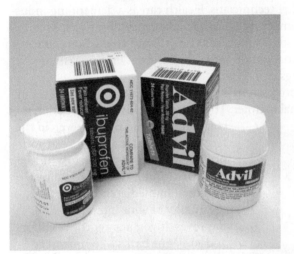

Pharmacy technicians can help customers read labels to compare generic and brand name OTC products.

Emergency Preparedness

At times of local, regional, or national emergencies or disasters, all pharmacy personnel may be called into action. If your pharmacy is interested in participation and planning, then a representative should contact the local health department. In addition to attending planning meetings, educational programs need to be completed for the pharmacy to participate fully.

If there is a serious epidemic, then what is the plan for your pharmacy? Many personnel may be out sick, and transportation and distribution networks may be seriously compromised. How can your wholesaler vendor get medications to you? How can patients at your pharmacy get needed medicine? What role can the pharmacy best serve in the community? Can it be a source of information and education for patients? Can the pharmacy share personnel with the department of public health? What type of protective gear will be available, and which personnel will receive vaccines or antiviral medications if dealing with the public? An interested technician could assist in the planning and communication with the health department.

Credentialing is the process for validating the qualifications of licensed professionals and may define what functions and roles pharmacists and pharmacy technicians can perform. If you have specialized training, such as CPR or ACLS certification or experience as an EMT or as a medic in the military, then you could be a valuable asset to your community in the time of a health crisis. Depending on your training and experience and the extent of the crisis, you may be triaging or screening injuries or illnesses in the field, providing CPR or necessary medications and supplies to medical personnel, or administering vaccines in times of a regional pandemic or epidemic.

Health Insurance Portability and Accountability Act

As discussed in Chapter 2, the **Health Insurance Portability and Accountability Act (HIPAA)** is a comprehensive federal law passed in 1996 to, among other things, protect patient private health information. All healthcare facilities (including pharmacies in all practice settings) that access, store, maintain, or transmit patient-identifiable medical information must comply with these regulations. Failure to do so can result in severe civil and criminal penalties. Although HIPAA covers many areas, the following are those related to security and patient confidentiality.

Patient Identifiers

A pharmacy is required by law to maintain the privacy of **protected health information (PHI).** Personal health information must be protected from unauthorized use and access. Obviously, a physician, nurse, pharmacist, and pharmacy technician have access to medical information to serve the needs of the patient. A pharmacy technician, for example, may be able to identify a medical diagnosis from the medications that are dispensed in the pharmacy (e.g., a patient receiving combination antiretroviral therapy most likely has an HIV infection). All health professionals are bound by law and ethics not to disclose this information outside the workplace.

To be in compliance, healthcare workers must remove or conceal from view any information that can identify the patient. **Patient identifiers** are defined as information that could identify the patient. Examples of patient identifiers are listed in Table 13.1.

A community pharmacy may use PHI to provide and coordinate the treatment, medications, and services that the patient receives. It may also be used to contact the insurer to determine the amount of medication covered by insurance and the resulting co-pay. PHI is occasionally used for quality assurance surveys or in response to a lawsuit. In most legal cases, the lawyer obtains written approvals from the patient to

TABLE 13.1 Patient Identifiers

■ name	■ health plan identification number
■ address and ZIP code	■ account number
■ relatives	■ vehicle identification
■ employer	■ certificate or license number
■ date of birth	■ uniform resource locater (URL) or Internet protocol (IP) address
■ telephone number or fax number	
■ e-mail address	■ fingerprint or voiceprint
■ social security number	■ photo
■ medical record number	

release his or her prescription records, or the pharmacy gets the approval of the patient. All requests for PHI other than by the patient should be directed to the pharmacist

In the pharmacy, shredding all patient-related information rather than discarding it in the trash is common practice. Even used prescription vials with patient-labeled information must be discarded appropriately (i.e., black out the patient name with a marking pen or peel the label from the vial and discard). As a technician, be extra vigilant and sensitive to maintaining patient confidentiality. In addition, be sure to understand the policy and procedures of your pharmacy. If you see potential violations, then bring them to the attention of your pharmacist supervisor. Maintaining the privacy and security of health information is an extremely important ethical and legal issue.

Patient Confidentiality

In the electronic age, all healthcare professionals must understand the importance of maintaining patient confidentiality. If a patient cannot trust the pharmacist or pharmacy technician with medical information, then both trust and a good customer may be lost. A pharmacy technician may be discussing sensitive medical issues with a patient in the course of trying to help identify or locate a product in the pharmacy. A patient may request a private conversation with a pharmacist to discuss a medical issue. Maintaining the security and privacy of a patient's medical information must remain a very high priority for the pharmacy technician. Every pharmacy is required to have a written policy on patient confidentiality that must be signed and recorded.

Security The issues of security and privacy are closely intertwined with patient confidentiality. Who should have access to what information internally or outside the pharmacy? How can unnecessary access to patient health information be limited, especially in large organizations such as hospitals, chain pharmacies, research sponsors, or insurance providers?

In the course of diagnosing or treating the patient, the physician and pharmacist (or their agents on their behalf) may exchange information without restriction or without the expressed written permission of the patient. For example, if a patient was receiving controlled narcotic prescriptions from several physicians, then the pharmacist may notify these physicians. In addition, some insurance reimbursement requires diagnostic codes from the physician for select diabetic and respiratory drugs; this information can be provided. In these examples, the permission of the patient is not necessary.

Other examples of situations in which some but not all health information is shared are investigational drug studies and communications between a patient's insurance provider and his or her employer. Studies must be designed so that patients cannot be individually identified.

How much information about the patient does the sponsor of an investigational drug study (often a pharmaceutical company) need to know? A minimum amount of information that directly relates to the study is exchanged with the sponsor per protocol approved by the Institutional Review Board or Human Use Committee. Investigational drug studies collate medical data such that PHI remains confidential.

An insurance company processing a prescription reimbursement has the right to know which drug and dose were dispensed, but it may not be necessary to share that information with the patient's employer. In the past, an insurance company occasionally shared medical information with an employer, resulting in employee job termination. No such information is shared with the employer under HIPAA today.

In other situations, the patient's permission must be obtained. A good example is a teenager who is receiving birth control pills from the family planning clinic; that information cannot be shared with her parents or anyone else without her permission. Or if a retail pharmacist wanted a copy of a recent hospital discharge summary or a copy of the patient's most recent laboratory results, then written permission by the patient may need to be obtained.

The electronic transmission of medical and insurance information improves the revenue of a community pharmacy (more prescriptions can be dispensed, more rapid reimbursement, fewer claims rejections), contains cost (fewer personnel needed for billing claims), and provides better patient care (more time to review patient profile and counsel patient). The efficiencies of transmitting medical information electronically must be balanced with the need to maintain security and protect patient confidentiality.

HIPAA also sets standards for the electronic submission of patient medical information and provides safeguards to protect the confidentiality of patient information. Access to some medical information (or fields of information) may be restricted to certain healthcare professionals. Frequent password renaming and resets are other ways to limit access.

Electronic transmission of data is common in the pharmacy. Every third-party insurance transaction involves the electronic submission of data with immediate online adjudication (as discussed in Chapter 7). A fax request for refill authorization to the physician's office is a common practice. Electronic prescriptions from handheld personal digital assistants (PDAs), as discussed in Chapter 12, may eventually replace written prescriptions in the near future. The Internet is usually not a completely secure place to transmit confidential medical information; therefore avoid sending e-mails containing patient identifiers (see Table 13.1) on the subject line.

You may also need to provide security by protecting your employer's proprietary information from competitors, including prescription volume, pricing issues, or policies and procedures in the pharmacy. If you are not sure, then ask a senior pharmacy technician or pharmacist.

Privacy In addition to HIPAA regulations, the pharmacy technician should use common sense, being sensitive and respectful of customer privacy as regards health information. Pharmacies sell many products related to private bodily functions and conditions (e.g., condoms and other contraceptives, feminine hygiene and menstrual products, suppositories, hemorrhoid remedies, enemas, adult diapers, catheters, bed pans, scabicides). Often customers find asking about such products embarrassing and have to work up the nerve to request assistance. If you find discussing such matters embarrassing, then you need to overcome your reservations quickly.

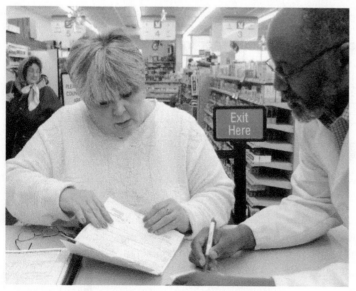

The pharmacy technician should make every effort to make the customer comfortable and to maintain customer privacy.

As a pharmacy employee, you are part of the healthcare profession and must adopt a helpful, no-nonsense, professional attitude toward the body and its functions. Responding to an inquiry about such a product with promptness, courtesy, respect, and a certain degree of nonchalance often relieves your customer's embarrassment and demonstrates your professionalism. Speak in a clear voice, but not so loudly that other customers or employees are privy to your private exchange with the customer.

In addition, often a patient's illness can be determined by his or her medication history. A patient receiving antiviral prescriptions for human immunodeficiency virus (HIV), antibiotics for gonorrhea, antivirals for herpes, antidepressants for depression, erectile dysfunction drugs, or chemotherapy for cancer requires the same amount of privacy as in a physician's office. This information cannot even be shared with a family member without the expressed written permission of the patient—you would not want information on your health to be made public! Violations of confidentiality of medical information can have serious legal ramifications (see the following section) and can potentially cost you your job and career as a pharmacy technician.

Privacy should be maintained as you update customer information. If, for example, you are stationed at the pharmacy window and need information for the customer's patient profile, then let the customer know why you need the information. Tell the customer, for example, "I need some information for your prescription profile so that we may better serve you. May I ask you a few questions? Thank you. What is your full name and address?" "Do you have any medication allergies or health conditions?" You may also need to verify insurance information; most customers are accustomed to presenting a card or proof of insurance regularly at the physician's office and are not upset once the procedure is explained.

When a patient is picking up a prescription, confirm his or her identity and what he or she is picking up. Keep your tone of voice low so as not to broadcast to nearby customers what the patient is receiving. Many pharmacies now have a private counseling area for prescription pickup, where the patient can have a higher degree of privacy. A customer may request that the technician print an annual prescription record for themselves and their spouse (for income tax calculations); permission must be given by the spouse before records can be released.

Policy on Security and Privacy A patient has the right to expect that medical information will be kept confidential. Each pharmacy is required to have a policy statement that defines patient privacy rights and how patient information will be used and

FIGURE 13.1
New Customer Information Form

Pharmacy New Customer Information
Confidential

Name: _____

Date of Birth: _____

Address: _____

City: _____ State: _____ ZIP Code: _____

Phone Numbers

Home: _____ Work: _____ Cell: _____

Drug Allergies: _____

Food Allergies: _____

I declare all of the above information to be accurate to the best of my knowledge. The signature below also gives this pharmacy permission to contact my physician and/or healthcare provider regarding my care. I also certify that this pharmacy has informed me of its privacy policy.

Signature: _____ Date: _____

protected by the pharmacy. These policy statements should be explained to all new pharmacy customers at the time that they first visit the pharmacy. To protect the pharmacy's interests, patients may be asked to sign a form to document that they have read and understood the pharmacy's privacy statement, called a **notice of privacy practices**. Figure 13.1 is an example of this information form.

This notice also includes the patient's health information rights. Parents can sign for their dependent minor children. Upon request, however, teenage minors may be treated as adults with respect to access and disclosure of health information records. A patient may give written permission to a personal representative (i.e., a son or daughter) to have access to health information and records.

Each pharmacy can develop its own mechanism to implement, communicate, audit, and document compliance with HIPAA regulations. Depending on the size of the pharmacy (i.e., independent, chain, hospital), formal training programs, with annual refresher courses, may be used. Each pharmacy should have a set of policy and procedures in its manual to cover the HIPAA regulations. Because a breach of confidentiality is often a sufficient reason for immediate termination, it behooves the technician to know and understand the policy.

Both state and federal law govern patient confidentiality. Generally, where conflict exists, the most stringent law is the one that should be followed. The pharmacy technician should know the laws in the state where he or she is practicing; if the technician moves to another state, then the regulations and laws may change. Many states have specific laws protecting patients with HIV or acquired immunodeficiency syndrome (AIDS).

Chapter Terms

appearance the overall outward look of an employee on the job, including dress and grooming

attitude the emotional stance or disposition that a worker adopts toward his or her job duties, customers, employer, and coworkers

closed-ended question a question that requires a yes or no answer

credentialing the process for validating the qualifications of licensed professionals, such as Basic Life Support (BLS) and ACLS (Advance Cardiac Life Support)

decorum proper or polite behavior that is in good taste

discrimination preferential treatment or mistreatment

etiquette unwritten rules of behavior

harassment mistreatment, whether sexual or otherwise

Health Insurance Portability and Accountability Act (HIPAA) a comprehensive federal law passed in 1996 to protect all patient-identifiable medical information

nonverbal communication communication without words—through facial expression, body contact, body position, and tone of voice

notice of privacy practices a written policy of the pharmacy to protect patient confidentiality, as required by HIPAA

open-ended question a question that requires a descriptive answer, not merely yes or no

patient identifiers any demographic information that can identify the patient, such as name, address, phone number, Social Security number, or medical identification number

policy and procedure manual a book outlining activities in the pharmacy, defining the roles of individuals and listing guidelines

protected health information (PHI) medical information that is protected by HIPAA, such as medical diagnoses, medication profiles, and results of laboratory tests

triage the assessment by the pharmacist of an illness or symptom; outcome may be to recommend an OTC product, or refer patient to a physician or emergency room

Chapter Summary

- Community pharmacies are returning to the concept of the small, customer-oriented neighborhood pharmacy of the past.
- Increased emphasis on personal service (i.e., attention to the needs of individual customers) requires the technician to consider carefully all interactions with pharmacy customers.
- Customer orientation involves dressing and grooming oneself neatly, maintaining a constant lookout for customers in need of assistance, knowing the layout of the store and the location of its merchandise, smiling and using courteous language, providing explanations to customers as necessary, being sensitive to language and cultural differences, following established policies and procedures, and referring requests for medical or pharmaceutical advice to competent professionals.
- Common courtesy should be used in all telephone communications and conversations with both patients and healthcare professionals.
- Providing customer care to a patient with a mental or physical disability may provide a challenge to the technician.
- A no-tolerance policy exists with regard to discrimination and harassment in the pharmacy workplace.
- A request for information about dosage, adverse effects, and drug interactions should always be referred to a supervising pharmacist.
- A pharmacy technician must be sensitive to maintaining patient privacy, confidentiality of medical information, and compliance with all state and federal HIPAA regulations.

Chapter Review

Checking Your Understanding

Choose the best answer from those provided.

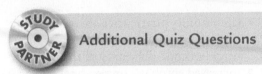

Additional Quiz Questions

1. The emphasis in retail pharmacy today is on
   a. discount pricing.
   b. customer care.
   c. extensive drug inventory.
   d. expansion of non-drug merchandising.

2. The emotional stance that a worker adopts toward his or her job duties is called
   a. tone.
   b. mood.
   c. attitude.
   d. appearance.

3. Which of the following is the primary rule of retail merchandising?
   a. Always dress and groom yourself neatly.
   b. Respect the customer's privacy.
   c. Explain necessary interactions to the customer.
   d. At all times you are representing your company to the customer.

4. Decorum is
   a. proper or polite behavior, or behavior that is in good taste.
   b. dissatisfaction with services provided.
   c. lack of understanding of the options available.
   d. ability to negotiate for goods and services.

5. A pharmacy technician should never
   a. waste time walking a customer across the store to show him or her the location of an item on the shelves.
   b. dispense advice regarding the use of a medication.
   c. attempt to speak to a customer in the customer's native language.
   d. take a written prescription from a customer.

6. When asking a customer for information for the patient profile, the pharmacy technician should explain
   a. how and when the prescription should be administered.
   b. why the pharmacy needs this information.
   c. the parts of the label of the prescription.
   d. the differences between the payment policies of various third-party insurance providers.

7. Preferential treatment or mistreatment based on age, gender, ethnicity, or other criteria is known as
   a. harassment.
   b. discrimination.
   c. innuendo.
   d. decorum.

8. When answering a drugstore telephone, a person should identify himself or herself and the name of the
   a. supervising pharmacist.
   b. pharmacy.
   c. customer.
   d. prescribing physician.

9. An underage teenager is on a birth control pill. All of the following can review this medical information at the pharmacy except the
   a. parent.
   b. physician.
   c. pharmacist.
   d. technician.

10. HIPAA involves all the following except
    a. medication profile.
    b. medical diagnoses.
    c. insurance provider.
    d. laboratory results.

Thinking Like a Pharmacy Tech

1. In a small group, recall your own experiences visiting drugstores or pharmacies. Make a list of problems that you have encountered in pharmacies (e.g., slow service, lack of a comfortable place in which to wait while a prescription was being filled, lack of private counseling area, difficulty in finding an item). As a group, brainstorm some ways to solve such problems and to improve customer service.

2. With other students in a small group, brainstorm a list of positive experiences you have had in retail merchandising establishments of all kinds. Using this list, draw up a list of recommendations for making a customer's experience in a pharmacy retail establishment a positive one.

3. Imagine that you are a drugstore manager who operates a 24 hour pharmacy in a big city in an urban neighborhood with the following demographics:

   10% Vietnamese-speaking customers
   26% Spanish-speaking customers
   16% Korean-speaking customers
   32% English-speaking customers
   16% customers who speak other languages (e.g., Thai, Laotian, Hmong, Russian, Latvian, Polish, and so forth)

   With other students, brainstorm a list of steps you might take to meet the needs of the customers whom you serve.

Communicating Clearly

1. As a class, identify four students to play the following roles: a customer, a physician, a pharmacy technician, and a supervising pharmacist. Have them act out some typical telephone calls to the pharmacy, including a customer calling to find out when a prescription will be ready, a physician calling in a prescription, a customer asking medical advice, a customer asking for signs of an overdose, and a customer with a complaint. Demonstrate both open-ended and closed-ended questions. After each call, critique what was said and done by the technician taking the telephone call.

2. Conduct the following role-play activities with other students: (1) a male who is obviously embarrassed asks a female technician for information on condoms; (2) a female who is obviously embarrassed asks a male technician for information on feminine hygiene products. Perform other scenarios with other products until each student has played a role. After each scenario is played out, critique the technician's response. Discuss the kinds of problems that can arise in such situations and how they might be avoided.

3. Tone of voice can communicate many types of feelings. Consider how to say the following sentences out loud to communicate the feeling listed in parentheses.
   a. I love my job. (Nobody else may love it, but *I* do.)
   b. I love my job. (I more than *like* my job—I love it.)
   c. I love my job. (I may not like anything *else*, but I love my job.)
   d. I love my job. (I don't like my *boss*, but I like my job.)
   e. I love my job. (You have *got* to be kidding!)

Try repeating the sentence using your own feelings, and see whether your classmates can interpret your true feelings about your job. Ask yourself whether you know how you sound.

4. The culture of the United States is changing constantly and becoming more diversified. Patients are often influenced by a wide variety of factors in their culture, religion, and community. Explain in writing why a pharmacist and the pharmacy employees should get to know individual patients, their families, and their cultural beliefs. Include three examples or case illustrations in your explanation.

Researching on the Web

1. Visit the Keirsey Web site at www.keirsey.com, register (free), and take the Temperament Sorter II self-evaluation test to discover your personality type.
   a. According to Keirsey Temperament Theory, there are four basic temperament groups that describe human behavior. Keirsey's four temperaments are referred to as Artisans™, Guardians™, Rationals™, and Idealists™. What type of person are you?
   b. Were the descriptions of your personality type accurate?
   c. How can knowing your own type and the type of your coworkers assist your communication skills?
   d. Which personality types do you communicate with easily, and which are more difficult for you to communicate with?

2. Do an Internet search to identify the laws of your state relating to patient confidentiality of medical information and how they affect community pharmacy practice. How do they differ from HIPAA? Are they more or less stringent than HIPAA?

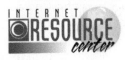

For further study of chapter-related topics, explore the Web links in the Web Center at www.emcp.net/pharmpractice4e.

Your Future in Pharmacy Practice

14

Learning Objectives

- Identify a variety of strategies for successful adaptation to the work environment.
- Define and differentiate the terms *licensure*, *certification*, and *registration*.
- Describe and contrast the format and content of the PTCB and ICPT certification examinations.
- Explain the criteria for recertification for pharmacy technicians by PTCB and ICPT.
- Discuss the importance of technician involvement in professional organizations and networking with colleagues in the profession.
- Make a plan for a successful job search.

- Write a résumé and a cover letter.
- Prepare for and successfully complete an interview.
- Define ethics and discuss characteristics of ethical behavior.
- Identify ethical dilemmas that may occur in pharmacy practice.
- Discuss some trends for the future of the pharmacy profession and their impact on pharmacy technicians.

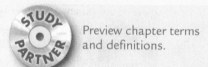

Preview chapter terms and definitions.

The past four decades have seen dramatic changes in the pharmacy profession, especially as the roles of the pharmacist and technician expand and become integral to modern-day practice. Exciting changes are afoot, including an increasing movement toward national and specialty certification and more formalized training and education of pharmacy technicians. Pharmacy technicians are finding more opportunities for placement in new roles and for responsibilities in community, hospital, managed care, home health, and specialty practices. This chapter presents useful information on these trends and provides information to prepare you better for becoming a pharmacy technician.

Increasing Your Employability

As you have learned in previous chapters, the pharmacy technician career field continues to undergo dramatic changes. The occupational outlook for the pharmacy paraprofessional is quite bright. A **paraprofessional** is one who is qualified and trained to assist a professional. A **professional** is defined as someone with recognized expertise in a field who is expected to use his or her knowledge and skills to benefit others and to operate ethically with some autonomy. Throughout the country, pharmacy technicians are gaining recognition for the vital role that they play in providing a wide range of pharmaceutical services in various employment settings.

Adjusting to the Work Environment

If you have not worked before or if your work experience has been sporadic, then getting used to your job as a technician might seem like getting used to life in a foreign country. You have to adjust to a new work culture, to different behaviors, to unfamiliar customs, and even to a new language—the technical jargon of the profession. The following list provides some advice for making your adjustment to the job a more comfortable one.

- Attitude: Do not give in to the temptation to behave in ways that are elitist or superior. Remember that you are part of a healthcare team, and cooperation is extremely important.
- Reliability: Health care, like teaching, is one of those industries in which standards for reliability are very high. You cannot, for example, show up late for work or take days off arbitrarily without good reason and supervisor approval. Unreliable employees in the healthcare industry do not keep their jobs for long, so make sure that your employer can always depend on you to arrive at work on time. Staying late does not make up for a tardy arrival. Tardiness can play havoc with other people's work schedules and workloads. Finish dressing, grooming, and eating before you enter your work area.
- Accuracy and responsibility: In a pharmacy, you rarely have the leeway to be partially correct. As discussed in Chapter 12, a medication error, even if a small one, can have dire consequences for a patient or customer, as well as for the pharmacy. Develop work habits to ensure accuracy, and expect to be held responsible for what you do on the job. Work steadily and methodically. Keep your attention on the task at hand, and always double-check everything you do.

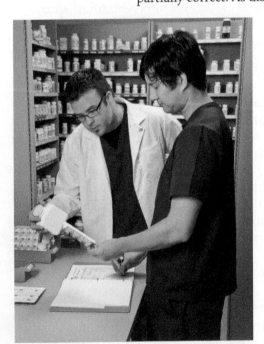

Feel comfortable in asking questions to improve your knowledge and understanding of the pharmacy operations.

- Relating to your supervisor: Always show your supervisor a reasonable degree of deference and respect. Ask your supervisor how he or she prefers to be addressed. Be respectful of your supervisor's experience and knowledge. If tensions arise between you and your supervisor, then take positive steps to lessen them. Your supervisor has power over your raises, promotions, benefits, and references for future employment. When you disagree with him or her, discuss these differences in private.
- Personality: Surprisingly, personality is one of the greatest predictors of job success. Be positive, cooperative, self-confident, and enthusiastic.
- Performance: Demonstrate that you can get things done and that you put the job first. Employers expect you to devote your full attention to your responsibilities for the entire length of your shift. Rushing through a task because it is close to the end of your shift places patient

care at risk. Maintaining attentiveness and accuracy is always important, even close to quitting time.

- **Questioning:** Sometimes people are afraid to ask questions because doing so might make them appear less intelligent or less knowledgeable. Nothing could be further from the truth.
- **Dress:** Follow the dress code of the company or institution for which you work.
- **Receptivity:** Listen to the advice of others who have been on the job longer. Accept criticism gracefully. If you make a mistake, then own up to it. If you are criticized unfairly, then adopt a non-defensive tone of voice and explain your view of the matter calmly and rationally. This behavior is part of performing with integrity, an important part of being a professional.
- **Etiquette:** Every workplace has its unique culture. Especially at first, pay close attention to the details of that culture. Pick up on the habits of interaction and communication practiced by other employees, and model the best of these.
- **Alliances:** In all organizations, two kinds of power systems exist: (1) formal, or organizational, ones and (2) informal ones, based on alliances. Cultivate alliances on the job, but make sure that you are not seen as part of a clique or an exclusive group. Even as a new employee, begin to build power through making alliances. If a problem or an opportunity arises, then you will probably hear about it first through your allies on the job. If a change in the workplace affects you, then advance notice may give you the necessary time to plan a strategic response.
- **Reputation:** Many people assume that if they work hard and are loyal, then they will be rewarded. This is often but not necessarily always true. Management personnel may be so involved with their own concerns that you remain little more than a face in the crowd. Being pleasant to others helps you to be noticed, as does making helpful or useful suggestions. Do not keep your professional qualifications a secret. Join professional organizations. Volunteer to serve on committees within the institution. Make yourself indispensable to the organization! When you have won an award or achieved some other success, see that your name is publicized in institutional newsletters, community newspapers, or the newsletters of professional organizations. Give presentations at professional meetings, civic groups, churches, or synagogues. Write articles for publication in professional publications. In short, avoid hiding your light under a bushel basket.
- **Luck:** Most of the big lucky breaks in life come through knowing the right people at the right time. By cultivating alliances, you can control your luck more than you might expect.
- **Crisis:** When a crisis occurs, do not overreact. Take time, if you can, to think and then act, and do not keep the crisis a secret from your supervisor.
- **Learning:** Pharmacy is a rapidly changing field. Staying current on new drugs, dosage forms, laws, and regulations is important. Accept the idea of continuing education (CE) as a way of life. CE may include reading pharmacy journals and newsletters or attending workshops and professional meetings. You may need to take formal course work or attend CE programs every year to maintain your certification and keep current on the latest trends. Think of your job-related learning as a regular "information workout," as necessary to your employment fitness as aerobic workouts are to your physical fitness.
- **Expertise:** How can you become a person who makes things happen? Become highly knowledgeable about a specialty within your field, such as sterile or nonsterile compounding, preparing hazardous drugs, inventory control, and so on. Be the most expert technician that you can be in that area; then move on and

master another area. Soon, others will be asking your advice, and your reputation will grow.

- Reflectiveness about your career: There will never be a time in your career to coast and relax. Good career chances can come your way at any time in life, so make a regular habit of taking the time to think about your career and where you are headed. Planning lends structure and substance to your career management.

Professionalism and the Technician

Just as pharmacists are required to obtain credentials—such as graduating from an accredited pharmacy school, sitting for a licensure examination, and perhaps completing a residency—pharmacy technicians are increasingly asked to seek credentials. A **credential** is defined simply as a *documented piece of evidence of one's qualifications.* Credentials for the pharmacy technician may include licensure and/or certification. This documentation of qualifications is moving the role of technicians forward in the profession of pharmacy. Nowadays, being a pharmacy technician is not simply having a job in a pharmacy; rather, it is a chosen career path in which the technician is recognized as a paraprofessional.

As a paraprofessional in healthcare, technicians have specific expectations for job performance. Technicians are part of the pharmacy profession, and professionals are expected to do the following.

- be qualified to perform the duties required
- use their specific knowledge and skills to perform the duties required
- adhere to a code of ethical conduct

These expectations are held for all healthcare professionals, elevating their job responsibilities beyond that of an hourly paid employee. Patients come to trust healthcare professionals and paraprofessionals. This trust obligates pharmacy technicians to serve the public good and benefit the lives of patients. Pharmacy technicians may be trained by virtue of on-the-job training at a pharmacy or in the military, or they may complete a formalized training program in a community college.

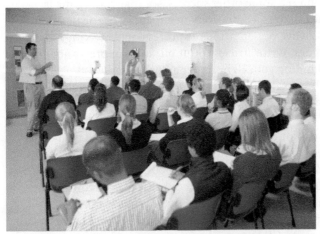

The combination of experience and formalized training should assist you in passing the necessary exams in order to become a certified pharmacy technician.

It is important to define and contrast three terms commonly used with pharmacists and pharmacy technicians. **Licensure** refers to the granting of a license by the state; it is usually required to work in a particular profession in order to ensure that the public is not harmed by the incompetence of the practitioners. People become licensed through training and/or passing an exam. Licensure is usually renewable and is often dependent on keeping current on knowledge and skills.

Certification is the process by which a nongovernmental association grants recognition to an individual who has met certain predetermined qualifications specified by that association; unlike licensure, certification is seldom mandatory in order to practice legally.

Whether required by the state or not, both hospitals and community pharmacies are increasingly calling for technicians to become certified by taking a technician

FIGURE 14.1
**States
Regulating
Pharmacy
Technicians**

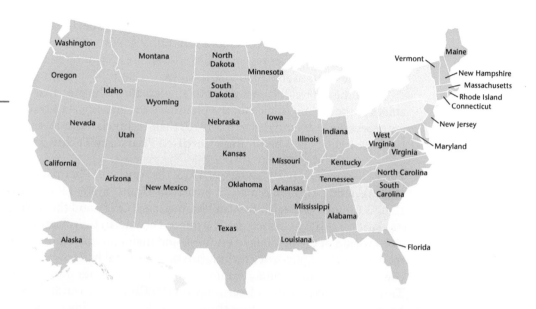

certification exam. Often certification is a requirement for initial employment or strongly encouraged within the first year of employment. The cost of taking the certification exam is commonly reimbursed by the employer. Financial incentives are often in place for technicians to become certified once they are employed.

Registration generally means that an individual is required to sign up or register with a state agency, such as the State Board of Pharmacy, before starting practice. Registration means that individuals working in a pharmacy as technicians must submit information on where they live and work to the state board of pharmacy. It usually does not require additional training or education, although certification may be required; registration allows the state board to more easily track any individuals with felony, theft, or drug diversion histories.

Although the type and length of technician education and training vary widely, certification as a pharmacy technician is quickly becoming preferred or even required for employment in many areas. Sometimes certification is required for newly hired technicians. Many states recognize national technician certification. Some states, such as Arizona, Louisiana, Massachusetts, Montana, New Mexico, Oregon, South Carolina, Texas, Utah, Virginia, and Wyoming, require certification to work as a technician in that state. Unlike licensure or registration, certification is generally valid and transferable to all states.

Other states recognize a pharmacy technician through state regulations such as registration or licensure (see Figure 14.1). If you are a certified technician who moves to another state, then you may be required to be licensed or registered in that new state prior to starting employment. Many states stipulate a maximum ratio of technicians (including pharmacy interns) to pharmacists, which may vary from 2:1 to 4:1; the ratio may be dependent on the number of employed certified pharmacy technicians. For instance, Colorado and Kansas pharmacies may use a higher technician-to-pharmacist ratio if at least one technician is certified. Renewal of licensure or registration is required in three-fourths of U.S. states.

Some states are also beginning to recognize the value of formal technician education. For instance, South Carolina now requires completion of an accredited technician education program in addition to certification by the Pharmacy Technician Certification Board (PTCB) and 1000 hours of work experience to be a certified pharmacy technician. Some organizations within the profession, including the Pharmacy

Technician Educators Council (PTEC), are calling for the development of a 2 year associate degree standard for technician training. With these new requirements, technicians are given greater responsibilities—they are even allowed to check the work of other technicians in some practice settings.

All of these developments point to an increase in the presence, responsibilities, and status of the technician within the pharmacy community. As a result, today's employers expect more of (and deliver more to) their technician employees. Two examinations are available for becoming a **Certified Pharmacy Technician (CPhT)**.

PTCB Examination In January of 1995, the American Pharmacists Association (APhA)—along with the American Society of Health-System Pharmacists (ASHP), the Illinois Council of Health-System Pharmacists (ICHP), and the Michigan Pharmacists Association (MPA)—created the Pharmacy Technician Certification Board (PTCB). The mission of the PTCB is to establish and maintain criteria for certification and recertification of pharmacy technicians on a national basis. A nonprofit testing company, the Professional Examination Service (PES), administers the **Pharmacy Technician Certification Examination (PTCE)**, which candidates must pass to become certified and to receive the title of CPhT. According to the PTCB, over 275,000 technicians have become certified since its inception.

Anyone who does not have a felony conviction and has graduated from high school (or has a general equivalency diploma [GED] or has obtained the foreign equivalent) is eligible to sit for the examination. The goal of the PTCE is to verify the candidate's knowledge and skill base for activities performed by pharmacy technicians under the supervising pharmacist. It is comprehensive in its scope; no specific pharmacy setting or specialty is emphasized. Skills and knowledge from both the community and institutional settings are required to pass this examination, including basic compounding knowledge and skills. No previous education, training, or work experience is required before taking the examination, but experience and/or formal training can greatly assist a candidate in preparing for it.

The exam is now taken online by computer-based testing (CBT). The PTCB recommends that persons taking the examination be familiar with the material in "any of the basic pharmacy technician training manuals." A practice exam and a pharmacy technician study book to prepare for the exam are available from APhA.

TABLE 14.1 PTCE Content

Exam Category	Description	Exam Weighting
I. Assisting the Pharmacist in Serving Patients	prescription interpretation, patient profile maintenance, prescription filling and processing, compounding, calculations, and customer service	66%
II. Maintaining Medication and Inventory Control Systems	ordering pharmaceuticals and devices, maintaining records and drug stock, repackaging, and quality control measures	22%
III. Participating in the Administration and Management of Pharmacy Practice	working with third-party payers, operating computer and automated dispensing technology, and maintaining federal laws and practice standards	12%

The questions are organized into three sections, each of which is weighted differently. Table 14.1 details the content of the examination as specified by the PTCB.

The most current blueprint for the examination is listed at the PTCB Web site. Candidates for certification are given 2 hours to complete the examination. The PTCE is a multiple-choice examination containing a total of 100 multiple-choice questions with four possible choices for each question. A student should answer every question, because the final score is based on the total number of questions correct rather than the percentage of correct answers. Educated guesses are encouraged! Candidates must receive a score of 650 or higher to pass and receive certification. So far, the PTCB reports that 77% to 82% of examination takers pass the test each year. More specifically, 80% of those who have taken the examination have passed. A technician may retake the examination as many times as is necessary to achieve a passing score; however, an application fee applies each time.

Recertification is required by the PTCB every 2 years. To be recertified, you must earn a total of 20 hours of credit in pharmacy-related continuing education, with at least 1 hour in pharmacy law. Certified technicians receive notification of the need for recertification approximately 60 days before their certification lapses. Pharmacy-related continuing education may be provided by professional organization meetings and Web sites, employers, and professional journals.

ICPT Examination   The Institute for the Certification of Pharmacy Technicians (ICPT) is an organization operated by pharmacists for the pharmacy profession. The mission of ICPT is to recognize pharmacy technicians who are proficient in the knowledge and skills needed to assist pharmacists to prepare and dispense prescriptions safely, accurately, and efficiently, and to promote high standards of practice for pharmacy technicians.

Since 2005, the ICPT also offers an online examination for pharmacy technicians, the **Exam for Certification of Pharmacy Technicians (ExCPT)**. The purpose of the exam is to determine whether an individual has achieved a certain minimum level of competency. The ExCPT is being offered in all 50 states and the District of Columbia and is available to pharmacy technicians from all practice settings. The ExCPT is recognized by several national pharmacy organizations as a valid instrument for pharmacy technician certification. The exam prepares a pharmacy technician to practice in either a community or hospital pharmacy environment.

Eligibility requirements are similar to those for the PTCB exam. ExCPT is a computer-based online test, consisting of 110 multiple choice questions from a large test bank, which must be completed within a 2 hour time frame. The content for the exam is weighted approximately 25% on regulations and technician duties, 23% on drugs and drug products (Top 200 Rx and Top 100 OTC products), and 52% on the dispensing process. Pharmacy technicians who successfully pass the ExCPT are considered Certified Pharmacy Technicians and receive a certificate (CPhT) that is recognized in most states.

In 2008, ICPT designed a practice and math self-assessment and training manual and test to help pharmacy technicians prepare for national certification. The test offers questions that are similar in content and style to those on the ExCPT. Candidates who do not pass the ExCPT are allowed to retake the exam after 4 weeks.

Certification expires after 2 years. During the 2 year period prior to recertification, certified pharmacy technicians must participate in at least 20 hours of continuing education (CE), including at least 1 hour of pharmacy law. To be approved, CE credit must be related to pharmacy technician practice. Acceptable topics include drug distribution, inventory control, managed healthcare, drug products, therapeutic issues, patient interaction, communication and interpersonal skills, pharmacy operations, prescription compounding, calculations, pharmacy law, preparation of sterile products, and drug repackaging.

Certificates of participation must be obtained for each CE program. CE programs offered by national and state pharmacy associations and pharmacy technician associations are generally acceptable if related to pharmacy technician practice. Applicable college courses with a grade of "C" or better may also be eligible for CE credit.

Hierarchy of Technician Positions

Because of expanded recognition of technician credentials, a hierarchy of pharmacy technician job descriptions has evolved, especially in institutional settings. Although specific job descriptions vary between organizations, many institutions have different levels of technician responsibilities. If certification is not required for an entry-level technician, then it is usually required for higher levels. Often, corresponding job titles are Technician I and II or Entry-Level Technician and Technician Specialist or Senior Technician. The difference in responsibility (and reward) grows and expands as the technician moves up the company ladder. For higher levels, added job responsibilities beyond basic competence for an entry-level technician may include the following.

- prioritization of work
- demonstrated initiative and ability to work independently
- troubleshooting and critical thinking
- supervision of others
- staff training responsibilities
- advanced communication skills (e.g., writing, word processing, taking refill requests if allowed)
- advanced computer application skills
- advanced calculations
- billing and documentation procedures
- inventory ordering and purchasing

In some cases, sterile and nonsterile compounding and nuclear pharmacy duties may be reserved for higher-level technicians because of new regulations and standards implemented by the Joint Commission, the United States Pharmacopeia (i.e., USP Chapter 797 and Chapter 795), and other national organizations. These technicians may be required to complete additional specialty certifications to practice within these areas.

Professional Organizations

Being part of a profession means taking an active role in advancing the profession. As a paraprofessional in pharmacy, technicians have an obligation and a vested interest to make their views heard in the local, state, and national forums that discuss issues facing their field. The future of the technician role is in the hands of those within the profession. This self-governance, something that is increasing for technicians, is one characteristic of a professional. As the status and role of pharmacy technicians increase, those within the profession should get involved in the decisions and movements affecting it.

Ways to get involved vary widely. Some examples include the following.

- volunteering to serve on a committee of your local, state, or national pharmacy organization (most of which have technician representation), such as the American

Society of Health System Pharmacists (ASHP), National Association of Boards of Pharmacy (NABP), or Pharmacy Technician Certification Board (PTCB).

- ASHP: The Pharmacy Technician Advisory Group is charged with advising ASHP's staff and Board of Directors about ASHP actions, products, and services pertaining to pharmacy technicians.
- NABP: Each of the state chapters welcomes technician input and participation.
- PTCB: The Stakeholder Policy and Certification Councils have opportunities for pharmacy technicians at the national level.
- running for office in your local chapter of the National Pharmacy Technician Association (NPTA) or American Association of Pharmacy Technicians (AAPT)
- serving on a committee for your state pharmacy association or participating in your state's annual pharmacy legislative day activities
- attending a national pharmacy technician conference

After attending local, state or national meetings, report what you learn to your employer and fellow technicians at work. Learning about and voicing concern for issues facing technicians and taking ownership in decisions made to advance their roles gives technicians control over their own destinies. Attending local, state, and professional organizations can also provide needed CE credits for recertification.

Current issues that face technicians are standardization of technician training or education, expansion of technician responsibilities to assist with the projected shortages in pharmacy workforces, salary and benefits, and implementation of state requirements for national certification. Locate your local technician organizations and inquire about how you can participate in decisions affecting the future practice of pharmacy in your state.

Job Search

Before you can implement the excellent strategies introduced in the preceding section, you must find the right job. Many people find the prospect of job hunting overwhelming but avoid such negative thinking. To help you be successful in your job search, break the process down into the steps identified and explained in this section.

What characteristics do pharmacy and human resources managers look for in a pharmacy technician? First of all, they consider customer service. As discussed in Chapter 13, good communication and interpersonal skills are essential for a pharmacy technician, who interacts with pharmacy coworkers, patients, and other healthcare professionals on a daily basis. The pharmacy technician must also enjoy performing precise work (math calculations, computer prescription entry), where accuracy can be a matter of life or death. Pharmacy technicians must also be able to maintain this accuracy even in stressful situations. Finally, all employers want dependable employees who show up for work on time. Are you willing to work weekends or nights if the position requires?

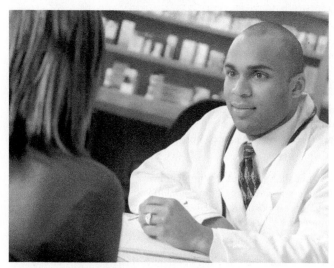

During the interview, be confident, polite, poised, and enthusiastic, and focus on your strengths.

Clarify Your Career Goals

Finding a job is difficult if you are not sure what you are looking for. Do you want to work in a community pharmacy? Do you want to work in a hospital, a long-term care facility, or a home infusion pharmacy? If you have uncertainties about the setting in which you wish to work, then arrange to interview pharmacists or technicians who work in these settings. In addition, do some thinking about what you want out of the job. Are you interested in jobs with opportunities for advancement in retail management? Are you more interested in customer care or prescription dispensing? Do you want to master the preparation of sterile products, the compounding of nonsterile products, or ordering, inventory, and billing? Can you balance your new job with your personal life, child care, and so on? Think about what you want to do; then look for jobs that suit your ambitions. Many programs have career counselors who can help you answer such questions. Check with your teacher or make an appointment to visit and talk to a career counselor, or go to the Internet or the library to obtain more background information.

TABLE 14.2   The Parts of a Résumé

Heading	Give your full name, address, and telephone number. Include your ZIP code in the address, area code in the phone number (and cell phone), and your e-mail address so that a potential employer can contact you.
Employment Objective	This is the first thing that an employer wants to know. The objective should briefly describe the position you are seeking and some of the abilities you would bring to the job. Identify the requirements of the position that you are applying for; then tailor the employment objective to match those requirements. Are you interested in part-time or full-time employment?
Education	Give your high school or college, city, state, degree, major, date of graduation, and additional course work related to the job, to the profession, or to business in general. State your cumulative grade point average (GPA) if it helps to sell you (3.0 or higher). List any honors or recognitions received in high school or college.
Experience	In reverse chronological order, list your work experience, including on-campus and off-campus work. Do not include jobs that would be unimpressive to your employer. Be sure to include cooperative education experience. For each job, indicate your position, employer's name, the location of the employment, the dates employed, and a brief description of your duties. Always list any advancements, promotions, or supervisory responsibilities. Be sure to include any certifications, registrations, or licensures on your résumé.
Skills	If you do not have a lot of relevant work experience, then include a skills section that details the skills that you can use on the job. Doing so is a way of saying, "I'm really capable. I just haven't had much opportunity to show it yet." If you have foreign language or computer software skills, then be sure to emphasize them.
Related Activities	Include any activities that show leadership, teamwork, or good communication skills. Include any club or organizational memberships, as well as professional or volunteer community activities that may help sell your skills. Hobbies and interests may be listed to demonstrate your more personal side.
References	State that these are available on request. Speak to former employers about using them as a reference and then have a list of references available when an interview is granted.

FIGURE 14.2
**Sample
Résumé**

BOBBIE KING
1700 Beltline Blvd.
My Town, GA 30107
(345) 555-3245

Objective: Position as pharmacy technician that makes use of my training in dispensing and compounding medications, ordering and inventory, patient profiling, third-party billing, and other essential functions

Education	Diploma in Health Science—Pharmacy	August 20XX–May 20XX
	My Town Technical College in My Town, GA	
	Program Accredited by American Society of Health-System Pharmacists (ASHP)	
	Dean's List	
Certification	(awaiting results)	July 20XX
	National Pharmacy Technician Certification Exam	
Skills	Converting units of measure	
	Setting up ratios and proportions for proper performance of pharmacy calculations	
	Preparing aseptic intravenous (IV) solutions	
	Proper interpretation of prescriptions and physician's orders	
	Proper interpretation and updating of prescription records	
	Attention to clerical detail	
	Operation of pharmacy computer systems and software	
	Preparation of compounded prescription products	
	Conversational Spanish	
Employment	Clerk	January 20XX–present
	Arborland Pharmacy in Erewhon, GA	
	Duties included customer service, operating cash register, and stocking inventory.	
	Sales Associate	September 20XX–January 20XX
	Brenda's Sporting Goods in My Town, GA	
	Duties included customer service and operating a cash register.	

References available on request.

Write a Good Résumé

Make use of some of the excellent résumé-writing software now available, or contact a résumé-writing service. A résumé is a brief written summary of what you have to offer an employer. It is a marketing tool, and the product you are selling is yourself. A résumé is an opportunity to present your work experience, your skills, and your education to an employer. Table 14.2 outlines the general topics to be included in a chronological résumé.

Make sure that your résumé follows a consistent, standard format such as the one shown in Figure 14.2. Limit it to a single page; type it or print it on a high-quality printer, using high-quality 8½ × 11 inch paper. Many special résumé papers are available from stationery and office supply shops; however, ordinary opaque or off-white paper is acceptable. Although unusual colors and textures may seem unique and serve to set you apart, they are usually viewed as unprofessional. Remaining conservative when selecting stationery is best to ensure that your résumé conveys a professional image.

Be sure to check your résumé carefully for errors in spelling, grammar, usage, punctuation, capitalization, and form. No one wants to hire a sloppy technician. Mistakes on your résumé may affect your prospective employer's confidence in the accuracy of your work. Once your résumé is complete, always have another person read through it and check for readability and for errors in spelling, grammar, and vocabulary—it is easy to overlook such things.

Establish a Network

Tell everyone you know that you are looking for a job. Identify faculty, acquaintances, friends, and relatives who can assist you in your job search. Identify persons within employers' organizations who can give you insight into their needs. If you complete any rotations or internships as part of your schooling, then ask your supervisors and coworkers about anticipated openings. If you perform well as a student-in-training, then you will be viewed as a good potential employee. Even previous graduates of your educational program can provide valuable information about hiring practices. Join state and national professional associations, attend meetings, and network with colleagues and potential employers.

Identify and Research Potential Employers

Your school may have a career placement office. If so, then use the services of that office. Check the classified ads in newspapers. Go to a career library and look up employers in directories. Look up potential employers in telephone directories. Make use of career opportunities posted on Web sites and job search Web sites; many local hospitals also have a Web site that is used to post job vacancies.

TABLE 14.3	Suggested Format for Cover Letters
First Paragraph	In your initial paragraph, state why you are writing, what specific position or type of work you are seeking, and how you learned of the opening (e.g., from the placement office, the news media, a friend). If you learned of the opening through networking, then be sure to mention who told you about the position. It may help get the employer's attention.
Second Paragraph	Explain why you are interested in the position, the organization, or the organization's products and services. This may take some investigation, but it shows desire and thoroughness. State how your academic background makes you a qualified candidate for the position. If you have had some practical experience, then point out your specific achievements.
Third Paragraph	Refer the reader to the enclosed résumé: a summary of your qualifications, training, and experience. If specific items on your résumé require a special explanation, then tactfully and positively point them out; you can include work experience from outside of pharmacy, but be sure that it relates to skills that you will use as a technician.
Fourth Paragraph	Indicate your desire for a personal interview and your flexibility as to the time and place. Repeat your telephone number (and cell phone number), as well as the best times to reach you, in the letter. If you use e-mail as a preferred method of communication, then let the employer know that. Close your letter with a statement or question to encourage a response, or take the initiative by indicating a day and date on which you will contact the employer to set up a convenient time for a personal meeting.

FIGURE 14.3
Sample Cover Letter in Block Style

February 1, 20XX

James Green, PharmD
Pharmacy Manager
Main Street Community Pharmacy
1500 Main Street
My Town, GA 30107

Dear Dr. Green:

I learned of Main Street Community Pharmacy's need for a pharmacy technician through the placement office at My Town Technical College. I was pleased to learn of an opening for a technician at the very pharmacy that my family has frequented for years.

I believe that my education and experience would be an asset to Main Street Community Pharmacy. In May, I graduated from My Town Technical College's pharmacy technician training program, and I just took the National Pharmacy Technician Certification Examination. I would welcome the opportunity to apply what I have learned to a career with your pharmacy. I bring to the job a number of assets, including a 3.4 grade point average, commitment to continuing development of my skills as a technician, a willingness to work hard, and a desire to be of service.

As you can see from my enclosed résumé, I already have some experience in pharmacy as a clerk. I am a responsible person, concerned with accuracy and accountability, and someone whom you can depend upon to carry out the technician's duties reliably. I also have plenty of experience—although not in pharmacy directly—dealing with customers in my position as a sales associate. Working with the public is something I am quite comfortable with and something I greatly enjoy.

I would appreciate an opportunity to discuss the position with you. I will call next week to inquire about a meeting. Thank you for considering my application.

Sincerely,

Brenda Collins
1700 Beltline Blvd.
My Town, GA 30107

Enc.: résumé

Write a Strong Cover Letter

The cover letter, or letter of application, is the first communication that you send to an employer in response to a job advertisement or posting. Your résumé should accompany the cover letter. Both the cover letter and the résumé should be typed or printed on the same kind of paper, and both should be placed in a matching business envelope addressed by means of typing or printing on a laser printer. The letter should be single-spaced, using a block or modified block style. In the block style, all items in the letter begin at the left margin. In the modified block style, the sender's address, the complimentary close, and the signature are left-aligned from the center of the paper, and all other parts of the letter begin at the left margin.

The cover letter should highlight your qualifications and call attention to your résumé, preferably in a one-page format. A sloppy cover letter detracts from even the most professional résumé. As with your résumé, proofread the cover letter carefully for errors in spelling, grammar, usage, punctuation, capitalization, and form. Address the letter, when possible, to a particular person by name and by title, and make sure to identify the position for which you are applying. Sometimes it takes extra investigation to find out these details, but it shows initiative and professionalism when the letter is addressed to the specific person (with his or her correct degree and title) who is doing the hiring. A letter addressed "To whom it may concern" does not get the same reception as one addressed to the actual pharmacist (or human resources) manager in charge of hiring. Pharmacists may have various degrees or titles: Registered Pharmacist (RPh), Bachelor of Science in Pharmacy (BS Pharm), or Doctor of Pharmacy (PharmD). If necessary, call the secretary at the employer's office to get the correct spelling (and title if necessary) of the recipient's name. Do not make assumptions. No one likes to receive correspondence with his or her name spelled incorrectly. Use the format shown in Table 14.3 for your letter. Figure 14.3 shows a sample cover letter.

Prepare for the Interview

Review your research on the employer and role-play an interview situation. Get plenty of sleep, and eat well on the day before as well as the day of the interview. Find out everything that you can about the company or institution before you go for an interview. Better yet, do this work before you write the cover letter that you

TABLE 14.4 Guidelines for Job Interviews

1. Find out the exact place and time of the interview. Get directions or information on parking if necessary.
2. Know the full name of the company and its address and the interviewer's full name with its correct pronunciation. Call the employer, if necessary, to get this information.
3. Know something about the company's operations.
4. Be courteous to the receptionist, if one exists, and to other employees. Any person with whom you meet or speak may be in a position to influence your employment.
5. Bring to the interview your résumé and the names, addresses, and telephone numbers of people who have agreed to provide references.
6. Arrive 10 to 15 minutes before the scheduled time for the interview.
7. Wear clothing and shoes appropriate to the job.
8. Greet the interviewer and call him or her by name. Introduce yourself at once. Shake hands only if the interviewer offers to do so. Remain standing until invited to sit down.
9. Be confident, polite, poised, and enthusiastic.
10. Look the interviewer in the eye.
11. Speak clearly and loudly enough to be understood. Be positive and concise in your comments. Do not exaggerate, but remember that an interview is not an occasion for modesty.
12. Focus on your strengths. Be prepared to enumerate these, using specific examples as evidence to support the claims that you make about yourself.
13. Do not hesitate to ask about the specific duties associated with the job. Show keen interest as the interviewer tells you about these.
14. Avoid bringing up salary requirements until the employer broaches the subject.
15. Do not chew gum or smoke.
16. Do not criticize former employers, coworkers, or working conditions.
17. At the close of the interview, thank the interviewer for his or her time and for the opportunity to learn about the company.

send with your résumé. Knowing details about a potential employer can help you assess whether the employer is right for you and can win you points in your cover letter or interview.

During the interview, follow the guidelines provided in Table 14.4 and be prepared to answer the questions in Table 14.5. Rehearse answers to these questions before the interview. Rehearsing out loud can help you identify wording choices and avoid mixing up words during the actual interview. When coming up with answers to such questions, bear in mind the employer's point of view. Imagine what you would want if you were the employer, and then take the initiative during the interview to explain to the employer how you can meet those needs.

Some interviewers pose hypothetical situations and ask for your response, or they may ask you to describe a past experience and how you handled it. These types of questions require you to think on your feet and talk about your problem-solving skills. At the least, be ready to describe a situation or two from your past where you had to deal with a difficult coworker or member of the public. Choose a situation

---

TABLE 14.5 Interview Questions

1. Why did you apply for a job with this company?
2. What part of the job interests you most and why?
3. What do you know about this company?
4. What are your qualifications?
5. What did you like the most and the least about your work experience? (Note: Explaining what you liked least should be done in as positive a manner as possible. For example, you might say that you wish that the job had provided more opportunity for learning about this or that and then explain that you made up the deficiency by study on your own. Such an answer indicates your desire to learn and grow and does not cast your former employer in an unduly negative light.)
6. Why did you leave your previous job? (Avoid negative responses. Find a positive reason for leaving, such as returning to school or pursuing an opportunity.)
7. What would you like to be doing in five years? How much money would you like to be making? (Keep your answer reasonable, and show that you have ambitions consistent with the employer's needs.)
8. What are your weak points? (Say something positive such as, "I am an extremely conscientious person. Sometimes I worry too much about whether I have done something absolutely correctly, but that can also be a positive trait.")
9. Why do you think that you are qualified for this position?
10. Would you mind working on the weekends or overtime? How do you feel about traveling?
11. Do you prefer working with others or by yourself? Do you prefer a quiet or a noisy environment?
12. If you could have any job you wanted, then what would you choose, and why?
13. Tell me a little about yourself.
14. What are your hobbies and interests?
15. Why did you attend the college that you attended?
16. Why did you choose this field of study?
17. What courses did you like best? What courses did you like least? (State your responses to both questions in positive ways.)
18. What have you learned from your mistakes?
19. What motivates you to put forth your greatest efforts?
20. Do you plan to continue your education?

where you were pleased with how you responded, and describe the measures you took to improve the end result. Interviewers should not ask you questions about your religion, marital status, or if you have or plan to have children. You are not obligated to answer questions such as these. If the opportunity arises toward the end of the interview, then be sure to ask any questions that you may have—such as typical work schedule, weekends, vacation, benefits, and so on.

After the interview, follow up with a note thanking the interviewer for seeing you and (within an appropriate time) with a telephone call. Be persistent but not pushy. If you did not get the position, then thank the employer for the opportunity to interview and request that the company keep your cover letter and résumé on file for future positions.

Ethics in Pharmacy Practice

Ethics is the study of standards of conduct and moral judgment that outline the right or wrong of human conduct and character. Ethics is a process for reflection and analysis of behavior when the proper course of action is unclear. It is the basis on which to make judgments. In addition, it is the system or code of conduct of a particular person, group, or profession. It is not necessarily part of religious beliefs; even those who subscribe to no religion per se can have a sense of right and wrong conduct. However, religion often has an influence on personal ethics.

The most important benefit of studying ethics is to internalize a framework or set of guidelines based on high professional standards that guide your decision making and actions. Be aware of situations in which you may find yourself while working in health care, and examine and discuss how to react and behave when faced with those situations. By determining ahead of time the ethical choice in such situations, you can avoid the paralyzing quandary of being confronted with questionable circumstances.

Everyone faces hundreds of situations in which moral beliefs seem unfounded, uninformed, and anything but a foundation on which to base a moral decision. Through ethical study, an individual can make decisions using a moral compass and can understand and respect the viewpoints of others. Pharmacy technicians, working side by side with pharmacists, must recognize and adopt the accepted ethical standards of pharmacy practice.

Not all behaviors in pharmacy practice are done solely because of the law. Moral obligations exist that are not legal obligations and vice versa. Using the best-priced medication within choices of generics, making true disclosures of prescription wait times, and providing accurate information on out-of-stock situations are examples of these obligations. Laws and regulations governing the practice of pharmacy do not always dictate the proper behavior in every situation that is encountered in pharmacy.

Codes of Behavior

Ethical codes are based on the belief that a relationship of trust exists between a professional (i.e., the pharmacist) and a client (i.e., the patient). Two reasons for this exist. First, professional service is not standardized; it is unique and personal. These essential qualities cannot be specified in a contract or purchased. Second, the patient often hardly knows what to ask for, let alone how it can be provided. Therefore the patient is vulnerable to the services provided by the pharmacist.

Employees categorized as professional are held to high standards of conduct. As paraprofessionals, pharmacy technicians are also, by extension, held to high standards of conduct in their everyday practice. To be considered professionals, they must meet selected criteria. First, professionals hold a specialized body of knowledge, which enables the practitioner to perform a highly useful social function. A pharmacist is considered a professional not because he or she can type or dispense medications but because of his or her knowledge about drugs and how to help patients make the best use of medicine. Technicians also have a duty to maintain their competence and continually enhance their knowledge of practice, even if not required for recertification.

A second characteristic of a professional is that the individual has a set of attitudes that influence his or her professional behavior. The basic attitude is an unselfish concern for the welfare of others, called *altruism*. A pharmacy technician must be empathetic, because many patients whom they come in contract with on a daily basis feel ill or have serious diseases.

Finally, a third characteristic of a professional is social sanction. More than licensing, social sanction also creates trust between society (i.e., patients) and professionals (i.e., pharmacists). Social sanction rewards the professional with status, income, and power. The trust that a pharmacist has with society has been transferred more and more to the pharmacy technician. It is important to do what is right for the patient—at times, that may mean loaning the patient a few doses of prescription for a heart or blood pressure medicine at night or on the weekend, even though the patient has no refills remaining.

Codes of ethics statements regarding professional behavior are often written as formal documents and supported by professional organizations. These statements provide language to aid in the decision-making process when an ethical issue presents itself in pharmacy practice.

Dilemmas and Questions Facing Healthcare Professionals

A code of ethics assists a healthcare professional in choosing the most appropriate course of action to handle an ethical dilemma. An **ethical dilemma** is a situation that calls for a judgment between two or more solutions, not all of which are necessarily wrong. Deciding what action to take when faced with an ethical dilemma in the pharmacy requires consideration of the circumstances, choosing an action, and justifying the action. To do this, you should ask questions such as the following.

- What is the dilemma?
- What pharmaceutical alternatives apply?
- What is the best alternative, and can it be justified on moral grounds?

Pharmacy technicians must recognize and accept the ethical standards of pharmacy practice and apply them when working side by side with pharmacists. They must also understand decision-making processes and become personally involved in obtaining facts that are relevant to a dilemma, evaluating the alternatives, and determining the correct solutions. The following are examples that a pharmacist or technician may face in everyday practice.

- OTC emergency contraceptives may be entirely valid and legal. However, some pharmacists (and technicians) may reserve the right to refuse to dispense such medication because they consider it morally or ethically unsound based on their religious beliefs.
- You receive a legal narcotic prescription but, because you are a local, you know that the individual is selling the drugs on the street. Do you tell the pharmacist and refuse to fill the prescription or contact the physician?
- You are asked to fill narcotic or sedative prescriptions for patients who are obviously physically addicted or dependent on the drugs.

- Although the physician wrote a prescription for three tablets a day of a cholesterol medication, after conferring with the patient, you find out that he or she is only taking one tablet a day as directed. You realize that the order is being made to take unfair advantage of the insurance company.
- You are selling insulin syringes to an out-of-town customer. Is he or she diabetic or requesting the needles for using illegal drugs?
- You are selling OTC pseudoephedrine products to an out-of-state customer. Does he or she have self-limited cold symptoms or is he or she purchasing the product for an illegal methamphetamine laboratory?

As modern pharmacy practice continues to evolve, new questions will arise that challenge pharmacy personnel in new decision-making deliberations. Advances in medical health, pharmaceutical delivery systems, and new medication development change how pharmacists and pharmacy technicians conduct their daily work. The answers to such ethical practice questions deserve both individual and profession-wide debate. As with any politically, professionally, and emotionally charged topic, a variety of opinions will surface. When those differences occur, the pharmacy technician, whether working in a team or with an individual patient, must learn to respect differences without prejudice.

Trends in Pharmacy Practice

One of the wonderful things about a career in pharmacy is that it is a dynamic profession, changing continually. Consider how different the average community pharmacy of today is from the druggist's shop at the turn of the century, in which premanufactured medicines were novelties and rows of bottled tonics and elixirs vied for customers' attention with open barrels of hard candies. Doubtless the profession will change as much or more in the next 30 years as it did in the past 100 years, and that is a lot of change. The following are but a few of the exciting developments that lie in store for the profession.

Workforce Issues

As the volume of prescriptions rises and reliance on drug therapy increases, the need for qualified personnel in the pharmacy profession continues to grow. The number of prescriptions filled in 2008 was 4 billion, and some estimate that this volume will double over the next 5 to 15 years. Consequently, the need for pharmacists to handle this increased workload is expected to double as well. By 2020, up to 400,000 pharmacists may be needed to handle the increased prescription volume. The number of pharmacists, however, is expected to increase only 30% (from less than 200,000 to 260,000) over that same period. Therefore the need for well-trained, qualified technicians to bridge the gap between the volume of work to be done and the personnel available to do it will be critical.

As the pace of work in pharmacies around the country increases, the demands on pharmacists for more direct patient care, drug therapy assessment, and cognitive duties also expand. Pharmacists are increasingly called out of the pharmacy to handle patient care situations and consultations with prescribers. Technicians must step in to manage the workflow and prescription-processing system to keep up with these new demands on the pharmacists' time. Employment opportunities for pharmacy technicians look extremely good, especially for technicians with formal training or previous experience.

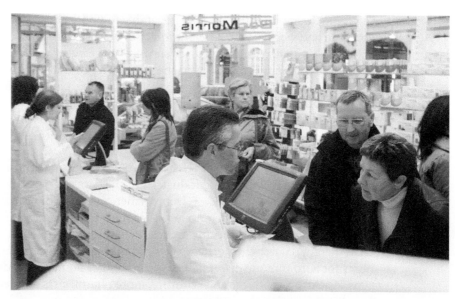

Demand for pharmacy technicians is expected to continue to grow through the year 2010 because of the increased pharmaceutical needs of a larger and older population.

Increased Emphasis on Mail-Order Pharmacies Mail order grew throughout the 1990s as plan sponsors continued to embrace its use, based on claims of cost savings. To contain rising healthcare costs, many employers mandate mail order or provide financial incentives to participate. Few studies, however, have proven a cost savings. Mail order has been the fastest growing distribution channel almost every year since 2000. Mail order accounted for $20.3 billion in sales in 2001; by 2004, sales at mail-order pharmacies had grown to $33.9 billion—a 67% increase in 3 years. Mail order now represents over 14% of all U.S. prescription sales, with projections of 25% of the market by 2011. The typical patient who uses mail order is at or near retirement age and consumes many medications for the many chronic illnesses of aging. A mail-order pharmacy is typically a warehouse operation, using the latest automation, with the capacity to dispense 6000 prescriptions per hour 24 hours per day (large national mail-order pharmacies have the capacity to fill 2 million prescriptions per week). Personnel needs for both pharmacists and pharmacy technicians will expand to oversee these operations and meet the expected growth in this area of practice.

Increased Emphasis on Managed Care Managed care has been applying fiscal conservation to the healthcare system since the early 1990s. The increased emphasis on primary and preventative care with attention to cost-effective medical services that managed care introduced has, in effect, revolutionized the healthcare system. As such, the practice of pharmacy has felt the squeeze. Pharmacy is increasingly called upon to provide the most appropriate drug therapy at the lowest possible cost. Technicians will find new opportunities available in support roles with pharmacists who work closely with programs and efforts to encourage smart but inexpensive drug use. The nature of this work may differ greatly in its day-to-day, hands-on time with drug products. Increased communication, writing, and computer application skills will be necessary for technicians specializing in managed care settings.

Increased Geriatric Applications As the population of the United States ages, the importance and volume of dispensing medications will increase. The aging of the population will place great financial burdens on the healthcare system as a whole and on pharmacy in particular, leading inevitably to political decisions that will affect the workload and work place of the pharmacist and the technician. Pharmacists and technicians will increasingly provide services to the population of older adults in the community pharmacy, as well as in the nursing home and the home health setting.

In addition, with Medicare Part D drug insurance, patients who are older adults will have some coverage for prescription costs, whereas they did not before. Although this is good news, the program is complex and can be confusing to a population that already finds navigating the Internet and the healthcare system difficult.

Increased Emphasis on Home Healthcare The home healthcare industry is one of the most rapidly growing of all industries in the developed world. The reasons behind this growth include reduced cost, improvements in technology that make home care more practical, and the preference of individuals for remaining under treatment at home rather than in institutions. Examples may include home TPN therapy, HIV/AIDS therapy, cancer chemotherapy, home antibiotic infusions, and biogenetic treatments for autoimmune diseases. The growth of the home care industry shows no signs of abating; therefore, in the future, more pharmacists and technicians will find themselves servicing this industry.

Growth in Clinical Applications The pharmaceutical care movement continues to grow. In the future, more of the pharmacy professional's time and energies will be given to educational and counseling functions. For instance, more pharmacies offer specialty services in education and management for patients who have diabetes or asthma. Pharmacists are commonly administering vaccinations in their communities. Managed care pharmacists may specialize in areas such as anticoagulation control and cholesterol management of patients with high risk for heart disease. In the hospital, pharmacists may specialize in total parenteral nutrition, pharmacokinetics, infectious disease, neonatology, and so on. This growth in clinical applications by the pharmacist requires increasing support by pharmacy technicians in the routine functions of medication preparation and dispensing.

Increased Technician Responsibility and Specialization Some states are already experimenting with allowing trained technicians to check the work of other technicians. Other states allow the pharmacy technician to accept new prescriptions from a physician's office. In the future, you can expect technicians to be given ever more responsibility; more technicians will become specialized in particular areas of service, such as sterile and nonsterile compounding and diabetic education. Technicians could find themselves working more on a one-on-one basis with patients to help them choose and use a glucose meter or a blood pressure monitor.

New Medicines and New Drug Development Technologies

Every day, new medicines come to market, many involving new drug development technologies such as genetic engineering. To work in pharmacy is to be at the front line when new medications are introduced to combat acquired immunodeficiency syndrome (AIDS), cancer, heart disease, cystic fibrosis, and other challenging diseases. Automation in every facet of drug distribution will play an increasingly important role in the profession. What the future holds is anyone's guess, but the one certainty is that new dosage forms, delivery mechanisms, and technologies will continue to evolve and emerge.

New Dosage Forms and Drug Delivery Mechanisms New dosage forms and drug delivery mechanisms are not introduced as often as new drugs, but the pace of innovation is increasing rapidly. In the past few years, such innovations as additional transdermal medications, ocular inserts, long-acting medications lasting more than a month, liposomes, and monoclonal antibodies have been introduced. In the near future, wearable intravenous (IV) infusion pumps may be combined with continuous sensory meters, creating, in effect, an artificial pancreas.

Robotics Robotic machinery, which is commonplace in mail-order pharmacies, is already used in many institutional settings for unit dose repackaging and for IV and TPN mixing procedures. It is being installed in the community pharmacy setting with greater frequency. Robotics will likely play a larger role in the future pharmacy, providing, for example, automated compounding, filling, labeling, and recordkeeping in a single device. The increased emphasis of e-prescribing and eMAR will continue in all practice settings. The use of bar coding and scanning has increased in both hospital and community pharmacies to maximize efficiency and minimize medication errors.

Increased Healthcare and Drug Costs

The United States spends a higher percentage of its gross national product (or GNP) on health care than any other country in the world. However, the United States is not among the leaders in average life span: this may be because of risky health behavior (diet, lack of exercise, smoking, alcohol excess, and so on) and the fact that more than 47 million citizens are without health insurance.

The costs for caring for patients who are enrolled in both government and private insurance programs are expected to outpace inflation over the next decade as the Baby Boomers enter their retirement years. The costs for Medicare (age greater than 65 years) are projected to more than double, from $427 billion to $884 billion, by 2017. The costs for Medicaid (for individuals who are poor or disabled) are projected to more than double, from $338 billion to $717 billion, by 2017. The costs for nursing home care are projected to increase 55% by 2016 and the costs for home healthcare by 100%. The net costs of the Medicare Part D drug insurance program are projected to increase from $60.3 billion in 2008 to $126.7 billion in 2015. The costs of healthcare spending are expected to consume over 20% of the GNP of the United States by 2017.

As patients spend more on health care in the United States, employers who offer health insurance as a benefit are paying more and thus experiencing greater drains on their bottom lines. As they ask employees to share in the financial burden of these increased costs, patients themselves are becoming more sensitive to the costs of health care and prescription drugs. The trend for employers and individuals alike is for more consumer-driven health insurance plans with higher deductibles in order to cope, at least partially, with rising healthcare costs and insurance premiums. Pharmacy staff need to work with these patients, as well as those without prescription insurance, to identify the most cost-effective and affordable options for drug therapy.

Chapter Terms

certification the process by which a professional organization grants recognition to an individual who has met certain predetermined qualifications

Certified Pharmacy Technician (CPhT) a pharmacy technician who has passed the PTCE or ExCPT examination

credential a documented piece of evidence of one's qualifications

ethical dilemma a situation that calls for a judgment between two or more solutions, not all of which are necessarily wrong

ethics the study of standards of conduct and moral judgment that outlines the right or wrong of human conduct or character

Exam for Certification of Pharmacy Technicians (ExCPT) an examination developed by the Institute for the Certification of Pharmacy Technicians (ICPT) that technicians must pass to be certified and receive the title of CPhT

licensure the granting of a license by the state, usually to work in a profession, in order to protect the public

paraprofessional a trained person who assists a professional person

Pharmacy Technician Certification Examination (PTCE) an examination developed by the Pharmacy Technician Certification Board (PTCB) that technicians must pass to be certified and receive the title of CPhT

professional someone with recognized expertise in a field who is expected to use his or her knowledge and skills to benefit others and to operate ethically with some autonomy

recertification the periodic updating of certification

registration mandatory signing up or registering with the State Board of Pharmacy before starting to practice

Chapter Summary

- The occupational outlook for the pharmacy technician is very promising. Increasingly, states are requiring national certification and possibly formal education.
- Preparing to work in an institutional or community-based pharmacy requires serious thought about one's attitude, reliability, accuracy, responsibility, personal appearance, organizational skills, and ability to relate to others.
- Technicians will have increasing opportunities for job advancement as requirements for certification and training increase.
- Certification for pharmacy technicians is offered through the Pharmacy Technician Certification Board (PTCB) and the Institute for Certification of Pharmacy Technicians (ICPT).
- Active involvement in professional organizations is important for establishing a network of colleagues and professional advancement.
- Writing a comprehensive, attractive résumé and cover letter is an important part of a carefully planned job search.
- Preparing for a job interview is integral to obtaining a desirable technician position.
- Society holds the pharmacy technician, as a paraprofessional, to a high code of ethics.
- New trends in the pharmacy workforce, in technologies, and in healthcare costs will have a positive impact on the role of technicians.

Chapter Review

Checking Your Understanding

Choose the best answer from those provided.

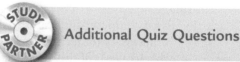 **Additional Quiz Questions**

1. The organization that certifies pharmacy technicians is the
   a. Pharmacy Technician Certification Board (PTCB).
   b. Institute for Certification of Pharmacy Technicians (ICPT).
   c. Both a and b are correct
   d. State Board of Pharmacy.

2. The format for the PTCE and ExCPT examinations is
   a. essay.
   b. multiple choice.
   c. true or false.
   d. on-site laboratory assessment.

3. How many pharmacy technicians have passed the certification examination in the United States?
   a. 25,000
   b. 75,000
   c. 160,000
   d. 275,000

4. To be eligible to take a technician certification exam, a candidate must meet all of the following requirements *except*
   a. being at least 18 years of age.
   b. having a high school diploma or GED.
   c. working 50 hours in a community or hospital pharmacy.
   d. having never been convicted of a felony.

5. Once a technician becomes certified (i.e., a CPhT), he or she can be recertified every two years by obtaining how many continuing education credits/hours?
   a. 2
   b. 15
   c. 20
   d. 60

6. Which of the following statements regarding the code of ethics for pharmacy technicians is true?
   a. The basis for the code of ethics is built entirely on laws and regulations governing pharmacy practice.
   b. Technicians have a duty to maintain competence and continually enhance their knowledge of practice.
   c. A technician's first consideration is to engage in the support of organizations that promote the profession of pharmacy and the role of technicians.
   d. All of the above

7. A standard résumé generally does *not* list
   a. the job objective.
   b. employment history.
   c. name, address, and telephone number of the applicant.
   d. names, addresses, and telephone numbers of references.

8. A candidate without a great deal of work experience can compensate for this deficiency by emphasizing the
   a. employment history section of the résumé.
   b. references section of the résumé.
   c. job objective section of the résumé.
   d. skills section of the résumé.

9. The cover letter sent with a résumé should highlight your
   a. qualifications.
   b. personality.
   c. network of connections.
   d. need for the job.

10. The increased emphasis and needs of the geriatric population will affect pharmacy technicians most specifically in which of the following ways?
    a. Increased computer application skills will be necessary for technicians to deal with the demands of this particular patient population.
    b. Robotics will play a larger role in the pharmacy, and technicians will have to work more closely with them to serve this population.
    c. Technicians will have to become familiar with Medicare Part D to assist these patients in gaining needed information about this drug coverage program.
    d. Technicians must step in to manage prescription-processing systems as pharmacists are increasingly called upon to provide greater clinical services.

Thinking Like a Pharmacy Tech

1. Using reference texts and the Internet, compile a list of three potential employers of pharmacy technicians in each of the following areas in your state: community pharmacy, hospital pharmacy, long-term care, and home infusion. Each list should include the name of the employer, the address, the telephone number, and a contact person. Collect the lists prepared by students in the class to make a master list.

2. Choose one potential employer of pharmacy technicians and find more information about the employer. Write a brief report providing information that might be of interest to a potential employee of this pharmacy or institution. Write a résumé and cover letter that you might use to apply for a job as a pharmacy technician.

3. Consider the following ethical dilemma facing pharmacy personnel: a pharmacist's religious beliefs preclude him or her from dispensing an emergency contraceptive prescription. Write a brief report on how this applies to the technician working under the supervision of this pharmacist. What would you do in such a situation if presented with a prescription for emergency contraception?

Communicating Clearly

1. Practice role-playing an interview situation with other students in your class. Use the interview questions supplied in this chapter. Develop or update your résumé. Share your résumé with another student. Ask that student to critique and identify your strengths, based on your résumé.

2. Debate with another student whether border states should encourage illegal drug importation from outside the United States (e.g., from Canada).

Researching on the Web

1. Visit the Web site of the Institute for the Certification of Pharmacy Technicians (ICPT) at www.icpt.org and view the registration and certification requirements for pharmacy technicians in your state. Include your state's maximum allowed ratio of technicians to pharmacists, CE requirements, and status of ExCPT.

2. Write a letter to the PTCB or ICPT requesting the information needed to take a certification exam.

3. Search the Web for the American Association of Pharmacy Technicians (AAPT). Some areas have a local chapter with a Web site. Locate the contact person's name, the next meeting dates, and times.

4. Search the Internet for news on which states allow "right-to-die" or physician-assisted suicide prescriptions. Report on what procedures must be taken to fill such a prescription in the pharmacy. What ethical dilemma might pharmacy personnel encounter in a state where such prescriptions are legal?

5. The ethical implications of the Human Genome Project are very serious and involve the pharmacy directly. Physicians may someday be able to diagnose instantly a disease that is based on the patient's genetic makeup. In addition, drug therapies may be designed specifically for a patient, based on his or her genetic makeup. Physicians, pharmacists, and many members of the healthcare team will need to access a patient's genetic information. Consider some of the ethical implications of this project, and prepare for a class discussion by listing some of the pros and cons of genetic testing. Poll the class: how many are for genetic testing and how many are against?

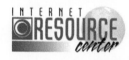

For further study of chapter-related topics, explore the Web links in the Web Center at www.emcp.net/pharmpractice4e.

Appendix A

Most Commonly Prescribed Drugs

Generic Name	Pronunciation	Category	Brand Name
acetaminophen	a-seat-a-MIN-oh-fen	analgesic	Tylenol
acetaminophen-codeine	a-seat-a-MIN-oh-fen KOE-deen	analgesic	Phenaphen With Codeine, Tylenol With Codeine
acyclovir	ay-SYE-kloe-veer	systemic antifungal	Zovirax
albuterol	al-BYOO-ter-ole	bronchodilator	Proventil, Proventil HFA, Ventolin HFA, ProAir HFA
alendronate	a-LEN-droe-nate	bone resorption inhibitor	Fosamax, Fosamax Plus D
alfuzosin	al-FYOO-zoe-sin	alpha blocker	Uroxatral
allopurinol	al-oh-PURE-i-nawl	antigout agent	Zyloprim
alprazolam	al-PRAZ-oh-lam	antianxiety agent, sleep agent	Xanax
amitriptyline	a-mee-TRIP-ti-leen	antidepressant	Elavil
amlodipine	am-LOE-di-peen	antihypertensive	Norvasc
amlodipine-benazepril	am-LOE-di-peen ben-AYE-ze-pril	antihypertensive	Lotrel
amlodipine-atoravastatin	am-LOE-di-peen a-tor-va-STAT-in	antihypertensive-statin	Caduet
amoxicillin	a-mox-i-SIL-in	systemic antibacterial	Amoxil, Trimox
amoxicillin-clavulanate	a-mox-i-SIL-in klav-yoo-LAN-ate	systemic antibacterial	Augmentin
aripiprazole	air-i-PIP-ra-zole	antipsychotic	Abilify
aspirin-dipyridamole	AS-pir-in dye-peer-ID-a-mole	stroke prevention agent	Aggrenox
atenolol	a-TEN-oh-lawl	antihypertensive	Tenormin
atenolol-hydrochlorothiazide	a-TEN-oh-lawl hye-droe-klor-oh-THYE-a-zide	beta-blocker-diuretic	Tenorectic
atomoxetine	at-oh-MOX-e-teen	ADHD therapy agent	Strattera
atorvastatin	a-tor-va-STAT-in	antihyperlipidemic	Lipitor
azithromycin	az-ith-roe-MYE-sin	systemic antibacterial	Zithromax

Note: This table, reformatted and organized by brand name, is available on this textbook's Internet Resource Center at www.emcp.net/pharmpractice4e.

Generic Name	Pronunciation	Category	Brand Name
benazepril	ben-AZ-eh-pril	antihypertensive	Lotensin
benazapril-hydrochlorothiazide	ben-AZ-eh-pril hye-droe-klor-oh-THYE-a-zide	antihypertensive-diuretic	Lotensin HCTZ
bisoprolol-hydrochlorothiazide	bis-OE-proe-lawl hye-droe-klor-oh-THYE-a-zide	beta-blocker-diuretic	Ziac
brimonidine	bri-MOE-ni-deen	antiglaucoma agent	Alphagan P
budesonide	byoo-DES-oh-nide	antiasthmatic	Entocort EC, Pulmicort Respules, Pulmicort Turbuhaler, Rhinocort
bupropion	byoo-PROE-pee-on	antidepressant, smoking cessation adjunct	Wellbutrin, Zyban
buspirone	byoo-SPYE-rone	antianxiety	BuSpar
calcitonin-salmon	kal-si-TOE-nin SAM-en	bone resorption inhibitor	Miacalcin
candesartan	kan-de-SAR-tan	antihypertensive	Atacand
carisoprodol	kar-eye-soe-PROE-dawl	skeletal muscle relaxant	Soma
carvedilol	KAR-ve-dil-ole	antihypertensive	Coreg
cefdinir	sef-DI-neer	systemic antibacterial	Omnicef
cefprozil	sef-PROE-zil	systemic antibacterial	Cefzil
celecoxib	sel-a-KOX-ib	analgesic, antirheumatic NSAID	Celebrex
cephalexin	sef-a-LEX-in	systemic antibacterial	Keflex
cetirizine	se-TEER-a-zeen	antihistaminic, H_1 receptor	Zyrtec
cetirizine-pseudoephedrine	se-TEER-a-zeen soo-doe-e-FED-rin	antihistaminic, H_1 receptor–decongestant	Zyrtec-D
ciprofloxacin	sip-roe-FLOX-a-sin	ophthalmic antibacterial	Occuflox, Ciprodex, Ciloxan
		systemic antibacterial	Cipro
citalopram	sye-TAL-oh-pram	antidepressant	Celexa
clarithromycin	kla-rith-roe-MYE-sin	systemic antibacterial, antimycobacterial	Biaxin
clindamycin	klin-da-MYE-sin	antibiotic	Cleocin
clonazepam	kloe-NAZ-e-pam	anticonvulsant	Klonopin
clonidine	KLON-i-deen	antihypertensive	Catapres, Catapres-TTS Duraclon
clopidogrel	kloh-PID-oh-grel	antithrombotic, platelet aggregation inhibitor	Plavix
clotrimazole-betamethasone	kloe-TRIM-a-zole bay-ta-METH-a-sone	antifungal, corticosteroid	Lotrisone

Generic Name	Pronunciation	Category	Brand Name
conjugated estrogen	CON-ju-gate-ed ES-troe-jen	antineoplastic, systemic estrogen, osteoporosis prophylactic, ovarian hormone therapy agent	Cenestin, Enjuvia, Premarin
conjugated estrogen–medroxyprogesterone	CON-ju-gate-ed ES-troe-jen me-DROX-ee-proe-JES-te-rone	estrogen-progestin, osteoporosis prophylactic, ovarian hormone therapy agent	Premphase, Prempro
cyclobenzaprine	sye-kloe-BEN-za-preen	skeletal muscle relaxant	Flexeril
desloratadine	des-lor-AT-a-deen	antihistaminic, H_1 receptor	Clarinex
dextroamphetamine-amphetamine	dex-troe-am-FET-a-meen am-FET-a-meen	CNS stimulant, ADHD therapy	Adderall
diazepam	dye-AZ-e-pam	amnestic, antianxiety agent, anticonvulsant, antipanic agent, anti-tremor agent, sedative-hypnotic, skeletal muscle relaxant adjunct	Valium
diclofenac-misoprostol	dye-KLOE-fen-ak mye-soe-PROST-awl	NSAID	Arthrotec
digoxin	di-JOX-in	antiarrhythmic, cardiotonic	Lanoxicaps Lanoxin
diltiazem	dil-TYE-a-zem	antianginal, antiarrhythmic, antihypertensive	Cardizem Dilacor XR
divalproex	dye-VAL-pro-ex	anticonvulsant, antiman-ic, migraine headache prophylactic	Depakote
donepezil	don-EP-a-zil	dementia symptoms treatment adjunct	Aricept
doxycycline	dox-i-SYE-kleen	systemic antibacterial, antiprotozoal	Vibramycin, Oracea, Adoxa, Doryx
enalapril	e-NAL-a-pril	antihypertensive, vasodilator	Vasotec
escitalopram	es-sye-TAL-oh-pram	antianxiety agent, antidepressant	Lexapro
esomeprazole	es-oh-MEP-ray-zole	gastric acid pump inhibitor, antiulcer agent	Nexium
estradiol	es-tra-DYE-awl	estrogen only hormone replacement	Alora, Climara, Elestrin, Eselim, Estrace, Estraderm, Estrasorb, Estring, Evamist, Femring, Menostar, Vivelle, Vivelle Dot
eszopiclone	es-zo-PIK-lone	hypnotic	Lunesta

Generic Name	Pronunciation	Category	Brand Name
ethinyl estradiol–desogestrel	ETH-in-il es-tra-DYE-awl des-oh-JES-trel	antiendometriotic, systemic contraceptive, gonadotropin inhibitor	Cyclessa, Desogen, Kariva, Mircette, Ortho-Cept
ethinyl estradiol–drospirenone	ETH-in-il es-tra-DYE-awl droh-SPYE-re-none	systemic contraceptive	Yasmin, Yaz
ethinyl estradiol–levonorgestrel	ETH-in-il es-tra-DYE-awl LEE-voe-nor-jes-trel	antiendometriotic, systemic postcoital contraceptive, systemic contraceptive, estrogen progestin, gonadotropin inhibitor	Aviane, Levlen, Lybrel, Nordette, Seasonale, Tri-Levlen, Triphasil, Trivora-28
ethinyl estradiol–norelgestromin	ETH-in-il es-tra-DYE-awl nor-el-JES-troe-min	systemic contraceptive	Ortho Evra
ethinyl estradiol–norethindrone	ETH-in-il es-tra-DYE-awl nor-eth-IN-drone	antiacne agent, antiendometriotic, systemic contraceptive, estrogen progestin, gonadotropin inhibitor	Estrostep Fe, femhrt, Loestrin Fe, Loestrin 24 Fe Ovcon
ethinyl estradiol–norgestimate	ETH-in-il es-tra-DYE-awl nor-JES-ti-mate	antiacne agent, antiendometriotic, systemic contraceptive, estrogen progestin, gonadotropin inhibitor	Ortho Tri-Cyclen, Ortho Tri-Cyclen Lo
ethinyl estradiol-norgestrel	ETH-in-il es-tra-DYE-awl nor-JES-trel	antiacne agent, antiendometriotic, systemic contraceptive, estrogen progestin, gonadotropin inhibitor	Lo/Ovral, Low-Ogestral, Ovral
ezetimibe	ee-ZET-e-mib	antihyperlipidemic	Zetia
ezetimbe-simvastatin	ee-ZET-e-mib sim-va STAT-in	antihyperlipidemic-statin	Vytorin
famotidine	fa-MOE-ti-deen	H-2 Histamine receptor antagonist	Pepcid
fenofibrate	fen-oh-FYE-brate	antihyperlipidemic	TriCor
fentanyl	FEN-ta-nil	analgesic	Duragesic
		analgesic, anesthesia adjunct	Actiq, Sublimaze
fexofenadine	fex-o-FEN-a-deen	antihistaminic, H_1 receptor	Allegra
fexofenadine-pseudoephedrine	fex-o-FEN-a-deen soo-doe-e-FED-rin	antihistaminic, H_1 receptor–decongestant	Allegra-D
finasteride	fin-AS-tur-ide	benign prostatic hyperplasia therapy agent, hair growth stimulant	Propecia, Proscar
fluconazole	floo-KOE-na-zole	systemic antifungal	Diflucan
fluoxetine	floo-OX-e-teen	antidepressant, antiobsessional agent, antibulemic agent	Prozac, Sarafem

Generic Name	Pronunciation	Category	Brand Name
fluticasone	floo-TIK-a-sone	steroidal nasal anti-inflammatory, nasal corticosteroid	Flonase, Flovent
fluticasone-salmeterol	floo-TIK-a-sone sal-ME-te-role	antiasthmatic, inhalation anti-inflammatory, bronchodilator	Advair Diskus
furosemide	fur-OH-se-mide	antihypercalcemic, antihypertensive, renal disease diagnostic aid adjunct, diuretic	Lasix
gabapentin	gab-a-PEN-tin	anticonvulsant, antineuralgic	Neurontin
gemfibrozil	jem-FI-broe-zil	antihyperlipidimic	Lopid
glimepiride	GLYE-me-pye-ride	antidiabetic	Amaryl
glipizide	GLIP-i-zide	antidiabetic	Glucotrol, Glucotrol XL
glyburide	GLYE-byoo-ride	antidiabetic	DiaBeta, Glynase, Micronase
glyburide-metformin	GLYE-byoo-ride met-FOR-min	antidiabetic	Glucovance
guaifenesin	gwye-FEN-e-sin	expectorant	Mucinex
guaifenesin-codeine	gwye-FEN-e-sin KOE-deen	expectorant	Robitussin A-C
guaifenesin-pseudoephedrine	gwye-FEN-e-sin soo-doe-e-FED-rin	expectorant-decongestant	Mucinex D
hydrochlorothiazide	hye-droe-klor-oh-THYE-a-zide	antihypertensive, diuretic, antiurolithic	Esidrix
hydrocodone-acetaminophen	hye-droe-KOE-done a-seat-a-MIN-oh-fen	analgesic	Lortab, Vicodin
hydrocodone-chlorpheniramine	hye-droe-KOE-done klor-fen-EER-a-meen	antihistaminic, H_1 receptor–antitussive	Tussionex
ibandronate	eye-BAN-droh-nate	bone resorption inhibitor	Boniva
ibuprofen	eye-byoo-PROE-fen	analgesic	Advil, Motrin
insulin glargine	IN-soo-lin GLARE-jeen	antidiabetic	Lantus
insulin lispro	IN-soo-lin LYE-sproe	antidiabetic	Humalog
insulin regular	IN-soo-lin re-gyoo-lar	antidiabetic	Humilin R, Novolin R
ipratropium	i-pra-TROE-pee-um	antiasthmatic	Atrovent
ipratropium-albuterol	i-pra-TROE-pee-um al-BYOO-ter-ole	antiasthmatic-bronchodilator	Combivent
irbesartan	ir-be-SAR-tan	antihypertensive	Avapro
irbesartan-hydrochlorothiazide	ir-be-SAR-tan hye-droe-klor-oh-THYE-a-zide	antihypertensive, diuretic	Avalide
isosorbide-hydralazine	eye-soe-SOR-bide hye-DRAL-a-zeen	vasodilator	BiDil

Generic Name	Pronunciation	Category	Brand Name
lamotrigine	la-MOE-tri-jeen	anticonvulsant	Lamictal
lansoprazole	lan-SOE-pra-zole	gastric acid pump inhibitor, antiulcer agent	Prevacid
latanoprost	la-TAN-oe-prost	antiglaucoma agent, ocular antihypertensive	Xalatan
levofloxacin	lee-voe-FLOX-a-sin	systemic antibacterial	Levaquin
levothyroxine, T$_4$	lee-voe-thye-ROX-een	antineoplastic, thyroid function diagnostic aid, thyroid hormone	Levothroid, Synthroid
lisinopril	lyse-IN-oh-pril	antihypertensive, vasodilator	Prinivil, Zestril
lisinopril-hydrochlorothiazide	lyse-IN-oh-pril hye-droe-klor-oh-THYE-a-zide	antihypertensive, diuretic	Zestoretic
lorazepam	lor-AZ-e-pam	amnestic, antianxiety agent, anticonvulsant, antiemetic, antipanic agent, antitremor agent, sedative-hypnotic, skeletal muscle relaxant	Ativan
losartan	loe-SAR-tan	angiotensin II–receptor antagonist, antihypertensive	Cozaar
losartan-hydrochlorothiazide	loe-SAR-tan hye-droe-klor-oh-THYE-a-zide	antihypertensive-diuretic	Hyzaar
lovestatin	loe-ve-STAT-in	lipid-lowering agent	Mevacor
meclizine	MEK-li-zeen	antiemetic, antivertigo agent	Antivert
meloxicam	mel-OX-i-kam	antirheumatic (NSAID)	Mobic
memantine	MEM-an-teen	treatment of dementia	Namenda
metaxalone	me-TAX-a-lone	skeletal muscle relaxant	Skelaxin
metformin	met-FOR-min	antihyperglycemic	Glucophage, Riornet
methylphenidate	meth-il-FEN-i-date	CNS stimulant, ADHD therapy	Concerta, Daytrana, Metadate, Metadate ER, Methylin, Ritalin-SR, Ritalin
methylprednisolone	meth-il-pred-NIS-oh-lone	steroidal anti-inflammatory, corticoid steroid, immunosuppressant	Medrol, Solu-Medrol
metoclopromide	met-oh-KLOE-pra-mide	anti-emetic	Reglan
metolazone	me-TOLE-a-zone	thiazide diuretic	Zaroxolyn
metronidazole	me-tro-NYE-da-zole	systemic antibiotic	Flagyl

Generic Name	Pronunciation	Category	Brand Name
metoprolol	met-TOE-proe-lawl	antiadrenergic, antianginal, antianxiety therapy adjunct, antiarrhythmic, antihypertensive, antitremor agent, hypertrophic cardiomyopathy therapy adjunct, myocardial infarction therapy, neuroleptic-induced akathisia therapy, pheochromocytoma therapy adjunct, thyrotoxicosis therapy adjunct, vascular headache prophylactic	Lopressor, Toprol-XL
minocycline	mi-noe-SYE-kleen	systemic antibacterial	Minocin Soladyne
mirtazapine	meer-TAZ-a-peen	antidepressant	Remeron
mometasone	moe-MET-a-sone	nasal steroidal anti-inflammatory, nasal corticosteroid	Nasonex
montelukast	mon-te-LOO-kast	antiasthmatic, leukotriene receptor antagonist	Singulair
moxifloxacin	mox-i-FLOX-a-sin	ophthalmic antibacterial	Vigamox
		systemic antibacterial	Avelox
mupirocin	myoo-PEER-oe-sin	topical antibacterial	Bactroban
naproxen	na-PROX-en	analgesic, nonsteroidal anti-inflammatory, antidysmenorrheal, antigout agent, antipyretic, nonsteroidal anti-inflammatory antirheumatic, vascular headache prophylactic, vascular headache suppressant	Aleve, Anaprox, Naprosyn
nifedipine	nye-FED-i-peen	antianginal, antihypertensive	Procardia
nisolidipine	nye-SOLE-di-peen	calcium channel blocker	Sular
nitrofurantoin	nye-troe-fyoor-AN-toyn	systemic antibacterial	Macrobid, Macrodantin
nitroglycerin	nye-troe-GLISS-er-in	antianginal, congestive heart failure vasodilator	Minitran, Nitrolingual, Nitrostat, NitroDur
olanzapine	oh-LAN-za-peen	antipsychotic	Zyprexa
olmesartan	ohl-me-SAR-tan	Angiotensin II receptor antagonist	Benicar
olopatadine	oh-loe-PAT-a-deen	ophthalmic antihistaminic, H_1 receptor; ophthalmic mast cell stabilizer; ophthalmic antiallergic	Patanol

Generic Name	Pronunciation	Category	Brand Name
omeprazole	oh-MEP-ra-zole	gastric acid pump inhibitor, antiulcer agent	Prilosec, Prilosec OTC
oxybutynin	ox-i-BYOO-ti-nin	urinary tract antispasmodic	Ditropan, Oxytrol
oxycodone	ox-i-KOE-done	analgesic	OxyContin
oxycodone-acetaminophen	ox-i-KOE-done a-seat-a-MIN-oh-fen	analgesic	Endocet, Percocet, Tylox
pantoprazole	pan-TOE-pra-zole	gastric acid pump inhibitor, antiulcer agent	Protonix
paroxetine	pa-ROX-e-teen	antianxiety agent, antidepressant, antiobsessional agent, antipanic agent, posttraumatic stress disorder agent, social anxiety disorder agent	Paxil
penicillin V	pen-i-SIL-in V	systemic antibacterial	Veetids
phenytoin	FEN-i-toyn	antiarrhythmic, anticonvulsant, trigeminal neuralgic antineuralgic, skeletal muscle relaxant	Dilantin
pimecrolimus	pim-e-KROW-li-mus	immunomodulator	Elidel
pioglitazone	pye-oh-GLIT-a-zone	antidiabetic	Actos
polyethylene glycol	pol-ee-ETH-il-een GLYE-kawl	hyperosmotic laxative	MiraLax
potassium chloride	poe-tass-EE-um KLOR-ide	antihypokalemic, electrolyte replenisher	Klor-Con
pravastatin	PRA-va-sta-tin	antihyperlipidemic, HMG-CoA reductase inhibitor	Pravachol
prednisone	PRED-ni-sone	steroidal inflammatory, cancer chemotherapy antiemetic, corticosteroid, immunosuppressant	Deltasone
pregabalin	pree-GAB-a-lin	antiseizure	Lyrica
promethazine	proe-METH-a-zeen	antiemetic; antihistaminic, H_1 receptor; antivertigo agent; sedative-hypnotic	Phenergan
promethazine-codeine	proe-METH-a-zeen KOE-deen	antihistaminic, H_1 receptor-antitussive	Phenergan with codeine
propoxyphene-acetaminophen	proe-POX-i-feen a-seat-a-MIN-oh-fen	analgesic	Darvocet-N 100

Generic Name	Pronunciation	Category	Brand Name
propranolol	proe-PRAN-oh-lawl	antiadrenergic, antianginal, antianxiety therapy adjunct, antiarrhythmic, antihypertensive, antitremor agent, hypertrophic cardiomyopathy therapy adjunct, myocardial infarction prophylactic, myocardial infarction therapy, neuroleptic-induced akathisia therapy, pheochromocytoma therapy adjunct, thyrotoxicosis therapy adjunct, vascular headache prophylactic	Inderal
quetiapine	kwe-TYE-a-peen	antipsychotic	Seroquel
quinapril	KWIN-a-pril	antihypertensive, vasodilator	Accupril
rabeprazole	ra-BEP-ra-zole	gastric acid pump inhibitor, antiulcer agent	Aciphex
raloxifene	ral-OX-i-feen	selective estrogen receptor modulator, osteoporosis prophylactic	Evista
ramipril	RA-mi-pril	antihypertensive, vasodilator	Altace
ranitidine	ra-NIT-i-deen	histamine H_2-receptor antagonist, antiulcer agent, gastric acid secretion inhibitor	Zantac, Zantac 75
risedronate	ris-ED-roe-nate	bone resorption inhibitor	Actonel
risperidone	ris-PAIR-i-done	antipsychotic	Risperdal
ropinirole	ro-PIN-a-role	anti-parkinson agent	ReQuip
rosiglitazone	ros-e-GLIT-a-zone	antidiabetic	Avandia
rosurvastatin	roe-soo-va-STAT-in	HmgCoA reductase inhibitor	Crestor
sertraline	SER-tra-leen	antianxiety agent, antidepressant, antiobsessional agent, antipanic agent, posttraumatic stress disorder therapy agent, premenstrual dysphoric disorder therapy agent	Zoloft
sildenafil	sil-DEN-a-fil	systemic impotence therapy agent	Viagra
simvastatin	SIM-va-STAT-in	antihyperlipidemic, HMG-CoA reductase inhibitor	Zocor

Generic Name	Pronunciation	Category	Brand Name
spironolactone	speer-on-oh-LAK-tone	aldosterone antagonist, antihypertensive, antihypokalemic, primary hyperaldosteronism diagnostic aid, diuretic	Aldactone
sulfamethoxazole-trimethoprim	sul-fa-meth-OX-a-zole trye-METH-oh-prim	systemic antibacterial, antiprotozoal	Bactrim, Bactrim DS, Cotrim, Cotrim DS, Septra, Septra DS
sumatriptan	soo-ma-TRIP-tan	antimigraine agent	Imitrex
tadalafil	tah-DAL-a-fil	male impotence	Cialis
tamsulosin	tam-SOO-loh-sin	benign prostatic hyperplasia therapy agent	Flomax
telmisartan	tel-me-SAR-tan	Antihypertensive - ARB	Micardis
temazepam	tem-AZ-e-pam	sedative-hypnotic	Restoril
terazosin	ter-AYE-zoe-sin	antihypertensive, benign prostatic hyperplasia therapy agent	Hytrin
timolol	TYE-moe-lawl	ophthalmic antiglaucoma agent	Timoptic
tiotropium	tye-oh-TRO-pee-um	bronchodilator	Spiriva
tobramycin-dexamethasone	toe-bra-MYE-sin dex-a-METH-a-sone	ophthalmic corticosteroid, ophthalmic steroidal anti-inflammatory, ophthalmic antibacterial	TobraDex
tolterodine	tole-TAIR-oh-deen	urinary bladder antispasmodic	Detrol
topiramate	toe-PYRE-a-mate	anticonvulsant, antimigraine headache	Topamax
tramadol	TRA-ma-dawl	analgesic	Ultram
tramadol-acetaminophen	TRA-ma-dawl a-seat-a-MIN-oh-fen	analgesic	Ultracet
trandolapril-verapamil	tran-DOE-la-pril ver-AP-a-mil	calcium channel blocker	Tarka
trazodone	TRAZ-oh-done	antidepressant, antineuralgic	Desyrel
triamcinolone	trye-am-SIN-oh-lone	inhalation anti-inflammatory, antiasthmatic	Azmacort
		nasal steroidal anti-inflammatory, nasal corticosteroid	Aristocort, Nasacort AQ
triamterene-hydrochlorothiazide	trye-AM-ter-een hye-droe-klor-oh-THYE-a-zide	antihypertensive, antihypokalemic, diuretic	Dyazide, Maxzide
valacyclovir	val-ay-SYE-kloe-veer	systemic antiviral	Valtrex
valproic acid	val-PRO-ik AS-id	anticonvulsant	Depakene
valsartan	val-SAR-tan	antihypertensive	Diovan

Generic Name	Pronunciation	Category	Brand Name
valsartan-hydrochlorothiazide	val-SAR-tan hye-droe-klor-oh-THYE-a-zide	antihypertensive	Diovan HCT
venlafaxine	ven-la-FAX-een	antidepressant, antianxiety agent	Effexor
verapamil	ver-AP-a-mil	antianginal, antiarrhythmic, antihypertensive, hypertrophic cardiomyopathy therapy adjunct, vascular headache prophylactic	Calan, Covera HS, Verelan Isoptin
warfarin	WOR-far-in	anticoagulant	Coumadin
zolpidem	ZOLE-pi-dem	sedative hypnotic	Ambien

Source: Adapted from RxList, The Top 200 Prescriptions for 2007 by Number of U.S. Prescriptions Dispensed (www.rxlist.com, accessed 11/17/08). Category information from the U.S. National Library of Medicine and National Institutes of Health MedlinePlus Web site Lexicom 2008-2009 (www.nlm.nih.gov/medlineplus, accessed 11/17/08).

Appendix B

Look-Alike and Sound-Alike Medications

Although manufacturers have an obligation to review new trademarks for error potential before use, there are some things that prescribers, pharmacists, and pharmacy technicians can do to help prevent errors with products that have look- or sound-alike names. The following recommendations are designed to prevent dispensing errors and are based on recommendations from the Institute for Safe Medication Practices (ISMP) (www.ismp.org).

- **Use electronic prescribing** to prevent confusion with handwritten drug names.
- **Encourage physicians to write prescriptions that clearly specify the dosage form, drug strength, and complete directions.** They should include the product's indication on all outpatient prescriptions and on inpatient *prn* orders. With name pairs known to be problematic, reduce the potential for confusion by writing prescriptions using both the brand and generic names. Listing both names on medication administration records and automated dispensing cabinet computer screens also may be helpful.
- **Whenever possible, determine the purpose of the medication** before dispensing or administering it. Many products with look-alike or sound-alike names are used for different purposes.
- **Accept verbal or telephone orders only when truly necessary.** Require staff to read back all orders, spell product names, and state their indication. Like medication names, numbers can sound alike, so staff should read the dosage back in numerals (e.g., "one five" for 15 mg) to ensure clear interpretation of dose.
- **When feasible, use magnifying lenses and copyholders under good lighting** to keep prescriptions and orders at eye level during transcription to improve the likelihood of proper interpretation of look-alike product names.
- **Change the appearance of look-alike product names** on computer screens, pharmacy and patient care unit shelf labels, and bins (including automated dispensing cabinets), pharmacy product labels, and medication administration records by highlighting—through boldface, color, and/or capital letters—the parts of the names that are different (e.g., hydrOXYzine, hydrALAzine).
- **Install a computerized reminder** (also placed on automated dispensing cabinet screens) for the most serious confusing name pairs so that an alert is generated when entering prescriptions for either drug. If possible, make the reminder auditory as well as visual.
- **Affix "name alert" stickers** in areas where look-alike or sound-alike products are stored (available from pharmacy label manufacturers).
- **Store products with look-alike or sound-alike names in different locations.** Avoid storing both products in the fast-mover area. Use a shelf sticker to help locate the product that is moved.
- **Continue to employ an independent check in the dispensing process** (one person interprets and enters the prescription into the computer, and another reviews the printed label against the original prescription and the product).

449

- **Open the prescription bottle or the unit dose package in front of the patient** to confirm the expected product appearance and review the indication. Caution patients about error potential when taking products that have a look-alike or sound-alike counterpart. Take the time to fully investigate the situation if a patient states that he or she is taking an unknown medication.
- **Monitor reported errors caused by look-alike and sound-alike medication names**, and alert staff to mistakes.
- **Look for the possibility of name confusion when a new product is added to the formulary.** Have several clinicians handwrite the product name and directions as they would appear in a typical order. Ask frontline nurses, pharmacists, technicians, unit secretaries, and physicians to view the samples of the written product name, as well as pronounce it, to determine whether it looks or sounds like any other drug product or medical term. It may be helpful to have clinicians first look at the scripted product name to determine how they would interpret it before the actual product name is provided to them for pronunciation. Once the product name is known, clinicians may be less likely to see more familiar product names in the written samples. If the potential for confusion with other products is identified, then take steps to avoid errors as listed here.
- **Encourage reporting of errors and potentially hazardous conditions** with look-alike and sound-alike product names, and use the information to establish priorities for error reduction. Also maintain awareness of problematic product names and error prevention recommendations provided by the ISMP (www.ismp.org and also listed in the quarterly *Action Agenda*), FDA (www.fda.gov), and USP (www.usp.org).
- **Review the following table for look-alike and sound-alike drug name pairs in use at your practice location.** Decide what actions might be warranted to prevent medication errors. Stay current with alerts from the ISMP, FDA, and USP in case new problematic name pairs emerge. Note that many sound-alike medications are indeed the same medication but in a different dosage form or drug delivery system (i.e., Metformin, Metformin XL).

Medication Name	Look- or Sound-Alike Name
Accupril	Aciphex
Aciphex	Aricept
Activase	TNKase
Actonel	Actos
Adderall	Inderal
Aldara	Alora
Alkeran	Leukeran, Myleran
Allegra	Viagra
alprazolam	lorazepam
Amaryl	Reminyl
amoxicillin	amoxicillin/clavulanate
Antivert	Axert
aripiprazole	rabeprazole
Asacol	Os-Cal
Avinza	Evista
Bicillin C-R	Bicillin L-A
Brethine	Methergine

Medication Name	Look- or Sound-Alike Name
camphorated tincture of opium (paregoric)	opium tincture
carboplatin	cisplatin
Cedax	Cidex
Celexa	Zyprexa, Celebrex
Claritin-D	Claritin-D 24
Cozaar	Zocor
Denavir	Indinavir
Depakote	Depakote ER
Depo-Medrol	Solu-Medrol
Desyrel	desipramine
DiaBeta	Zebeta
Diovan	Zyban
Diprivan	Ditropan
Ditropan	Ditropan LA
dobutamine	dopamine
doxorubicin hydrochloride	liposomal doxorubicin (Doxil)
Effexor	Effexor XR
Endocet	Indocin, Ultracet
epinephrine	ephedrine
Estratest	Estratest H.S.
Femara	Femhrt
folic acid	folinic acid (leucovorin calcium)
Foradil	Toradol
Granulex	Regranex
Humalog	Humulin
Humalog Mix 75/25	Humulin 70/30
Humulin	Humalog
Humulin 70/30	Humalog Mix 75/25
hydralazine	hydroxyzine
infliximab	rituximab
Isordil	Plendil
isotretinoin	tretinoin
K-Phos Neutral	Neutra-Phos K
Kaletra	Keppra
Lamictal	Lamisil
lamivudine	lamotrigine
Lasix	Luvox
leucovorin calcium	Leukeran
Levbid	Levisin
Lotronex	Protonix
Maxzide	Microzide
Metadate ER	Metadate CD
metformin	Metformin ER, metronidazole
Micronase	Microzide
mifepristone	misoprostol
Miralax	Mirapex
morphine, oral liquid concentrate	morphine, non-concentrated oral liquid
MS Contin	OxyContin
Mucinex	Mucomyst

Medication Name	Look- or Sound-Alike Name
Neurontin	Noroxin
Occlusal-HP	Ocuflox
OxyContin	oxycodone
Paxil	Taxol, Plavix
Prilosec	Prozac
propylthiouracil	Purinethol
quinine	quinidine
Reminyl	Robinul
Retrovir	ritonavir
Ritalin LA	Ritalin-SR
Roxanol	Roxicodone Intensol, Roxicet
Sarafem	Serophene
sumatriptan	zolmitriptan
Tegretol	Tegretol XR
Tequin	Tegretol, Ticlid
Tiazac	Ziac
TNKase	t-PA
Tobradex	Tobrex
Topamax	Toprol-XL
tramadol hydrochloride	trazodone hydrochloride
Tylenol	Tylenol PM
Ultracet	Duricef
Varivax	VZIG
Viagra	Allegra
vinblastine	vincristine
Viokase	Viokase 8
Viracept	Viramune
Wellbutrin SR	Wellbutrin XL
Xeloda	Xenical
Yaz	Yasmin
Zantac	Zyrtec, Xanax
Zebeta	Zetia
Zestril	Zetia, Zyprexa
Zocor	Zyrtec
Zostrix	Zovirax
Zovirax	Zyvox
Zyprexa	Zyrtec

This list of confused drug names is based on information reported in the *ISMP Medication Safety Alert! AcuteCare Edition*, published by the Institute for Safe Medication Practices (www.ismp.org). This master is used with permission of ISMP.

Category	English	Categoría	Español
Greetings and Courtesies	Good morning.	**Saludos y Cortesía**	Buenos días.
	Good afternoon.		Buenas tardes.
	Good evening.		Buenas noches.
	Good night.		Buenas noches.
	Hello.		Hola.
	Please.		Por favor.
	Thank you.		Gracias.
	You are welcome.		De nada.
	May I help you?		¿En qué puedo ayudarle?
	Do you need to speak to the pharmacist?		¿Necesita usted hablar con el/la farmacéutico/a?
	Do you want to wait?		¿Quiere usted esperar?
	When would you like to pick this up?		¿Cuándo quiere recoger su pedido?
	Do you want this delivered?		¿Quiere que se lo envíen a su casa?
	Yes.		Sí.
	No.		No.
	Do you speak Spanish?		¿Habla usted español?
	I speak a little Spanish.		Yo hablo un poco de español.
	Please speak slower.		Por favor, hable despacio.
	Please repeat that again.		Por favor, repita lo que dijo.
	I am sorry.		Lo siento.
	Do you speak English?		¿Habla usted inglés?
	Do you have someone who can help translate?		¿Tiene usted a alguien que le traduzca?
	Yes, you have ___ refills left. Would you like a refill on your prescription?		Sí, le quedan ___ dosis de relleno. ¿Le gustaría ordenar una dosis de relleno para su receta?
	I will check on that.		Voy a verificar eso.
	Your prescription is not ready yet.		Su receta (orden) aún no está lista.
	It will only be a few more minutes.		Sólo se tardará unos minutos.
Patient Replies	Yes.	**Respuestas del Paciente**	Sí.
	No.		No.
	Do I have refills?		¿Tengo rellenos con esta receta?

Category	English	Categoría	Español
Patient Replies (continued)	I do not speak English.	**Respuestas del Paciente** (continued)	Yo no hablo inglés.
	I do not understand.		No entiendo.
	May I speak to the pharmacist?		¿Podría hablar con el/la farmacéutico/a?
	Is my prescription ready?		¿Ya está lista mi receta (orden)?
	How much is this?		¿Cuánto cuesta esto?
	Where will I find ____?		¿Dónde puedo encontrar ____?
	Will you help me?		¿Puede usted ayudarme?
	Thank you.		Muchas gracias.
Numbers	none (zero)	**Números**	nada (cero)
	one		uno
	two		dos
	three		tres
	four		cuatro
	five		cinco
	six		seis
	seven		siete
	eight		ocho
	nine		nueve
	ten		diez
	twenty		veinte
	thirty		treinta
	forty		cuarenta
	fifty		cincuenta
	one hundred		cien
	one-half		medio/a
	one-quarter		un cuarto
	three-quarters		tres cuartos
Days of the Week	Sunday	**Días de la Semana**	domingo
	Monday		lunes
	Tuesday		martes
	Wednesday		miércoles
	Thursday		jueves
	Friday		viernes
	Saturday		sábado
Time	15 minutes	**La Hora**	quince minutos
	1 hour		una hora
	morning		en la mañana / por la mañana
	noon		mediodía / al mediodía

Category	English	Categoría	Español
Time (continued)	afternoon	**La Hora (continued)**	en la tarde / por la tarde
	bedtime		antes de acostarse
	tomorrow morning		mañana en la mañana / mañana por la mañana
	tomorrow afternoon		mañana en la tarde / mañana por la tarde
Verbs	take	**Verbos**	tomar
	apply		aplicar
	place		colocar
	swish and swallow		enjuagar y tragar
	swish and spit		enjuagar y escupir
	inhale		inhalar
	dissolve		disolver
	insert		insertar
	remove		quitar / remover
	inject		inyectar
Dosage Forms	tablet	**Dosificación**	tableta
	capsule		cápsula
	caplet		tableta
	suspension		suspensión
	solution		solución
	suppository		supositorio
	cream		crema
	ointment		ungüento
	sublingual tablet		tableta para poner debajo de la lengua
	vaginal insert		para insertar vaginalmente
	patch		parche
Common Directions	Take 1 tablet daily.	**Indicaciones Generales**	Tomar 1 tableta diaria.
	Take 1 tablet two times a day.		Tomar 1 tableta dos veces al día.
	Take 1 tablet three times a day.		Tomar 1 tableta tres veces al día.
	Take 1 tablet four times a day.		Tomar 1 tableta cuatro veces al día.
	Take 1 tablet weekly.		Tomar 1 tableta por semana.
	Take 1 tablet monthly.		Tomar 1 tableta por mes.
	Take 1 tablet every hour.		Tomar 1 tableta cada hora.
	Take 1 tablet every 4 hours.		Tomar 1 tableta cada 4 horas.
	Take 1 tablet every 6 hours.		Tomar 1 tableta cada 6 horas.
	Take 1 tablet every 8 hours.		Tomar 1 tableta cada 8 horas.
	Take 1 tablet every 12 hours.		Tomar 1 tableta cada 12 horas.
	Take 1 capsule daily.		Tomar 1 cápsula diaria.

Category	English	Categoría	Español
Common Directions (continued)	Take 1 capsule two times a day.	Indicaciones Generales (continued)	Tomar 1 cápsula dos veces al día.
	Take 1 capsule three times a day.		Tomar 1 cápsula tres veces al día.
	Take 1 capsule four times a day.		Tomar 1 cápsula cuatro veces al día.
	Insert 1 suppository rectally every 4 to 6 hours as needed for nausea.		Insertar rectalmente 1 supositorio cada 4 a 6 horas cuando sea necesario por náusea.
	Inhale 2 sprays by mouth four times a day.		Inhalar 2 rociadas por la boca cuatro veces al día.
	Apply 1 patch to a hairless area of skin every morning.		Aplicar cada mañana un parche en un área de la piel que no tenga pelo (bello).
	Remove at bedtime.		Quitarse a la hora de dormir.
	Apply topically to the skin as directed.		Aplicar en la piel como se indica.
	Dissolve 1 tablet under the tongue as needed for chest pain. Call physician if no relief.		Disolver una tableta debajo de la lengua cuando sea necesario por dolores en el pecho. Llame a su médico/a si no siente mejoría.
	Place 1 drop in both eyes at bedtime.		Aplicar 1 gota en cada ojo antes de acostarse.
	Take after meals and at bedtime with a snack.		Tomarse después de las comidas y a la hora de dormir con algo de comer.
	Take 30 minutes before each meal.		Tomar 30 minutos antes de las comidas.
	As needed for _____.		A medida que lo necesite para ____.
	1 teaspoonful		1 cucharadita
	2 teaspoonsful		2 cucharaditas
	1 tablespoonful		1 cucharada
	2 tablespoonsful		2 cucharadas
	1 fluid ounce		1 onza fluida
	5 milliliters		5 mililitros
	10 milliliters		10 mililitros
	30 milliliters		30 mililitros
Warning Labels	Take this medication until finished.	Etiquetas de Advertencias	Tomar esta medicina hasta terminarla.
	Take on an empty stomach.		Tomarse con el estómago vacío.
	Take with 8 fluid ounces of water.		Tomarse con 8 onzas de agua.
	Shake it well.		Agítelo/a bien.
	Keep refrigerated.		Mantenga esta medicina refrigerada.
	Store in the freezer.		Mantenga esta medicina en el congelador.
	Do not freeze.		No se debe congelar.

Category	English	Categoría	Español
Warning Labels (continued)	Store in a cool, dry place.	**Etiquetas de Advertencias (continued)**	Guardar en un lugar fresco y seco.
	May cause drowsiness.		Puede producir somnolencia.
	Take with food.		Tomarse con comida.
	Avoid prolonged exposure to sunlight.		Evitar la exposición prolongada al sol.
	May discolor urine or feces.		Puede cambiar el color de la orina y de las heces.
	Do not drink alcohol when taking this medication.		No beber alcohol mientras se toma esta medicina.
	This is the generic for ____.		Ésta es una medicina genérica de _____.
	Do not take with calcium, iron, or dairy products.		No se debe tomar con calcio, hierro o productos lácteos.
	Do not chew.		No masticarla.
	Do not crush.		No machacarla.
	May blur vision.		Puede provocar visión borrosa.
	Federal law prohibits the use of this medication for anyone other than the patient it was prescribed for.		La ley federal prohíbe el uso de esta medicina por cualquier persona que no sea el paciente a quien se le recetó.
	Discard used patches out of reach of children and pets.		Desechar los parches usados fuera del alcance de los niños y animales.
	Keep out of reach of children.		Manténgase fuera del alcance de los niños.
Rationales	pain	**Fundamento**	dolor
	sinus infection		sinusitis
	urinary tract infection		infección en las vías urinarias
	nausea and vomiting		nausea y vómito
	high blood pressure		presión arterial alta
	chest pain (angina)		dolor de pecho (angina)
	for sleep		para dormir
	for anxiety		para la ansiedad
	for breathing		para respirar
Routes of Administration	orally (by mouth)	**Formas de Aplicación**	de manera oral (por la boca)
	topically		para uso externo / para aplicase en la piel
	in the ear		en el oído
	in the eye		en el ojo
	in the rectum		en el recto
	in the vagina		en la vagina / vaginalmente
	inject		inyectado
	in the nose		en la nariz

Category	English	Categoría	Español
Patient Information	What is your name?	Información del (de la) Paciente	¿Cómo se llama usted? / ¿Cuál es su nombre?
	What relationship are you to the patient?		¿Cuál es su relación con el (la) paciente?
	How do you spell that?		¿Cómo se deletrea?
	What is your address?		¿Cuál es su dirección?
	What is your date of birth?		¿Cuál es su fecha de nacimiento?
	What is the patient's date of birth?		¿Cuál es la fecha de nacimiento del (de la) paciente?
	Are you pregnant?		¿Está usted embarazada?
	Is the patient pregnant?		¿Está embarazada la paciente?
	What is your doctor's name?		¿Cuál es el nombre de su médico/a?
	What is your telephone number?		¿Cuál es su número de teléfono?
	Do you have insurance?		¿Tiene usted seguro médico?
	Do you have any drug allergies?		¿Es alérgico/a a alguna medicina?
	What happens when you take that drug?		¿Qué le sucede cuando usted toma esa medicina?
	What prescription medications do you take?		¿Está tomando alguna medicina recetada?
	What vitamins, herbals, or over-the-counter medicines do you take?		¿Cuáles vitaminas, medicinas naturales o sin necesidad de receta médica está tomando usted?
	Is there any other information we should have on file?		¿Hay alguna información que debamos tener en archivo?
	Do you want childproof caps on your vials?		¿Quiere sus envases con tapas a prueba de niños?
Common Drug Allergies	penicillin	Reacciones Alérgicas	penicilina
	aspirin		aspirina
	acetaminophen (Tylenol)		acetaminofen (Tylenol)
	codeine		codeína
	morphine		morfina
	no known allergies		alergias no conocidas
Common Side Effects	rash	Efectos Secundarios	sarpullido
	shortness of breath		falta de aire
	stomach upset		malestar estomacal
	drowsiness		somnolencia
	hyperactivity		hiperactividad
	insomnia		insomnio
	headache		dolor de cabeza
	Contact your physician immediately if experiencing an unexpected reaction.		Contacte inmediatamente a su médico/a si tiene una reacción inesperada.

Category	English	Categoría	Español
Colors and Shapes	green	**Colores y Formas**	verde
	blue		azul
	yellow		amarillo/a
	red		rojo/a
	white		blanco/a
	brown		marrón / café
	peach		color melocotón
	pink		rosado/a
	black		negro/a
	orange		anaranjado
	purple		morado/a
	round		redondo/a
	square		cuadrado/a
	oval		ovalado/a
	oblong		rectangular
	triangular		triangular
	diamond shaped		rombo
Body Parts	mouth	**Las Partes del Cuerpo**	la boca
	stomach		el estómago
	ankle		el tobillo
	arm		el brazo
	back		la espalda
	rectum		el recto
	vagina		la vagina
	breast		los senos
	head		la cabeza
	liver		el hígado
	kidneys		los riñones
	heart		el corazón
	skin		la piel
Store Directions	That is in aisle number __.	**Direcciones**	Lo encuentra en el pasillo número __.
	on the left		a la izquierda
	on the right		a la derecha
	top shelf		en el estante de arriba
	bottom shelf		en el estante de abajo
	I will help you find that.		Permítame le ayudo a encontrar eso.
	This is a less expensive generic equivalent.		Ésta es un equivalente genérico que cuesta menos.

Category	English	Categoría	Español
Pharmacy Products	analgesics/pain relievers	**Productos Farmacéuticos**	analgésicos / contra el dolor
	cough/cold products		productos contra la tos y el resfriado
	feminine hygiene		higiene femenina
	vitamins		vitaminas
	first aid products		productos de primeros auxilios
	band-aids		curas
	condoms		condones
	antacids		antiácidos
	diabetic supplies		productos para diabéticos
	needles and syringes		agujas y jeringas
	blood sugar test strips		tiras para examinar el azúcar en la sangre
	alcohol swabs		hisopos con alcohol
Paying	Would you like to talk to the pharmacist about your prescription?	**Pago**	¿Quiere hablar con el/la farmacéutico/a acerca de su receta?
	Will this be cash, credit, or store charge?		¿Pagará en efectivo, con tarjeta de crédito o lo quiere cargar a su cuenta?
	Would you like a receipt?		¿Quiere un recibo?
	Please sign here.		Por favor, firme aquí.
	Do you have any questions?		¿Tiene alguna pregunta?
	Would you like to charge this?		¿Quiere cargar esto a su cuenta de crédito?
	You owe ___.		Usted debe pagar ___.
	Thank you. Come again.		Gracias. Regrese pronto.
	Please call if you have any questions.		Por favor, llame si tiene alguna pregunta.
	Good bye.		Adiós.
Miscellaneous Problems	The pharmacists needs to call your doctor. It may take a few minutes longer.	**Problemas Varios**	El/la farmacéutico/a necesita llamar a su doctor(a), se va a tardar unos minutos más.
	You will need a prescription for that medication.		Usted necesitará una receta para esa medicina.
	Please read and sign this document; it guarantees your right to privacy.		Por favor, lea y firme este documento que le garantiza el derecho a su privacidad.
	Your insurance will not cover this medicine.		Su seguro médico no cubre esta medicina.
	Do you still want to fill the prescription?		¿Quiere aún que se le ordene su receta?
	Would you like the pharmacist to call your doctor?		¿Quiere que el/la farmacéutico/a llame a su médico/a?
	We need to order this; it will be in on ____.		Necesitamos poner una orden para esta medicina y la tendremos el ____.

Glossary

A

abbreviated new drug application (aNDA) the process by which applicants must scientifically demonstrate to the FDA that their generic product is bioequivalent to or performs in the same way as the innovator drug

accreditation the stamp of approval of the quality of services of a hospital by the Joint Commission

active ingredient the biochemically active component of the drug that exerts a desired therapeutic effect

addiction compulsive and uncontrollable use of controlled substances, especially narcotics

admitting order a medication order written by a physician on admission of a patient to the hospital; may or may not include a medication order

adverse drug reaction (ADR) a negative consequence to a patient from taking a particular drug

aerosol a pressurized container with propellant used to administer a drug through oral inhalation into the lungs

alchemy the European practice during the Middle Ages that combined elements of chemistry, metallurgy, physics, and medicine with astrology, mysticism, and spiritualism such as turning ordinary metals into silver and gold

allergy a hypersensitivity to a specific substance, manifested in a physiological disorder

alligation the compounding of two or more products to obtain a desired concentration

ampule a single-dose-only drug container; it contains no preservative

ante area the area of the IV room used for hand washing and donning protective garments, among other high-particulate-generating activities

antibiotic a chemical substance that is used in the treatment of bacterial infectious diseases and has the ability to either kill or inhibit the growth of certain harmful microorganisms

antibody the part of the immune system that neutralizes antigens or foreign substances in the body

anticipatory compounding preparing excess product (besides an individual compound prescription) in reasonable quantities; these preparations must be labeled with lot numbers

antineoplastic drug a cancer-fighting drug

appearance the overall outward look of an employee on the job, including dress and grooming

aromatic water a solution of water containing oils or other substances that have a pungent, and usually pleasing, smell and are easily released into the air

asepsis the absence of disease-causing microorganisms

aseptic technique the manipulation of sterile products and devices in such a way as to avoid disease-causing organisms

assumption error an error that occurs when an essential piece of information cannot be verified and is guessed or presumed

attitude the emotional stance or disposition that a worker adopts toward his or her job duties, customers, employer, and coworkers

autoclave a device that generates heat and pressure to sterilize

automated compounding device (ACD) a programmable, automated device to make complex IV preparations such as TPNs

auxiliary label a supplementary label added to a medication container at the discretion of the pharmacist that provides additional directions

average wholesale price (AWP) the average price that wholesalers charge the pharmacy for a drug

B

bacterium a small, single-celled microorganism that can exist in three main forms, depending on type: spherical (i.e., cocci), rod-shaped (i.e., bacilli), and spiral (i.e., spirochetes)

beyond-use dating the documentation of the date after which a compounded preparation expires and should no longer be used

bioequivalent a generic drug that delivers approximately the same amount of active ingredient into a healthy volunteer's bloodstream in the same amount of time as the innovator or brand name drug

biotechnology the field of study that combines the sciences of biology, chemistry, and immunology to produce synthetic, unique drugs with specific therapeutic effects

black box warning a warning statement required by the FDA indicating a serious or even life-threatening adverse reaction from a drug; the warning statement is on the product package insert (PPI) for the pharmacy staff and in the MedGuide for consumers

blending the act of combining two substances

body surface area (BSA) a measurement related to a patient's weight and height, expressed in meters squared (m^2), and used to calculate patient-specific dosages of medications

brand name the name under which the manufacturer markets a drug; also known as the *trade name*

brand name medically necessary a designation on the prescription by the physician indicating that a generic substitution by the pharmacist is not allowed; commonly seen on prescriptions for thyroid medication; often abbreviated as "brand necessary"

buccal route of administration oral administration in which a drug is placed between the gum and the inner lining of the cheek; also called transmucosal route of administration

buffer area the area of the IV room used for the storage of components and supplies (such as IV bags and administration sets) that are used for compounding CSPs; also area for hand hygiene and donning protective gloves

C

cannula the barrel of a syringe or bore area inside the syringe that correlates with the volume of solution

caplet a hybrid solid dosage formulation sharing characteristics of both a tablet and a capsule

capsule the dosage form containing powder, liquid, or granules in a gelatin covering

capture error an error that occurs when focus on a task is diverted elsewhere and therefore the error goes undetected

cart fill list a printout of all unit dose profiles for all patients

catheter a device inserted into a vein for direct access to the blood vascular system

Celsius temperature scale the temperature scale that uses zero degrees (i.e., 0 °C) as the temperature at which water freezes at sea level and 100 °C as the temperature at which it boils

Centers for Disease Control and Prevention (CDC) a governmental agency that provides guidelines and recommendations on health care, including infection control

central venous catheter (CVC) a catheter placed into a large vein deep into the body; also called a central line

certificate of medical necessity form to be completed and signed by the prescriber for insurance payment for diabetic supplies

certification the process by which a professional organization grants recognition to an individual who has met certain predetermined qualifications

Certified Pharmacy Technician (CPhT) a pharmacy technician who has passed the PTCE or ExCPT examination

chain pharmacy a community pharmacy that consists of several similar pharmacies in the region (or nation) that are corporately owned

chemo venting pin a device used to equalize pressure in the preparation of hazardous drugs

chewable tablet a solid oral dosage form meant to be chewed that is readily absorbed; commonly prescribed for school-age children

child-resistant container a medication container with a special lid that cannot be opened by 80% of children but can be opened by 90% of adults; a container designed to prevent child access in order to reduce the number of accidental poisonings

civil law the areas of the law that concern U.S. citizens and the crimes they commit against one another

Class III prescription balance a two-pan balance used to weigh material (120 g or less) with a sensitivity rating of +/–6 mg; also known as a Class A balance

clean room an area that includes the buffer and staging areas and the sterile, direct compounding area (DCA) of the IV compounding lab

closed system transfer device (CSTD) a needleless delivery system by which medications are aseptically activated and added to an IV minibag at patient bedside

closed-ended question a question that requires a yes or no answer

co-insurance a percentage-based insurance plan whereby the patient must pay a certain percentage of the prescription price

cold flow the tendency of a clamp on an IV administration set to return slowly to a more open position, with an increase in fluid flow

colloid the dispersion of ultrafine particles in a liquid formulation

comminution the act of reducing a substance to small, fine particles, including trituration, levigation, pulverization, spatulation, sifting, and tumbling

common law the system of precedents established by decisions in cases throughout legal history

community pharmacy any independent, chain, or franchise pharmacy that dispenses prescription medications to outpatients; also called a *retail pharmacy*

compounded preparation a patient-specific medication prepared on-site by the technician, under the direct supervision of the pharmacist, from individual ingredients

compounded sterile preparation (CSP) a sterile product that is prepared outside the pharmaceutical manufacturer's facility, typically in a hospital or compounding pharmacy

compounding the process of preparing a prescribed medication for an individual patient from bulk ingredients created by a pharmacist in order to treat a specified medical condition according to a prescription by a licensed prescriber

compounding log a printout of the prescription for a specific patient, including the amounts or weights of all ingredients and instructions for compounding; used by the technician to prepare a compounded medication for a patient

compounding pharmacy a pharmacy that specializes in the preparation of nonsterile (and sometimes sterile) preparations that are not commercially available

compounding slab a flat, hard, nonabsorbent surface used for mixing compounds; also known as an ointment slab

computer an electronic device for inputting, storing, processing, and/or outputting information

conjunctival route of administration the placement of sterile ophthalmic medications in the conjunctival sac of the eye(s)

continuation order a medication order written by a physician to continue treatment; like a refill of medication

continuous quality improvement (CQI) a process of written procedures designed to identify problems and recommend solutions

controlled substance a drug with potential for abuse; organized into five schedules that specify the way the drug must be stored, dispensed, recorded, and inventoried

Controlled Substances Act (CSA) laws created to combat and control drug abuse

controlled-release dosage form the dosage form that is formulated to release medication over a long duration of time; also called delayed release

coordination of benefits (COB) online billing of both a primary and a secondary insurer

co-payment (co-pay) the amount that the patient is to pay for each prescription

coring the act of introducing a small chunk of the rubber closure into the solution while removing medication from a vial

counterbalance a two-pan balance used for weighing material up to 5 kg with a sensitivity rating of +/−100 mg

cream a cosmetically acceptable oil-in-water (O/W) emulsion for topical use on the skin

credential a documented piece of evidence of one's qualifications

credentialing the process for validating the qualifications of licensed professionals, such as Basic Life Support (BLS) and ACLS (Advance Cardiac Life Support)

credit card a method of online payment that is a type of loan, either paid totally at the end of the month or partially with a finance charge added

creep the tendency of a clamp on an IV administration set to return to its previous position

cytotoxic drug a hazardous drug that must be handled and prepared with extra precautions; such a drug may be used in cancer chemotherapy, an antiviral drug for a patient with HIV, a biological hormone, a bioengineered drug, or a radioactive pharmaceutical

D

database management system (DBMS) application that allows one to enter, retrieve, and query records

days supply the duration of time (number of days) a dispensed medication will last the patient and often required on drug claims submitted for insurance billing

DEA number an identification number assigned by the Drug Enforcement Administration (DEA) to identify someone authorized to handle or prescribe controlled substances within the United States

debit card a method of online cash payment that instantly deducts the cost of the purchase from the customer's bank account

decimal any number that can be written in decimal notation using the integers 0 through 9 and a point (.) to divide the "ones" place from the "tenths" place (e.g., 10.25 is equal to 10¼)

decorum proper or polite behavior that is in good taste

deductible an amount that must be paid by the insured before the insurance company considers paying its portion of a medical or drug cost

defendant one who defends against accusations brought forward in a lawsuit

denominator the number on the bottom part of a fraction that represents the whole

deoxyribonucleic acid (DNA) the helix-shaped molecule that carries the genetic code

destructive agent a drug that kills bacteria, fungi, viruses, or even normal or cancer cells

diet supplement a category of nonprescription drugs that includes vitamins, minerals, and herbals that are not regulated by the FDA

digital electronic analytical balance a single-pan balance that is more accurate than Class III balances or counterbalances; it has a capacity of 100 g and sensitivity as low as +/-1 mg

diluent an inert filler substance added as an inactive ingredient in tablets and capsules; also a sterile fluid added to a powder to reconstitute, dilute, or dissolve a medication

diluent powder an inactive ingredient that is added to the active drug in compounding a tablet or capsule

direct compounding area (DCA) the sterile, compounding area of the IV room, in which the concentration of airborne particles is controlled with a HEPA filter providing ISO Class 5 air quality

director of pharmacy the chief executive officer of the pharmacy department

discount a reduced price

discrimination preferential treatment or mistreatment

disinfectant a chemical applied to an object or topically to the body for sterilization purposes, such as rubbing alcohol

diskus a nonaerosolized powder that is used for inhalation

dispense as written (DAW) a notation indicating on a prescription that a brand name drug is necessary or that a generic substitution is not allowed; DAW2 is often used to indicate patient preference for a brand name drug

dispersion a liquid dosage form in which undissolved ingredients are mixed throughout a liquid vehicle

dosage form the physical manifestation of a drug (e.g., capsule, tablet)

doughnut hole insurance coverage gap in Medicare Part D programs by which the patient must pay 100% of the cost of the medication

drop set the calibration in drops per milliliter on IV sets

dropper a measuring device used to accurately dose medication for infants

drug any substance taken into or applied to the body for the purpose of altering the body's biochemical functions and thus its physiological processes

drug delivery system a design feature of the dosage form that affects the delivery of the drug; such a system may protect the stomach or delay the release of the active drug

Drug Enforcement Administration (DEA) the branch of the U.S. Justice Department that is responsible for regulating the sale and use of drugs with abuse potential

drug recall the process of withdrawing a drug from the market by the FDA or the drug manufacturer for serious adverse effects or other defects in the product

drug seeker a customer who requests early refills on medications or gets prescriptions from multiple physicians for controlled substances in order to obtain more than the normally prescribed amount of medication

drug tolerance a situation that occurs when the body requires higher doses of a drug to produce the same therapeutic effect

drug utilization review (DUR) a procedure built into pharmacy software designed to help pharmacists check for potential medication errors in dosage, drug interactions, allergies, and so on

dumb terminal a computer device that contains a keyboard and a monitor but does not contain its own storage and processing capabilities

durable medical equipment (DME) medical equipment such as hospital beds, wheelchairs, canes, or crutches that may be covered under Medicare Part B insurance

E

effervescent salts granular salts that release gas and dispense active ingredients into solution when placed in water

electrolyte a dissolved mineral salt, commonly found in IV fluids

electronic medication administration record (eMAR) documents the administration time of each drug to each patient often using bar-code technology

elixir a clear, sweetened, flavored solution containing water and ethanol

eMAR an electronic medication administration record, used to minimize medication errors

emulsion the dispersion of a liquid in another liquid varying in viscosity

enteric-coated tablet (ECT) a tablet coated in a way designed to resist destruction by the acidic pH of the gastric fluids and to delay the release of the active ingredient

e-prescribing the transmission of a prescription via electronic means

estrogen replacement therapy (ERT) treatment consisting of some combination of female hormones

ethical dilemma a situation that calls for a judgment between two or more solutions, not all of which are necessarily wrong

ethics the study of standards of conduct and moral judgment that outlines the right or wrong of human conduct or character

etiquette unwritten rules of behavior

Exam for Certification of Pharmacy Technicians (ExCPT) an examination developed by the Institute for the Certification of Pharmacy Technicians (ICPT) that technicians must pass to be certified and receive the title of CPhT

expiration date the date after which a manufacturer's product should not be used

extended-release (XL) dosage form a tablet or capsule designed to reduce frequency of dosing compared with immediate-release and most sustained-release forms

extra dose error an error in which more doses are received by a patient than were prescribed by the physician

extract a potent dosage form derived from animal or plant sources from which most or all the solvent has been evaporated to produce a powder, an ointment-like form, or a solid

F

Fahrenheit temperature scale the temperature scale that uses 32 °F as the temperature at which water freezes at sea level and 212 °F as the temperature at which it boils

FDA Online Orange Book an online reference that provides information on the generic and therapeutic equivalence of drugs that may have many different brand names or generic manufacturer sources

film-coated tablet (FCT) a tablet coated with a thin outer layer that prevents serious GI side effects

filter a device used to remove contaminants such as glass, paint, fibers, rubber cores, and bacteria from IV fluids

Flex card a medical and prescription insurance credit card

floor stock medications stocked in a secured area on each patient care unit

fluidextract a liquid dosage form prepared by extraction from plant sources and commonly used in the formulation of syrups

Food and Drug Administration (FDA) the agency of the federal government that is responsible for ensuring the safety and efficacy of food and drugs prepared for the market

forceps an instrument used to pick up small objects, such as pharmacy weights

formulary a list of drugs that have been pre-approved for use by a committee of health professionals; used in hospitals, in managed care, and by many insurance providers

fraction a portion of a whole that is represented as a ratio

franchise pharmacy a small chain of professional community pharmacies that dispense and prepare medications but are independently owned; sometimes called an *apothecary*

fungus a single-celled organism similar to human cells; marked by the absence of chlorophyll, a rigid cell wall, and reproduction by spores; feed on living organisms (or on dead organic material)

G

gel a dispersion containing fine particles for topical use on the skin

generic drug a drug that contains the same active ingredients as the brand name product and delivers the same amount of medication to the body in the same way and in the same amount of time; a drug that is not protected by a patent

generic name a common name that is given to a drug regardless of brand name; sometimes denotes a drug that is not protected by a trademark; for example, acetaminophen is the generic drug name for Tylenol

genetic engineering process of utilizing DNA biotechnology to create a variety of drugs

genome the entire DNA in an organism, including its genes

geometric dilution method the gradual combining of drugs using a mortar and pestle

germ theory of disease the idea that microorganisms cause diseases

glycerogelatin a topical preparation made with gelatin, glycerin, water, and medicinal substances

good compounding practices (GCP) USP standards in many areas of practice to ensure high-quality compounded preparations

graduate cylinder a flask used for measuring liquids

gram the metric system's base unit for measuring weight

granules a dosage form larger than powders that are formed by adding very small amounts of liquid to powders

gross profit the difference between the purchase price and the selling price; also called markup

H

hand hygiene the use of special dry, alcohol-based rinses, gels, or foams that do not require water

hand washing the use of plain or antiseptic soap and water with appropriate time and technique

harassment mistreatment, whether sexual or otherwise

health insurance coverage of incurred medical costs such as physician visits, laboratory costs, and hospitalization

Health Insurance Portability and Accountability Act (HIPAA) a comprehensive federal law passed in 1996 to protect all patient-identifiable medical information

health maintenance organization (HMO) an organization that provides health insurance using a managed care model

high-efficiency particulate air (HEPA) filter a device used with laminar flow hoods to filter out most particulate matter to prepare parenteral products safely and aseptically

home healthcare the delivery of medical, nursing, and pharmaceutical services and supplies to patients at home

home healthcare pharmacy a pharmacy that dispenses, prepares, and delivers drugs and medical supplies directly to the home of the patient

homeopathic medications very small dilutions of natural drugs claimed to stimulate the immune system

horizontal laminar airflow workbench (LAFW) a special biological safety cabinet used to prepare IV drug admixtures, nutrition solutions, and other parenteral products aseptically

hormone replacement therapy (HRT) therapy consisting of some combination of estrogen and progestin (female) and androgen (male) hormones

hospital pharmacy an institutional pharmacy that dispenses and prepares drugs and provides clinical services in a hospital setting

human failure an error generated by failure that occurs at an individual level

hypertonic solution a parenteral solution with a greater number of particles than the number of particles found in blood (greater than 285 mOsm/L); also called hyperosmolar, as in a TPN solution

hypotonic solution a parenteral solution with a fewer number of particles than the number of particles found in blood (less than 285 mOsm/L); also called hypoosmolar

I

independent pharmacy a community pharmacy that is privately owned by the pharmacist

inert ingredient an inactive chemical that has little or no physiological effect that is added to one or more active ingredients to improve drug formulations such as fillers, preservatives, colorings, and flavorings; also called inactive ingredient

infection control committee (ICC) a committee of the hospital that provides leadership in relation to infection control policies

informed consent written permission by the patient to participate in an IRB-approved research study in terms understandable to the lay public

injection the administration of a parenteral medication into the bloodstream, muscle, or skin

inpatient drug distribution system a pharmacy system to deliver all types of drugs to a patient in the hospital setting; commonly includes unit dose, repackaged medication, floor stock, and IV admixture and TPN services

inscription the part of the prescription listing the medication or medications prescribed, including the drug names, strengths, and amounts

Institute for Safe Medication Practices (ISMP) a nonprofit healthcare agency whose primary mission is to understand the causes of medication errors and to provide time-critical error reduction strategies to the healthcare community, policymakers, and the public

institutional pharmacy a pharmacy that is organized under a corporate structure, following specific rules and regulations for accreditation

institutional review board (IRB) a committee of the hospital that ensures that appropriate protection is provided to patients using investigational drugs; sometimes referred to as the human use committee

International Organization for Standardization (ISO) a classification system to measure the amount of particulate matter in room air; the lower the ISO number, the less particulate matter is present in the air

intrarespiratory route of administration the administration of a drug by inhalation into the lungs; also called inhalation

intrauterine device a device to deliver medication to prevent conception or to treat cancer within the uterus

intravenous (IV) infusion the process of injecting fluid or medication into the veins, usually over a prolonged period of time

inventory the entire stock of products on hand for sale at a given time

inventory value the total value of the entire stock of products on hand for sale on a given day

investigational drugs drugs used in clinical trials that have not yet been approved by the FDA for use in the general population or drugs used for nonapproved indications

irrigating solution any solution used for cleansing or bathing an area of the body, such as the eyes or ears

isotonic solution a parenteral solution with an equal number of particles as blood cells (285 mOsm/L); 0.9% normal saline is isotonic

IV administration set a sterile, pyrogen-free disposable device used to deliver IV fluids to patients

IV admixture service a centralized pharmacy service that prepares IV and TPN solutions in a sterile, germ-free work environment

IV piggyback (IVPB) a small-volume IV infusion (50 mL, 100 mL, 250 mL) containing medications

IV push (IVP) the rapid injection of a medication in a syringe into an IV line or catheter in the patient's arm; also called bolus injection

J

jelly a gel that contains a higher proportion of water in combination with a drug substance, as well as a thickening agent

Joint Commission an independent, not-for-profit group that sets the standards by which safety and quality of health care are measured and accredits hospitals according to those standards; previously called the Joint Commission on Accreditation of Healthcare Organizations (JCAHO)

just-in-time (JIT) purchasing involves frequent purchasing in quantities that just meet supply needs until the next ordering time

L

large-volume parenteral (LVP) an IV fluid of more than 250 mL that may contain drugs, nutrients, or electrolytes

law a rule that is designed to protect the public and usually enforced through local, state, or federal governments

law of agency and contracts the general principle that allows an employee to enter into contracts on the employer's behalf

leading zero a zero that is placed in the ones place in a number less than zero that is being represented by a decimal value

legend drug a drug that requires a prescription from a licensed provider for a valid medical purpose

levigation a process usually used to reduce the particle size of a solid during the preparation of an ointment

licensure the granting of a license by the state, usually to work in a profession, in order to protect the public

liniment a medicated topical preparation for application to the skin, such as Ben Gay

liter the metric system's base unit for measuring volume

local effect the site-specific application of a drug

long-term care facility an institution that provides care for geriatric and disabled patients; includes extended-care facility (ECF) and skilled-care facility (SCF)

lotion a liquid for topical application that contains insoluble dispersed solids or immiscible liquids

lozenge a medication in a sweet-tasting formulation that is absorbed in the mouth

M

magma a milklike liquid colloidal dispersion in which particles remain distinct, in a two-phase system; for example, milk of magnesia

mail-order pharmacy a large-volume centralized pharmacy operation that uses automation to fill and mail prescriptions to a patient

malpractice a form of negligence in which the standard of care was not met and was a direct cause of injury

managed care a type of health insurance system that emphasizes keeping the patient healthy or diseases controlled in order to reduce healthcare costs

manufactured products products prepared off-site by a manufacturer

markup the difference between the purchase price and the selling price; also called gross profit

master control record a recipe for a compound preparation that lists the name, strength, dosage form, ingredients and their quantities, mixing instructions, and beyond-use dating

Material Safety Data Sheet (MSDS) contains important information on hazards and flammability of chemicals used in compounding and procedure for treatment of accidental ingestion or exposure

MedGuide written patient information mandated by the Federal Drug Administration (FDA) for select high-risk drugs; also known as a patient medication guide

Medicaid a state government health insurance program for low-income and disabled citizens

medical error any circumstance, action, inaction, or decision related to health care that contributes to an unintended health result

Medicare Part D a voluntary insurance program that provides partial coverage of prescriptions for patients who are eligible for Medicare

medication administration record (MAR) a form in the patient medical chart used by nurses to document the administration time of all drugs

medication container label a label containing the dosage directions from the physician, affixed to the container of the dispensed medication; the technician may use this hard copy to select the correct stock bottle and to fill the prescription

medication error any preventable event that may cause or lead to inappropriate medication use or patient harm while the medication is in the control of the health care professional, patient, or consumer

Medication Error Reporting Program (MERP) a USP program designed to allow healthcare professionals to report medication errors directly to the Institute for Safe Medication Practices (ISMP)

medication order a prescription written in the hospital setting

medication special a single dose preparation not commercially available that is repackaged and made for a particular patient

MEDMARX an Internet-based program of the USP for use by hospitals and healthcare systems for documenting, tracking, and identifying trends for adverse events and medication errors

MedWatch a voluntary program run by the FDA for reporting serious adverse events for medications and medical devices; serves as a clearinghouse for information on safety alerts and drug recalls

meniscus the moon-shaped or concave appearance of a liquid in a graduate cylinder used in measurement

meter the metric system's base unit for measuring length

metered-dose inhaler (MDI) a device used to administer a drug in the form of compressed gas through the mouth into the lungs

metric system a measurement system based on subdivisions and multiples of 10; made up of three basic units: meter, gram, and liter

microemulsion a clear formulation that contains one liquid of extremely fine size droplets dispersed in another liquid; for example Haley's M-O

military time a measure of time based on a 24 hour clock in which midnight is 0000, noon is 1200, and the minute before midnight is 2359; also referred to as international time

mortar and pestle equipment used for mixing and grinding pharmaceutical ingredients

multiple compression tablet (MCT) a tablet formulation on top of a tablet or a tablet within a tablet, produced by multiple compressions in manufacturing

N

nasal route of administration the placement of sprays or solutions into the nose

National Association of Boards of Pharmacy (NABP) an organization that represents the practice of pharmacy in each state and develops pharmacist licensure exams

National Drug Code (NDC) number a unique number assigned to a brand name, generic, or OTC product to identify the manufacturer, drug, and packaging size

nebulizer a device used to deliver medication in a fine-mist form to the lungs; often used in treating asthma

negligence a tort for not providing the minimum standard of care

new drug application (NDA) the process through which drug sponsors formally propose that the FDA approve a new pharmaceutical for sale and marketing in the United States

nonpyrogenic the state of being free from microorganisms; a description of a packaged IV set

nonsterile compounding the preparation of a medication, in an appropriate quantity and dosage form, from several pharmaceutical ingredients in response to a prescription written by a physician, such as tablets, capsules, ointments, or creams; sometimes referred to as extemporaneous compounding

nonverbal communication communication without words—through facial expression, body contact, body position, and tone of voice

nosocomial infection an infection caused by bacteria found in the hospital from any source that causes a patient to develop an infectious disease; also called healthcare-associated infection (HAI)

notice of privacy practices a written policy of the pharmacy to protect patient confidentiality, as required by HIPAA

nuclear pharmacy a specialized practice that compounds and dispenses sterile radioactive pharmaceuticals to diagnose or treat disease

numerator the number on the upper part of a fraction that represents the part of the whole

O

ocular route of administration the placement of ophthalmic medications into the eye

oil-in-water (O/W) emulsion an emulsion containing a small amount of oil dispersed in water, as in a cream

ointment a semisolid emulsion for topical use on the skin

omission error an error in which a prescribed dose is not given

online adjudication real-time insurance claims processing via wireless telecommunications

open-ended question a question that requires a descriptive answer, not merely yes or no

oral disintegrating tablet (ODT) a solid oral dosage form designed to dissolve quickly on the tongue for oral absorption

oral route of administration the administration of medication through swallowing for absorption along the GI tract into systemic circulation

oral syringe a needleless device for administering medication to pediatric or older adult patients unable to swallow tablets or capsules

organizational failure an error generated by failure of organizational rules, policies, or procedures

orphan drug a medication approved by the FDA to treat rare diseases

osmolarity a measure of the milliosmoles of solute per liter of solution (mOsm/L)

osmotic pressure the pressure required to maintain an equilibrium, with no net movement of solvent; for example, the osmotic pressure of blood is 285 mOsm/L; often referred to as tonicity for IV solutions

otic route of administration the placement of solutions or suspensions into the ear

out of stock (OOS) a medication not in stock in the pharmacy; a drug that must be specially ordered from a drug wholesaler

over-the-counter (OTC) drug a medication that the FDA has approved for sale without a prescription

P

paraprofessional a trained person who assists a professional person

parenteral route of administration the injection or infusion of fluids and/or medications into the body, bypassing the GI tract

parenteral solution a product that is prepared in a sterile environment for administration by injection

partial fill a supply dispensed to hold the patient until a new supply is received from the wholesaler because insufficient inventory in the pharmacy prevents completely filling the prescription

paste a water-in-oil (W/O) emulsion containing more solid material than an ointment

pasteurization a sterilization process designed to kill most bacteria and mold in milk and other liquids

pathophysiology the study of disease and illnesses affecting the normal function of the body

patient identifiers any demographic information that can identify the patient, such as name, address, phone number, Social Security number, or medical identification number

patient information sheet a leaflet printed from the prescription software and provided to patients on each medication dispensed; the tech may use this hard copy to select the correct drug stock bottle and fill the prescription

patient profile a record kept by the pharmacy listing a patient's identifying information, insurance information, medical and prescription history, and prescription preferences

patient-controlled analgesia (PCA) infusion device a device used by a patient to deliver small doses of medication to the patient for chronic pain relief

percent the number or ratio per 100

percentage of error the acceptable range of variation above and below the target measurement; used in compounding and manufacturing

perpetual inventory record unit-by-unit accountability, often required for Schedule II controlled inventory records

pH value the degree of acidity or alkalinity of a solution; less than 7 is acidic and more than 7 is alkaline; the pH of blood is 7.4

pharmaceutical alternative drug product a drug product that contains the same active therapeutic ingredient but contains different salts or different dosage forms; cannot be substituted without prescriber authorization

pharmaceutical care a philosophy of care that expanded the pharmacist's role to include appropriate medication use to achieve positive outcomes with prescribed drug therapy

pharmaceutical elegance the physical appearance of the final compound preparation

pharmaceutical weights measures of various sizes made of polished brass, often used with a two-pan Class III prescription balance; available in both metric and apothecary weights

pharmaceutically equivalent drug product a drug product that contains the same amount of active ingredient in the same dosage form and meets the same USP–NF compendial standards (i.e., strength, quality, purity, and identity); can be substituted without contacting the prescriber

pharmaceutics the study of the release characteristics of specific drug dosage forms

pharmacist one who is licensed to prepare and dispense medications, counsel patients, and monitor outcomes pursuant to a prescription from a licensed health professional

pharmacodynamic agent a drug that alters body functions in a desired way

pharmacognosy the study of medicinal functions of natural products of animal, plant, or mineral origins

pharmacokinetics individualized doses of drugs based on absorption, distribution, metabolism, and elimination

pharmacology the scientific study of drugs and their mechanisms of action

pharmacy and therapeutics (P&T) committee a committee of the hospital that reviews, approves, and revises the hospital's formulary of drugs and maintains the drug use policies of the hospital

Pharmacy Compounding Accrediting Board (PCAB) an organization that provides quality standards for a compounding pharmacy through voluntary accreditation

pharmacy technician an individual working in a pharmacy who, under the supervision of a licensed pharmacist, assists in activities not requiring the professional judgment of a pharmacist; also called the *pharmacy tech* or *tech*

Pharmacy Technician Certification Examination (PTCE) an examination developed by the Pharmacy Technician Certification Board (PTCB) that technicians must pass to be certified and receive the title of CPhT

physical dependence taking a drug continuously such that physical withdrawal symptoms like restlessness, anxiety, insomnia, diarrhea, vomiting, and "goose bumps" occur if not taken

pipette a long, thin, calibrated hollow tube used for measuring liquids less than 1.5 mL

plaintiff one who files a lawsuit for the courts to decide

plaster a solid or semisolid, medicated or nonmedicated preparation that adheres to the skin

policy and procedure manual a book outlining activities in the pharmacy, defining the roles of individuals and listing guidelines

posting the process of reconciling the invoice and updating inventory

powder volume (pv) the amount of space occupied by a freeze-dried medication in a sterile vial, used for reconstitution; equal to the difference between the final volume (fv) and the volume of the diluting ingredient, or the diluent volume (dv)

powders fine particles of medication used in tablets and capsules

prescription an order written by a qualified, licensed practitioner for a medication to be filled by a pharmacist for a patient in order to treat a qualified medical condition

prescription benefits manager (PBM) a company that administers drug benefits from many insurance companies

prescription record a computer-generated version of the compounding log that documents the compounding recipe for a specific prescription and patient

prime vendor purchasing an agreement made by a pharmacy for a specified percentage or dollar volume of purchases

priming the act of flushing out the small particles in the tubing's interior lumen prior to medication administration and letting fluid run through the tubing so that all of the air is flushed out

prior authorization (PA) approval for coverage of a high-cost medication or a medication not on the insurer's approved formulary, obtained after a prescriber calls the insurer to justify the use of the drug; must be obtained before the drug is dispensed by the pharmacy in order to be covered by insurance

prior authorization (PA) approval for coverage of a high-cost medication or a medication not on the insurer's approved formulary, obtained after a prescriber calls the insurer to justify the use of the drug; must be obtained before the drug is dispensed by the pharmacy in order to be covered by insurance

product package insert (PPI) scientific information supplied to the pharmacist and technician by the manufacturer with all prescription drug products; the information must be approved by the FDA

professional someone with recognized expertise in a field who is expected to use his or her knowledge and skills to benefit others and to operate ethically with some autonomy

professional standards guidelines of acceptable behavior and performance established by professional associations

profit the amount of revenue received that exceeds the expense of the sold product

prophylactic agent a drug used to prevent disease

proportion a comparison of equal ratios; the product of the means equals the product of the extremes

protected health information (PHI) medical information that is protected by HIPAA, such as medical diagnoses, medication profiles, and results of laboratory tests

protozoa a single-celled organism that inhabits water and soil

psychological dependence taking a drug on a regular basis because it produces a sense of well-being; if the drug is stopped suddenly, anxiety withdrawal symptoms can result

pulverization the process of reducing particle size, especially by using a solvent

punch method a method for filling capsules in which the body of a capsule is repeatedly punched into a cake of medication until the capsule is full

purchasing the ordering of products for use or sale by the pharmacy

pyrogen a fever-producing by-product of microbial metabolism

Q

quality assurance (QA) program a feedback system to improve care by identifying and correcting the cause of a medication error or improper technique

R

radiopharmaceutical a drug containing radioactive ingredients, often used for diagnostic or therapeutic purposes

ratio a comparison of numeric values

receipt a printout that is a proof of purchase

receiving a series of procedures for accepting the delivery of products to the pharmacy

recertification the periodic updating of certification

reciprocation the administrative process for relicensure of pharmacists in another state

rectal route of administration the delivery of medication via the rectum

refill an approval by the prescriber to dispense the prescribed medication again without the need for a new prescription order

registration mandatory signing up or registering with the State Board of Pharmacy before starting to practice

regulation a written rule and procedure that exists to carry out a law of the state or federal government

regulatory law the system of rules and regulations established by governmental bodies

remote computer a minicomputer or a mainframe that stores and processes data sent from a dumb terminal

repackaging control log a form used in the pharmacy when drugs are repackaged from manufacturer stock bottles to unit doses; the log contains the name of the drug, dose, quantity, manufacturer lot number, expiration date, and the initials of the pharmacy technician and pharmacist

ribonucleic acid (RNA) an important component of the genetic code that arranges amino acids into proteins

root-cause analysis a logical and systematic process used to help identify what, how, and why something happened, in order to prevent recurrence

route of administration a way of getting a drug onto or into the body, such as orally, topically, or parenterally

S

safety paper a special tamper-proof paper required in many states for C-II prescriptions to minimize forgeries

Schedule II drug administration record a manual or electronic form on the patient care unit to account for each dose of each narcotic administered to a patient

Schedule V drug a medication with a low potential for abuse and a limited potential for creating physical or psychological dependence; available in most states without a prescription

selection error an error that occurs when two or more options exist and the incorrect option is chosen

semisynthetic drug a drug that contains both natural and synthetic components

sentinel event an unexpected occurrence involving death or serious physical or psychological injury or the potential for occurrences to happen

sharp a used needle, which can be a source of infection

sifting a process used to blend powders through the use of a sieve

signa ("sig") the part of the prescription that indicates the directions for the patient to follow when taking the medication

small-volume parenteral (SVP) an IV fluid of 250 mL or less commonly used for infusion of drugs; with medication, also called an IV piggyback

smart terminal a computer that contains its own storage and processing capabilities

solute an ingredient dissolved in a solution or dispersed in a suspension

solution a liquid dosage form in which the active ingredients are completely dissolved in a liquid vehicle

solvent the vehicle that makes up the greater part of a solution

spatula a stainless steel, plastic, or hard rubber instrument used for transferring or mixing solid pharmaceutical ingredients

spatulation a process used to blend ingredients, often used in the preparation of creams and ointments

specific gravity the ratio of the weight of a substance compared to an equal volume of water when both have the same temperature

spike the sharp plastic end of IV tubing that is attached to an IV bag of fluid

spirit an alcoholic or hydroalcoholic solution containing volatile, aromatic ingredients

spray the dosage form that consists of a container with a valve assembly that, when activated, emits a fine dispersion of liquid, solid, or gaseous material

stability the extent to which a compounded product retains the same physical and chemical properties and characteristics it possessed at the time of preparation

standard a set of criteria to measure product quality or professional performance against a norm

standard of care the usual and customary level of practice in the community

stat order a medication order that is to be filled and sent to the patient care unit immediately

sterile compounding the preparation of a parenteral product in the hospital, home healthcare, nuclear, or community pharmacy setting; an example is an intravenous antibiotic

sterilization a process that destroys the microorganisms in a substance, resulting in asepsis

sublingual route of administration oral administration in which a drug is placed under the tongue and is rapidly absorbed into the bloodstream

subscription the part of the prescription that lists instructions to the pharmacist about dispensing the medication, including information about compounding or packaging instructions, labeling instructions, refill information, and information about the appropriateness of dispensing drug equivalencies

sugar-coated tablet (SCT) a tablet coated with an outside layer of sugar that protects the medication and improves both appearance and flavor

suppository a solid formulation containing a drug for rectal or vaginal administration

suspension the dispersion of a solid in a liquid

sustained-release (SR) dosage form a delayed-release dosage form that allows less frequent dosing than an immediate-release dosage form

synthetic drug a drug that is artificially created but in imitation of naturally occurring substances

syringe a device used to inject a parenteral solution into the bloodstream, muscle, or under the skin

syrup an aqueous solution thickened with a large amount of sugar (generally sucrose) or a sugar substitute such as sorbitol or propylene glycol

systemic effect the distribution of a drug throughout the body by absorption into the bloodstream

T

tablet the solid dosage form produced by compression and containing one or more active and inactive ingredients

tablet splitter a device used to manually split or score tablets

technical failure an error generated by failure because of location or equipment

therapeutic agent a drug that prevents, cures, diagnoses, or relieves symptoms of a disease

therapeutic effect the desired pharmacological action of a drug on the body

therapeutics the study of applying pharmacology to the treatment of illness and disease states

tiered co-pay an escalating cost or co-pay for a generic drug, a preferred brand name drug, and a nonpreferred brand name drug

tincture an alcoholic or hydroalcoholic solution of extractions from plants

topical route of administration the administration of a drug on the skin or any mucous membrane such as the eyes, nose, ears, lungs, vagina, urethra, or rectum; usually administered directly to the surface of the skin

tort the legal term for personal injuries that one citizen commits against another in a lawsuit

total parenteral nutrition (TPN) a specially formulated parenteral solution that provides nutritional needs intravenously (IV) to a patient who cannot or will not eat

transdermal dosage form a formulation designed to deliver a continuous supply of drug into the bloodstream by absorption through the skin via a patch or disk

triage the assessment by the pharmacist of an illness or symptom; outcome may be to recommend an OTC product, or refer patient to a physician or emergency room

Tricare a federal government health insurance program for active and retired military and their dependents

trituration the process of rubbing, grinding, or pulverizing a substance to create fine particles, generally by means of a mortar and pestle

tumbling a process used to combine powders by placing them in a bag or container and shaking it

U

unit dose an amount of a drug that has been prepackaged or repackaged for a single administration to a particular patient at a particular time

unit dose cart a movable storage unit that contains individual patient drawers of medication for all patients on a given patient care unit

unit dose profile the documentation that provides the information necessary to prepare the unit doses, including patient name and location, medication and strength, frequency or schedule of administration, and quantity for each order

unit of use a fixed number of dose units in a drug stock container, usually consisting of a month's supply, or 30 tablets or capsules

United States Pharmacopeia (USP) the independent scientific organization responsible for setting official quality standards for all drugs sold in the United States as well as standards for practice

United States Pharmacopeia–National Formulary (USP–NF) a book that contains U.S. standards for medicines, dosage forms, drug substances, excipients or inactive substances, medical devices, and dietary supplements

universal precautions procedures followed in healthcare settings to prevent infection as a result of exposure to blood or other bodily fluids

urethral route of administration the administration of a drug by insertion into the urethra

USP Chapter 797 guidelines on the sterility and stability of CSPs developed by the United States Pharmacopeia (USP) that have become standards for hospital accreditation

V

vaccine a substance introduced into the body in order to produce immunity to disease

Vaccine Adverse Event Reporting System (VAERS) a postmarketing surveillance system operated by the FDA and CDC that collects information on adverse events that occur after immunization

vaginal route of administration the administration of a drug by application of a cream or insertion of a tablet into the vagina

vertical laminar airflow workbench (LAFW) a special biological safety cabinet used to prepare hazardous drugs, such as cancer chemotherapy drugs, aseptically

virus a minute infectious agent that does not have all of the components of a cell and thus can replicate only within a living host cell

W

water-in-oil (W/O) emulsion an emulsion containing a small amount of water dispersed in an oil, such as an ointment

weighing paper a special paper that is placed on a weighing balance pan to avoid contact between pharmaceutical ingredients and the balance tray; also called powder paper

wholesaler purchasing the ordering of drugs and supplies from a local vendor who delivers the product to the pharmacy on a daily basis

workers' compensation insurance provided for a patient with a medical injury from a job-related accident; also called workers' comp

wrong dosage form error an error in which the dosage form or formulation is not the accepted interpretation of the physician order

wrong dose error an error in which the dose is either above or below the correct dose by more than 5%

wrong time error a medication error in which a drug is given 30 minutes or more before or after it was prescribed, up to the time of the next dose, not including as needed orders

Y

Y-site a rigid piece of plastic with one arm terminating in a resealable port that is used for adding medication to the IV

Index

Note: Page numbers in italics refer to figures and photos and those followed by a "*t*" indicate that the reference is to a table.

Photo Credits: Cover Paul Skelcher-Rainbow, Science Faction, Getty Images; **4** *top*, © Front cover of 'L 'Egypte' by G. Ebers, published in Paris, 1880 (red leather and gold), French School, 19th century, Bibliotheque des Arts Decoratifs, Paris, France, Archives Charmet, The Bridgeman Art Library; *bottom*, © Ms 1229 Sultan Ahmet III (1673-1736) with one of his disciples, from 'De Materia Medica' by Dioscorides (gouache on paper), Turkish School, Topkapi Palace Museum, Istanbul, Turkey, The Bridgeman Art Library; **5** © Claudius Galenus (c.130-c.201 AD) (oil on canvas), French School, 17th century, Bibliotheque de la Faculte de Medecine, Paris, France, Archives Charmet, The Bridgeman Art Library; **6** IMS Health National Sales Perspective, April 2008; **7** © AP Images, Steven Senne; **8** © Larry Mulvehill, Corbis; **9** Courtesy